Network Pharmacology: Drug Discovery and Development

Network Pharmacology: Drug Discovery and Development

Editor: Brianna Willis

AMERICAN
MEDICAL PUBLISHERS
www.americanmedicalpublishers.com

AMERICAN
MEDICAL PUBLISHERS
www.americanmedicalpublishers.com

Cataloging-in-Publication Data

Network pharmacology : drug discovery and development / edited by Brianna Willis.
p. cm.
Includes bibliographical references and index.
ISBN 979-8-88740-300-7
1. Pharmacology--Data processing. 2. Drugs--Design. 3. Drug development.
4. Pharmacology--Computer network resources. 5. Pharmacology--Computer simulation.
6. Bioinformatics. 7. Information storage and retrieval systems--Pharmacology. 8. Pharmaceutical te
I. Willis, Brianna.
RM301 .N483 2023
615.1--dc23

American Medical Publishers,
41 Flatbush Avenue,
1st Floor, New York,
NY 11217, USA

ISBN 979-8-88740-300-7 (Hardback)

Contents

Preface VII

Chapter 1 **The Yin-Yang Property of Chinese Medicinal Herbs Relates to Chemical Composition but not Anti-Oxidative Activity: An Illustration Using Spleen-Meridian Herbs** 1
Yun Huang, Ping Yao, Ka Wing Leung, Huaiyou Wang, Xiang Peng Kong, Long Wang, Tina Ting Xia Dong, Yicun Chen and Karl Wah Keung Tsim

Chapter 2 **IMCC: A Novel Quantitative Approach Revealing Variation of Global Modular Map and Local Inter-Module Coordination among Differential Drug's Targeted Cerebral Ischemic Networks** 18
Pengqian Wang, Yanan Yu, Jun Liu, Bing Li, Yingying Zhang, Dongfeng Li, Wenjuan Xu, Qiong Liu and Zhong Wang

Chapter 3 **Network Pharmacology-Based Analysis on the Potential Biological Mechanisms of Sinisan Against Non-Alcoholic Fatty Liver Disease** 33
Xiaoyi Wei, Weixin Hou, Jiajun Liang, Peng Fang, Bo Dou, Zisong Wang, Jiayang Sai, Tian Xu, Chongyang Ma, Qiuyun Zhang, Fafeng Cheng, Xueqian Wang and Qingguo Wang

Chapter 4 **A Computational Systems Pharmacology Approach to Investigate Molecular Mechanisms of Herbal Formula Tian-Ma-Gou-Teng-Yin for Treatment of Alzheimer's Disease** 47
Tianduanyi Wang, Zengrui Wu, Lixia Sun, Weihua Li, Guixia Liu and Yun Tang

Chapter 5 **Network Pharmacology and Experimental Assessment to Explore the Pharmacological Mechanism of Qimai Feiluoping Decoction Against Pulmonary Fibrosis** 63
Yingying Yang, Lu Ding, Tingting Bao, Yaxin Li, Jing Ma, Qingwei Li, Zezheng Gao, Siyu Song, Jing Wang, Jiachao Zhao, Ziyuan Wang, Daqing Zhao, Xiangyan Li, Zeyu Wang, Linhua Zhao and Xiaolin Tong

Chapter 6 **Network Pharmacology Databases for Traditional Chinese Medicine** 79
Runzhi Zhang, Xue Zhu, Hong Bai and Kang Ning

Chapter 7 **The Key Target and Molecular Mechanism of the Volatile Component of *Scutellaria baicalensis* Georgi in Acute Lung Injury Based on Network Pharmacology** 93
Guosong Zhu, Jiaqiang Zhang, Yali Yang, Haoran Zhang, Wenwen Jin, Fangchu Su, Junting Liang, Kaiwei Wang, Jianhua Zhang and Chuanliang Chen

Chapter 8 **Systems Pharmacology for Investigation of the Mechanisms of Action of Traditional Chinese Medicine in Drug Discovery** 104
Wenjuan Zhang, Ying Huai, Zhiping Miao, Airong Qian and Yonghua Wang

Chapter 9 **WTD Attenuating Rheumatoid Arthritis *via* Suppressing Angiogenesis and Modulating the PI3K/AKT/mTOR/HIF-1α Pathway** **126**
Xin Ba, Ying Huang, Pan Shen, Yao Huang, Hui Wang, Liang Han, Wei Ji Lin, Hui Jia Yan, Li Jun Xu, Kai Qin, Zhe Chen and Sheng Hao Tu

Chapter 10 **Anti-Endometriosis Mechanism of *Jiawei Foshou San* Based on Network Pharmacology** **143**
Yi Chen, Jiahui Wei, Ying Zhang, Wenwei Sun, Zhuoheng Li, Qin Wang, Xiaoyu Xu, Cong Li and Panhong Li

Chapter 11 **Analysis of Antidepressant Activity of Huang-Lian Jie-Du Decoction Through Network Pharmacology and Metabolomics** **157**
Shu-Yue Qu, Xiao-Yue Li, Xia Heng, Yi-Yu Qi, Ping-Yuan Ge, Sai-jia Ni, Zeng-Ying Yao, Rui Guo, Nian-Yun Yang, Yi Cao, Qi-Chun Zhang and Hua-Xu Zhu

Chapter 12 ***Cyclocarya paliurus* Leaves Tea Improves Dyslipidemia in Diabetic Mice: A Lipidomics-Based Network Pharmacology Study** **174**
Lixiang Zhai, Zi-wan Ning, Tao Huang, Bo Wen, Cheng-hui Liao, Cheng-yuan Lin, Ling Zhao, Hai-tao Xiao and Zhao-xiang Bian

Chapter 13 **Network Pharmacology-Based Analysis and Experimental Exploration of Antidiabetic Mechanisms of Gegen Qinlian Decoction** **186**
Yu Xu, Jihan Huang, Ning Wang, Hor-Yue Tan, Cheng Zhang, Sha Li, Guoyi Tang and Yibin Feng

Chapter 14 **Mechanisms Underlying the Action of Ziziphi Spinosae Semen in the Treatment of Insomnia: A Study Involving Network Pharmacology and Experimental Validation** **201**
Zhenhua Bian, Wenming Zhang, Jingyue Tang, Qianqian Fei, Minmin Hu, Xiaowei Chen, Lianlin Su, Chenghao Fei, De Ji, Chunqin Mao, Huangjin Tong, Xiaohang Yuan and Tulin Lu

Chapter 15 **Anti-Inflammatory Effect of a TCM Formula Li-Ru-Kang in Rats with Hyperplasia of Mammary Gland and the Underlying Biological Mechanisms** **216**
Yingying Wang, Shizhang Wei, Tian Gao, Yuxue Yang, Xiaohua Lu, Xuelin Zhou, Haotian Li, Tao Wang, Liqi Qian, Yanling Zhao and Wenjun Zou

Permissions

List of Contributors

Index

Preface

Network pharmacology reveals pharmacological mechanisms of drugs for outlining the development and discovery of drugs along with clinical treatment. It combines clinical, experimental and computational investigation, while creating favorable conditions for investigating the features of traditional medicine. The aim of network pharmacology is to reveal and reflect on the biological foundations of various complex diseases and effects of drugs by the application of network based understanding. It is useful in drug discovery and development, as it combines system biology and genomic technologies through computational biological tools. It is capable of elucidating complex relations amidst biological systems, diseases and drugs. It emphasizes on systems level modeling of mechanism of drugs, by integrating protein-protein interaction, drug-target interaction along with other type of interactome data. This book explores all the important aspects of network pharmacology in the present day scenario. It presents researches and studies performed by experts across the globe. As this field is emerging at a rapid pace, the contents of this book will help the readers to understand drug discovery and development within network pharmacology.

The information shared in this book is based on empirical researches made by veterans in this field of study. The elaborative information provided in this book will help the readers further their scope of knowledge leading to advancements in this field.

Finally, I would like to thank my fellow researchers who gave constructive feedback and my family members who supported me at every step of my research.

Editor

1

The Yin-Yang Property of Chinese Medicinal Herbs Relates to Chemical Composition but not Anti-Oxidative Activity: An Illustration Using Spleen-Meridian Herbs

Yun Huang[1,2], Ping Yao[2], Ka Wing Leung[1,2], Huaiyou Wang[1,2], Xiang Peng Kong[1,2], Long Wang[2†], Tina Ting Xia Dong[1,2], Yicun Chen[2,3] and Karl Wah Keung Tsim[1,2]*

[1] Shenzhen Key Laboratory of Edible and Medicinal Bioresources, Shenzhen Research Institute, Shenzhen, China, [2] Division of Life Science and Center for Chinese Medicine, The Hong Kong University of Science and Technology, Clear Water Bay, Hong Kong, [3] Department of Pharmacology, Shantou University Medical College, Shantou, China

Correspondence:
Karl Wah Keung Tsim
botsim@ust.hk

"Yin-Yang" and "Five Elements" theories are the basis theories of Traditional Chinese Medicine (TCM). To probe and clarify the theoretical basis of these ancient Chinese wisdoms, extensive efforts have been taken, however, without a full success. In the classification of TCM herbs, hot, cold and neutral herbs are believed to possess distinct profile of chemical compositions of which the compounds should have different polarity and mass: this view provides a new perspective for further illustration. To understand the chemical properties of TCMs in the classification of "Yin-Yang" and "Five Elements," 15 commonly used herbs attributed to spleen-meridian were selected for analyses. Chemically standardized water extracts, 50% ethanol extracts and 90% ethanol extracts were prepared and subjected to different analytic measurements. Principle component analysis (PCA) of full spectrum of HPLC, NMR and LC-MS of the extracts were established. The results revealed that the LC-MS profile showed a strong correlation with the "Yin-Yang" classification criterion. The Yang-stimulating herbs generally contain more compounds with lower molecular weight and less polar property. Additionally, a comprehensive anti-oxidative profiles of selected herbs were developed, and the results showed that its correlation with cold and hot properties of TCM, however, was rather low. Taken together, the "Yin-Yang" nature of TCM is closely related to the physical properties of the ingredients, such as polarity and molecular mass; while such classification has little correlation with anti-oxidative property. Therefore, the present results provide a new direction in probing the basic principle of TCM classification.

Keywords: Yin-Yang classification criterion, cold and hot properties, principle component analysis, chemical composition, anti-oxidative activity

INTRODUCTION

In the theoretical basis of TCM clinical application, "Yin-Yang" and "Five Elements" theories could further differentiate into secondary classification principles, e.g., four natures and five flavors, meridian tropism, floating and sinking (Li et al., 2008; Fu et al., 2009, 2015; Mohd et al., 2013; Qiu, 2015). Having a long history of clinical experience, these TCM theories are aiming to merge with each other and achieve unity gradually. As the "Yin-Yang" attribution is not only specified to the description of patient symptoms ("Zheng" or syndrome), but also defines the nature of herbal medicines. Thus, the exact relationship between these two identification systems of TCM, i.e., "Yin-Yang" versus chemical composition, remains as a puzzle (Zhou et al., 2009; Ma et al., 2010; Li, 2012). In order to maintain a homeostasis in our body, the herbs with cold nature, also known as Yin-stimulating herbs, were generally used to treat hot diseases like inflammation, while the herbs with nature of warm and hot, belonging to Yang-stimulating herbs, were good for various types of deficiency (Fu et al., 2017a). In recent years, the works on chemical properties of TCMs has made a significant progress, and new ideas have been proposed, e.g., molecular drug hypothesis (Fu et al., 2017b), biodynamics (Yang et al., 2017), genetic hypothesis (Rezapour-Firouzi, 2017), transient receptor potential channel hypothesis (Bishnoi et al., 2018). Indeed, many of these newly proposed methods have been adopted and improved, including micro-calorimetry (Gao et al., 2014), mathematical modeling (Ramirez-Rodrigues et al., 2011), biophoton detection (Han et al., 2011; Zhao and Han, 2013). These methods are mainly derived from the collation of ancient books (Wang et al., 2010), pharmacological effects (Liang et al., 1988; Xu et al., 2011; Xiong et al., 2011), structure of components (Wang and Zhou, 2006) and thermodynamics (Yang et al., 2010). However, these studies are still lacking a co-relationship of the current TCM theory with the chemical composition of different classes of herbs.

Having highly developed analytical techniques and various novel chemometrics methods today, the study on relationship between TCM herb properties with their chemical composition has become possible. The widely employed analytical techniques, including HPLC, NMR and LC-MS, enabled researchers to establish robust methods to qualitative and quantitative determination of almost all kinds of compounds in biological matrices (Kuang et al., 2012). According to clinical application and experimental basis, the major ingredients corresponding to property and taste of TCM herbs are expected to be different. For example, volatile oil and polysaccharide are major bioactive components of pungent and sweet herbs; while alkaloid, glycoside and phenolic acid are generally abundant in bitter and acid herbs (Ung et al., 2007). In addressing these problems being encountered in TCM research, the omics techniques play a key role due to its advantage in solving information-rich puzzles and providing comprehensive and holistic results (Wiklund et al., 2008). Among the most commonly used multivariate statistical and visualization tools, principal component analysis (PCA) is a bilinear decomposition method that reduces original data to a few principal components and reserves the features contributing to variance (Kuang et al., 2012).

According to the concept of "Yin-Yang" nature of herbal medicine, the property of Chinese medicinal herbs was mainly summarized based on the efficacy and cognitive experience gained from patients' response. Some pharmacological studies supported the notion that cold and hot properties of TCM herbs were closely related to excitability of nervous system and endocrine (Li et al., 2008; Fu et al., 2009), mitochondrial ATP generation, and immunomodulatory function (Ko et al., 2004, 2006; Ko and Leung, 2007). On the other hand, the potential relationship between "Yin-Yang" properties and redox system of herbs have been proposed (Ou et al., 2003). Nevertheless, the physical meaning behind the criteria of "Yin-Yang" classification is still missing (Szeto and Benzie, 2006; Wong et al., 2006). Moreover, previous research has mainly focused on chemically based of anti-oxidative activity in TCM herbs; however, the relationship of anti-oxidative property with chemical nature of herbs is still missing. PCA analysis of full spectrum of HPLC, NMR and LC-MS of different classes of herbs were conducted to provide a multi-angle and multi-dimensional perspectives of the connection between the "Yin-Yang" properties and their chemical composition. In addition, the possible relationship between "Yin-Yang" nature and anti-oxidant of various herbs was clarified.

MATERIALS AND METHODS

Chemicals and Preparation of Herbal Extracts

HPLC-grade acetonitrile and ethanol were from Merck (Darmstadt, Germany). Ultra-pure water was obtained from a Milli-Q purification system (Millipore, Molsheim, France). Deuterium oxide (D_2O), 3-(4,5-dimethylthiazol-2-yl)-2,5-diphenyltetra-zolium bromide (MTT), gallic acid, 1,1-Diphenyl-2-picrylhydrazyl radical 2,2-diphenyl-1-(2,4,6-trinitrophenyl) hydrazyl (DPPH), *tert*-butyl hydroperoxide (tBHP), vitamin C, 2′,7′-dichlorodihydrofluorescein diacetate (DCFH-DA), β-galactosidase, dimethyl sulfoxide (DMSO) and Hank's Balanced Salt Solution (HBSS) were purchased from Sigma-Aldrich (St. Louis, MO, United States). Lipofectamine 3,000 was bought from Invitrogen (Waltham, MA, United States) and Triton X-100 was from BDH Tech (Marshalltown, IA, United States). The pARE-Luc DNA construct was obtained from Promega (Madison, WI, United States).

Three batches of 15 spleen-meridian herbs (**Table 1**) and a batch of Quinquefolium Radix, Rehmanniae Radix and Rehmanniae Radix Praeparata were collected from their production sites or pharmacy. The collected samples were first authenticated by Dr. Tina Dong and stored in dry and clean container before further analysis. The authentication of these herbs was according to Hong Kong Materia Medica Standards including morphology, microscopy, chemical fingerprint and chemical assay. The voucher specimens were stored in Centre for Chinese Medicine R&D at the university.

A unified extraction method was developed. Water extract, 50% ethanol extract and 90% ethanol extract of each herb were prepared to obtain extracts having different polarities. The specific extraction procedure was as following. First, the herbal samples were milled and passed through a No. 2 sieve and mixed well. Then, 4 g of the powdered sample was extracted in 100 mL distilled water, 50% ethanol and 90% ethanol, respectively, for 2 h by reflux, and the herbs were extracted twice. For the second extraction, the residue from the first extraction was filtered, and the same extraction condition was applied onto the filtered

TABLE 1 | The pharmacological action, origin and extracting yields of the tested 15 spleen-meridian herbs.

Attributes	Herbs	Major Composition	Actions	Origin/Drugstore	Yield (%, W/E50/E90)[a]
Yang herbs (hot, warm)	Codonopsis Radix	Polysaccharide, saponins, volatile oils, alkaloids, etc	To fortify spleen and replenish lung, **nourish blood**[b]	Gansu	27.8/23.6/18.5
				Gansu	23.6/24.1/16.4
				Gansu	22.2/21.8/14.6
	Atractylodis Macrocephalae Rhizoma	Volatile oil, saponins, polysaccharide, etc.	To fortify spleen and **check diarrhea**	Hengxing Pharmacy	12.8/9.77/11.7
				Zhejiang	14.7/13.1/16.7
				Yong Sheng Hang	17.4/12.4/17.2
	Angelicae Sinensis Radix	Volatile oil, flavonoids, organic acids, polysaccharide, amino acids, etc.	To **nourish** and active **blood**	Gansu	16.5/23.7/26.2
				Gansu	18.6/27.6/25.2
				Gansu	17.5/31.1/27.1
	Astragali Radix	Saponins, flavonoids, polysaccharide, etc.	To tonify qi, uprise yang and **nourish blood**	Shanxi	25.2/17.5/14.3
				Gansu	25.9/15.2/15.3
				Gansu	26.1/15.8/15.4
	Jujubae Fructus	Nutrients, flavonoids and phenolic acids, triterpenic acids, etc.	To tonify the middle energizer, **nourish blood**	Shandong	4.75/4.34/3.56
				Henan	4.78/3.66/3.33
				Ningxia	5.66/3.54/2.85
	Ginseng Radix	Ginsenosides, polysaccharide, volatile oils, etc.	To **tonify** the original **qi** and tonify spleen	Jilin	16.8/15.7/8.42
				Rong Chang Hang	15.8/14.6/7.38
				Jilin	14.8/13.2/8.38
	Amomi Fructus	Volatile oil, saponins, flavonoid glycosides, organic acid, etc.	Warm the spleen to **check diarrhea**	Hengxing Pharmacy	1.22/1.28/2.41
				Guangxi	1.32/1.22/2.53
				Yong Sheng Hang	1.04/1.21/1.91
	Aucklandiae Radix	Volatile oil, sesquiterpenes, amino acids, etc.	To move qi and **promote digestion**	Hengxing Pharmacy	1.15/2.45/5.44
				Sichuan	1.21/2.13/4.11
				Sichuan	1.17/2.02/3.02
	Areca Catechu	Alkaloids, flavonoids, tannins, triterpenes and steroids, fatty acids, etc.	To move qi and **check diarrhea**	Hengxing Pharmacy	3.04/3.89/4.24
				Hainan	2.43/3.33/4.51
				Yong Sheng Hang	1.49/2.48/4.42

(Continued)

TABLE 1 | Continued

Attributes	Herbs	Major Composition	Actions	Origin/Drugstore	Yield (%, W/E50/E90)[a]
Neutral herbs (Plain)	Dioscoreae Ahizoma	Polysaccharide, Saponins, etc.	To tonify spleen and stomach, **check diarrhea**	Hengxing Pharmacy	7.46/8.38/5.36
				Henan	9.49/7.43/7.45
				Henan	8.76/5.78/5.33
	Lablab Semen Album	Volatile oil, phytic acid, polyphenols, tannins, etc.	To fortify spleen, **check diarrhea** and resolve dampness	Hengxing Pharmacy	4.65/3.76/3.13
				Hunan	5.68/3.88/6.87
				Yong Sheng Hang	4.93/3.99/5.49
	Poria Cocos	Polysaccharide, triterpenoids, etc.	To fortify spleen and **calm the heart**	Hengxing Pharmacy	1.33/1.23/1.01
				Yunnan	1.32/1.34/1.11
				Yong Sheng Hang	1.42/1.46/1.31
Yin herbs (cool, cold)	Nelumbinis Semen	Alkaloids, flavonoids, amino acids, fatty acid, etc.	To tonify spleen, **check diarrhea** and **calm the heart**	Hengxing Pharmacy	5.65/4.33/3.22
				Jiangxi	5.54/3.56/2.32
				Hunan	6.86/4.55/3.58
	Coicis Semen	Esters, triglycerides, polysaccharide, sterols, alkaloids, etc.	Fortify the spleen to **check diarrhea**	Hengxing Pharmacy	2.64/1.51/0.49
				Hunan	3.32/1.67/1.11
				Yong Sheng Hang	2.63/1.21/1.01
	Crataegi Fructus	Flavonoids, triterpenoids, etc.	To **promote digestion** and invigorate the stomach, move qi	Hengxing Pharmacy	12.8/9.24/13.7
				Guangdong	11.5/7.46/13.2
				Shandong	16.5/6.65/15.3

[a]W, water extract; E50, 50% ethanol extract; E90, 90% ethanol extract. [b]Pharmacological effects were based on the Chinese Pharmacopoeia. The bold words are to emphasize the main pharmacological effects of the TCM.

residue. Then, the extracts were combined, dried under vacuum and stored at 4°C.

The preparation of wine-treated Angelica Sinensis Radix was according to previous research (Zhan et al., 2011). To be specific, 30 g of the dried roots were sliced and sprayed with 3 mL of 15% ethanol and then processed in an oven at 80°C for 90 min with 3 flipping. Then 4 g of processed Angelica Sinensis Radix was weighed and prepared as the extraction procedure mentioned above.

HPLC Fingerprint Analysis of Herbal Extracts

The fingerprint analysis of herbal extracts was performed on an Agilent HPLC 1200 series system (Agilent, Waldbronn, Germany), which was equipped with a degasser, a binary pump, an auto sampler, a thermostated column compartment and a DAD. The samples were separated on a Waters Symmetry C18 column (4.5 mm × 250 mm, 5 μm i.d.) after filtered with a guard column. The mobile phase was composed of acetonitrile (A) and water (B) according to the pre-set gradient program: 0–50 min, linear gradient 0–70% (A); 50–55 min, linear gradient 70–100% (A); 55–60 min, isocratic elution. A pre-balance period of 5 min was used between each run. The injection volume was 10 μL, and the flow rate was set at 1 mL/min. To get the fingerprints of herbal extracts, the wavelength of UV detector was set to 254 nm with full spectral scanning from 190 to 400 nm.

NMR Spectrum Profiling

The ^{1}H NMR experiments were conducted to the extracts in revealing high abundance chemicals. Fifty mg of the dried extract was dissolved in 400 μL of D_2O. All particulate materials were removed by centrifugation at 13,000 × *g* for 1 min, and the supernatant was transferred to a standard 5-mm NMR tube. NMR spectra were acquired on a Varian 300 MHz NMR spectrometer, operating at 300.13 MHz ^{1}H NMR frequency at 298 K. Gradient shimming was used to improve the magnetic field homogeneity prior to all acquisition. ^{1}H NMR spectra of the samples were acquired using a 1D CPMG pulse sequence (RD-90°-t1-90°-tm- 90°-acquire) to generate a spectrum with a reduced residual solvent peak. The experiment time for each sample was around 10 min.

LC-MS Spectrum Profiling

The LC-MS profiles of extracts were established on the Xevo G2-XS® Quadrupole Time-of-Flight (Q-TOF) Mass Spectrometer coupled with an integrated ACQUITY UPLC® I-Class System. The analysis column is ACQUITY UPLC® BEH C18 column (2.1 mm × 50 mm, 1.7 μm). The mobile phase condition was recorded as follows: acetonitrile (A) and water (B), 0–0.5 min, isocratic gradient 5% (A); 0.5-8 min, linear gradient 5–50% (A); 8–12 min, linear gradient 50–90% (A); 12–14 min, linear gradient 90–100% (A); 14–16 min, isocratic gradient 100% (A). The flow rate was set at 0.4 mL/min with injection volume of 5 μL. The column temperature was 25°C. The effluent was further analyzed by Xevo G2-XS® Quadrupole Time-of-Flight (Q-TOF) Mass Spectrometer with an ESI ion source in positive mode. The acquisition range was 50–1200 Da with 0.1 s scan rate. These analytic settings were aiming to reveal most of the chemicals within the herbal extracts.

Cell Culture

RAW264.7 cell, a mouse blood macrophage cell line, was obtained from American Type Culture Collection (ATCC, Manassas, VA, United States). Cells were cultured in Dulbecco's modified Eagles medium supplemented with 100 U/mL penicillin, 100 μg/mL of streptomycin and 10% heat in-active fetal bovine serum in a humidified CO_2 (5%) incubator at 37°C. When the cells reached 80% confluence, they were harvested from plate with a scraper (Corning Incorporated, Corning, NY, United States).

Cell Viability

Cell viability was measured by MTT assay. Cells were seeded in 96-well plates at a density of 1×10^4 cells per well. After 24 h drug treatment, cells in each well were incubated with 10 μL MTT (5 mg/mL) at a final concentration of 0.5 mg/mL for 2 h at 37°C. After the solution was removed, DMSO was used to re-suspend the purple precipitate inside the cells, and the absorbance was detected at 570 nm. The cell viability was calculated as percentage of absorbance value of control (without drug treatment) while the value of control was 100%.

Folin-Ciocalteu Assay

Total phenolic content of herbal extracts was measured with Folin-Ciocalteu assay. To be specific, 20 μL of each extract together with 40 μL 10% (*v*/*v*) Folin-Ciocalteu reagent was added into each well of 96-well microplate. Then, 160 μL Na_2CO_3 (700 mM) was added into each well. The assay plates were incubated at room temperature in dark for 2 h and then the absorbance at 765 nm were recorded. Here, gallic acid (Sigma-Aldrich, > 98%) was used as the reference compound, and the total phenolic contents of each extract were expressed as the value compared with gallic acid.

DPPH Radical Scavenging Assay

Free radical scavenging activity of herbal extracts was measured with DPPH radical scavenging assay. Briefly, 50 μL of each extract with different concentrations (0–8 mg/mL) was mixed with 150 μL DPPH solution in each well of 96-well microplate. After standing for 10 min, the absorbance at 517 nm was recorded. The DPPH free radical scavenging activity was calculated as an inhibition percentage based on the following equation: Inhibition (%) = $[(A_0 - A_1)/A_0] \times 100$, where A_0 is the absorbance of the control, and A_1 is the absorbance of the RA sample aliquot. Here, gallic acid (0–100 μM) was used as a positive control.

tBHP-Induced Oxidative Stress Assay

The dose of tBHP (150 μM; Sigma-Aldrich) and positive control (vitamin C, 1 mM) were optimized with MTT assay as previously reported (Huang et al., 2018a,b). Similar to the cell viability assay, the cells were cultured in 96-well plate first. After drug treatments for 24 h, tBHP (150 μM) were added into the wells for 3 h before MTT at a final concentration of 0.5 mg/mL was added. After the solution was removed, the purple precipitate inside the cells was re-suspended in DMSO and then measured at 570 nm absorbance.

ROS Formation Assay

The measurement of ROS content in cell cultures was performed by using DCFH-DA, an oxidation-sensitive dye. Cultured RAW264.7 cells (1×10^4 cells/well) in a 96-well plate were pre-treated with herbal extracts or standard compounds for 24 h, and the cells were labeled with 100 μM DCFH-DA (Sigma-Aldrich) in HBSS (Sigma-Aldrich) for 1 h at 37°C. After washing three times with HBSS, the cells were then treated with 150 μM tBHP for 1 h at 37°C. Then the amount of intracellular tBHP-induced ROS formation was detected by fluorometric measurement with excitation at 485 nm and emission at 530 nm.

Assay for Anti-oxidant Response Element

To reveal the transcriptional activation of anti-oxidant response element (ARE), the pARE-Luc DNA construct, containing four copies of ARE (5′-TGACnnnGCA-3′) that drives transcription of the luciferase reporter gene luc2P (*Photinus pyralis*), was transfected into cultured RAW264.7 cells by Lipofectamine 3000 (Invitrogen) according to the manufacturer's instructions. Transfected RAW264.7 cells were treated with various concentrations of ginseng extracts for 1 day. Then, the medium was aspirated, and the cultures were lysed by a buffer containing 100 mM potassium phosphate buffer (pH 7.8), 0.2% Triton X-100 and 1 mM DTT at 4°C. After centrifugation at 16,100 × *g* for 5 min, the supernatant was collected and used to perform luciferase assay. The activity was normalized as absorbance (up to 560 nm) per mg of protein.

Statistical Analysis

HPLC profile processing were conducted using Agilent MassHunter workstation software version B.01.00. The ^{1}H

NMR spectra obtained from each sample were phased, baseline-corrected, calibrated and integrated using MestReNova 6.1.1 software. LC-MS profile were analyzed with Waters MassLynx V4.1 SCN923. The data were then formatted in XML for importing into PCA software SIMCA-P+ version 12.0 (Umetrics, Sweden). All data were expressed as the mean ± SEM for $n = 3$–5, unless otherwise specified. Statistical tests were performed by one-way ANOVA with multiple comparisons using Dunnett's test. Differences were considered significant at $p < 0.05$.

RESULTS

Chemical Composition of Herbal Extracts

By reflux, the water extracts and ethanol extracts of individual herbs were prepared with the consideration of their common usage and historical preparation of a herbal decoction in TCM. The origin of herbs and its extracting yields are shown in **Table 1**. The extracting yield of Codonopsis Radix, Astragali Radix, Jujubae Fructus, Ginseng Radix, Nelumbinis Semen and Coicis Semen suggested that the water-soluble ingredients in these herbs were relatively abundant; while Angelicae Sinensis Radix, Amomi Fructus, Aucklandiae Radix and Areca Catechu contained less water-soluble ingredients (**Figure 1**). Among the tested herbs, Codonopsis Radix, Angelicae Sinensis Radix and Astragali Radix possessed the highest yield of extraction up to ~25% per dried weight. In contrast, the yields of water and ethanol extracts of Amomi Fructus, Poria Cocos and Coicis Semen were less than 3%.

The HPLC fingerprints of water and ethanol extracts showed that there were plenty of trace compounds (**Figure 2**). By comparing the HPLC profiles, the 90% ethanol extracts in general contained higher amounts of trace compounds, recognized by the number of peaks, as compared to that of water and 50% ethanol extracts. The distribution of peaks in HPLC profiles showed apparent migration in accord to decreasing polarity of extracting solvent, i.e., more peaks at the end of run in ethanol extracts (**Figure 2**). The ^{1}H NMR experiment was conducted to reveal those high abundance compounds in aforementioned herbal extracts. Similar to HPLC fingerprint, the NMR profile showed close similarity between herbs extracted with the same solvents, and generally the 90% ethanol extracts showed higher content of chemical composition, as compared with that of other extracts (**Figure 3**).

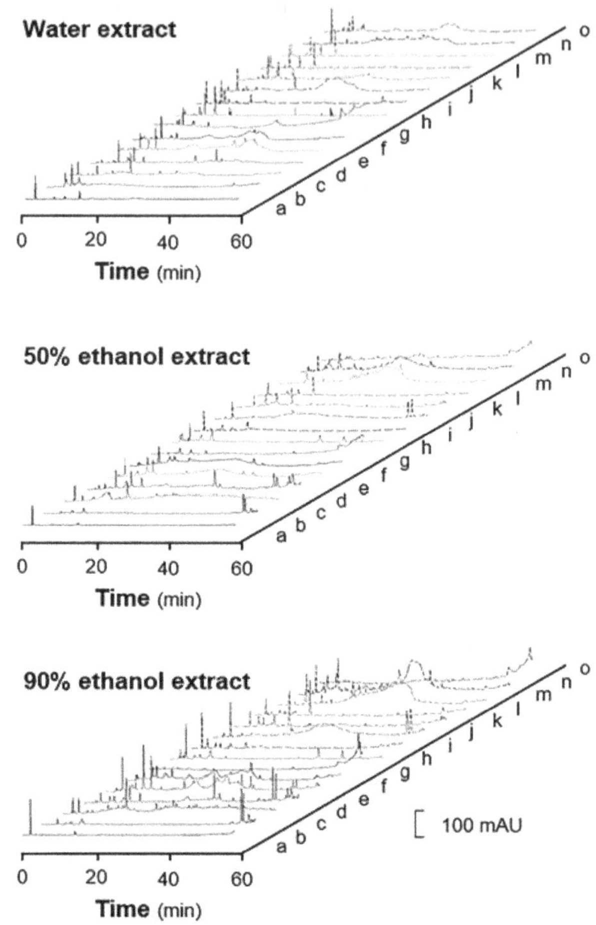

FIGURE 2 | HPLC profiles of herbal extracts from the 15 collected herbs. The fingerprints were obtained with an Agilent HPLC 1200 series system (Agilent, Waldbronn, Germany) and a Waters Symmetry C18 column (4.5 mm × 250 mm, 5 μm i.d.). The mobile phase was composed of acetonitrile and water, and the wavelength of UV detector was set to 254 nm with full spectral scanning from 190 to 400 nm. The extracting solvents are indicated. The extracts from 3 batches of herbs were subjected to analysis, a representative profile was shown. a, Codonopsis Radix; b, Atractylodis Macrocephalae Rhizoma; c, Angelicae Sinensis Radix; d, Astragali Radix; e, Jujubae Fructus; f, Ginseng Radix; g, Amomi Fructus; h, Aucklandiae Radix; i, Areca Catechu; j, Dioscoreae Ahizoma; k, Lablab Semen Album; l, Poria Cocos; m, Nelumbinis Semen; n, Coicis Semen; o, Crataegi Fructus.

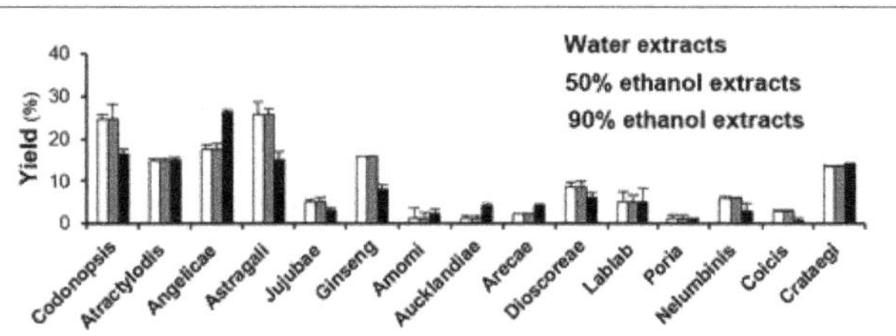

FIGURE 1 | The yields of water extract, 50% ethanol extract and 90% ethanol extract of 15 spleen-meridian herbs. The herbal extracts were prepared with distilled water, 50% ethanol and 90% ethanol by refluxing twice and each time for 2 h. The yields were calculated as the percentage of the weight of dried extracts to herbal powders. All values are in Mean ± SD, $n = 3$. The detailed yield and origin of each batch were shown in **Table 1**.

High resolution mass spectrometry was established in analyzing the herbal extracts. The LC-MS profiles could be displayed in two forms: total ion chromatogram (TIC) and mass spectrum. **Figure 4** shows a typical profile of 90% ethanol extract of Ginseng Radix. The distribution of trace ingredients with different polarity and molecular mass were shown. A list of mass spectrum with intensity was obtained for the herbal extracts. The LC-MS profiles of 15 spleen-meridian

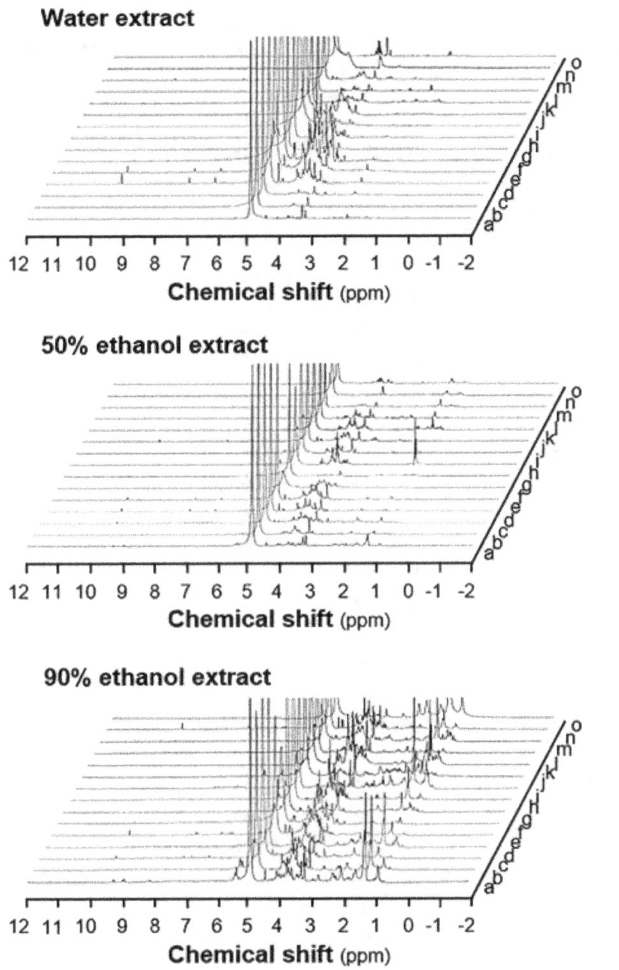

FIGURE 3 | ^{1}H NMR profiles of herbal extracts from the 15 spleen-meridian herbs. The extracts (50 mg) were dissolved in 400 μL of D_2O and centrifuged at 13,000 × *g* for 1 min before transferred to a standard 5-mm NMR tube. The ^{1}H NMR experiment were conducted on a Varian 300 MHz NMR spectrometer, operating at 300.13 MHz ^{1}H NMR frequency at 298 K. The spectra were acquired using a 1D CPMG pulse sequence (RD-90°-t1-90°-tm-90°-acquire) to generate a spectrum with a reduced residual solvent peak. The range of chemical shift was set from −2 to 12 ppm, and the deuterated solvent peak at 4.8 was set as calibration. The extracting solvents are indicated. The extracts from 3 batches of herbs were subjected to analysis, a representative profile was shown. a, Codonopsis Radix; b, Atractylodis Macrocephalae Rhizoma; c, Angelicae Sinensis Radix; d, Astragali Radix; e, Jujubae Fructus; f, Ginseng Radix; g, Amomi Fructus; h, Aucklandiae Radix; i, Areca Catechu; j, Dioscoreae Ahizoma; k, Lablab Semen Album; l, Poria Cocos; m, Nelumbinis Semen; n, Coicis Semen; o, Crataegi Fructus.

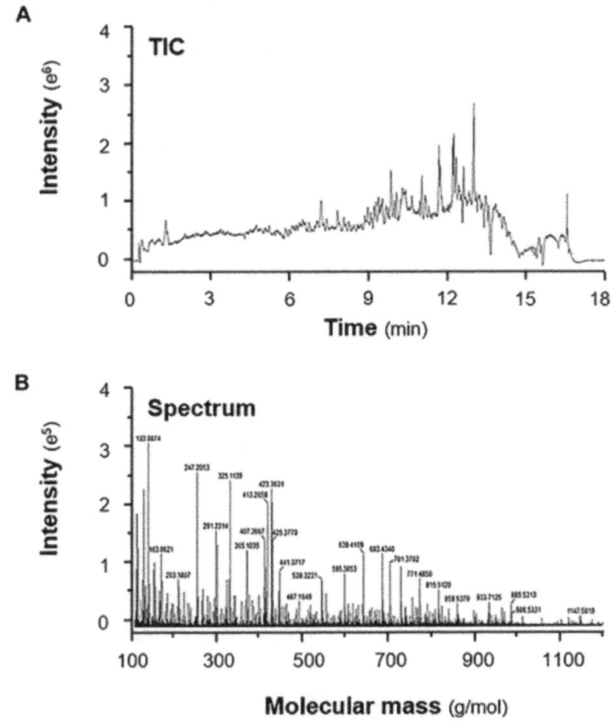

FIGURE 4 | A typical total ion chromatogram (TIC) and mass spectrum. The 90% ethanol extract of Ginseng was served as an example. **(A)** Total ion chromatogram (TIC) and **(B)** mass spectrum of the Ginseng extracts are shown. The X-axis of TIC is time (min); while the X-axis of spectrum is mass (Da). Both profiles were obtained with a Xevo G2-XS® Quadrupole Time-of-Flight (Q-TOF) Mass Spectrometer coupled with an integrated ACQUITY UPLC® I-Class System. The mobile phase was composed of acetonitrile and water, and the effluent was analyzed with an ESI ion source in positive mode. The acquisition range was set from 50 to 1200 Da with 0.1 s scan rate to reveal most of the chemicals within the herbal extracts. The extracts from 3 batches of herbs were subjected to analysis, a representative profile was shown.

herbs were established, and the data processing was performed on Waters MassLynx V4.1 SCN923. With MassLynx, each chromatographic peak was identified by a mass-to-charge ratio (m/z) and retention time, as illustrated in **Supplementary Figure 1**. As shown in **Table 2**, 65 compounds in 15 herbs were identified with unique relative molecular mass of $[M + H]^+$, $[M + Na]^+$ or $[2M + H]^+$ within acceptable experimental error, which therefore could be used for the purpose of chemical authentication.

Principal Component Analysis of Chemical Composition Profiles

To determine the similarities and differences among the herbal extracts, PCA analyses of chemical profiles deriving from HPLC, NMR and LC-MS were conducted. PCA is a chemometrics method to determine the possible relationship of different samples. The general procedure of PCA on full spectrum was shown in **Figure 5**. The spectrums were firstly divided into bins according to the resolution of analytic methods, i.e., 9,000 bins for HPLC, 1,200 bins for NMR, 10,800 bins for TIC and 230,000 bins for mass spectrum, with analytic softwares, e.g., Agilent MassHunter workstation software version B.01.00 for HPLC, Waters MassLynx V4.1 SCN923 for LC-MS and MestReNova 6.1.1 for NMR. The intensity of each bin was extracted and arranged. The obtained excel or txt files were further imported into PCA software (SIMCA-P+ version 14.1) for chemometrics analysis.

According to the TCM theory, the selected 15 spleen-meridian herbs could not only be divided into three different groups

TABLE 2 | The compounds identified from the herbal extracts.

Herbs	Retention time (t_R, min)	Identification	$[M + H]^+$ (m/z)	Molecular weight (Da)	Formula	Mass error (ppm)
Codonopsis Radix	0.942	Codonopsine	268.1614	267.1549	$C_{14}H_{21}NO_4$	5.4
	2.323	Vanillic acid	169.0581	168.0494	$C_8H_8O_4$	4.5
	3.565	Tryptophan sulfate	286.0615	285.054	$C_{11}H_{12}N_2O_5S$	1.5
	5.932	Ferulic acid	196.0743	195.0665	$C_{10}H_{10}O_4$	0.7
	9.921	Atractylenolide II	234.1618	233.1538	$C_{15}H_{20}O_2$	0.3
	9.936	Codonopyrrolidium A	351.4372	350.429	$C_{19}H_{28}NO_5$	0.7
Atractylodis Macrocephalae Rhizoma	5.903	Icariside D1	417.1715	416.1687	$C_{19}H_{28}O_{10}$	12.4
	7.382	Atractylenolide III	271.1321[a]	248.1417	$C_{15}H_{20}O_3$	2.2
	7.749	Atractylenolactam	230.1557	229.1471	$C_{15}H_{19}ON$	2.9
	8.087	Atractyloside A	449.2399	448.2313	$C_{21}H_{36}O_{10}$	1.5
	8.145	Atractyloside B	473.2363[a]	450.246	$C_{21}H_{38}O_{10}$	1.1
	8.796	β-sitosterol	415.3944	414.3867	$C_{29}H_{50}O$	0.6
	11.231	Atractylenolide I	233.1544	232.1467	$C_{15}H_{20}O_2$	1
	12.26	Atractylenolide II	231.1381	230.1311	$C_{15}H_{18}O_2$	4.1
	12.26	Atractylenolide VI	203.1807	202.1726	$C_{15}H_{22}$	0.8
Angelicae Sinensis Radix	9.583	Ferulic acid	196.0759	195.0659	$C_{10}H_{10}O_4$	10.6
	10.797	Levistolide A	382.2154	381.2066	$C_{24}H_{28}O_4$	2.3
	12.256	Linoleic acid	280.2395	279.2314	$C_{18}H_{32}O_2$	0.6
Astragali Radix	4.453	Calycosin	285.2673	284.2634	$C_{16}H_{12}O_5$	14.2
	4.608	Wogonin	285.2673	284.2636	$C_{16}H_{12}O_5$	14.9
	5.987	Formononetin	269.2712	268.264	$C_{16}H_{12}O_4$	2.8
	6.001	Astragaloside II	828.0103	827.0069	$C_{43}H_{70}O_{15}$	5.5
	6.339	Astragaloside IV	785.9793	784.9702	$C_{41}H_{68}O_{14}$	1.5
	7.03	Soyasaponin I	944.1336	943.1221	$C_{48}H_{78}O_{18}$	3.8
	9.821	Isorhamnetin	317.2684	316.2623	$C_{16}H_{12}O_7$	5.8
	10.274	Astragaloside VII	948.1183	947.1108	$C_{47}H_{78}O_{19}$	0.5
	10.275	Soyasaponin II	914.1056	913.0961	$C_{47}H_{76}O_{17}$	1.7
	11.724	Medicarpin	271.2863	270.28	$C_{16}H_{14}O_4$	6.1
Jujubae Fructus	2.154	Coclaurine	286.1543	285.1443	$C_{17}H_{19}NO_3$	7.2
	2.334	Magnoflorine	342.1794	341.1705	$C_{20}H_{24}NO_4$	2.8
	4.154	Juzirine	282.1187	281.113	$C_{17}H_{15}NO_3$	8
	4.636	Spinosin	609.1878	608.1819	$C_{28}H_{33}O_{15}$	3.4
Ginseng Radix	2.705	Ginsenoside Rg_2	785.5016	784.4973	$C_{42}H_{72}O_{13}$	4.6
	5.27	Ginsenoside Rh_2	623.4571	622.4445	$C_{36}H_{62}O_8$	7.5
Amomi Fructus	3.126	Isoquercitrin	465.3867	464.38	$C_{21}H_{20}O_{12}$	2.7
	3.508	Quercetin	449.3878	448.3769	$C_{21}H_{20}O_{11}$	6.6
Aucklandiae Radix	6.439	β-caryophyllene	205.3671	204.36	$C_{15}H_{24}$	4.1
	9.936	Alantolactone	233.3176	232.31	$C_{15}H_{20}O_2$	1.5
Areca Catechu	8.087	Catechin	291.2758	290.27	$C_{15}H_{14}O_6$	7.4
	13.009	Epigallocatechin	307.2769	306.27	$C_{15}H_{14}O_7$	3.4
Dioscoreae Ahizoma	13.135	Pseudoprotodioscin	1031.507	1030.5	$C_{51}H_{82}O_{21}$	3.4
Lablab Semen Album	9.77	Arachidic acid	313.3159	312.3028	$C_{20}H_{40}O_2$	3.4
Poria Cocos	6.666	Dehydrotumulosic acid	485.3644	484.3553	$C_{31}H_{48}O_4$	2.4
	7.087	Mechylcis-9-hexadecenoate	269.4418	268.4348	$C_{17}H_{32}O_2$	3.5
	9.184	Hederagenin	473.3619	472.3553	$C_{30}H_{48}O_4$	2.8
	9.202	Pachymic acid	529.3865	528.3815	$C_{33}H_{52}O_5$	5.6
	10.994	Dehydropachymic acid	527.3738	526.3658	$C_{33}H_{50}O_6$	0.1
Nelumbinis Semen	10.36	Naringenin	273.0734	272.0685	$C_{15}H_{12}O_5$	11.2
Coicis Semen	2.618	1,3-diolein	621.9989	620.986	$C_{39}H_{72}O_5$	8
	13.502	Trilinolein	880.3988	879.384	$C_{57}H_{98}O_6$	7.8
	14.544	Triolein	886.4386	885.432	$C_{57}H_{104}O_6$	1.5

(Continued)

TABLE 2 | Continued

Herbs	Retention time (t_R, min)	Identification	$[M + H]^+$ (*m/z*)	Molecular weight (Da)	Formula	Mass error (ppm)
Crataegi Fructus	2.661	Quercetin 3-*O*-(6-*O*-rhamnosyl-glucoside) (rutin)	611.1526	610.1458	$C_{27}H_{30}O_{16}$	1.9
	2.677	Quercetin 3-*O*-(2, 6-di-*O*-rhamnosyl-glucoside)	757.2094	756.2037	$C_{33}H_{40}O_{20}$	3
	2.846	(epi)afzelechin-(epi)catechin	563.1459	562.1402	$C_{30}H_{26}O_{11}$	4
	3.097	Quercetin	303.0414	302.0349	$C_{15}H_{10}O_7$	4.8
	4.636	Diosmetin 7-*O*-rutinoside (diosmin)	609.1737	608.1665	$C_{28}H_{32}O_{15}$	1.2
	4.64	Quercetin 3-*O*-rhamnoside (quercitrin)	448.0975	447.0928	$C_{21}H_{20}O_{11}$	7.2
	9.3	Pectolinarin	623.1901	622.1827	$C_{29}H_{34}O_{15}$	0.9
	9.767	Apigenin 7-*O*-glucoside	433.1032	432.0979	$C_{21}H_{20}O_{10}$	6.1
	10.314	Quinic acid	193.0655	192.0561	$C_7H_{12}O_6$	7.6
	10.343	Epicatechin	291.0789	290.0716	$C_{15}H_{14}O_6$	2.2
	10.512	Isorhamnetin-*O*-hexoside	479.1131	478.1036	$C_{22}H_{22}O_{12}$	3.3
	10.994	Phloretin 2′-*O*-glucoside (phlorizin)	437.1365	436.1294	$C_{21}H_{24}O_{10}$	1.9
	11.724	3-*O*-caffeoylshikimic acid	337.0856	336.0773	$C_{16}H_{16}O_8$	1.1
	12.361	*p*-coumaric acid-*O*-hexoside	327.1006	326.0927	$C_{15}H_{18}O_8$	0.1

[a]*Mass-to-charge ratio (m/z) is* $[M + Na]^+$.

according to their "Yin-Yang" nature, and which also could be divided into four groups according to their pharmacological activities (**Table 1**). In clinical application, these herbs nourish the blood, calm the heart and promote the digestion. By characterizing the relationship between the distributions of herbal extracts in score scatter plots with their identified pharmacological activities, the correlation between chemical composition basis and known pharmacology could be clarified. Although the score scatter plots of HPLC fingerprints (**Figure 6A**) and NMR profiles (**Figure 6B**) possessed acceptable first principal component (58.9%, 50.2%) and second principal component (14.1%, 13.2%), the distribution of herbal extracts showed no apparent regular pattern among different groups. The results indicated that HPLC and NMR profiles might not able to distinguish the herbal extracts with different pharmacological properties.

The LC-MS profiles, including TIC and mass spectrum obtained from UPLC/Q-TOF, were further analyzed with the same procedures as that of HPLC and NMR profiles. Both score scatter plots possessed acceptable first principal component and second principal component, especially in the scenario of two principal components of mass spectrum accounting for 97.7% of total variance (**Figures 7A,B**). These results therefore could be an outcome of ultra-high resolution of UPLC/Q-TOF. The two PCA scoring plots showed similar distribution according to their identified pharmacological activities, indicating that the polarity of herbal compounds might have positive correlation with their mass, at least to certain degree. Moreover, the herbal extracts having similar pharmacological activities showed a clustering effect. In the clustering analysis, the blood nourishing herbs could be distinguished obviously from other herbs (**Figure 7**). Thus, the plots showed a strong correlation between distribution of herbal extracts with their pharmacological activities, which was in line with the hypothesis that the bioactivities of herbal extracts should be strongly related to their chemical composition.

The relationship between "Yin-Yang" nature and distribution of the herbal extracts in scoring plots were determined. The distribution of Yin, Yang and neutral herbs were significantly identified to be different, in particular the right part of score scatter plots contained only the Yang-stimulating herbs (**Figures 8A,C**). To clarify the chemical basis of distinct distribution, the variables in loading scatter plots could be divided into three clustering groups, according to their retention time and molecular mass. From the distribution of herbal extracts in score scatter plot, the contents of compounds eluted between 6 and 12 min showed greater impacts in the "Yin-Yang" distinction of herbal extracts (**Figure 8B**). Similarly, the lighter molecules, i.e., less than 900 g/mol, were distributed in marginal positions in the loading scatter plots (**Figure 8D**), indicating that these compounds might have obvious influence

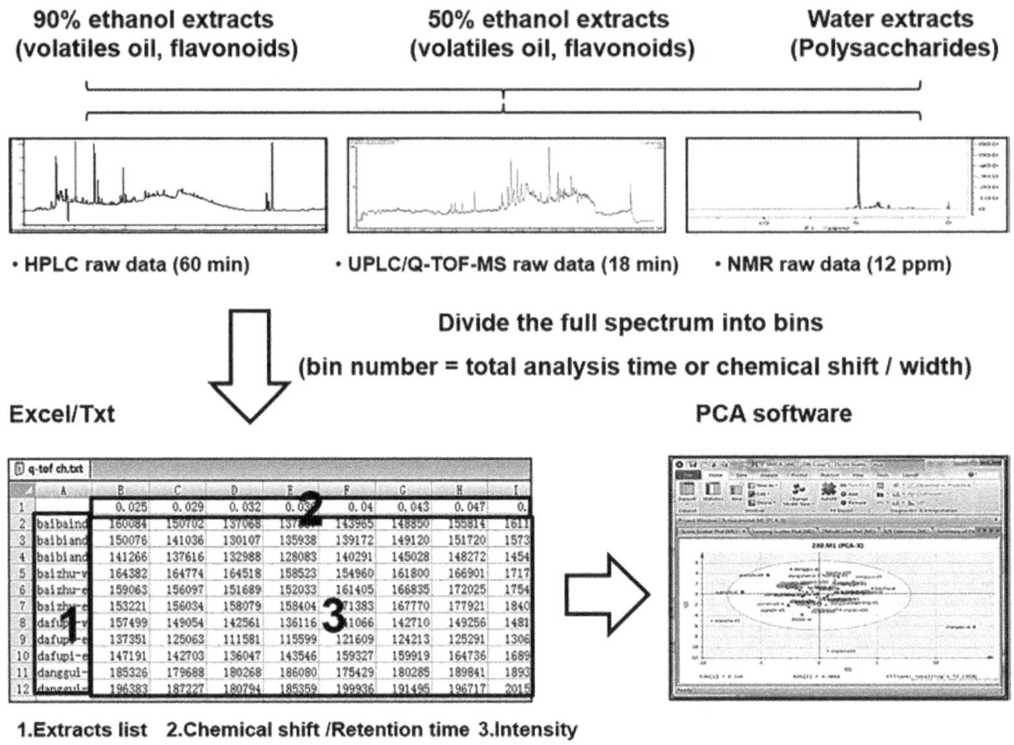

FIGURE 5 | The procedure of full spectrum principle component analysis. The spectrums were firstly divided into bins according to the resolution of analytic methods with its corresponding softwares (Agilent MassHunter workstation software version B.01.00 for HPLC, Waters MassLynx V4.1 SCN923 for LC-MS and MestReNova 6.1.1 for NMR). The intensity of each bin was extracted and arranged as the figure showed. The obtained excel or txt file was further subjected into PCA software (SIMCA-P+ version 12.0, Umetrics, Sweden).

to the herbs' properties. Moreover, it could be deduced that the Yang-stimulating herbs were shown to contain more compounds, i.e., the compounds with higher polarity and lower molecular mass. These results not only illustrated the chemical basis in classify "Yin-Yang" nature of TCM, and which also suggested the polarity and molecular mass of ingredients in the herbs could be two major influencing factors.

To determine applicability of present analytic methods, three pair-herbs having typical cold and hot properties, as recorded in TCM practice, were subjected into our developed PCA analysis. Ginseng Radix and Rehmanniae Radix Praeparata are considered as hot and warm herbs aiming to tonify qi and to nourish blood; while Quinquefolium Radix and Rehmanniae Radix are cold herbs used to clear heat aiming to promote fluid production (Yu et al., 2001; Zhang et al., 2008). Angelica Sinensis Radix is a typical herb in invigorating blood in TCM therapy. However, the treatment of Angelica Sinensis Radix with wine reduces the amount of volatile oil, and this treatment could directly minimize the hot property of Angelica Sinensis Radix (Zhan et al., 2011). These three paired-herbs have the same or similar origin, and however, they have opposite functions. From the PCA score scatter plots of TIC and spectrum, the distribution of herbal extracts with hot or warm properties (i.e., Ginseng Radix and Rehmanniae Radix Praeparata) were significantly different from the herbs having cold or cool properties (i.e., Quinquefolium Radix and Rehmanniae Radix) (**Figures 9A,B**). As expected, the polarity and molecular mass of major components in the extracts of pair-herbs were different, accordingly. Although the difference between Angelica Sinensis Radix and wine-treated Angelica Sinensis Radix in pharmacological properties was not as obvious as other paired-herbs, as mentioned above, the distribution of the two herbal extracts could also be distinguished significantly in the score scatter plots (**Figures 9A,B**). The result strongly supported the precision applicability of the present established analytical model.

Anti-oxidative Profile of Spleen-Meridian Herbs

To elucidate the connection between the "Yin-Yang" nature and redox system, a series of *in vitro* assays were conducted to measure the anti-oxidative properties of herbal extracts. Folin-Ciocalteu assay was used to determine total phenolic compounds in herbal extracts. Phenolic compounds, highly abundant in plant, generally have unstable electrons in the phenolic hydroxyl groups, and which protect cells from being oxidized by directly neutralizing free radicals or decomposing peroxides. The content of total phenolic compounds in the selected herbs were rather similar (**Figure 10** and **Table 3**). In exception, the water and 50% ethanol extracts of Lablab Semen Album contained much less of total phenolic content (**Figure 10**). In contrast, Arecae Pericarpium and Crataegi Fructus possessed relative higher contents, as compared with

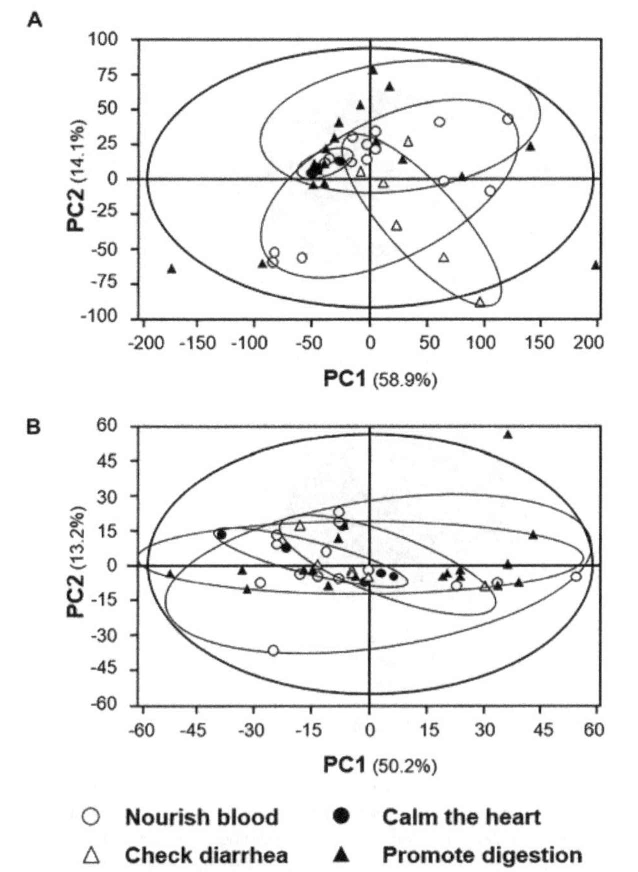

FIGURE 6 | PCA analyses of **(A)** HPLC and **(B)** ^{1}H NMR profiles of signals from the 15 spleen-meridian herbs. The distribution of each herbal extract in score scatter plots was calculated according to its correlation with the major components. The classification of herbal extracts was according to the proposed pharmacological activity, as described in TCM practice. The results showed very low discrimination between different types of herbal extracts.

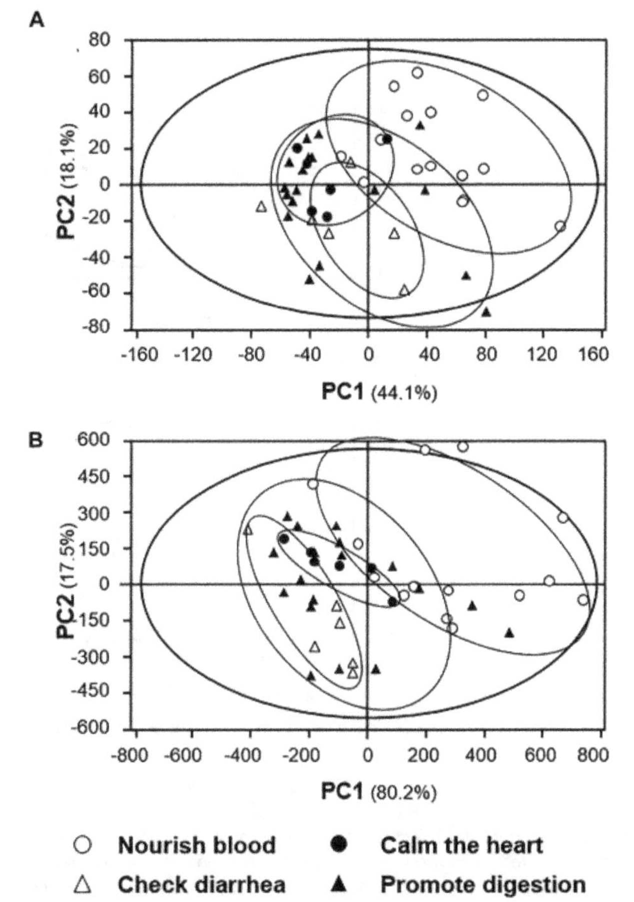

FIGURE 7 | PCA analyses of **(A)** TIC and **(B)** spectrum profiles of signals from the 15 spleen-meridian herbs. Similarly, the distribution of each herbal extract in score scatter plots was calculated according to its correlation with the major components. The classification of the herbal extracts was according to the proposed pharmacological activity, as described in TCM practice. The results showed relatively higher discrimination between different types of extracts.

other herbs. The 50% ethanol extracts of herbs contained higher amounts of phenolic compounds in general, except in the scenario of Aucklandiae Radix and Nelumbinis Semen (**Figure 10**).

The free radical scavenging activity of the polyphenolic compounds in herbal extracts was measured with DPPH radical scavenging assay. DPPH, having stable free radicals, was used to detect radical-scavenging ability of herbal extracts. Here, the EC50 of each herbal extract was determined (**Figure 10**). The DPPH radical scavenging activity of most extracts were similar (**Figure 10** and **Table 3**). Among all the herbs, Lablab Semen Album showed the largest value of EC50, indicating the weakest anti-oxidant. In contrary, Arecae Pericarpium and Crataegi Fructus showed stronger DPPH radical scavenging activity: the outcome was consistent with the result of Folin-Ciocalteu assay (**Figure 10**).

To reveal the protective effect, the herbal extract was applied onto the tBHP-treated RAW264.7 macrophages. RAW264.7 murine cell was chosen because of its high breeding speed and stability. A stress inducer, tBHP, was chosen to damage the macrophage, which induced cell death in a dose-dependent manner. Vitamin C served as a positive control (Huang et al., 2018a,b). A series of concentrations was employed, and the 15 herbs were divided into four groups, according to their efficiency (**Supplementary Figure 2**). After the optimization of dose of herbal extracts with MTT assay, the protective effects of the extracts to tBHP-induced cell cytotoxicity were determined. As shown in **Supplementary Figure 3**, the extracts protected the cells from oxidative damage in a dose-dependent manner. The protective effects and EC50 of the herbal extracts were summarized in **Figure 10** and **Table 3**. The extracts of Angelicae Sinensis Radix and Ginseng Radix possessed the best protection effects to more than 50%, as compared to the control. In contrast, Aucklandiae Radix, Nelumbinis Semen and Coicis Semen provided significantly lower protective effects at around 20% (**Figure 10**).

The formation of ROS is one of the vital causes in inducing cell death. By determining the inhibition effects of herbal extracts to tBHP-induced ROS formation, the protective effect of herbal

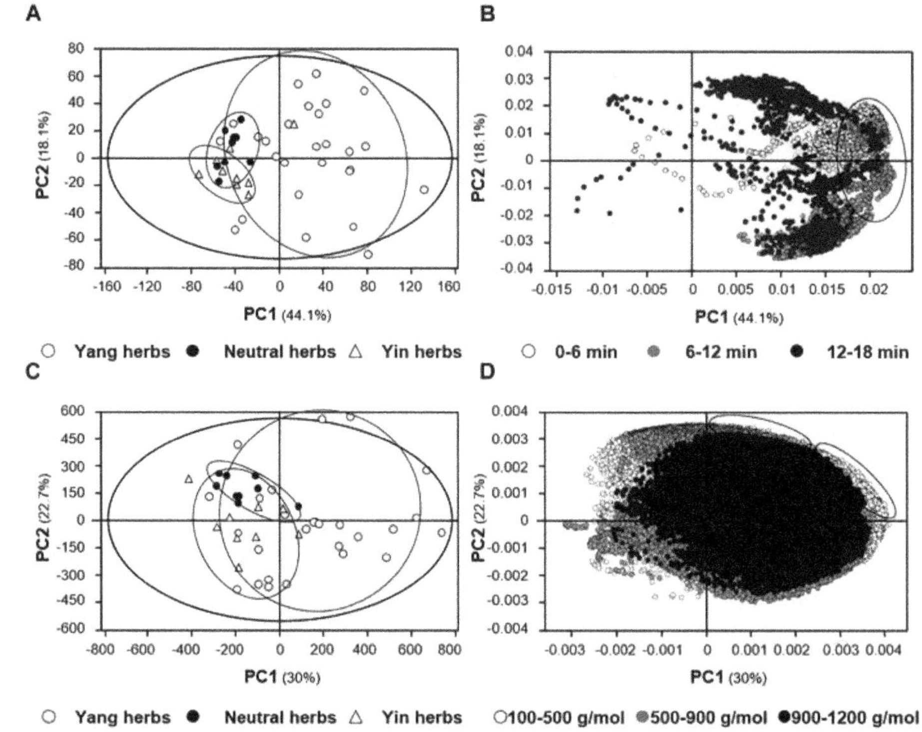

FIGURE 8 | PCA analyses of LC-MS profiles of signals from the 15 spleen-meridian herbs. **(A)** Scoring plots of TIC. **(B)** Loading scatter plots of TIC. **(C)** Scoring plots of spectrum. **(D)** Loading scatter plots of spectrum. The distribution of each herbal extract in score scatter plots was calculated according to its correlation with the major components. The classification of herbal extracts was according to the "Yin-Yang" nature of herbs, i.e., Yin, neutral and Yang herbs, according to TCM practice. The results showed very obvious discrimination between herbal extracts with different properties. Each dot in the loading scatter plots represents a variable. Dots in **(B)** represent time intervals for 0.1 s, and dots in **(D)** represent mass intervals of 0.005 Da.

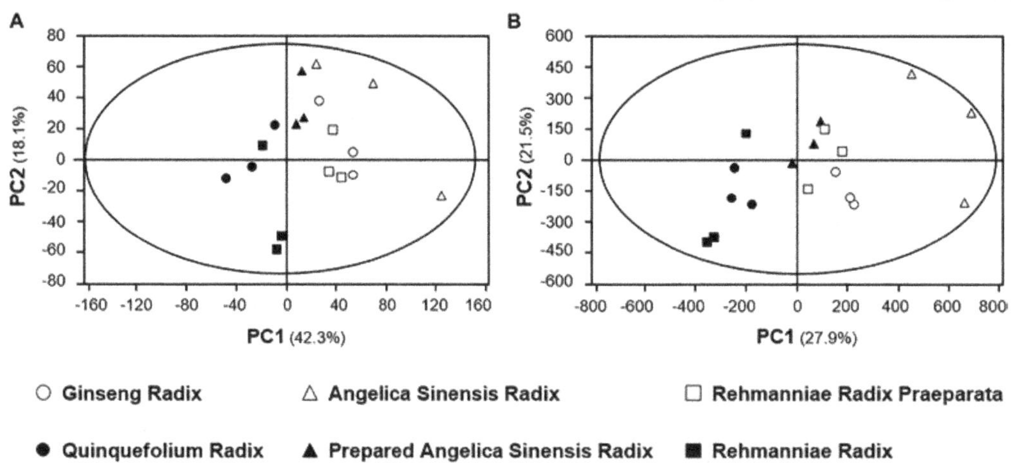

FIGURE 9 | PCA analyses of **(A)** TIC and **(B)** spectrum profiles of three paired-herbs with typical cold or hot property, i.e., Ginseng Radix-Quinquefolium Radix, Angelica Sinensis Radix-Prepared Angelica Sinensis Radix, Rehmanniae Radix Praeparata-Dried Rehmanniae Radix. The distribution of each herbal extract in score scatter plots was calculated according to its correlation with the major components.

extracts was further compared and analyzed. As shown in **Table 3**, the inhibition effects to ROS formation were positively related with the protective effects to cell viability. The 50% ethanol extracts of Atractylodis Macrocephalae Rhizoma, Angelicae Sinensis Radix, Jujubae Fructus possessed the best effect having over 50% of inhibition, as compared to the control (**Figure 10**). Moreover, the luciferase-reporter construct (i.e., pARE-Luc) containing four ARE DNA regulatory elements deriving from the promoters of anti-oxidative genes, tagged upstream of a luciferase gene, was transfected into cultured RAW264.7 cells.

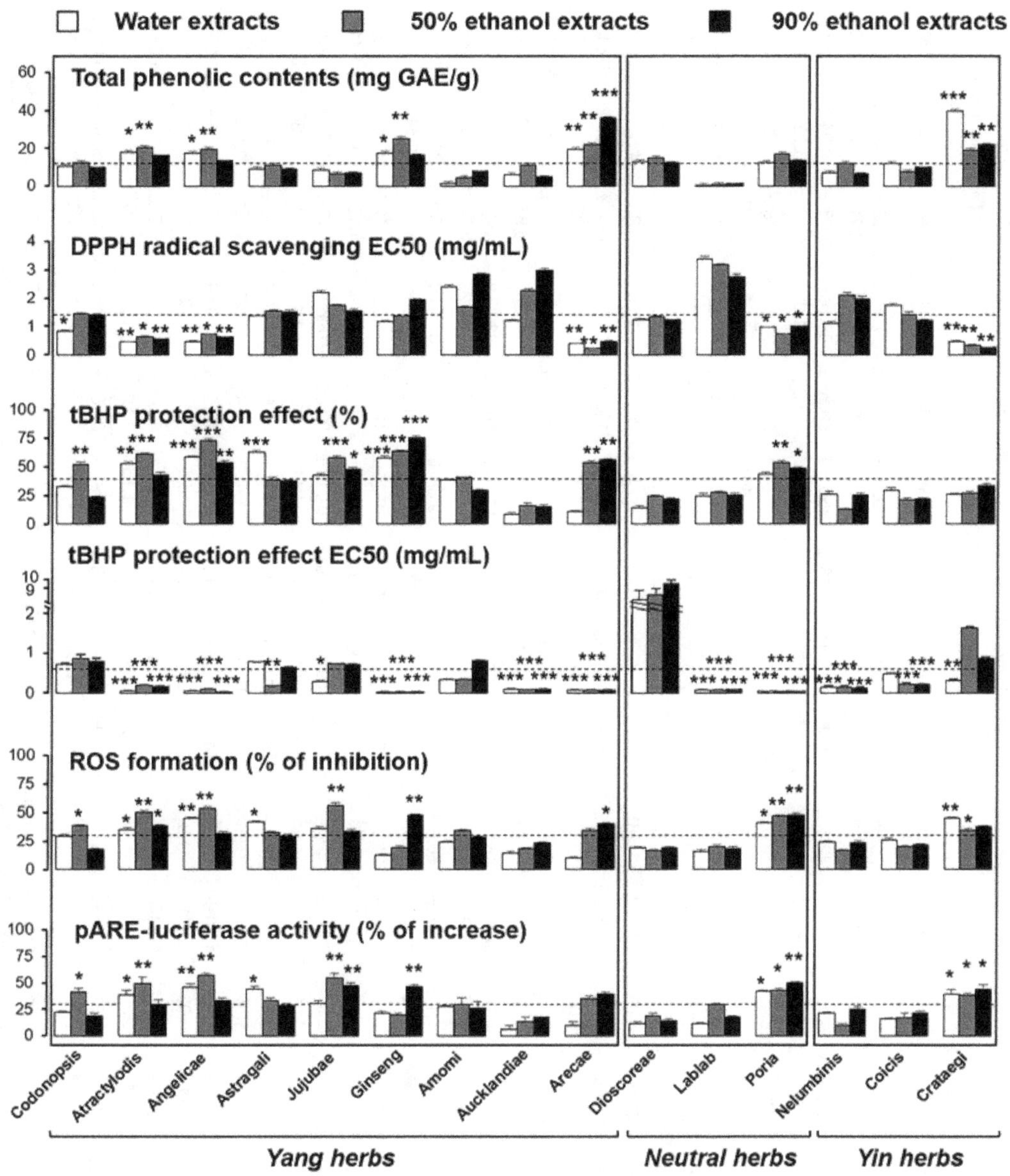

FIGURE 10 | The correlation between anti-oxidative profiles of the spleen-meridian herbs with the "Yin-Yang" classification criterion. Values are expressed as Mean ± SD, where $n = 4$, each with triplicate samples. Statistical comparison was made with mean value. The mean value of total phenolic compounds was 12.87 mg GAE/g; mean value of DPPH radical scavenging EC50 was 1.38 mg/mL; mean value of tBHP protection effect was 37.9%; mean value of tBHP protection effect at IC50 was 0.65 mg/mL; mean value of inhibition effects to ROS formation was 30.5%; mean value of pARE-luciferase activity increase was 29.6%. $^{*}p < 0.05$; $^{**}p < 0.01$; $^{***}p < 0.001$.

The activation of pARE-Luc, triggered by herbal extracts, showed the same pattern as the result of ROS formation. Again, the 50% ethanol extracts of Atractylodis Macrocephalae Rhizoma, Angelicae Sinensis Radix, Jujubae Fructus exhibited the best inhibition effects of over 50% (**Figure 10** and **Table 3**).

Correlation Between Yin-Yang Attributes With Anti-oxidative Profile

After establishment of anti-oxidative profiles of spleen-meridian herbs, the correlation of this activity with the "Yin-Yang" classification criterion was determined. By comparing the specific anti-oxidative data of herbal extracts with the mean value of 45 extracts, the statistical tests were performed by one-way ANOVA with multiple comparisons using Dunnett's test (**Figure 10** and **Table 3**). According to the comparison results, the differences between species were relatively higher than that from different herbal extracts. Moreover, the correlation between the anti-oxidative profiles of the spleen-meridian herbal extracts with the "Yin-Yang" classification criterion was rather weak in the tested parameters. Poria Cocos is a plain medicine used to fortify spleen, while Crataegi Fructus is classified as Yin herb due to its acid flavor. These herbs contain abundant phenolic compounds

TABLE 3 | The correlation between anti-oxidant profiles of the spleen-meridian herbs with the "Yin-Yang" classification criterion.

Attributes	Herbs	Total phenolics (mg GAE/g)[b]			DPPH radical scavenging EC50 (mg/mL)			tBHP protection(%)			tBHP protection EC50 (mg/mL)			ROS formation (% of inhibition)			pARE-luciferase activity (% of increase)		
		W[c]	E50	E90	E90	E50	E90	W	E50	E90	W	E50	E90	W	E50	E90	W	E50	E90
Yang herbs	CR[a]	10.21 ± 0.32[d]	12.25 ± 0.22	9.71 ± 0.21	0.82 ± 0.03*	1.44 ± 0.04	1.39 ± 0.05	32.7 ± 0.97	51.8 ± 2.34**	23.6 ± 0.92	0.72 ± 0.05	0.88 ± 0.1	0.8 ± 0.1	29.72 ± 1.22	38.37 ± 1.41*	17.41 ± 1.18	21.82 ± 1.72	40.94 ± 4.09*	18.21 ± 2.82
	AMR	17.91 ± 0.32*	20.31 ± 0.24**	16.19 ± 0.23	0.46 ± 0.01**	0.64 ± 0.02*	0.55 ± 0.02**	53 ± 1.65**	61.3 ± 0.67***	42.8 ± 2.53	0.05 ± 0.01***	0.2 ± 0***	0.18 ± 0***	35.28 ± 1.39*	50.36 ± 1.89**	38.14 ± 1.3*	38.68 ± 4.19*	49.04 ± 6.19**	29.82 ± 3.8
	ASR	17.61 ± 0.22*	19.5 ± 0.26**	13.25 ± 0.11	0.47 ± 0.02**	0.72 ± 0.02*	0.62 ± 0.03*	58.4 ± 1.21***	73.1 ± 1.63***	53.6 ± 1.71**	0.06 ± 0.01***	0.1 ± 0***	0.03 ± 0.01***	45.01 ± 1.46**	53.61 ± 1.57**	31.89 ± 1.33	45.75 ± 3.15**	57.02 ± 2.57**	32.62 ± 3.26
	AsR	9.02 ± 0.21	10.93 ± 0.31	8.92 ± 0.21	1.36 ± 0.02	1.52 ± 0.04	1.5 ± 0.06	62.5 ± 1.87***	38.7 ± 2.39	37.6 ± 0.82	0.8 ± 0.01	0.19 ± 0**	0.67 ± 0	41.72 ± 1.44*	32.46 ± 1.33	29.63 ± 1.29	43.72 ± 2.37*	33.48 ± 1.85	28.86 ± 1.89
	JF	8.45 ± 0.31	6.18 ± 0.11	7.02 ± 0.21	2.19 ± 0.08	1.75 ± 0.03	1.53 ± 0.06	42.5 ± 1.93	57.7 ± 1.92***	47.8 ± 1.28*	0.3 ± 0.01*	0.75 ± 0	0.74 ± 0.01	36.12 ± 1.3	56.49 ± 1.75**	33.37 ± 1.48	30.33 ± 3.03	54.54 ± 4.54**	47.64 ± 2.48**
	GR	17.21 ± 0.33*	24.91 ± 0.43**	16.23 ± 0.43	1.17 ± 0.03	1.36 ± 0.02	1.94 ± 0.03	57.7 ± 1.76***	63.3 ± 1.45***	75.6 ± 1.13***	0.04 ± 0.01***	0.04 ± 0.01***	0.04 ± 0.01***	12.47 ± 1.12	19.44 ± 1.2	47.46 ± 1.47**	21.67 ± 1.22	19.82 ± 1.4	46.81 ± 1.57**
	AF	1.11 ± 0.02	4.17 ± 0.03	7.89 ± 0.07	2.41 ± 0.05	1.66 ± 0.05	2.83 ± 0.06	38.4 ± 1.08	40.7 ± 0.57	29.6 ± 0.81	0.34 ± 0	0.36 ± 0.01	0.83 ± 0	24.16 ± 1.27	34.03 ± 1.29	28.13 ± 1.26	27.47 ± 0.87	29.38 ± 6.29	26.28 ± 5.55
	AuR	5.94 ± 0.23	11.06 ± 0.36	5.03 ± 0.27	1.19 ± 0.05	2.27 ± 0.07	2.98 ± 0.07	8.5 ± 1.45	16.3 ± 1.91	15.2 ± 1.91	0.1 ± 0***	0.1 ± 0***	0.1 ± 0***	14.56 ± 1.14	18.55 ± 1.17	23.23 ± 1.22	5.63 ± 3.63	13.63 ± 3.98	17.4 ± 0.67
	AC	19.28 ± 0.32**	21.73 ± 0.34**	35.97 ± 0.46***	0.39 ± 0.01**	0.22 ± 0.01**	0.48 ± 0.02**	11.1 ± 0.27	53.4 ± 1.85**	56.3 ± 0.36**	0.09 ± 0***	0.08 ± 0***	0.08 ± 0***	9.88 ± 1.1	34.71 ± 1.34	39.94 ± 1.39*	9.59 ± 3.96	34.4 ± 3.44	39.17 ± 2
Neutral herbs	DA	12.79 ± 0.44	15.1 ± 0.54	12.45 ± 0.52	1.24 ± 0.01	1.34 ± 0.02	1.23 ± 0.01	14 ± 1.65	24.2 ± 0.51	21.4 ± 1.44	4.43 ± 0.07	5.04 ± 0.06	6.5 ± 0.06	19.26 ± 1.12	16.84 ± 1.19	19.06 ± 1.14	11.74 ± 1.12	19.06 ± 1.91	14.13 ± 1.41
	LSA	0.14 ± 0.01	0.72 ± 0.02	1.14 ± 0.03	3.39 ± 0.09	3.17 ± 0.05	2.74 ± 0.09	24.4 ± 2.05	27.5 ± 0.92	25 ± 1.94	0.09 ± 0***	0.09 ± 0***	0.09 ± 0***	16.32 ± 1.11	20.56 ± 1.3	18.65 ± 1.18	11.42 ± 1.01	29.54 ± 0.9	17.73 ± 0.77
	PC	12.57 ± 0.54	16.84 ± 0.51	13.31 ± 0.41	0.95 ± 0.01*	0.74 ± 0.01*	0.99 ± 0.01*	43.7 ± 1.52	53.4 ± 2.2**	48.6 ± 0.85*	0.04 ± 0.01***	0.04 ± 0.01***	0.04 ± 0***	40.81 ± 1.42*	46.67 ± 1.43**	47.86 ± 1.5**	41.88 ± 0.82*	43.03 ± 1.93*	49.92 ± 0.8**
Yin herbs	NS	6.97 ± 0.32	12.09 ± 0.34	6.58 ± 0.42	1.11 ± 0.06	2.12 ± 0.09	1.98 ± 0.08	26.2 ± 1.92	12.6 ± 0.71	25.2 ± 1.8	0.14 ± 0.05***	0.14 ± 0.04***	0.13 ± 0.04***	24.26 ± 1.21	16.54 ± 1.1	23.84 ± 1.25	21.03 ± 0.81	10.02 ± 1.1	24.88 ± 2.49
	CS	12.07 ± 0.44	7.47 ± 0.32	9.9 ± 0.37	1.72 ± 0.02	1.41 ± 0.01	1.19 ± 0.01	29.7 ± 1.33	20.8 ± 2.08	21.4 ± 1.47	0.49 ± 0.03	0.21 ± 0.04***	0.21 ± 0.04***	26.31 ± 1.16	20.06 ± 1.17	21.73 ± 1.21	15.7 ± 1.16	17.18 ± 3.72	21.37 ± 1.53
	CF	39.72 ± 0.11***	19.14 ± 0.17**	21.94 ± 0.21**	0.48 ± 0.08**	0.34 ± 0.08**	0.26 ± 0.05**	25.8 ± 2.25	26.5 ± 1.89	33.4 ± 1.44	0.32 ± 0.02**	1.65 ± 0.04	0.88 ± 0.03	44.91 ± 1.49**	34.68 ± 1.19	37.36 ± 1.14*	39.12 ± 4.91*	38.57 ± 1.86*	44.06 ± 4.04*

[a]*CR, Codonopsis Radix; AMR, Atractylodis Macrocephalae Rhizoma; ASR, Angelicae Sinensis Radix; AsR, Astragali Radix; JF, Jujubae Fructus; GR, Ginseng Radix; AF, Amomi Fructus; AuR, Aucklandiae Radix; AC, Areca Catechu; DA, Dioscoreae Ahizoma; LSA, Lablab Semen Album; PC, Poria Cocos; NS, Nelumbinis Semen; CS, Coicis Semen; CF, Crataegi Fructus.* [b]*GAE, gallic acid equivalent.* [c]*W, water extract; E50, 50% ethanol extract; E90, 90% ethanol extract.* [d]*Values are expressed as Mean ± SD, where n = 4, each with triplicate samples. Statistical comparison was made with mean value (mean value of total phenolics is 12.87 mg GAE/g; mean value of DPPH radical scavenging EC50 is 1.38 mg/mL; mean value of tBHP protection effect is 37.9%; mean value of tBHP protection effect EC50 is 0.65 mg/mL; mean value of inhibition effects to ROS formation is 30.5%; mean value of pARE-luciferase activity increase is 29.6%).* $*p < 0.05$; $**p < 0.01$; $***p < 0.001$.

and possess appreciable anti-oxidative activity, resulting in better protective effects to oxidative stressed cells than that from Yang herbs, e.g., Amomi Fructus, Aucklandiae Radix (**Figure 10**).

Furthermore, the PCA analysis of anti-oxidative profiles was conducted. As shown in **Figure 11**, the two principal components of the mass spectrum accounted for 86.9% of total variance, which is enough to support the credibility of the results. The distribution of Yang, neutral and Yin herbs could not be distinguished in the score scatter plot, indicating there are no significant difference between anti-oxidative profiles of these herbs (**Figure 11A**). This insignificant distinction could also be predicted from the loading scatter plot (**Figure 11B**). Having the parameters of tBHP-protected effect (%), ROS formation (% of inhibition) and pARE-luciferase activity (% of increase) at similar locations, there should be insufficient variables to distinguish the samples. Thus, the anti-oxidative properties of herbal extract were not equivalent to its "Yin-Yang" properties of herbal medicine.

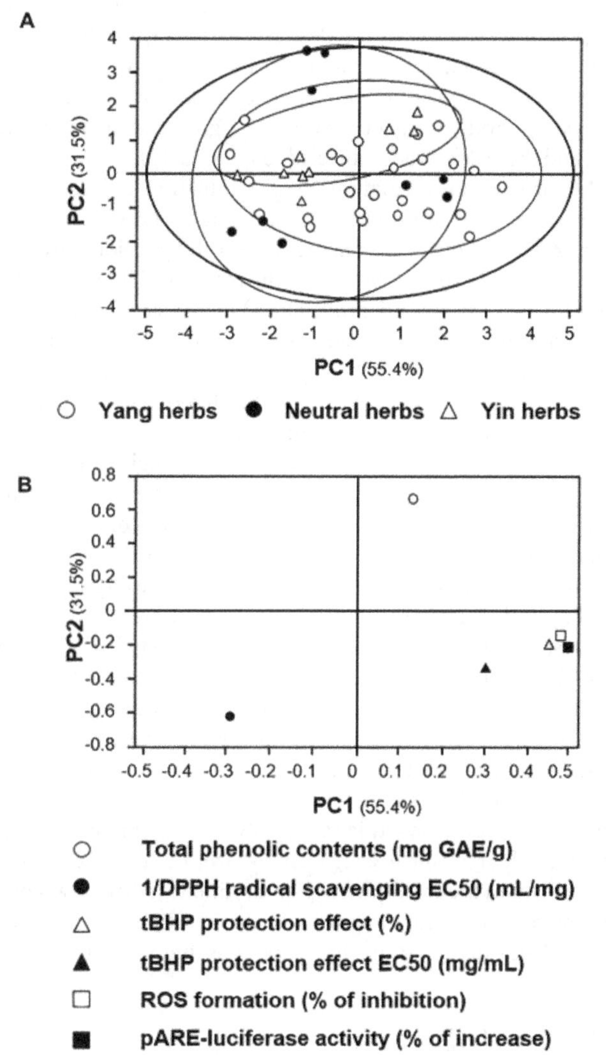

FIGURE 11 | PCA analyses of anti-oxidative profiles of signals from the 15 spleen-meridian herbs. **(A)** Scoring plots. **(B)** Loading scatter plots. The distribution of each herbal extract in score scatter plots was calculated according to its correlation with the major components. The classification of the herbal extracts was according to the "Yin-Yang" nature of herbs, i.e., Yin-stimulating, neutral and Yang-stimulating herbs, according to TCM practice. The results showed low discrimination between herbal extracts with anti-oxidative properties. Each dot in the loading scatter plots **(B)** represents a variable, i.e., the parameters reflecting the anti-oxidant of extracts.

DISCUSSION

The concept of four natures and five flavors of TCM herb is accumulated from long-term medical practice, and this theory plays a key role in clinical medication. To clarify the modern physiological meaning of the "Yin-Yang" properties, 15 spleen-meridian herbs were selected for the illustration of such classification. In accordance to TCM clinical practice, we have chosen different types of herbs that are known to have certain pharmacological functions: (i) herbs to fortify spleen and promote digestion, e.g., Aucklandiae Radix and Crataegi Fructus; (ii) herbs to keep digestion system in normal state by resolving dampness and treating diarrhea, e.g., Atractylodis Macrocephalae Rhizoma, Amomi Fructus, Areca Catechu, Dioscoreae Ahizoma, Lablab Semen Album, Nelumbinis Semen and Coicis Semen; (iii) herbs to replenish Qi and nourish blood, e.g., Codonopsis Radix, Angelicae Sinensis Radix, Astragali Radix, Jujubae Fructus and Ginseng Radix; and (iv) herbs to calm the heart and soothe the nerves, e.g., Poria Cocos and Nelumbinis Semen. Apart from the classification according to their pharmacological activity, these herbs could also be further divided into three groups, Yin, Yang and neutral herbs. Thus, the herbs chosen in present study is trying to cover the most commonly used TCM in treating spleen-related unwell.

Identifying chemical composition in herbal extract is the key to probe the properties of TCM herbs. However, the natural products always accompany with a huge amount of chemical variables, which greatly shake the credibility of any outcome (Kuang et al., 2012). Here, we employed standard methods, i.e., HPLC fingerprinting, NMR profiling and LC-MS profiling, as to reduce the variables in herbal extracts. Generally, HPLC fingerprinting is adopted to show all compounds with ultraviolet absorption; ^{1}H-NMR profiling is able to display all compounds with active hydrogen; while LC-MS profiling is capable to show trace compounds (Zhao et al., 2005; Crockford et al., 2006). To obtain information of the components as much as possible, the detection wavelength of HPLC was set from 190 to 400 nm, and the gradient elution programs covered 0–100% acetonitrile. The chemical shift range was set from −2 to 12 ppm covering active hydrogen in almost all kinds of organic matters. Furthermore, the identified signals were subjected to full spectrum PCA determination, and which did not request the true nature of identified chemicals and could therefore reduce the possible variation (Savorani et al., 2010; Lu et al., 2014).

According to previous research, the herbal compounds associated with cold nature generally possess more polar structures; in contrast the compounds associated with hot nature have lower molecular weight; and the neutral compounds have a higher polar surface area (Fu et al., 2017a). The cold and hot properties of TCM are defined according to the impacts to human physiological condition, indicating the importance of chemical composition of herbal extracts. By using various analytic methods, we generated a large group of chemometrics data, and these data were subjected to PCA analysis. The results of LC-MS profile showed that the Yang-stimulating herbs contained more compounds of lower molecular weight and with less polar structures. This result is consistent with the previous proposed notion (Fu et al., 2017a). However, the results of HPLC and NMR profiles were not able to prove above conclusion, which might due to low resolution and similar chemical shift of most of the organic compounds.

Apart from the chemical basis, the differences of biological effects are always the most concern issues in studying the four natures of TCM herbs. Due to the high similarity of the opposition and interdependence relationship in "Yin-Yang" theory and redox system, the study on their connection was continuously. By using an oxygen radical absorbance capacity (ORAC) assay to compare the free radical-scavenging activity of Yin- and Yang-tonic herbs, Ou et al. (2003) was among the first groups to provide physical meaning of "Yin and Yang" in relating to biochemical processes. The result revealed that the amount of total phenolic compounds in Yin-tonic herbs were generally higher, and meanwhile which possessed a higher antioxidant activity than the Yang-tonic herbs. Thus, the authors deduced that Yin-tonic represents anti-oxidation, and Yang-tonic represents oxidation involved in energy metabolism. However, their result was against by Szeto and Benzie (2006): they measured the 1,1-diphenylpicrylhydrazyl radical-scavenging activity of Yin- and Yang-tonic herbs and found that most of the 'Yang-invigorating' herbs possess higher anti-oxidative activity. However, their conclusion was still not finalized due to different selection criterions, and the thoughtful analytic methods were not used. To set up a more credible and convincing antioxidant profiles, our present approach adopted various common assays at different levels, as to evaluate anti-oxidative properties of unknown herbal samples. Accompanied with PCA method, the current results showed that the correlation between "Yin-Yang" and anti-oxidative properties was relatively low, indicating the connection between these two systems might not be closely related, at least in ours 15 spleen-meridian herbs.

AUTHOR CONTRIBUTIONS

KT and TD conceived and designed the experiments. YH, LW, and PY performed the experiments, analyzed the results, and made figures and tables. KL, HW, XK, and YC contributed to scientific discussions. KT and YH wrote the paper.

FUNDING

This study was supported by Hong Kong RGC Theme-based Research Scheme (T13-607/12R), Innovation Technology Fund (UIM/288, UIM/302, UIM/340, UIT/137, ITS/022/16FP), TUYF15SC01, Shenzhen Science and Technology Committee Research Grant (CKFW2,016,082,916,015,476; JCYJ20,170,413, 173,747,440; JCYJ20,160,229,205,726,699; JCYJ20,160,229,205, 812,004; JCYJ20,160,229,210,027,564; ZDSYS201,707,281,432,317; and 20,170,326).

REFERENCES

Bishnoi, M., Khare, P., Brown, L., and Panchal, S. K. (2018). Transient receptor potential (TRP) channels: a metabolic TR(i)P to obesity prevention and therapy. *Obes. Rev.* 19, 1269–1292. doi: 10.1111/obr.12703

Crockford, D. J., Holmes, E., Lindon, J. C., Plumb, R. S., Zirah, S., Bruce, S. J., et al. (2006). Statistical heterospectroscopy, an approach to the integrated analysis of NMR and UPLC-MS data sets: application in metabonomic toxicology studies. *Anal. Chem.* 78, 363–371. doi: 10.1021/ac051444m

Fu, J. L., Pang, J. X., Zhao, X. L., and Han, J. X. (2015). The quantitative ideas and methods in assessment of four properties of Chinese medicinal herbs. *Cell. Biochem. Biophys.* 71, 1307–1312. doi: 10.1007/s12013-014-0349-y

Fu, X., Mervin, L. H., Li, X., Yu, H., Li, J., Mohamad Zobir, S. Z., et al. (2017a). Toward understanding the cold, hot, and neutral nature of Chinese medicines using in silico mode-of-action analysis. *J. Chem. Inf. Model.* 57, 468–483. doi: 10.1021/acs.jcim.6b00725

Fu, X., Song, X. X., Li, X. B., Wong, K. K., Li, J. Y., Zhang, F. C., et al. (2017b). Phylogenetic tree analysis of the cold-hot nature of traditional Chinese marine medicine for possible anticancer activity. *Evid. Based Complementary Altern. Med.* 2017:4365715. doi: 10.1155/2017/4365715

Fu, X. J., Liu, H. B., Wang, P., and Guan, H. S. (2009). A study on the antioxidant activity and tissues selective inhibition of lipid peroxidation by saponins from the roots of *Platycodon grandiflorum*. *Am. J. Chin. Med.* 37, 967–975. doi: 10.1142/S0192415X09007375

Gao, Y. S., Zheng, F. J., Li, X., Xu, H., Zhang, S. J., and Li, Y. H. (2014). A microcalorimetric research on the effect of traditional Chinese medicine on the growth and metabolism of E. *coli*. *J. Yunnan Univ. Tradit. Chin. Med.* 37, 10–13.

Han, J. X., Yang, M., and Yu, C. (2011). Quantum: may be a new-found messenger in biological systems. *Biosci. Trends* 5, 89–92. doi: 10.5582/bst.2011.v5.3.89

Huang, Y., Kwan, K. L., Leung, K. W., Wang, H. Y., Dong, T. T. X., and Tsim, K. W. K. (2018a). The extracts and major compounds derived from *Astragali* radix alter mitochondrial bioenergetics in cultured cardiomyocytes: comparison of various polar solvents and compounds. *Int. J. Mol. Sci.* 19:E1574. doi: 10.3390/ijms19061574

Huang, Y., Kwan, K. L., Leung, K. W., Yao, P., Wang, H. Y., Dong, T. T. X., et al. (2018b). Ginseng extracts modulate mitochondrial bioenergetics of live cardiomyoblasts: a functional comparison of different polar extracts. *J. Ginseng. Res.* doi: 10.1016/j.jgr.2018.02.002

Ko, K. M., Leon, T. Y. Y., Mak, D. H. F., Chiu, P. Y., Du, Y., and Poon, M. K. T. (2006). A characteristic pharmacological action of 'Yang-invigorating' Chinese tonifying herbs: enhancement of myocardial ATP-generation capacity. *Phytomedicine* 13, 636–642. doi: 10.1016/j.phymed.2006.02.007

Ko, K. M., and Leung, H. Y. (2007). Enhancement of ATP generation capacity, antioxidant activity and immunomodulatory activities by Chinese Yang and Yin tonifying herbs. *Chin. Med.* 2:3. doi: 10.1186/1749-8546-2-3

Ko, K. M., Mak, D. H. F., Chiu, P. Y., and Poon, M. K. T. (2004). Pharmacological basis of 'Yang-invigoration' in Chinese medicine. *Trends Pharmacol. Sci.* 25, 3–6. doi: 10.1016/j.tips.2003.11.002

Kuang, H. X., Wang, Y. Y., Wang, Q. H., Yang, B. Y., and Xia, Y. G. (2012). "Metabonomics research of the four properties in traditional Chinese medicine based on UPLC-QTOF-MS system," in *Recent Advances in Theories and Practice of Chinese Medicine*, ed. H. Kuang (London: IntechOpen Limited).

Li, P. P. (2012). Toward an integrative framework of indigenous research: the geocentric implications of Yin-Yang balance. *Asia Pac. J. Manag.* 29, 849–872. doi: 10.1007/s10490-011-9250-z

Li, W. F., Jiang, J. G., and Chen, J. (2008). Chinese medicine and its modernization demands. *Arch. Med. Res.* 39, 246–251. doi: 10.1016/j.arcmed.2007.09.011

Liang, Y. H., Wang, C. S., and Zhang, Y. J. (1988). A research of the mechanism and effect of cold and hot compound prescription and rhizoma anemarrhenae on sympathetic nervous system. *Chin. J. Chin. Mater. Medic* 13, 48–50.

Lu, Y. J., Gao, B. Y., Chen, P., Charles, D., and Yu, L. L. (2014). Characterisation of organic and conventional sweet basil leaves using chromatographic and flow-injection mass spectrometric (FIMS) fingerprints combined with principal component analysis. *Food Chem.* 154, 262–268. doi: 10.1016/j.foodchem.2014.01.009

Ma, T., Tan, C., Zhang, H., Wang, M., Ding, W., and Li, S. (2010). Bridging the gap between traditional Chinese medicine and systems biology: the connection of cold syndrome and NEI network. *Mol. Biosyst.* 6, 613–619. doi: 10.1039/B914024G

Mohd, F. F., Koutsoukas, A., Lowe, R., Joshi, K., Fan, T. P., Glen, R. C., et al. (2013). Chemogenomics approaches to rationalizing the mode-of-action of traditional Chinese and Ayurvedic medicines. *J. Chem. Inf. Model.* 53, 661–673. doi: 10.1021/ci3005513

Ou, B., Huang, D., Hampsch-Woodill, M., and Flanagan, J. A. (2003). When east meets west: the relationship between Yin-Yang and antioxidation-oxidation. *FASEB* 17, 127–129. doi: 10.1096/fj.02-0527hyp

Qiu, J. (2015). When the east meets the west: the future of traditional Chinese medicine in the 21st century. *Nat. Sci. Rev.* 2, 377–380. doi: 10.1093/nsr/nwv049

Ramirez-Rodrigues, M. M., Plaza, M. L., Azeredo, A., Balaban, M. O., and Marshall, M. R. (2011). Physicochemical and phytochemical properties of cold and hot water extraction from *Hibiscus sabdariffa*. *J. Food. Sci.* 76, 428–435. doi: 10.1111/j.1750-3841.2011.02091.x

Rezapour-Firouzi, S. (2017). "Herbal oil supplement with hot-nature diet for multiple sclerosis," in *Nutrition and Lifestyle in Neurological Autoimmune Diseases*, eds R. R. Watson and W. D. S. Killgore (Cambridge, MA: Academic Press), 229–245.

Savorani, F., Tomasi, G., and Engelsen, S. B. (2010). Icoshift: a versatile tool for the rapid alignment of 1D NMR spectra. *J. Magn. Reson.* 202, 190–202. doi: 10.1016/j.jmr.2009.11.012

Szeto, Y. T., and Benzie, I. F. F. (2006). Is the Yin-Yang nature of Chinese herbal medicine equivalent to antioxidation-oxidation? *J. Ethnopharmacol.* 108, 361–366. doi: 10.1016/j.jep.2006.05.033

Ung, C. Y., Li, H., Cao, Z. W., Li, Y. X., and Chen, Y. Z. (2007). Are herb-pairs of traditional Chinese medicine distinguishable from others? Pattern analysis and artificial intelligence classification study of traditionally defined herbal properties. *J. Ethnopharmacol.* 111, 371–377. doi: 10.1016/j.jep.2006.11.037

Wang, P., Zhang, Y. Q., and Wang, Z. G. (2010). The methodology framework of data analysis in the modern research of the theory of Chinese medicinal herbal property. *J. Shandong Univ. TCM* 34, 470–472.

Wang, P. X., and Zhou, C. X. (2006). An exploration into nature of Chinese drugs based on "polynary drug nature" hypothesis. *J. Nanjing Univ. Tradit. Chin. Med.* 22, 345–347.

Wiklund, S., Johansson, E., Sjostrom, L., Mellerowicz, E. J., Edlund, U., Shockcor, J. P., et al. (2008). Visualization of GC/TOF-MS-based metabolomics data for identification of biochemically interesting compounds using OPLS class model. *Anal. Chem.* 80, 115–122. doi: 10.1021/ac0713510

Wong, C. C., Li, H. B., Cheng, K. W., and Chen, F. (2006). A systematic survey of antioxidant activity of 30 Chinese medicinal plants using the ferric reducing antioxidant power assay. *Food Chem.* 97, 705–711. doi: 10.1016/j.foodchem.2005.05.049

Xiong, Q. P., Zhang, Q. H., and Shi, Y. Y. (2011). Research ideas and methods of material basis of Chinese medicine efficacy based on metabolomics. *Res. Pract. Chin. Med.* 25, 97–99.

Xu, H. Y., Tang, S. H., and Chen, J. X. (2011). Research ideas and strategies of Chinese medicine "group activity relationship" based on the metabolomics. *World Sci. Technol.* 13, 3–35.

Yang, H. B., Zhao, Y. L., and Li, B. C. (2010). Study on the chills and fever property of the stomach cold/hot syndrome pathology model mice based on the cold/hot plat differential methods. *J. Tradit. Chin. Med.* 51, 241–243.

Yang, J. M., Li, G., Wang, M., Jin, Y. X., Zheng, F. J., Sun, Y., et al. (2017). The Effects of natural Chinese medicine aconite root, dried ginger rhizome, and *Coptis* on rectal and skin temperatures at acupuncture points. *Evid. Based Complementary Altern. Med.* 2017:7250340. doi: 10.1155/2017/7250340

Yu, H. M., Liu, T. S., Xiao, X. H., Zhao, Y. L., Yuan, H. L., Jan, A. M., et al. (2001). Biothermodynamic study on four properties of Chinese traditional medicine-comparison of the properties of Radix ginseng and *Radix quinquefolium* by microcalorimetry. *Chin. J. Basic Med. Tradit. Chin. Med.* 7, 60–64.

Zhan, J. Y. X., Zheng, K. Y. Z., Zhu, K. Y., Bi, C. W. C., Zhang, W. L., Du, C. Y. Q., et al. (2011). Chemical and biological assessment of *Angelicae sinensis* Radix after processing with wine: an orthogonal array design to reveal the optimized conditions. *J. Agric. Food Chem.* 59, 6091–6098. doi: 10.1021/jf200728e

Zhang, R. X., Li, M. X., and Jia, Z. P. (2008). *Rehmannia glutinosa*: review of botany, chemistry and pharmacology. *J. Ethnopharmacol.* 117, 199–214. doi: 10.1016/j.jep.2008.02.018

Zhao, L. H., Huang, C. Y., Shan, Z., Xiang, B. R., and Mei, L. H. (2005). Fingerprint analysis of *Psoralea corylifolia* L. by HPLC and LC-MS. *J. Chromatogr. B* 821, 67–74. doi: 10.1016/j.jchromb.2005.04.008

Zhao, X. L., and Han, J. X. (2013). The connotation of the quantum traditional Chinese medicine and the exploration of its experimental technology system for diagnosis. *Drug. Discov. Ther.* 7, 225–232. doi: 10.5582/ddt.2013.v7.6.225

Zhou, C., Wang, J., Zhang, X., Zhao, Y., Xia, X., Zhao, H., et al. (2009). Investigation of the differences between the "cold" and "hot" nature of *Coptis chinensis* Franch and its processed materials based on animal's temperature tropism. *Sci. Chin. Ser. C Life Sci.* 52, 1073–1080. doi: 10.1007/s11427-009-0146-9

2

IMCC: A Novel Quantitative Approach Revealing Variation of Global Modular Map and Local Inter-Module Coordination among Differential Drug's Targeted Cerebral Ischemic Networks

Pengqian Wang[1†], *Yanan Yu*[2†], *Jun Liu*[2], *Bing Li*[2,3], *Yingying Zhang*[4], *Dongfeng Li*[4], *Wenjuan Xu*[5], *Qiong Liu*[2] *and Zhong Wang*[2*]

[1]*Institute of Chinese Materia Medica, China Academy of Chinese Medical Sciences, Beijing, China,* [2]*Institute of Basic Research in Clinical Medicine, China Academy of Chinese Medical Sciences, Beijing, China,* [3]*Institute of Information on Traditional Chinese Medicine, China Academy of Chinese Medical Sciences, Beijing, China,* [4]*Dongzhimen Hospital, Beijing University of Chinese Medicine, Beijing, China,* [5]*School of Mathematical Sciences, Peking University, Beijing, China,* [6]*School of Life Sciences, Beijing University of Chinese Medicine, Beijing, China*

***Correspondence:**
Zhong Wang
zhonw@vip.sina.com

[†]*These authors have contributed equally to this work*

Stroke is a common disease characterized by multiple genetic dysfunctions. In this complex disease, detecting the strength of inter-module coordination (genetic community interaction) and subsequent modular rewiring is essential to characterize the reactive biosystematic variation (biosystematic perturbation) brought by multiple-target drugs, whose effects are achieved by hitting on a series of targets (target profile) jointly. Here, a quantitative approach for inter-module coordination and its transition, named as IMCC, was developed. Applying IMCC to mouse cerebral ischemia–related gene microarray, we investigated a holistic view of modular map and its rewiring from ischemic stroke to drugs (baicalin, BA; ursodeoxycholic acid, UA; and jasminoidin, JA) perturbation states and locally identified the cooperative pathological module pair and its dissection. Our result suggested the global modular map in cerebral ischemia exhibited a characteristic "core–periphery" architecture, and this architecture was rewired by the effective drugs heterogeneously: BA and UA converged modules into an intensively connected integrity, whereas JA diverged partial modules and widened the remaining inter-module paths. Locally, the PMP dissociation brought by drugs contributed to the reversion of the pathological condition: the focus of the cellular function shift from survival after nervous system injury into development and repair, including neurotrophin regulation, hormone releasing, and chemokine signaling activation. The core targets and

Abbreviation: AKT, protein kinase B; ALS, amyotrophic lateral sclerosis; BA, baicalin; cAMP, cyclic adenosine monophosphate; CM, concha margaritifera; CT, consistency score; DIMC, direct inter-module connections; DR, dissociation rate; ECA, external carotid artery; GnRH, gonadotropin-releasing hormone; IIMC, indirect inter-module connections; IMASP, inter-module average shortest path, also named as inter-module average characteristic path length; IMCC, inter-module coordination coefficient; JA, jasminoidin; JS, Jaccard similarity; KEGG, Kyoto Encyclopedia of Genes and Genomes; LTP, long-term potentiation; MAPK, mitogen-activated protein kinase; MCAO, middle cerebral artery obstruction; mTOR, mammalian target of rapamycin; PCA, principal component analysis; PI3K: phosphoinositide 3-kinases; PMP, pathological module pair; PS, path strength; Rap1, Ras-proximate-1; SW, sum of inter-module weight; TTC, 4% 2,3,5-triphenyltetrazolium chloride; UA, ursodeoxycholic acid; VRCD, variation of ratio of characteristic path length and density mechanisms were validated by *in vivo* experiments. Overall, our result highlights the holistic inter-module coordination rearrangement rather than a target or a single module that brings phenotype alteration. This strategy may lead to systematically explore detailed variation of inter-module pharmacological action mode of multiple-target drugs, which is the principal problem of module pharmacology for network-based drug discovery.

Keywords: IMCC, modular map rewiring, inter-module coordination, multiple-target drug, cerebral ischemia

INTRODUCTION

Stroke is a common disease characterized by multiple genetic dysfunctions (Matthew et al., 2012; Zhou et al., 2018). The discovery of the multi-target therapeutic drugs is considered as a potential solution for reversing the biomolecular network of disease systematically to achieve homeostasis (Frantz, 2005; Roth et al., 2004; Wang et al., 2015a). How to clarify the "shotguns-like" action mode of multi-target drugs is still far from clear. Network-based drug analysis aims to harness explosion of high-throughput data to investigate the pharmacology of drugs, which makes it feasible to understand the intrinsic pharmacological mechanism of multi-target drugs (Cheng et al., 2019). As accumulated data from high-throughput technologies delineate a holistic view of intracellular molecular network, the major challenge in the post-genomic era is deciphering how these entities in the cell work together to execute sophisticated functions (Wang and Wang, 2013; Kim et al., 2014). The ongoing efforts have been made in decomposing a network into modules and identifying the targeted modules of drugs (Wang et al., 2012). This may help to decipher modularized function organization in targeted networks and reveal the pharmacological mechanisms of multi-target drugs.

However, inter-module connections, as the "backbone" contributing to functional coordination and information flow between modules in most biological processes, are ever important (Granovetter, 1973; Lin et al., 2012; Ma and Gao, 2012; Onnela et al., 2009; Levy et al., 2017). The inter-module connections, which are more transient and flexible than intra-module connections (Ma and Gao, 2012; Kim et al., 2014), could be considered as targets of drugs, since modular rearrangement brought by inter-module relationship transitions may provide more efficient ways for phenotype alteration (Amar et al., 2013; Meda et al., 2014) than genetic variation or modular allostery (Roguev et al., 2008; Bandyopadhyay et al., 2010; Costanzo et al., 2016). Such modular rewiring of conserved functional modules can be used as a network biomarker to characterize the dynamics of drug responses (Zeng et al., 2014), by identifying and evaluating the drug-conditional existence of collaborations between modules (Zeng et al., 2013). Especially for the multiple-target drugs, it is an extremely interesting and promising perspective to apply inter-module connectivity analysis to reveal the mechanism of pharmacology (Wang et al., 2011; Ding et al., 2015; Liu and Wang, 2015). A set of studies have referred the quantitative evaluation method for inter-module connections (Ulitsky et al., 2008; Missiuro et al., 2009; Hsu et al., 2011; Kelder et al., 2011; David and Ron, 2014); for example, the number of interactions or overlapping nodes between modules or community is commonly considered as the connections between modules (Yang et al., 2009; Bandyopadhyay et al., 2010; Tesson, et al., 2010; Kelder et al., 2011; Amar et al., 2013). Many of these addressed the problem of module detection and module-to-module interactions simultaneously but did not treat inter-module assessment as a main task. Algorithms for inter-module assessment are still far from perfect. Furthermore, it is pertinent to introduce biological function to measure reliability and validity of inter-module evaluations. And how to quantify transition of inter-module coordination related to pharmacological mechanisms remains unknown.

Baicalin (BA), ursodeoxycholic acid (UA), and jasminoidin (JA) are three major components contained in Qingkailing injection, an effective preparation widely prescribed to patients with ischemic stroke. Our previous studies showed that each of BA, UA, and JA significantly reduced the infarction volume in the ischemic brain and exerts neuroprotective effects by inhibiting inflammatory response in cerebral ischemia (Liu et al., 2012; Wang et al., 2015b; Wang et al., 2018). These studies provide "targeting section" of these multi-target drugs. Nevertheless, it is still unclear to characterize the overview of functional module rewiring response to distinct drug perturbations. The underlying mechanisms of these drugs regarding the inter-module coordination in modulating complex disease phenotypes are still to be explored.

In this study, we propose an integrated computational and experimental approach to the systematic discovery of differential transition of inter-module coordination that are causal determinants of phenotype alteration (**Figure 1**). Here, the gene expression profile of hippocampus from MCAO (middle cerebral artery obstruction) mice treated by BA, JA, and UA was analyzed by cDNA microarray, and the weighted gene co-expression network and modules are constructed accordingly. First, we integrated the quantitative methods and statistical analysis to construct an inter-module coordination coefficient (IMCC) to evaluate the module-to-module cooperation. Next, the inter-module coordination rewiring across treated condition to disease was evaluated and compared globally. Third, the most closely coordinating module pair was further analyzed using the dissection rate and KEGG pathway. Finally, the mechanism of BA, UA, and JA was validated by *in vivo* experiments.

MATERIALS AND METHODS

Animals Model and Drug Administration

All animal experiments conducted were approved by the Ethics Committee of China Academy of Chinese Medicine. The operation was performed according to NIH Guidelines for the Care and Use of Laboratory Animals for Experimental Procedures (National Research Council, 1996). A total of 126 mice were used to pharmacodynamic experiment and transcriptome data examination in this study. Animals were randomized into sham-operated, vehicle,

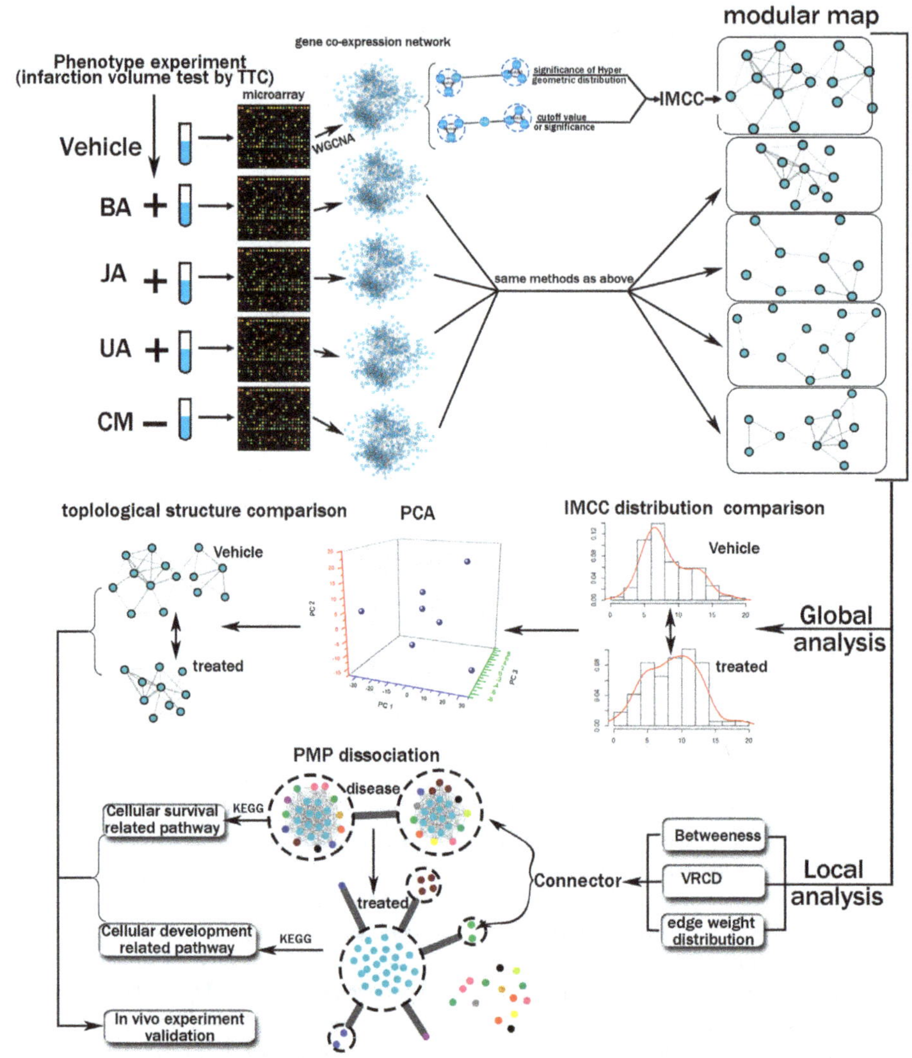

FIGURE 1 | Schematic diagram of the systematic strategies used to reveal variation of global modular map and local inter-module coordination.

BA-treated, JA-treated, UA-treated, and CM-treated groups. Except the sham-operated group, all animals were operated for middle cerebral artery obstruction to induce focal cerebral ischemia–reperfusion model. Briefly, the left middle cerebral artery was occluded using an intraluminal filament. The artery was ligated for 1.5 h, after that reperfused for about 24 h. For animals in the sham group, the external carotid artery (ECA) was sham-operated and prepared surgically without filament inserting. Drugs were injected into the tail vein for 2 ml/kg immediately after modeling. The concentration of drugs was BA in 5 mg/ml, JA in 25 mg/ml, UA in 7 mg/ml, and CM (concha margaritifera) in 50 mg/ml.

Drug Efficacy Examination and Transcriptome Data Analysis

For each group, nine mice were used to examine infarction volume by TTC (2, 3, 5-triphenyltetrazolium chloride staining). The volume of the infarct region was determined by Pathology Image Analysis System (Topica Inc.) and was recognized to reflect efficacy of drugs.

After reperfusion for 24 h, the hippocampus of 12 animals of each group was sliced and homogenized using TRIzol reagent, and total RNA was extracted and purified. Then, cDNA microarray consisted of a collection of 374 ischemia-related genes, including 114 genes related to stroke and 260 genes in pathways related to cerebral ischemia. Expression data of the 374 genes were uploaded to the public database ArrayExpress (http://www.ebi.ac.uk/arrayexpress/, E-TABM-662).

Co-Expression Network Construction and Module Detection

Based on the expression of aforementioned 374 genes, co-expression network was constructed and modules were identified using weighted gene co-expression network analysis (WGCNA) R package (Langfelder and Horvath, 2008). WGCNA can be used for finding clusters (modules) of highly correlated genes, for summarizing such clusters for relating modules to one another (Langfelder and Horvath, 2008). Correlation networks facilitate network-based gene screening methods that can be used to identify candidate therapeutic targets or further inter-module analysis (Langfelder and Horvath, 2008). Correlation network in different conditions was related to genes' expression pattern. In this study, we aim to calculate inter-module coordination, which may reflect the disease- and drug-conditional existence of collaborations between modules, to facilitate the further pharmacological investigation. Therefore, we employed the WGCNA to construct weighted gene co-expression network.

In brief, the weighted network was fully specified by its adjacency matrix, which was constructed between all pairs of probes across the measured samples by using appropriate adjacency function parameters (β) for each group (β = 8 for vehicle, seven for CM, four for BA, 12 for JA, and eight for UA) (Langfelder and Horvath, 2008; Li et al., 2016). The soft thresholds were selected when the network gets the best scale-free topology criterion. As a result, adjacency functions $a_{ij} \geq 0.02$ were used to construct weight gene co-expression network and further analysis.

The WGCNA identified gene modules using average linkage hierarchical clustering with topologic overlap measure and Dynamic Hybrid Tree Cut algorithm (Langfelder and Horvath, 2008); modules are subsequently assigned a color as names, and the details of the module detection were shown in our previous study (Li et al., 2016).

Inter-Module Coordination Analysis

According to the local structure, connections between two modules composed of edges between nodes from distinct modules were defined as direct inter-module connections (DIMC), and interactions mediated by genes that associate with both the two modules were classified as indirect inter-module connections (IIMC). We firstly calculated two types of correlation parameters: SW for DIMC; CT and PS for IIMC; then, we screened these parameters using hypergeometric distribution or cutoff value and integrated the identified parameters; finally, we optimized the integration weight according to KEGG database.

Parameters Calculations

For SW, we calculated the sum of weight of edges between pairs of modules:

$$SW(Mx, My) = \sum_{i \in Mx, j \in My} aij, \tag{1}$$

where M_x and M_y denote any two modules connected by at least one edge, i and j are a gene in M_x and M_y, respectively, and a_{ij} is the weight of edge between gene i and j. Using this formula, we calculated the direct inter-module connections for any module pair possessing one or more edges.

To decide whether the inter-module direct connections were statistically significant, we used the p value of the hypergeometric distribution (Lin et al., 2012), defined as

$$p = \sum_{k=x}^{n} \frac{\binom{M}{k}\binom{N-M}{n-k}}{\binom{N}{n}}, \tag{2}$$

where x is observed inter-module connections; k and n are the numbers of inter-module connections and all possible edges between two modules, respectively; and M and N represent the total numbers of inter-module connections and all combinational gene pairs between any two modules in a module-to-module network, respectively. If $p < 0.05$, the *SW* is defined as a valid direct measurement.

For indirect inter-module connections, we introduced two parameters: path strength (*PS*) and consistency score (*CT*).

In the light of the network, paths consisted of multiple vertexes and links between them (Kelder et al., 2011). To simplify the problem, we restricted the length of paths and only considered paths that consist of three nodes [outset (*o*), mediation (*m*), and end (*e*)] with two links.

$$PS(Mx, My) = \sum_{\substack{o \in Mx, e \in My \\ m \notin Mx, m \notin My}} \frac{Wm, o}{Wm} \bullet \frac{Wm, e}{Wm}. \tag{3}$$

The path strength (*PS*) of a path is defined as the product of the weighted probabilities that mediation chooses outset and end. The weighted probability from *m* to *o* is the ratio of the weight between *m* and *o* (W_m,o) to the sum of the weights between *m* (W_m) and its first neighbors, the same as *m* to *e*.

Hypergeometric distribution was also used to screen the statistically significant *PS*. However, different from *SW*, in **Eq. 2**, *x* is observed nodes connecting a pair of module; *k* and *n* are the numbers of nodes connecting a pair of modules and all possible nodes connecting the two modules, respectively; and *M* and *N* represent the total numbers of nodes connecting any pair of module and all possible nodes between any two modules in a module to module network, respectively.

We also employed consistency score (*CT*) to measure the inter-module connectivity as described in (Hsu et al., 2011).

$$CTscoreM_x, M_y = \sum_{i \in G}\left(Min\left\{\left(C_{M_x}, i - \frac{S}{C}CLi\right), \left(C_{M_y}, i - \frac{T}{C}CLi\right)\right\} \times \frac{C_{M_x}, i \times C_{M_y}, i}{CLi} \times Wi\right). \tag{4}$$

G is a gene set that consists of all genes in network, and *C* is the total number of genes in *G*. CL_i is the total number of links to gene *i*; W_i is the weight of gene *i* in network. *S* and *T* are the numbers of genes in modules M_x and M_y, respectively; $CM_{x,i}$ and $CM_{y,i}$ are the observed numbers of links connecting gene *i* and modules M_x and M_y, respectively. **Eq. 4** was used to compare the weights of genes correlated with a pair of modules with the weights of genes related to only one of the modules (Hsu et al., 2011). As the *CT* is a value after comparison with theoretical value, we set cutoff value (10) to screen out the valid *CT*.

Measurement Integration

To obtain a more accurate and objective relationship between modules, we merged *DIMC* and *IIMC*. First, we set *SW* of the inter-module connections, whose p-value of hypergeometric distribution was less than 0.05, as weight of *DIMC*. In the process of $IMCC_1$ integration, *SW* and *CT* were two parameters of different dimensions, so it was adopted to correct the two parameters to the value of 0–1 (**Supplementary Table S1**). We normalized the two measurements to be numbers between [0–1] by the follow formula:

$$f'_x = \frac{f_x - f_{\min}}{f_{\max} - f_{\min}}. \tag{5}$$

The two parameters were weighted using weighted coefficients α and β for *SW* and *CT*, respectively. The two weighted parameters were summed up, as follows:

$$IMCC_1 = \alpha \bullet SW + \beta \bullet CT. \tag{6}$$

We set α + β = 1 and coefficient ratio ρ = α/β. By adjusting ρ value, the effect of *SW* and *CT* on $IMCC_1$ would be altered. We calculated the $IMCC_1$ when ρ = 1/10, 1/8, 1/4, 1/2, 1/1, 2/1, 4/1, 8/1, and 10/1, respectively.

In the integration of *SW* and *PS*, both of them belonged to the same dimension, so we plus the two parameters without weighting (**Supplementary Table S2**), defined as:

$$IMCC_2 = SW + PS. \tag{7}$$

Optimization and Verification of Weighting Coefficient

In biological networks, the communication between certain modules is commonly mediated by component with important functions; for example, a gene might be a target regulated by two modules competitively. All the inter-module correlations summarized or predicted are presumed to contribute to biological functions. Therefore, it is imperative to introduce biological data to define the best weighting coefficient, in order to select the optimal *IMCC*. As a result, we employed the KEGG (Kyoto Encyclopedia of Genes and Genomes) database, according to which we calculated the Jaccard similarity of enriched pathways of each module pair.

$$JS = \frac{|A \cap B|}{|A \cup B|}. \tag{8}$$

A and *B* is the category of enriched KEGG terms in module M_x and M_y, respectively. Therefore, $A \cap B$ represents the number of identical categories of KEGG terms between *A* and *B*, and $A \cup B$ represents the number of all the categories of KEGG terms in both A and B. For example, if $A \cap B = 6$ and $A \cup B = 11$, then *JS* will be 0.54545. We presumed that modules enriched with the same KEGG categories might form more dense connections than those with different KEGG categories. We benchmarked the $IMCC_1$ of different ρ values based on *JS*, and the $IMCC_1$ scores were plotted vs. the observed *JS* for each module pair (**Supplementary Table S3**). Through nonlinear curve estimating and coefficient of determination (R^2) comparison, we quantitatively identified the best ρ value and the most fitting model. To obtain more precise results, we removed the outliers.

Our results suggested that the optimal ρ value was 1/1, and the most fitting model was logarithmic model with a R^2 of 0.616. Thus, the final formula for *IMCC* could be simplified as:

$$IMCC = SW + CT. \tag{9}$$

We also plotted the $IMCC_2$ against *JS* and compared R^2 of fitted curves of $IMCC_1$ and $IMCC_2$ to select the optimal integrative method.

Comparison and Verification of IMCC

As many established algorithms addressed the problem of inter-module interaction evaluation using sum of weight (*SW*) of inter-module interactions, we compared SW with *IMCC* by fitting the KEGG database coverage. We also compared IMCC with inter-module average shortest path (*IMASP*), also named as inter-module average characteristic path length, a topological parameter proposed to evaluate the distance of a module pair. *IMCC* was plotted vs. the *IMASP* (**Supplementary Table S4**), and determination coefficient of curve fitting was also calculated.

GLOBAL TRANSITION OF MODULE REWIRING AND LOCAL PATHOLOGICAL MODULE PAIRS

Global Transition of Module Rewiring

To access the transitions of inter-module coordination response to drug perturbation, we compared the distribution of IMCC score between the treated and untreated group by dividing these scores into four intervals by quartiles, through the chi-square test. Besides, the principal component analysis (PCA) was employed to evaluate the distance of IMCC distributions among these groups.

Local Pathological Module Pairs Identification

In order to further investigate the core factors of the modular map, we tried to identify the "connectors." We utilized three computational methods, that is, betweenness centrality, variation of ratio of characteristic path length and density (VRCD), and distribution of edge weight, to identify candidate connector modules from module networks. In the first method, the betweenness of each module in modular map was calculated, and the top 10% modules were selected as connectors. As for the second method, the VRCD was calculated to detect connectors. As the bridging modules constituted the channels between modules, their removal would lead to interruption of the inter-module connectivity (Missiuro et al., 2009; Yang et al., 2009; Zhu et al., 2014). Therefore, we removed nodes (module) in module map one by one and calculated the change ratio of characteristic path length and network density.

$$\eta = \Delta s / \Delta t, \tag{10}$$

$$\Delta s = \frac{CPLa - CPLo}{CPLo}, \tag{11}$$

$$\Delta t = \frac{Da - Do}{Do}. \tag{12}$$

Δs is the change ratio of characteristic path length of modular map. CPL_o is the origin characteristic path length. CPL_a is the altered characteristic path length of modular map after deleting a module. Δt is the change ratio of density of modular map. D_o is the origin density. D_a is the altered density of modular map after deleting a module. η is the ratio of Δs and Δt.

We set the double average η in each modular map as respondent cutoff. Thereby, the modules, whose η is more than cutoff, were identified as connectors based on *VRCD*.

In the edge weight distribution, the inter-module connections were distributed based on their weight. The modules, whose inter-module connection weight is more than 0.1, were selected as connectors.

The connectors identified by all the three methods were regarded as the characteristic modules in corresponding state. A pair of connector modules (blue and brown) in the vehicle group was identified as characteristic pathological inter-module connection, which was named as "pathological module pair (PMP)."

Calculation of Dissociation Rate of PMP

The dissociation rate (DR) of PMP was also calculated. We defined DR as the corrected ratio of the amount of modules before dissociation to that after dissociation. The formula of DR is as follows:

$$DR = \frac{n_B}{n_A} \bullet \frac{N_A}{N_B}. \tag{13}$$

n_A is number of modules in the initial state (disease state, $n_A = 2$); n_B is number of modules in the succeeding state (treated by drugs); and N_A and N_B are the total number of modules in initial and succeeding states, respectively.

In Vivo Experiments Validation

In order to verify the conclusion, we designed three validation assays using a rat MCAO model, which were introduced as the above section.

Western Blot

Twenty MCAO rats were divided into five groups: sham, vehicle, BA, JA, and UA group and administrated as before. The hippocampus of rats was removed from their brains. After protein extraction and protein quantitative analysis, protein concentration was adjusted for load. We separated proteins using sodium dodecyl sulfate–polyacrylamide gel electrophoresis (SDS-PAGE). After proteins electrotransferred to nitrocellulose membranes, blots were incubated with rabbit anti-Map2k6 antibody (1:2,000, Santa Cruz, CA, United States) for overnight at 4°C. Then, cyclic membrane was washed and stained by goat anti-rabbit IgG. The membranes were incubated with an electrochemiluminescence reagent, After exposure, the band density was determined with a GS-700 densitometer (Bio-Rad). Each measurement was taken in three replicates.

RT-PCR

All of 40 rats were grouped and administrated as mentioned in the earlier section. Total RNA from rats' hippocampus was isolated using TRIzol (Invitrogen, United States). Real-time PCR was performed using a ABI 7300 Real-Time PCR System. The relative expression of BBC3 and Bcl2l1 was analyzed using the relative content, through the $2^{-\Delta\Delta Ct}$ method normalized by GAPDH expression.

Co-Immunoprecipitation (Co-IP)

Co-IP was performed to prove the interaction between BBC3 and Bcl2l1 as described in (Wang et al., 2009). Briefly, tissues from animals were homogenized. The procedure of supernatants collection and separation is the same as Western blot. After protein extraction and protein quantitative analysis, rabbit anti-BBC3 (CST14570, Danvers, MA, United States) and anti-Bcl2l1 (CST2764, Danvers, MA, United States) at a concentration of 1:1,000 and 1:2,000, respectively, were coupled to SiezeX beads according to the protocol of kit parameters (Pierce). Finally, eluted proteins were separated in 12–15% SDS-PAGE and electrotransferred to nitrocellulose for immunoblots.

RESULTS

Drug Efficacy Variation in Ischemic Infarct Volume

According to the drug efficacy examination, BA, UA, and JA significantly reduced the ischemic infarct volume, whereas no significant change was detected in the CM group compared with vehicle. Therefore, we described BA, UA, and JA as effective drugs, and CM as an ineffective drug in the following section.

Construction and Evaluation of Inter-module Coordination Analysis

Based on the expression of above 374 genes, co-expression network was constructed and modules were identified using a WGCNA R package (Langfelder and Horvath, 2008). A total of 48, 23, 42, 15, and 24 modules were detected in the vehicle, BA, JA, UA, and CM groups, and the detailed process was described in our previous study (Li et al., 2016) (**Supplementary Figure S1**); the expression level of mRNA was shown in **Supplementary Material 1**. Inter-module coordination was achieved not only by direct interactions among modules but also through shared partners (Hsu et al., 2011) or between-module (or pathways) paths that consist of multiple proteins and interactions. In this study, we used the CT score and PS to evaluated inter-module relationship mediated by paths and SW for direct module-to-module interactions. For the false-positive levels inherent in the DNA microarray data, we introduced the hypergeometric distribution test, as a result, identified 28.35% SW and 31.74% PS with significance, and screened 22.07% valid CT score by cutoff value (**Figure 2A**; **Supplementary Tables S1, S2**). These CT scores and PS provided supplementary inter-module relationship: 64.42 and 146.01% more than SW (**Figure 2B**).

All the inter-module correlations summarized or calculated are presumed to contribute to biological function coordination. In this study, we employed KEGG signaling to optimize the IMCC (**Supplementary Table S3**). Our results (**Figures 2E,F**)

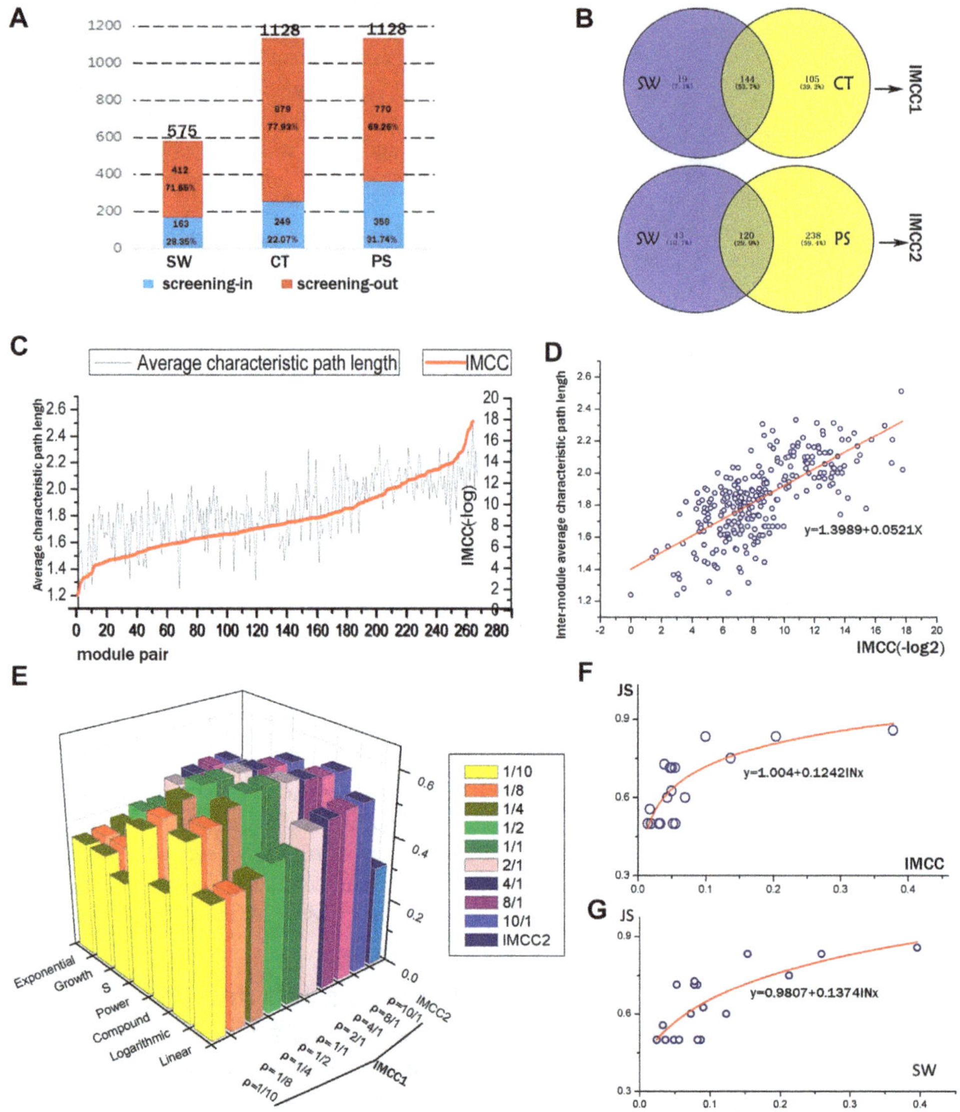

FIGURE 2 | Quantitative evaluation of the IMCC method. **(A)** The screening outcomes of the three inter-module connectivity parameters (SW, CT, and PS). The height of the column represents the total amount of SW, CT, and PS, respectively. Red and blue parts of the columns represent the screened out and the remaining parameters, respectively. **(B)** The overlapping condition of two parameters to be integrated as $IMCC_1$ and $IMCC_2$. **(C)** The IMCC value against the inter-module average characteristic path length (IMASP) of module pairs. **(D)** Scatter plot and linear fitting of log2 transformation of IMCC vs. IMASP. The formula is y = 0.0521x + 1.3989, with R^2 = 0.493. **(E)** The R^2 of multiple fitting models for IMCC and JS. **(F,G)** are the fitting curves of logarithmic model of JS and IMCC, JS, and SW.

suggested that the optimal ρ value in the $IMCC_1$ model was 1/1 and the most fitting model was the logarithmic model with R^2 reaching the peak of 0.616 with two sides sloping down to lower values: when ρ = 1/10 or ρ = 10/1, the minimum R^2 of each side was observed, respectively (**Supplementary Figure S2**). Therefore, it is proper to decide that the integrated parameter $IMCC_1$ is more consistent with the KEGG classification than any single index (SW or CT), which would provide more accurate evaluation of the relationship between modules. Using the same method, we compared the $IMCC_2$ with $IMCC_1$ and chose the $IMCC_1$ model as the optimal model with a ρ value of 1/1. This also indicated that the quantitative parameter $IMCC_1$ reflects the functional coordination of module pairs.

For comparison between SW and IMCC, the fitting model of SW was y = 0.1374ln(10) + 0.9807, with R^2 equal to 0.580, which is lower than 0.616 of IMCC (**Figure 2G**). The results indicate that IMCC achieved better performance on the weighted gene co-expression data. It also means that the results based on IMCC are more consistent with biological function than *SW*. This can be attributed to the adjustable parameters (weighted coefficient α and β) for SW and consistency score (CT), which make IMCC more likely to reach the optimal result in KEGG function coverage.

From the topological structure, the *IMCC* was generally consistent with inter-module average shortest path with coefficient of determination equal to 0.493 (**Figures 2C,D; Supplementary Table S4**).

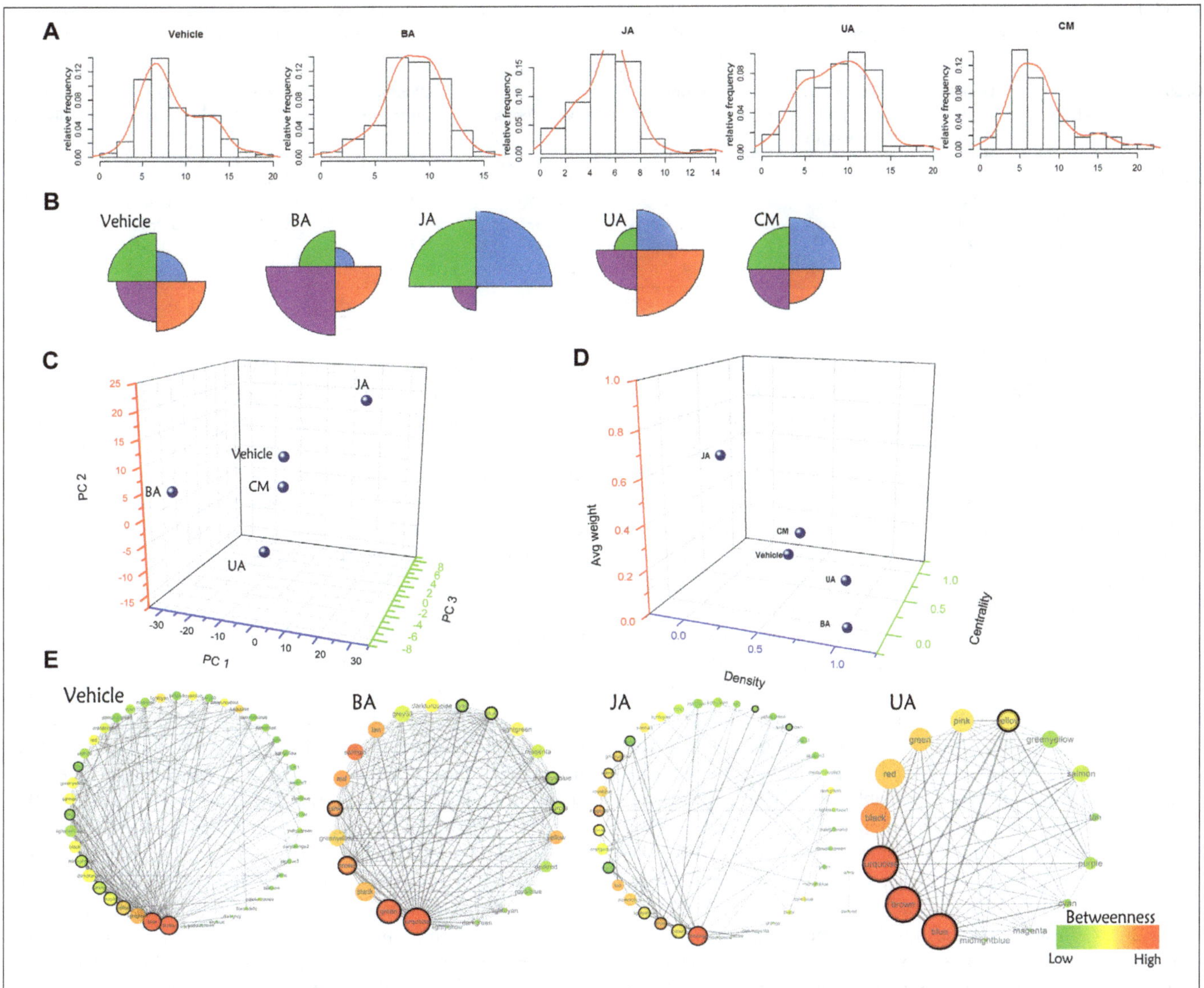

FIGURE 3 | Comparison of distribution of the IMCC score and global modular map rewiring. **(A)** The relative distribution of the IMCC score. The *X*-axis is the -log2 of the IMCC score. **(B)** Star graph of the relative account of the IMCC score distributing in four intervals (−∞, 5.2] (5.2–7.3] (7.3–10.2] (10.2–+∞]. These four intervals were indicated by black, red, green, and blue, respectively. **(C)** The principal component analysis of distribution of the IMCC score in each group. Each interval is set as variable, and relative frequencies in each interval are set as values of corresponding variables. **(D)** Euclidean distance of architecture of modular map in different groups. Three indexes (average weight, density, and centrality) were used to constitute the dimensions of space euclidean distance calculation. **(E)** Modular map based on IMCC across conditions. Each circle in modular map represents a module, the color of which indicates the betweenness in the corresponding modular map. Circles with black solid line around are connectors (modules) identified by edge weight distribution for further GO enrichment analysis.

GLOBAL MODULAR MAP REWIRING REVEALS THE PERTURBATION PATTERN OF DRUGS ON DISEASE

Drugs Destroyed the Characteristic "Core–periphery" Structure in Disease

Globally, the distribution of IMCC between disease and treated groups was obviously diverse (**Figures 3A,B**): BA-, JA-, and UA-treated groups were different compared to the vehicle group with significance (chi-square test, $p < 0.05$), whereas no statistical difference was noted between the ineffective (CM) group and the vehicle group (chi-square test, $p = 0.06374$). Besides, according to the distance in PCA, CM was the nearest to the vehicle (**Figure 3C**; **Supplementary Table S5**). This indicated that the transitions of inter-module coordination induced by the effective drugs were more thorough than those induced by the ineffective one.

Based on the IMCC, the modular map across condition was constructed in which modules were regarded as uniform nodes and the IMCC between any pair of modules as edges. As a result, the module map provided a holistic perspective of the inter-module coordination and framework extracted as "backbone" in disease and treated conditions. According to the topological analysis, the modular map in the disease exhibited a topical

TABLE 1 | Topological parameters of the module map in different groups. The symbols "↑" and "↓" represent "increase" and "decrease," respectively, compared with the vehicle group. The three highlighted parameters with red letter were selected as the representative index of the three types of parameters for further euclidean distance calculation.

Group	Avg. degree	Density	Characteristic path length	Diameter	Avg. betweenness	Cluster coefficient	Centrality	Avg. weight	Euclidean distance
Vehicle	11.911	0.271	1.848	4	0.0197	0.615	0.525	0.0213	–
BA	18.87↑	0.858↑	1.142↓	2↓	0.0068↓	0.867↑	0.156↓	0.0208↓	1.2655
JA	3.95↓	0.101↓	2.865↑	7↑	0.0493↑	0.281↓	0.271↓	0.081↑	0.9476
UA	11.333↓	0.81↑	1.19↓	2↓	0.0147↓	0.857↑	0.22↓	0.0357↑	1.0998
CM	8.571↓	0.429↑	1.71↓	4	0.0373↑	0.661↑	0.411↓	0.0409↑	0.4199

"core–periphery" structure, with the network centrality of the modular map of 0.525. Whereas this "core–periphery" structure collapsed in the treated groups, the network centrality was significantly decreased to 0.156, 0.271, and 0.22 (one-sample *t*-test, two-sided $p < 0.05$) in BA, JA, and UA groups, respectively (**Figures 3D,E**; **Table 1**).

It is indicated that from the mesoscopic perspective, network organization in stress exhibits a characteristic "core–periphery" architecture. In this architecture, the "periphery" is constituted of small well-defined communities; conversely, the "core" consists of highly interconnected larger modules harder to decompose (Bollobás, 1998; Lancichinetti et al., 2010; Han et al., 2013; Verma et al., 2016). According to results, in this "core–periphery" structure in disease condition, all the information propagation is of radial distribution around a couple of modules, and the integrity of the network is completely dependent on the modules at the center; thus, the system is liable to collapse under stress response. It is also suggested that when a biological network is on stress, the center of this "core–periphery" structure is a conserved and stable module, with crucial role for cell survival rather than development (Mihalik and Csermely, 2011; Kim et al., 2012; Han et al., 2013), to adapt to the novel situation. Accordingly, the modular map in disease state exhibits a characteristic "core–periphery" structure, core of which may contribute to cell survival. And this structure would be rewired and collapse in response to drug perturbation.

Aggregation and Dispersion of Modules: Two Allosteric Directions of Drugs

Although the network centrality decreased in all of the treated groups, we wondered if there were any distinct topological structures in different effective drug groups. Using analysis of neighborhood-based parameters in modular maps, we noted that the effective drugs showed two distinct regulatory directions. For one direction, in BA and UA groups, the inter-module connections were very dense and modules tended to aggregate. For example, the network density increased from 0.271 in vehicle to 0.858 (increased by 216.6%) and 0.81 (increased by 198.9%), the characteristic path length of the modular map decreased from 1.848 in vehicle to 1.142 (decreased by 38.2%) and 1.19 (decreased by 35.6%), in BA and UA groups, respectively. Generally, after treatment with BA and UA, the centrality of the modular map decreased, and the connections between noncentral modules increased (**Figures 3D,E** and **Table 1**). All these alterations drive the modular map into a clique-like structure, in which any module pairs are connected by edges. Such alterations indicated that information propagation was easier to be implemented. Such a structure is shown to have the highest integrity and the strongest robustness under perturbation. Overall, the modules in BA or UA groups aggregated into a more intensively connected integrity.

As for the opposite direction, in the JA group, the modular map altered into a sparser network, and the information propagation path was elongated: compared with vehicle, the network density decreased to 0.101 (decreased by 62.7%); and the characteristic path length and average betweenness centrality increased by 55 and 150%, to 2.865, and 0.0493, respectively. In general, after treatment with JA, the centrality of the modular map also decreased, which attributed to the disruption between central modules and noncentral modules. Thus, we assumed that the effect of JA on the module map included module dispersing. It should be noted that the average weight nearly quadrupled from 0.021 in vehicle to 0.081 in JA (**Figures 3D,E** and **Table 1**), indicating that the paths between modules became wider and smoother than those in disease state. Therefore, we inferred that the pharmacological effects of JA were decoupling partial inter-module paths and widening the remaining connectivity, which may consequently interrupt the pathological information transmission and enhance the remaining information transmission.

Both of module aggregation and dispersion effect of drugs destroyed the characteristic "core–periphery" architecture in disease, that means the importance of "core" for cell survival decreased in treated conditions, and the emphasis of the cell may turn from survival into development. We can infer that cerebral ischemia injury was repaired after treated by these drugs. Then, what is the biological function of the "core"? How is this "core" reversed by these drugs?

LOCAL DISSECTION OF COOPERATIVE PATHOLOGICAL MODULE PAIR INDICATED MECHANISMS

Identification and Dissection of Connectors

The topological structure analysis of modular map provides a landscape of the transition of inter-module connections from

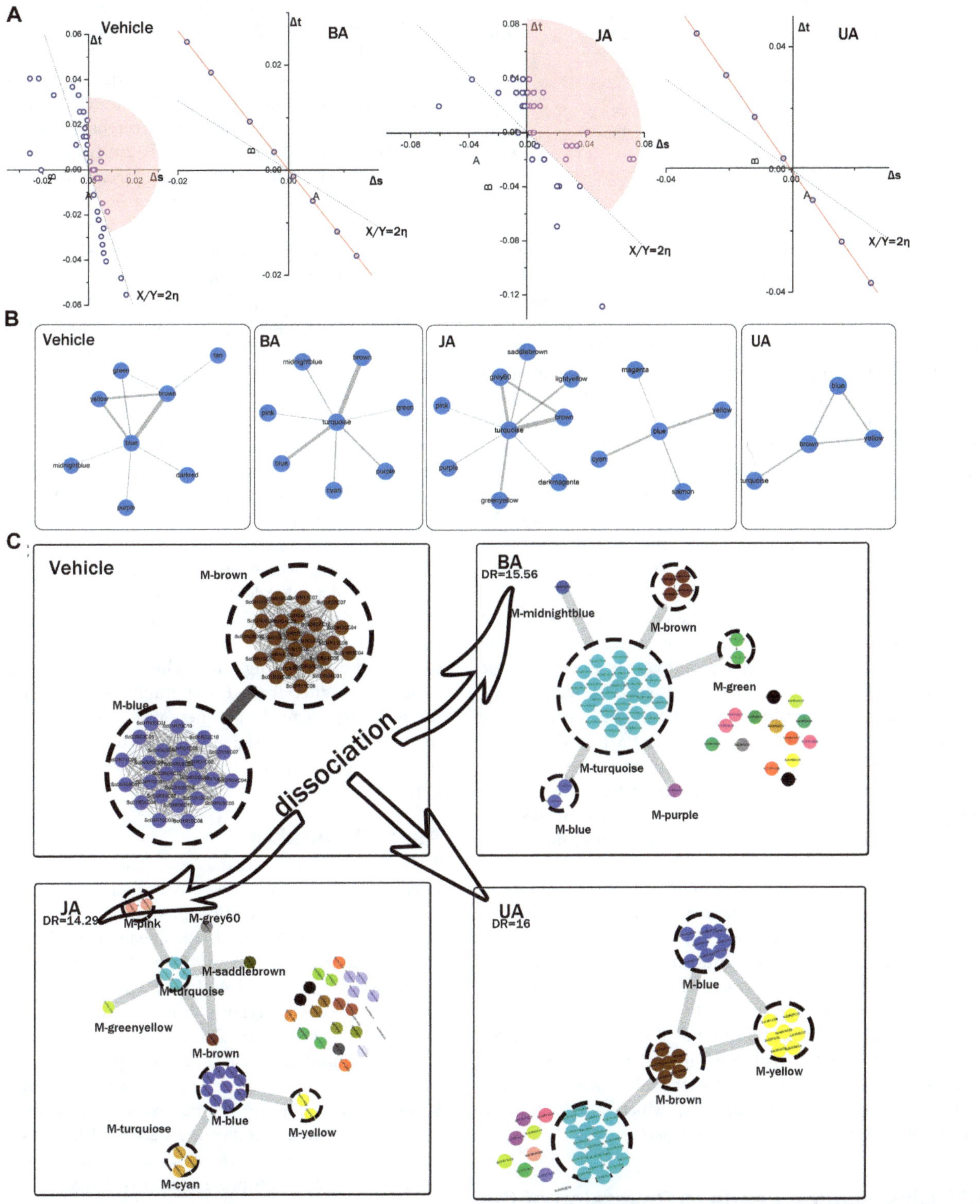

FIGURE 4 | Identification of connectors and dissociation of pathological module pair. **(A)** Connectors identified by variation of ratio of characteristic path length and density (VRCD). The Δs and Δt represent the variation ratio of characteristic path length to network density, η represents average ratio of Δs and Δt. The 2-fold change of η, shown as dotted linear, was set as cutoff. Modules in the pink sector domains were identified as connectors. None of modules were identified as connector in BA and UA groups for their clique-like structure with equal η of all modules (red line). **(B)** Connector sub-network identified by edge weight distribution. **(C)** Local dissection of cooperative pathological module pair (PMP). Genes of PMP in vehicle were scattered into different modules in BA-, JA-, and UA-treated groups. Each dashed circle represents a module; circles with the same color in the same region indicate genes in the same module; gray rough lines represent the inter-module connections; gray thread lines represent the interactions between genes.

TABLE 2 | Dissociation rate of the PMP in each treated group.

	BA	JA	UA	CM
nA	2	2	2	2
nB	15	25	10	11
NA	48	48	48	48
NB	23	42	15	23
DR	15.65	14.29	16	11.48

disease to treated conditions. In order to identify the modules contributing to information propagation in the modular map, we employed three methods to detect the "connectors" (**Figure 4A, Supplementary Tables S6, S7**), which were defined as modules bridging one community to another (Yu et al., 2007; Zhu et al., 2014) and controlling the information flow dissemination between modules. As a result, connector networks were detected in each group (**Figure 4B**). In the light of the disease condition, the module pair with the strongest coordination was identified as connectors, which can be regarded as "a broad bridge with heavy traffic, controlling essential pass." This pair of connectors can be treated as the "core" reflecting the characteristic pathological process in the disease condition (**Figure 4C**), so were named as "pathological module pair (PMP)."

To assess the allosteric communication of connectors from untreated to treated conditions, we investigated what had happened to the "core" after perturbation to reveal the pharmacological mechanisms of these drugs. Dissociation rate (DR) was proposed to evaluate how one modular pair in one condition scattered in other condition. The PMP in the vehicle group dispersed into several modules in different treated groups. The DR was 15.65, 14.29, and 16 in BA, JA, and UA, respectively (**Table 2**). As shown in **Figure 4C**, the effective drugs also displayed two distinct directions. In the BA group, more than one half of the nodes constituting PMP dispersed into one common module (turquoise). Similar to BA, 81.63% nodes in the PMP dispersed into four connectors (blue, brown, turquoise, and yellow) after treatment with UA. Nodes from the PMP aggregated into a compact integrity, like an intensely interacted module sub-network facilitating information communication. In the JA group, the nodes from the PMP scattered into 25 modules, the amount of which accounted for more than one half of the total 48 modules. This dispersion from an intimate interaction to more sparsely association was also noted in the modular map analysis, which would lead to interruption of some information propagation.

PMP Dissociation Leads to Reversion of the Pathological Processes

In order to understand how functions altered by PMP dispersion, we enriched KEGG pathways for each module of the PMP and modules that PMP nodes assembling in treated condition (**Table 3**).

All enriched KEGG pathways of the PMP in disease are related to the pathological process of the nervous system injury. For example, inhibition of MAPK signaling or mTOR signaling can effectively reduce cerebral ischemia reperfusion injury (Dennis et al., 2001; Sovan, 2013; Johansson et al., 2014; King et al., 2015; Yang et al., 2016). Ischemic long-term potentiation (i-LTP) increasing and vascular smooth muscle contraction are pathological changes following cerebral ischemic injury (Maddahi et al., 2009) (Orfila et al., 2014) (Wang et al., 2014). ALS is related to motor neurons degeneration in the cortex (Sathasivam et al., 2001); (Menzies et al., 2002); (Hristelina et al., 2009); (Jordi 2009 Giovanni 2009); (Ivanova et al., 2014). Prion disease may lead to neuronal death by oxidative stress and regulation of complement activation (McLennan et al., 2004). Notably, these pathways were all cross-talk with MAPK signaling: MAPK signaling pathway is the upstream signaling of mTOR signaling pathway and is involved in long-term potentiation and ALS and also acts as a critical factor to mediate vascular smooth muscle contraction. It is the inter-module structural connection in PMP that bridges the functional correlations among these nervous injury–related pathways, in which the MAPK signaling pathway plays a major role. Therefore, these pathways of PMP reflected the cell survival condition in the process of neural ischemia injury.

Whereas, in the treated groups, PMP was dissociated into several modules, accompanied with reversion of the pathological processes and a new adaptive balance of biological system. In BA and UA, the top 10 KEGG signaling concentrated in MAPK signaling, GnRH signaling, viral infection, cancer, neurotrophin signaling, and chemokine signaling pathway. That means, after treated, the emphasis of the cell shift from survival, represented by nervous injury–related pathways centered on MAPK signaling, into development and repair, such as neurotrophin regulation, chemokine signaling, and hormone releasing.

Assay Validation

To validate the PMP that is essential for the contribution of disease phenotype, we used MCAO rats to examine the core protein, genes, and interaction. First, we compared the expression of a protein (MAP2k6) of MAPK signaling by Western blot in the disease and treated groups. Second, in order to verify the regulatory direction of BA, JA, and UA, we used RT-PCR to examine the gene expression differences of a pair of genes from PMP, Bcl2l1, and BBC3. The interaction of the two genes was tested using immune co-immunoprecipitation (co-IP).

According to Western blot analysis (**Figures 5A,B, Supplementary Figure S3**), the expression of Map2k6 protein in mice brains was significantly decreased in the vehicle group than the sham group ($p < 0.05$, one-sided, paired *t*-test). Expression of Map2k6 protein increased significantly in the JA group compared with samples in the vehicle group ($p < 0.05$, one-sided, paired *t*-test). No statistically significant differences were found in other treated groups.

The BBC3 and Bcl2l1 mRNA were examined by RT-PCR (**Figures 5C,D**). The BBC3 mRNA expression was significantly increased in the JA group ($p < 0.05$, one-sided, paired *t*-test), but decreased slightly in BA and UA groups. Compared with vehicle, the expression of Bcl2l1 was significantly increased in the JA

TABLE 3 | Enriched KEGG pathways of the PMP in disease condition, and top 10 KEGG pathways of modules in BA and UA that PMP nodes scattered in.

	Enriched KEGG pathways	*p* value
Vehicle-blue	mmu04150: mTOR signaling pathway	0.010,800,621
	mmu04720: Long-term potentiation	0.017,728,358
	mmu04270: Vascular smooth muscle contraction	0.048,072,485
Vehicle-brown	mmu05014: Amyotrophic lateral sclerosis	3.13E-04
	mmu04010: MAPK signaling pathway	0.00308,276
	mmu05020: Prion diseases	0.00314,163
Top 10 signaling of BA-blue	mmu05200: Pathways in cancer	3.40E-16
	mmu04912: GnRH signaling pathway	4.48E-15
	mmu04010: MAPK signaling pathway	9.55E-14
	mmu05166: HTLV-I infection	4.56E-11
	mmu05161: Hepatitis B	2.49E-10
	mmu04722: Neurotrophin signaling pathway	1.95E-09
	mmu04062: Chemokine signaling pathway	2.59E-09
	mmu04668: TNF signaling pathway	4.82E-08
	mmu05203: Viral carcinogenesis	1.91E-07
	mmu05210: Colorectal cancer	3.01E-07
Top 10 signaling of UA-blue, brown, turquoise, and yellow	mmu05200: Pathways in cancer	3.40E-16
	mmu04912: GnRH signaling pathway	4.48E-15
	mmu04010: MAPK signaling pathway	9.55E-14
	mmu05166: HTLV-I infection	4.56E-11
	mmu05161: Hepatitis B	2.49E-10
	mmu05212: Pancreatic cancer	1.54E-10
	mmu04722: Neurotrophin signaling pathway	1.95E-09
	mmu04062: Chemokine signaling pathway	2.59E-09
	mmu04015: Rap1 signaling pathway	1.53E-09
	mmu04668: TNF signaling pathway	4.82E-08

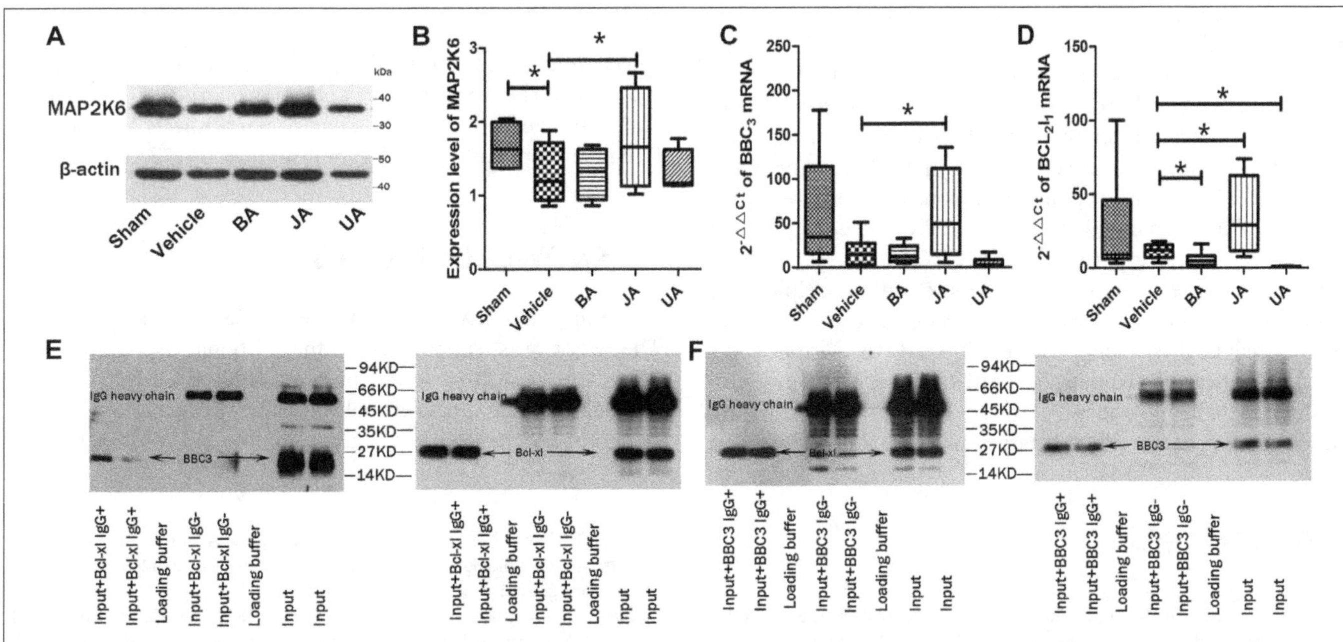

FIGURE 5 | Validation of core protein, genes, and interaction in PMP. **(A and B)** show expression of MAP2K6 of Western blot in distinct groups. **(C and D)** are relative contents of BBC3 and Bcl2l1 among different groups. $^*p < 0.05$. **(E and F)** represent the co-immunoprecipitation results of BBC3 and Bcl-xl.

group (p < 0.05, one-sided, paired t-test) but decreased significantly in BA and UA groups (p < 0.05, one-sided, paired t-test). The outcome of RT-PCR indicated that the regulatory effects of BA and UA showed opposite directions to that of JA.

Both Bcl-Xl and BBC3 were detected in precipitation products of BBC3 IgG or Bcl-Xl IgG (**Figures 5E,F**). There was an interaction between BBC3 protein and Bcl-XL protein. By searching the String database (String 10.0, http://www.string-db.org/), we found that BBC3 and Bcl2l1 were correlated with each other (correlation score = 0.999), remarked by reaction and binding.

DISCUSSION

In the current study, we proposed an integrated mathematical model for quantitative evaluation of the transition of inter-module coordination across conditions. Globally, we found the high centrality "core–periphery" modular map is a characteristic structure in cerebral ischemia condition. Furthermore, it is the rewiring of the interactions between modules and consequent architecture alteration in the modular map, rather than a single gene or a single module, that leads to phenotype alteration in response to drugs perturbation. Our result also indicated that BA, UA, and JA showed diversification of the pharmacological effect directions: the pharmacological mechanism of BA and UA can be attributed to aggregation of modules into a clique-like community, enhanced connections between noncentral modules, facilitation of paths for information communication between non-modules, and promotion of robustness in response to perturbation; the pharmacological mechanism of JA is ascribed to selective interruption of information transmission and enhancement of some specific information propagation. According to the local allosteric, the "core" of "core–periphery" structure is an interacting PMP, whose biological function focused on nervous injury pathways bridged by MAPK signaling pathway. BA and UA aggregated the dissociated nodes into a compact integrity, whereas JA dispersed the dissociated nodes from the PMP. PMP dissociation leading by drugs contributed to the reversion of the pathological condition: the focus of the cellular function shift from survival after nervous system injury into development and repair, including neurotrophin regulation, hormone releasing, and chemokine signaling activation. Finally, these results were validated by *in vivo* experiments of MCAO rats.

Ischemic stroke is a complex disease with multiple gene mutations. For this disease, a "from systematic to molecular levels" analytical strategy was established to decipher the pharmacological mechanism of multi-target drugs. Our result highlights the holistic inter-module coordination rearrangement rather than a target or a single module that brings phenotype alteration. That may indicate in the biological system, one kind of complex adaptive system composed of a set of basic units and interactions, rewiring of interactions between basic units lead to nonlinear phenomena: novel phenotype emergence to response to perturbation (Zhang et al., 2014). Therefore, complexity, in essence, is a science of emergence. The challenge is how to discover the primary principles of emergence, as a foundation, to quantify the interactions between basic units and their alterations across different conditions. Quantitative analysis of drug-induced transition in modular map was the principal problem for systematically elucidating the comprehensive pharmacological mechanisms of multi-target drugs and the inevitable choice for network-based drug discovery. Our strategy may help to map the detailed variations of inter-module pharmacological actions of multiple-target drugs and could be set as reference for other active ingredients.

AUTHOR CONTRIBUTIONS

ZW and PW designed the study and wrote the manuscript. PW, JL, YY, and WX performed the experiments. YZ, BL, and QL revised the manuscript. DL conducted the statistical data analysis.

FUNDING

I declare all sources of funding received for the research being submitted. The open access publication fees will be paid from National Science and Technology Major Projects "Major New Drug Development Project" (grant number 2017ZX09301–059).

ACKNOWLEDGMENTS

The authors thank Xiang Diao for helpful discussions and revision. The work was supported by the National Natural Science Foundation of China [grant number 81904064, 81673833] and National Science and Technology Major Projects "Major New Drug Development Project" [grant number 2017ZX09301–059].

REFERENCES

Amar, D., Safer, H., and Shamir, R. (2013). Dissection of regulatory networks that are altered in disease via differential co-expression. *Plos Comput. Biol.* 9, e1002955. doi:10.1371/journal.pcbi.1002955

Bandyopadhyay, S., Mehta, M., Kuo, D., Sung, M.-K., Chuang, R., Jaehnig, E. J., et al. (2010). Rewiring of genetic networks in response to DNA damage. *Science* 330, 1385–1389. doi:10.1126/science.1195618

Bollobás, B. (1998). *Modern graph theory*. Berlin, Germany: Springer.

Cheng, F., Kovács, I. A., and Barabási, A. L. (2019). Network-based prediction of drug combinations. *Nat. Commun.* 10, 1197. doi:10.1038/s41467-019-09186-x

Costanzo, M., VanderSluis, B., Koch, E. N., Baryshnikova, A., Pons, C., Tan, G., et al. (2016). A global genetic interaction network maps a wiring diagram of cellular function. *Science* 353, 6306. doi:10.1126/science.aaf1420

David, A., and Ron, S. (2014). Constructing module maps for integrated analysis of heterogeneous biological networks. *Nucleic Acids Res.* 42, 4208–4219. doi:10.1093/nar/gku102

Dennis, P. B., Jaeschke, A., Saitoh, M., Fowler, B., Kozma, S. C., and Thomas, G. (2001). Mammalian TOR: a homeostatic ATP sensor. *Science* 294, 1102–1105. doi:10.1126/science.1063518

Ding, F., Zhang, Q., Ung, C. O. L., Wang, Y., Han, Y., Hu, Y., et al. (2015). An analysis of chemical ingredients network of Chinese herbal formulae for the treatment of coronary heart disease. *PLos One* 10, e0116441. doi:10.1371/journal.pone.0116441

Frantz, S. (2005). Playing dirty. *Nature* 437, 942–943. doi:10.1038/437942a

Granovetter, M. S. (1973). The strength of weak ties. *Am. J. Sociol.* 78, 1360–1380. doi:10.1086/225469

Han, H. W., Ohn, J. H., Moon, J., and Kim, J. H. (2013). Yin and Yang of disease genes and death genes between reciprocally scale-free biological networks. *Nucleic Acids Res.* 41, 9209–9217. doi:10.1093/nar/gkt683

Hristelina, I., Magdalini, P., and Cleveland, D. W. (2009). Non-cell autonomous toxicity in neurodegenerative disorders: ALS and beyond. *J. Cel Biol* 187, 761–772. doi:10.1083/jcb.200908164

Hsu, J. T., Peng, C. H., Hsieh, W. P., Lan, C. Y., and Tang, C. Y. (2011). A novel method to identify cooperative functional modules: study of module coordination in the *Saccharomyces cerevisiae* cell cycle. *BMC Bioinformatics* 12, 1–22. doi:10.1186/1471-2105-12-281

Ivanova, M. I., Sievers, S. A., Guenther, E. L., Johnson, L. M., Winkler, D. D., Galaleldeen, A., et al. (2014). Aggregation-triggering segments of SOD1 fibril formation support a common pathway for familial and sporadic ALS. *Proc. Natl. Acad. Sci.* 111, 197–201. doi:10.1073/pnas.1320786110

Johansson, S. E., Larsen, S. S., Povlsen, G. K., and Edvinsson, L. (2014). Early MEK1/2 inhibition after global cerebral ischemia in rats reduces brain damage and improves outcome by preventing delayed vasoconstrictor receptor upregulation. *PLoS One* 9, e92417. doi:10.1371/journal.pone.0092417

Jordi, M., and Giovanni, M. (2009). Mitochondrial function, morphology, and axonal transport in amyotrophic lateral sclerosis. *Antioxid. Redox Signal.* 11, 1615–1626. doi:10.1089/ARS.2009.2604

Kelder, T., Eijssen, L., Kleemann, R., van Erk, M., Kooistra, T., and Evelo, C. (2011). Exploring pathway interactions in insulin resistant mouse liver. *BMC Syst. Biol.* 5, 1814–1817. doi:10.1186/1752-0509-5-127

Kim, D., Kim, M.-S., and Cho, K.-H. (2012). The core regulation module of stress-responsive regulatory networks in yeast. *Nucleic Acids Res.* 40, 8793–8802. doi:10.1093/nar/gks649

Kim, I., Lee, H., Han, S. K., and Kim, S. (2014). Linear motif-mediated interactions have contributed to the evolution of modularity in complex protein interaction networks. *Plos Comput. Biol.* 10, e1003881. doi:10.1371/journal.pcbi.1003881

King, D., Yeomanson, D., and Bryant, H. E. (2015). PI3King the lock. *J. Pediatr. Hematol. Oncol.* 37, 245–251. doi:10.1097/mph.0000000000000329

Lancichinetti, A., Kivelä, M., Saramäki, J., and Fortunato, S. (2010). Characterizing the community structure of complex networks. *PLos One* 5, e11976. doi:10.1371/journal.pone.0011976

Langfelder, P., and Horvath, S. (2008). WGCNA: an R package for weighted correlation network analysis. *BMC Bioinformatics* 9, 1–13. doi:10.1186/1471-2105-9-559

Levy, O., Knisbacher, B. A., Levanon, E. Y., and Havlin, S. (2017). Integrating networks and comparative genomics reveals retroelement proliferation dynamics in hominid genomes. *Sci. Adv.* 3, e1701256. doi:10.1126/sciadv.1701256

Li, B., Liu, J., Zhang, Y., Wang, P., Yu, Y., Kang, R., et al. (2016). Quantitative identification of compound-dependent on-modules and differential allosteric modules from homologous ischemic networks. *CPT Pharmacometrics Syst. Pharmacol.* 5, 575–584. doi:10.1002/psp4.12127

Lin, C. Y., Lin, Y. W., Yu, S. W., Lo, Y. S., and Yang, J. M. (2012). MoNetfamily: a web server to infer homologous modules and module-module interaction networks in vertebrates. *Nucleic Acids Res.* 40, 263–270. doi:10.1093/nar/gks541

Liu, J., Zhang, Z. J., Zhou, C. X., Wang, Y., Cheng, Y. Y., Duan, D. Y., et al. (2012). Outcome-dependent global similarity analysis of imbalanced core signaling pathways in ischemic mouse hippocampus. *CNS Neurol. Disord. Drug Targets* 11, 1070–1082. doi:10.2174/1871527311211080018

Liu, J., and Wang, Z. (2015). Diverse array-designed modes of combination therapies in Fangjiomics. *Acta Pharmacol. Sin* 36, 680–688. doi:10.1038/aps.2014.125

Ma, X., and Gao, L. (2012). Discovering protein complexes in protein interaction networks via exploring the weak ties effect. *BMC Syst. Biol.* 6, 1–15. doi:10.1186/1752-0509-6-s1-s6

Maddahi, A., Chen, Q., and Edvinsson, L. (2009). Enhanced cerebrovascular expression of matrix metalloproteinase-9 and tissue inhibitor of metalloproteinase-1 via the MEK/ERK pathway during cerebral ischemia in the rat. *BMC Neurosci.* 10, 1–12. doi:10.1186/1471-2202-10-56

Matthew, T., Martin, F., Holliday, E. G., Cathie, S., Hopewell, J. C., Cheng, Y. C., et al. (2012). Genetic risk factors for ischemic stroke and its subtypes (the meta stroke collaboration): a meta-analysis of genome-wide association studies. *Lancet Neurol.* 11, 951–962. doi:10.1016/S1474-4422(12)70234-X

McLennan, N. F., Brennan, P. M., McNeill, A., Davies, I., Fotheringham, A., Rennison, K. A., et al. (2004). Prion protein accumulation and neuroprotection in hypoxic brain damage. *Am. J. Pathol.* 165, 227–235. doi:10.1016/s0002-9440(10)63291-9

Meda, S. A., Ruaño, G., Windemuth, A., O'Neil, K., Berwise, C., Dunn, S. M., et al. (2014). Multivariate analysis reveals genetic associations of the resting default mode network in psychotic bipolar disorder and schizophrenia. *Proc. Natl. Acad. Sci. USA* 111, 2066–2075. doi:10.1073/pnas.1313093111

Menzies, F. M., Cookson, M. R., Taylor, R. W., Turnbull, D. M., Chrzanowska-Lightowlers, Z. M., Dong, L., et al. (2002). Mitochondrial dysfunction in a cell culture model of familial amyotrophic lateral sclerosis. *Brain* 125, 1522–1533. doi:10.1093/brain/awf167

Mihalik, Á., and Csermely, P. (2011). Heat shock partially dissociates the overlapping modules of the yeast protein-protein interaction network: a systems level model of adaptation. *Plos Comput. Biol.* 7, e1002187. doi:10.1371/journal.pcbi.1002187

Missiuro, P. V., Liu, K., Zou, L., Ross, B. C., Zhao, G., Liu, J. S., et al. (2009). Information flow analysis of interactome networks. *Plos Comput. Biol.* 5, 1000350. doi:10.1371/journal.pcbi.1000350

National Research Council (US) Institute for Laboratory Animal Research (1996). *Guide for the Care and Use of Laboratory Animals.* Washington (DC): National Academies Press (US).

Onnela, J. P., Saramäki, J., Hyvönen, J., Szabó, G., Lazer, D., Kaski, K., et al. (2009). Structure and tie strengths in mobile communication networks. *Proc. Natl. Acad. Sci. USA* 104, 7332–7336. doi:10.1073/pnas.0610245104

Orfila, J. E., Shimizu, K., Garske, A. K., Deng, G., Maylie, J., Traystman, R. J., et al. (2014). Increasing small conductance Ca2+-activated potassium channel activity reverses ischemia-induced impairment of long-term potentiation. *Eur. J. Neurosci.* 40, 3179–3188. doi:10.1111/ejn.12683

Roguev, A., Bandyopadhyay, S., Zofall, M., Zhang, K., Fischer, T., Collins, S. R., et al. (2008). Conservation and rewiring of functional modules revealed by an epistasis map in fission yeast. *Science* 322, 405–410. doi:10.1126/science.1162609

Roth, B. L., Sheffler, D. J., and Kroeze, W. K. (2004). Magic shotguns versus magic bullets: selectively non-selective drugs for mood disorders and schizophrenia. *Nat. Rev. Drug Discov.* 3, 353–359. doi:10.1038/nrd1346

Sathasivam, S., Ince, P. G., and Shaw, P. J. (2001). Apoptosis in amyotrophic lateral sclerosis: a review of the evidence. *Neuropathol. Appl. Neurobiol.* 27, 257–274. doi:10.1046/j.0305-1846.2001.00332.x

Sovan, S. (2013). Regulation of autophagy by mTOR-dependent and mTOR-independent pathways: autophagy dysfunction in neurodegenerative diseases and therapeutic application of autophagy enhancers. *Biochem. Soc. Trans.* 41, 1103–1130. doi:10.1042/BST20130134

Tesson, B. M., Breitling, R., and Jansen, R. C. (2010). DiffCoEx: a simple and sensitive method to find differentially coexpressed gene modules. *BMC Bioinformatics* 11, 497. doi:10.1186/1471-2105-11-497

Ulitsky, I., Shlomi, T., Kupiec, M., and Shamir, R. (2008). From E-MAPs to module maps: dissecting quantitative genetic interactions using physical interactions. *Mol. Syst. Biol.* 4, 173–178. doi:10.1038/msb.2008.42

Verma, T., Russmann, F., Arajo, N. A., Nagler, J., and Herrmann, H. J. (2016). Emergence of core-peripheries in networks. *Nat. Commun.* 7, 36–41. doi:10.1038/ncomms10441

Wang, J., Lou, H., Pedersen, C. J., Smith, A. D., and Perez, R. G. (2009). 14-3-3ζ contributes to tyrosine hydroxylase activity in MN9D cells. *J. Biol. Chem.* 284, 14011–14019. doi:10.1074/jbc.m901310200

Wang, N., Chen, L., Cheng, N., Zhang, J., Tian, T., and Lu, W. (2014). Active calcium/calmodulin-dependent protein kinase II (CaMKII) regulates NMDA receptor mediated postischemic long-term potentiation (i-LTP) by promoting the interaction between CaMKII and NMDA receptors in ischemia. *Neural Plast.* 2014, 827161. doi:10.1155/2014/827161

Wang, P.-q., Li, B., Liu, J., Zhang, Y.-y., Yu, Y.-n., Zhang, X.-x., et al. (2015a). Phenotype-dependent alteration of pathways and networks reveals a pure synergistic mechanism for compounds treating mouse cerebral ischemia. *Acta Pharmacol. Sin* 36, 734–747. doi:10.1038/aps.2014.168

Wang, Z., Duan, D., and Wang, Y.-Y. (2015b). Editorial (thematic issue): combination therapy of vascular diseases and fangjiomics: when west meets east in the era of phenomics. *Cvp* 13, 420–422. doi:10.2174/157016111304150722171221

Wang, P.-q., Liu, Q., Xu, W.-j., Yu, Y.-n., Zhang, Y.-y., Li, B., et al. (2018). Pure mechanistic analysis of additive neuroprotective effects between baicalin and jasminoidin in ischemic stroke mice. *Acta Pharmacol. Sin* 39, 961–974. doi:10.1038/aps.2017.145

Wang, Z., Liu, J., Cheng, Y., and Wang, Y. (2011). Fangjiomics: in search of effective and safe combination therapies. *J. Clin. Pharmacol.* 51, 1132–1151. doi:10.1177/0091270010382913

Wang, Z., Liu, J., Yu, Y., Chen, Y., and Wang, Y. 2012). Modular pharmacology: the next paradigm in drug discovery. *Expert Opin. Drug Discov.* 7, 667–677. doi:10.1517/17460441.2012.692673

Wang, Z., and Wang, Y. (2013). Navigating personalized medicine dependent on modular flexibility. *Trends Mol. Med.* 19, 393–395. doi:10.1016/j.molmed.2013.05.003

Yang, H., Li, L., Zhou, K., Wang, Y., Guan, T., Chai, C., et al. (2016). Shengmai injection attenuates the cerebral ischemia/reperfusion induced autophagy via modulation of the AMPK, mTOR and JNK pathways. *Pharm. Biol.* 54, 1–10doi:10.3109/13880209.2016.1155625

Yang, S. K., Wang, Y. C., Chao, C. C., Chuang, Y. J., Lan, C. Y., and Chen, B. S. (2009). Dynamic cross-talk analysis among TNF-R, TLR-4 and IL-1R signalings in TNFalpha-induced inflammatory responses. *BMC Med. Genomics* 3, 19. doi:10.1186/1755-8794-3-19

Yu, H., Kim, P. M., Sprecher, E., Trifonov, V., and Gerstein, M. (2007). The importance of bottlenecks in protein networks: correlation with gene essentiality and expression dynamics. *Plos Comput. Biol.* 3, e59. doi:10.1371/journal.pcbi.0030059

Zeng, T., Sun, S.-y., Wang, Y., Zhu, H., and Chen, L. (2013). Network biomarkers reveal dysfunctional gene regulations during disease progression. *FEBS J.* 280, 5682–5695. doi:10.1111/febs.12536

Zeng, T., Wang, D. C., Wang, X., Xu, F., and Chen, L. (2014). Prediction of dynamical drug sensitivity and resistance by module network rewiring-analysis based on transcriptional profiling. *Drug Resist. Updates* 17, 64–76. doi:10.1016/j.drup.2014.08.002

Zhang, Y., Azizalaou, M. A., Bertelle, C., Zhou, S., and Wang, W. (2014). Emergence of cooperation in non-scale-free networks. *J. Phys. A-math Theor.* 47, 801–811. doi:10.1088/1751-8113/47/22/225003

Zhou, X. Z., Lei, L., Liu, J., Halu, A., Zhang, Y. Y., Li, B., et al. (2018). A Systems Approach to Refine Disease Taxonomy by Integrating Phenotypic and Molecular Networks. *EBioMedicine* 31, 79–91. doi:10.1016/j.ebiom.2018.04.002

Zhu, F., Wang, W., Di, Z., and Fan, Y. (2014). Identifying and characterizing key nodes among communities based on electrical-circuit networks. *Plos One* 9, e97021. doi:10.1371/journal.pone.0097021

3

Network Pharmacology-Based Analysis on the Potential Biological Mechanisms of Sinisan Against Non-Alcoholic Fatty Liver Disease

Xiaoyi Wei[1], Weixin Hou[1], Jiajun Liang[1], Peng Fang[1], Bo Dou[1], Zisong Wang[2], Jiayang Sai[3], Tian Xu[4], Chongyang Ma[1], Qiuyun Zhang[1]*, Fafeng Cheng[4]*, Xueqian Wang[4]* and Qingguo Wang[4]*

[1]School of Traditional Chinese Medicine, Capital Medical University, Beijing, China, [2]Department of Traditional Chinese Medicine, Beijing Chaoyang Hospital, Capital Medical University, Beijing, China, [3]Department of Oncology, The Third Affiliated Hospital, Beijing University of Chinese Medicine, Beijing, China, [4]School of Traditional Chinese Medicine, Beijing University of Chinese Medicine, Beijing, China

***Correspondence:**
Chongyang Ma
chongyang@ccmu.edu.cn
Qiuyun Zhang
zhangqiuyun8202@aliyun.com
Fafeng Cheng
fafengcheng@gmail.com
Xueqian Wang
shirlyding@163.com

Non-alcoholic fatty liver disease (NAFLD) has become the most prevalent liver disease in China. Sinisan (SNS) is a traditional Chinese medicine formula that has been widely used in treating chronic liver diseases, including NAFLD. However, its underlying biological mechanisms are still unclear. In this study, we employed a network pharmacology approach consisting of overlapped terms- (genes or pathway terms-) based analysis, protein-protein interaction (PPI) network-based analysis, and PPI clusters identification. Unlike the previous network pharmacology study, we used the shortest path length-based network proximity algorithm to evaluate the efficacy of SNS against NAFLD. And we also used random walk with restart (RWR) algorithm and Community Cluster (Glay) algorithm to identify important targets and clusters. The screening results showed that the mean shortest path length between genes of SNS and NAFLD was significantly smaller than degree-matched random ones. Six PPI clusters were identified and ten hub targets were obtained, including STAT3, CTNNB1, MAPK1, MAPK3, AGT, NQO1, TOP2A, FDFT1, ALDH4A1, and KCNH2. The experimental study indicated that SNS reduced hyperlipidemia, liver steatosis, and inflammation. Most importantly, JAK2/STAT3 signal was inhibited by SNS treatment and was recognized as the most important signal considering the network pharmacology part. This study provides a systems perspective to study the relationship between Chinese medicines and diseases and helps to discover potential mechanisms by which SNS ameliorates NAFLD.

Keywords: network pharmacology, NAFLD, Sinisan, protein-protein interaction (PPI) network, topological analysis, JAK2/STAT3

Abbreviations: AGEs: advanced glycation end-products; ALT: alanine aminotransferase; AST: aspartate aminotransferase; FFA: free fatty acid; HDL-C: high-density lipoprotein cholesterol; IL1β: interleukin 1β; IL6: interleukin 6; LDL-C: low-density lipoprotein cholesterol; NAFLD: non-alcoholic fatty liver disease; NFκB: nuclear factor kappa-B; NASH: non-alcoholic steatohepatitis; PI3K: phosphatidylinositol 3-kinase; PPI: protein-protein interaction; RAGE: receptor for advanced glycation end-products; RWR: random walk with restart; STAT3: signal transducer and activator of transcription; TC: total cholesterol Line; TG: total triglyceride; TNFα: tumor necrosis factor alpha.

INTRODUCTION

Non-alcoholic fatty liver disease (NAFLD) is the most common liver disease with a global prevalence of 25% (Cotter and Rinella, 2020). Although NAFLD was traditionally considered as a benign condition and only patients with obesity had been more likely to receive medical care, recent evidence has shown it to be a far more complex disease. Increased NAFLD-related mortality has been observed in several studies from the past years (Allen et al., 2019; Targher et al., 2020). And even simple steatosis might finally result in increased all-cause mortality because of the progression of this disease after a follow-up observation over decades (Tilg and Targher, 2020). NAFLD includes various clinical phenotypes ranging from simple steatosis (a benign condition called fatty liver) to non-alcoholic steatohepatitis (NASH) and hepatic fibrosis. And these conditions increase the risks of liver-related complications, such as cirrhosis, liver failure, and hepatocellular carcinoma. NAFLD is also closely associated with important extra-hepatic manifestations, such as cardiovascular disease and chronic kidney disease, which further increases its disease burden. Therefore, it has to be acknowledged that control of this disease would have a major impact on the benefits of health care.

Sinisan (SNS), also called Shigyaku-san in Japan, is a classic Chinese medicine formula originating from the book of Treatise on Febrile Diseases (Shang Han Lun) of the Han Dynasty (200–201 AD) China. It comprises four botanical drugs: *Bupleurum chinense DC.* (Apiaceae; *Bupleuri radix*) (Chaihu), *Paeonia lactiflora Pall.* (Paeoniaceae; *Paeoniae radix alba*) (Shaoyao), *Gardenia jasminoides J. Ellis* (Rubiaceae; *Aurantii fructus immaturus*) (Zhishi), and *Glycyrrhiza uralensis Fisch.* (Leguminosae; *Glycyrrhizae radix et rhizoma*) (Gancao) with a dose proportion of 1:1:1:1. For centuries, SNS has been widely applied in treatment of chronic liver diseases in the clinic. Our previous study indicated that SNS decreased liver steatosis and inflammation in NAFLD rats (Mu et al., 2020). However, for the well-accepted multi-component and multi-target effects of TCM formulas, it is difficult to understand the potential biological mechanisms by the traditional pharmacology approach. Network pharmacology was a recently proposed TCM research strategy to use a "network target" as a mathematical and computable representation of various connections between botanical formulae and diseases (Li and Zhang, 2013; Li et al., 2014). Therefore, we used this system biology-based approach to describe the association of multiple components with multiple targets and multiple pathways and recovery of the potential mechanisms of SNS against NAFLD at a system level.

In the present work, we, firstly, investigated the effect of SNS against NAFLD in high fat diet- (HFD-) induced NAFLD rat

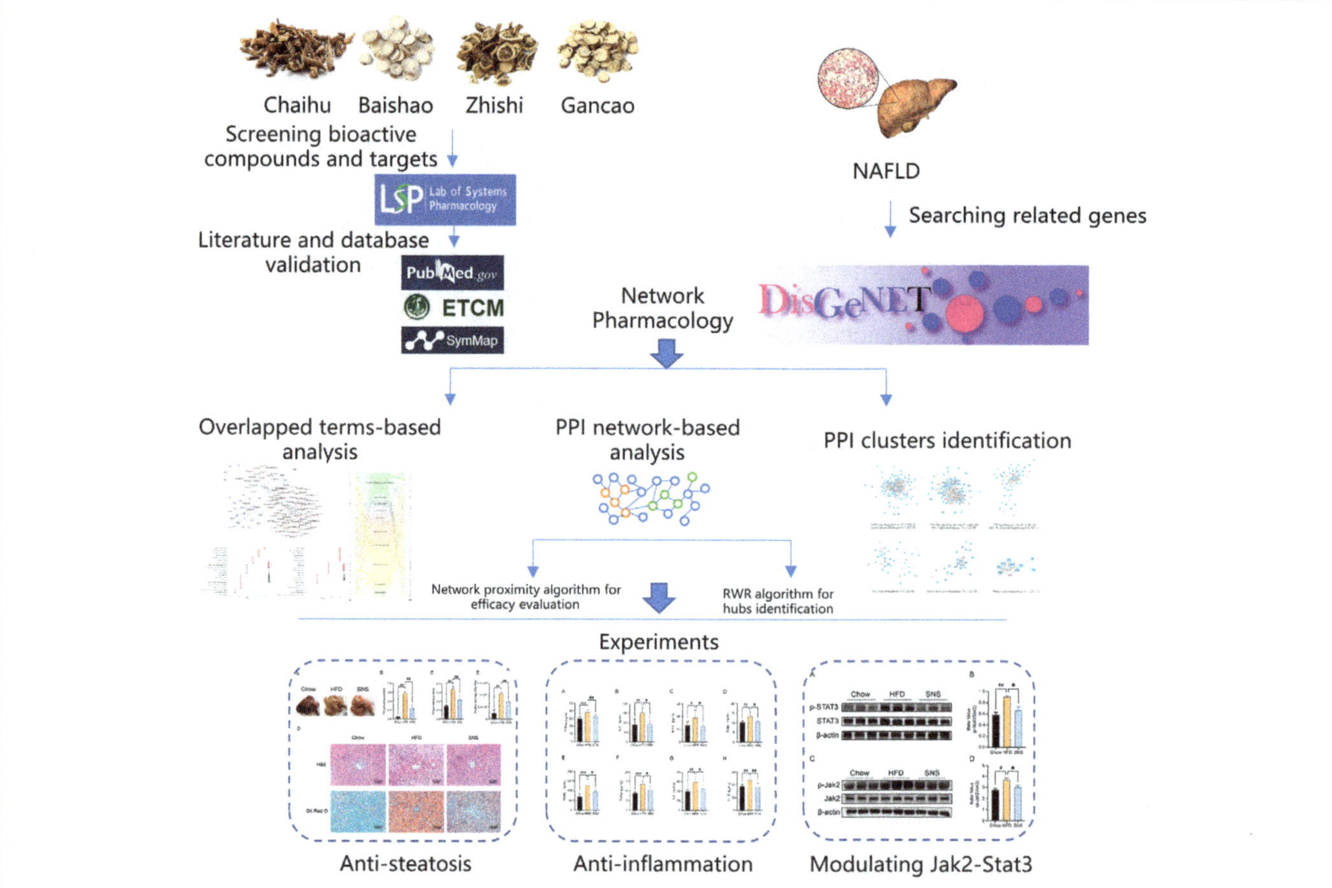

FIGURE 1 | Integrated workflow for discovery of the potential mechanisms of SNS against NAFLD.

TABLE 1 | Top 10 genes ranked by random walk with start algorithm.

Rank	Gene	Score
1	STAT3	0.005377152
2	CTNNB1	0.004535756
3	MAPK1	0.004386918
4	MAPK3	0.004010912
5	AGT	0.003464108
6	NQO1	0.002783255
7	TOP2A	0.002570216
8	FDFT1	0.00255187
9	ALDH4A1	0.002469136
10	KCNH2	0.002469136

model. Next, we collected information about compounds, compound-related targets, and NAFLD-related genes from extensive databases and identified important targets and pathways using a protein-protein interaction network-based method. Finally, a series of *in vivo* experiments were conducted to validate important targets of SNS against NAFLD (**Figure 1**).

METHODS

Collection of Bioactive Compounds and Prediction of Corresponding Targets

All compounds of SNS decoction and their corresponding absorption, distribution, metabolism, and excretion (ADME) parameters were obtained from the Traditional Chinese Medicine Systems Pharmacology Database and Analysis Platform (TCMSP). OB value (systemic bioavailability after oral absorption and distribution) ≥30% and DL value (structural similarity between compounds and clinically used drugs in the DrugBank database) ≥ 0.18 were employed as criteria to filter bioactive compounds. A total of 137 distinct bioactive compounds with literature or other database validation were identified for further analysis (**Table 1**). The putative targets of bioactive compounds in SNS decoction were predicted using TCMSP database as we previously mentioned. After removing duplicate genes, we obtained 155 SNS targets for further analysis.

Prediction of Non-Alcoholic Fatty Liver Disease Genes

Disease genes were obtained using the recently updated DisGeNET database with keywords "Non-alcoholic Fatty Liver Disease", "FATTY LIVER DISEASE, NONALCOHOLIC", "Nonalcoholic Steatohepatitis", and "Fibrosis, Liver" (Piñero et al., 2020). After removing BEFREE text mining genes, we obtained 306 unduplicated genes related to NAFLD and the details are provided in **Table 2**.

Construction of Protein-Protein Interaction Networks

We used two highly cited human protein-protein interaction data for background network constructions, dataset constructed by Professor Barabasi's team (Cheng et al., 2018) and the Search Tool for the Retrieval of Interacting Genes (STRING) database (Szklarczyk et al., 2019). The first dataset was derived from 15 commonly used databases with experimental evidence and the in-house confirmed data without inferred information. We constructed a PPI network containing 16,677 nodes and 243,603 edges and called it Bnet. The second dataset provided functional associations for proteins, which were sorted by a confidence score. Data only for "*Homo sapiens*" with a confidence score ≥0.9 was used for Snet construction, containing 9,941 nodes and 227,186 edges.

Network-Based Efficacy Evaluation of Sinisan Against Non-Alcoholic Fatty Liver Disease

Here, we used the network proximity index proposed by Prof. Barabasi's group to evaluate the efficacy of drugs against diseases in the background of Bnet (Cheng et al., 2019). Specifically, we marked T and V as the set of SNS genes and the set of NAFLD genes, respectively. We defined the shortest path length between nodes v ∈ V and t ∈ T in the network as **Equation 1**.

$$d_c(V,T) = \frac{1}{\|T\|}\sum_{t\in T} min_{v\in V} d(v,t). \quad (1)$$

We also compared the shortest path length between genes of SNS and NAFLD with the expected shortest path length between two random and size-matched groups of genes. As shown in **Equation 2**, we calculated the mean $\mu_{d(V,T)}$ and standard deviation $s_{d(V,T)}$ of the reference distribution and converted the absolute distance d_c to a relative distance Z_{dc}.

$$Z_{d_c} = \frac{d_c - \mu_{d_c(V,T)}}{\sigma_{d_c(V,T)}}. \quad (2)$$

Network-Based Important Genes Identification of Sinisan against Non-Alcoholic Fatty Liver Disease

In this study, the random walk with restart (RWR) algorithm, a classic ranking algorithm, was adopted to select important genes in the sub-network based on Snet. As shown in **Equation 3**, the vector p_0 is the initial probability distribution. Therefore, in p_0, only the seeds have values different from zero. After several iterations, the difference between the vectors p_{t+1} and p_t becomes negligible, the stationary probability distribution is reached, and the elements in these vectors represent a proximity measure from every graph node to the seeds. In this work, iterations are repeated until the difference between p_t and p_{t+1} falls below 10^{-10} (Valdeolivas et al., 2019).

$$p_{t+1}^{T} = (1-r)Mp_{t}^{T} + rp_{0}^{T}. \quad (3)$$

In detail, before the algorithm was executed, a sub-network of SNS genes and NAFLD genes was obtained from the Snet and

TABLE 2 | Identified bioactive compounds in SNS from UPLC-ESI-MS/MS Analysis.

ID	Name	Status	Ion mode
MOL000098	Quercetin	Confirmed	Positive
MOL000211	Mairin	Confirmed	Negative
MOL000239	Jaranol	Confirmed	Negative
MOL000354	Isorhamnetin	Confirmed	Negative
MOL000359	Sitosterol	Confirmed	Positive
MOL000392	Formononetin	Confirmed	Negative
MOL000417	Calycosin	Confirmed	Positive
MOL000422	Kaempferol	Confirmed	Negative
MOL000497	Licochalcone A	Confirmed	Positive
MOL000500	Vestitol	Confirmed	Negative
MOL001484	Inermine	Confirmed	Negative
MOL001792	DFV	Confirmed	Positive
MOL002311	Glycyrol	Confirmed	Positive
MOL002565	Medicarpin	Confirmed	Negative
MOL004328	Naringenin	Confirmed	Positive
MOL004841	Licochalcone B	Confirmed	Positive
MOL004848	Licochalcone G	Confirmed	Positive
MOL004855	Licoricone	Confirmed	Positive
MOL004879	Glycyrin	Confirmed	Positive
MOL004883	Licoisoflavone	Confirmed	Positive
MOL004884	Licoisoflavone B	Confirmed	Negative
MOL004885	Licoisoflavanone	Confirmed	Positive
MOL004908	Glabridin	Confirmed	Positive
MOL004910	Glabranin	Confirmed	Positive
MOL004911	Glabrene	Confirmed	Negative
MOL004912	Glabrone	Confirmed	Positive
MOL004915	Eurycarpin A	Confirmed	Positive
MOL004917	Glycyroside	Confirmed	Positive
MOL004948	Isoglycyrol	Confirmed	Negative
MOL004949	Isolicoflavonol	Confirmed	Positive
MOL004957	HMO	Confirmed	Positive
MOL004961	Quercetin der	Confirmed	Negative
MOL005000	Gancaonin G	Confirmed	Negative
MOL005020	Dehydroglyasperins C	Confirmed	Negative
MOL002776	Baicalin	Confirmed	Positive
MOL004609	Areapillin	Confirmed	Positive
MOL004702	Saikosaponin c_qt	Confirmed	Negative
MOL013187	Cubebin	Confirmed	Negative
MOL000492	(+)-Catechin	Confirmed	Negative
MOL001918	Paeoniflorgenone	Confirmed	Positive
MOL001921	Lactiflorin	Confirmed	Positive
MOL001924	Paeoniflorin	Confirmed	Negative
MOL001925	paeoniflorin_qt	Confirmed	Negative
MOL001928	albiflorin_qt	Confirmed	Positive
MOL001930	Benzoyl paeoniflorin	Confirmed	Positive
MOL000006	Luteolin	Confirmed	Positive
MOL001798	neohesperidin_qt	Confirmed	Negative
MOL001803	Sinensetin	Confirmed	Positive
MOL001941	Ammidin	Confirmed	Positive
MOL005100	5,7-Dihydroxy-2-(3-hydroxy-4-methoxyphenyl)chroman-4-one	Confirmed	Negative
MOL005828	Nobiletin	Confirmed	Positive
MOL005849	Didymin	Confirmed	Negative
MOL007879	Tetramethoxyluteolin	Confirmed	Positive
MOL013276	Poncirin	Confirmed	Negative
MOL013277	Isosinensetin	Confirmed	Positive
MOL013279	5,7,4′-Trimethylapigenin	Confirmed	Positive
MOL013352	Obacunone	Confirmed	Negative
MOL013428	Isosakuranetin-7-rutinoside	Confirmed	Negative

considered to be the core PPI network of SNS against NAFLD. The RWR algorithm was employed with seed genes as SNS genes and a restarting probability (r) of 0.75 by RandomWalkRestartMH R package, as in previous studies (Yang et al., 2020). The top 10 genes with the highest affinity scores were identified. The affinity score referred to the proximity between two nodes and the parameter "r" is the probability of moving to seed nodes.

Network Construction and Enrichment Analysis

Compound-gene networks and PPI networks were constructed by Cytoscape software (Version 3.8). To identify clusters of the sub-PPI network of SNS genes and NAFLD genes, ClusterMaker 2 plugin for Cytoscape was applied by the Community Cluster (Glay) algorithm (Morris et al., 2011). For gene enrichment analysis, gene ontology (GO) enrichment of these genes includes a biological process (BP), molecular function (MF), and cellular component (CC). For comparison between the SNS gene set and NAFLD gene set, the ClusterProfiler package of R 3.5.0 software is adopted to conduct GO enrichment (Yu et al., 2012). Kyoto Encyclopedia of Genes and Genomes (KEGG) pathway enrichment analysis of core targets is also carried out and visualized using the ggplot2 R package. P value < 0.05 was set to be significant. A suite of KEGG mapping tools, KEGG Mapper, was used for specific pathway visualization (Kanehisa and Sato, 2020).

Preparation of Sinisan

The mixture of Chaihu, Zhishi, Baishao, and Gancao (1:1:1:1) was purchased from Beijing Tongrentang (Beijing, China) and authenticated by our team. The mix was immersed in water for 30 min and extracted twice with boiling water as we previously mentioned (Wei et al., 2016). The extraction was filtered and concentrated in a rotary evaporator under reduced pressure. Ultimately, the dry powder was manufactured by a freeze dryer at a relatively low temperature condition (−80°C).

UPLC-ESI-MS/MS Analysis

To confirm the important bioactive compounds in SNS, the SNS samples were analyzed using a UPLC-ESI-MS/MS system (UPLC, SHIMADZU Nexera X2; MS, Applied Biosystems 6500 Q TRAP). An Agilent SB-C18 column (1.8 μm, 2.1 mm*100 mm) was used. The mobile phase was pure water with 0.1% formic acid (A) and acetonitrile with 0.1% formic acid (B). Sample measurements were performed with a gradient program that employed the starting conditions of 95% A, 5% B. Within 9 min, a linear gradient to 5% A, 95% B was programmed, and a composition of 5% A, 95% B was kept for 1 min. Subsequently, a composition of 95% A, 5% B was adjusted within 1.10 min and kept for 2.9 min. The flow rate was 0.35 ml/min, and 2 μl of the filtrate was injected into the system for analysis. The ESI source operation parameters were as follows: ion source, turbo spray; source temperature 550°C; ion spray voltage (IS) 5500 V (positive ion mode)/−4500 V (negative ion mode); ion source gas I (GSI), gas II(GSII), and curtain gas (CUR) set at 50, 60, and 25.0 psi, respectively; and the collision-activated dissociation (CAD) was high. Instrument tuning and mass calibration were performed with 10 and 100 μmol/L polypropylene glycol solutions in QQQ and LIT modes, respectively. QQQ scans were acquired as MRM experiments with collision gas (nitrogen) set to medium. DP and CE for individual MRM transitions were done with further DP and CE optimization. A specific set of MRM transitions were monitored for each period according to the metabolites eluted within this period.

Animals and Treatments

All animal experiments were approved by the Institutional Animal Care and Use Committee of the Department of Laboratory Animal Sciences, Capital Medical University. Animal Experimental Ethics number (AEEI-2020–165). Twenty-seven male Wistar rats (280–320 g) were purchased from Charles River Inc., (Vital River Ltd., Beijing, China) and kept at the SPF animal room of the Department of Laboratory Animal Sciences, Capital Medical University. All rats were randomly distributed into three groups after 1 week of acclimatization and were fed either standard chow (Chow group) or high fat diet (HFD and SNS group). After 4 weeks of feeding, rats in the SNS group (n = 9) were intragastrically administered with SNS exact per day (0.368 g/kg), and the Chow group (n = 9) and HFD group (n = 9) were given the same volume of distilled water to mimic the effects of oral gavage administration while remaining on the previous diet, respectively, for another 4 weeks. The dose of SNS was determined based on the body surface area index between humans and rats (Nair et al., 2018).

Sample Collection

At the end of 8 weeks, the final body weights of rats were recorded before sacrificing. After anesthetized with pentobarbital sodium (25 mg/kg; IP), blood was obtained from the abdominal aorta and separated by centrifugation (3,000 rpm, 15 min) for serum collection after being kept at room temperature for 30 min, and the serum was collected from the supernatant of blood and stored at −80°C for the further determination. The liver was quickly removed, weighed, and thoroughly washed with phosphate buffer saline (PBS). A portion of the liver was stored separately in a 4% paraformaldehyde for histopathological examination. The rest of the liver was snap-frozen using liquid nitrogen for further investigation.

Biochemical Indicators of Hepatic Function

The serum alanine aminotransferase (ALT), aspartate aminotransferase (AST), free fatty acids (FFA), total triglyceride (TG), total cholesterol (TC), low-density lipoprotein cholesterol (LDL-C), and high-density lipoprotein cholesterol (HDL-C) were detected by a Fully Automatic Biochemical Analyzer (Beckman Coulter, Indianapolis, IN, United States) according to manufacturer's protocol.

Measurement of Serum and Liver Cytokines

Serum and liver levels of TNFα, IL6, and IL1β were detected using ELISA kits of TNFα, IL6, and IL1β, following the manufacturer's instructions, respectively. Absorbance at 450 nm was measured using a microplate spectrophotometer (Thermo Scientific Multiskan GO). Total protein was used to normalize these cytokine levels in the liver.

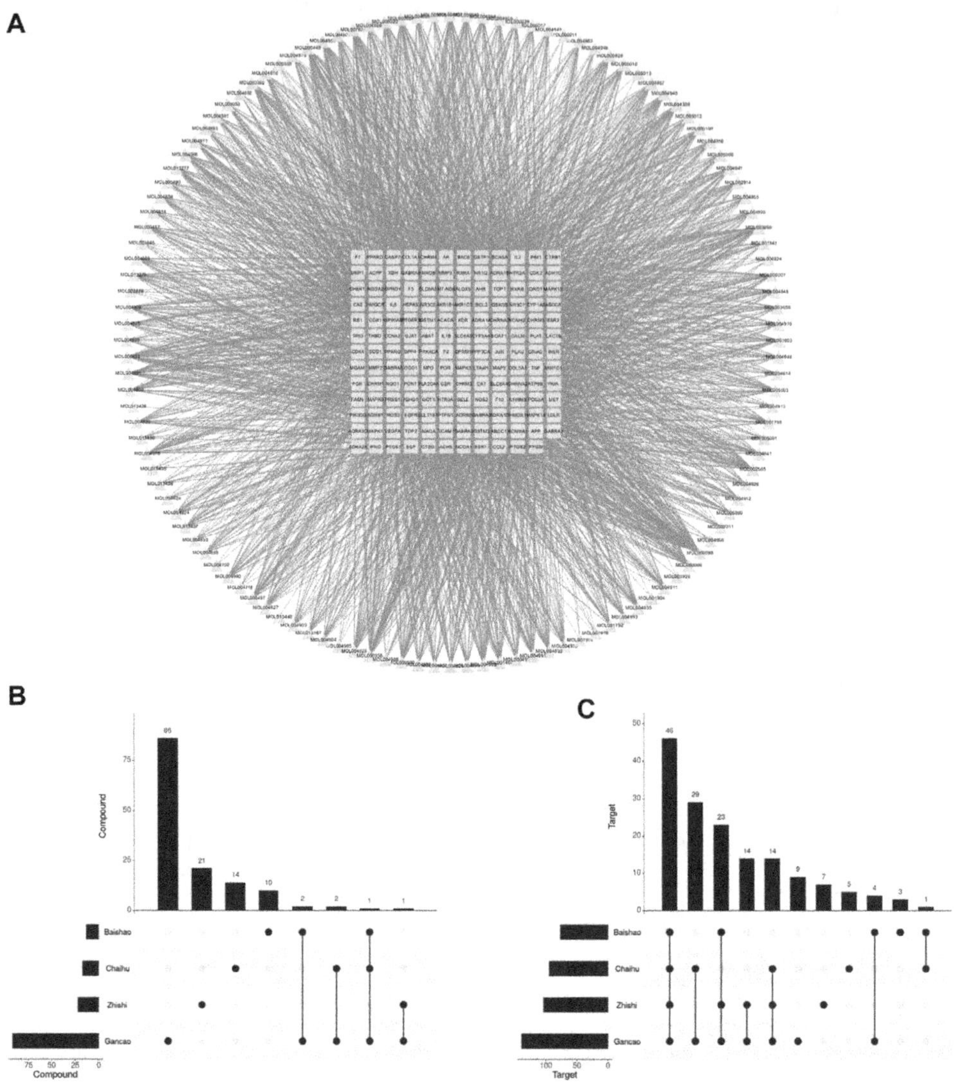

FIGURE 2 | Compounds in SNS and their corresponding targets. **(A)** Compound-target network of SNS. **(B)** The SNS compound amount in each botanical drug. **(C)** The SNS target amount in each botanical drug.

Measurement of Advanced Glycation End-Products and Receptor for Advanced Glycation End-Products

Serum and liver levels of AGEs and RAGE were detected using ELISA kits of AGEs and RAGE, following the manufacturer's instructions, respectively. Absorbance at 450 nm was measured using a microplate spectrophotometer (Thermo Scientific Multiskan GO). Total protein was used to normalize these levels in the liver.

Histological Examination

The liver was immediately fixed in 4% paraformaldehyde overnight at room temperature, washed with ddH_2O, rehydrated with gradient ethanol solutions, and embedded in paraffin for Hematoxylin–Eosin (H&E) staining. For the detection of lipids, frozen liver sections were stained with Oil Red O.

Triglyceride and Cholesterol Evaluation in Liver

Liver samples of appropriate weight were homogenized with RIPA lysis buffer; homogenate was collected to assay intrahepatic triglyceride and cholesterol using commercial kits (Applygen, China). Triglyceride and cholesterol values were normalized by total protein contents.

Immunoblotting Analysis

The liver tissues were homogenized with lysis buffer (Applygen, China) according to the manufacturer's protocol. The protein extracts were separated by 8% SDS-PAGE electrophoresis and

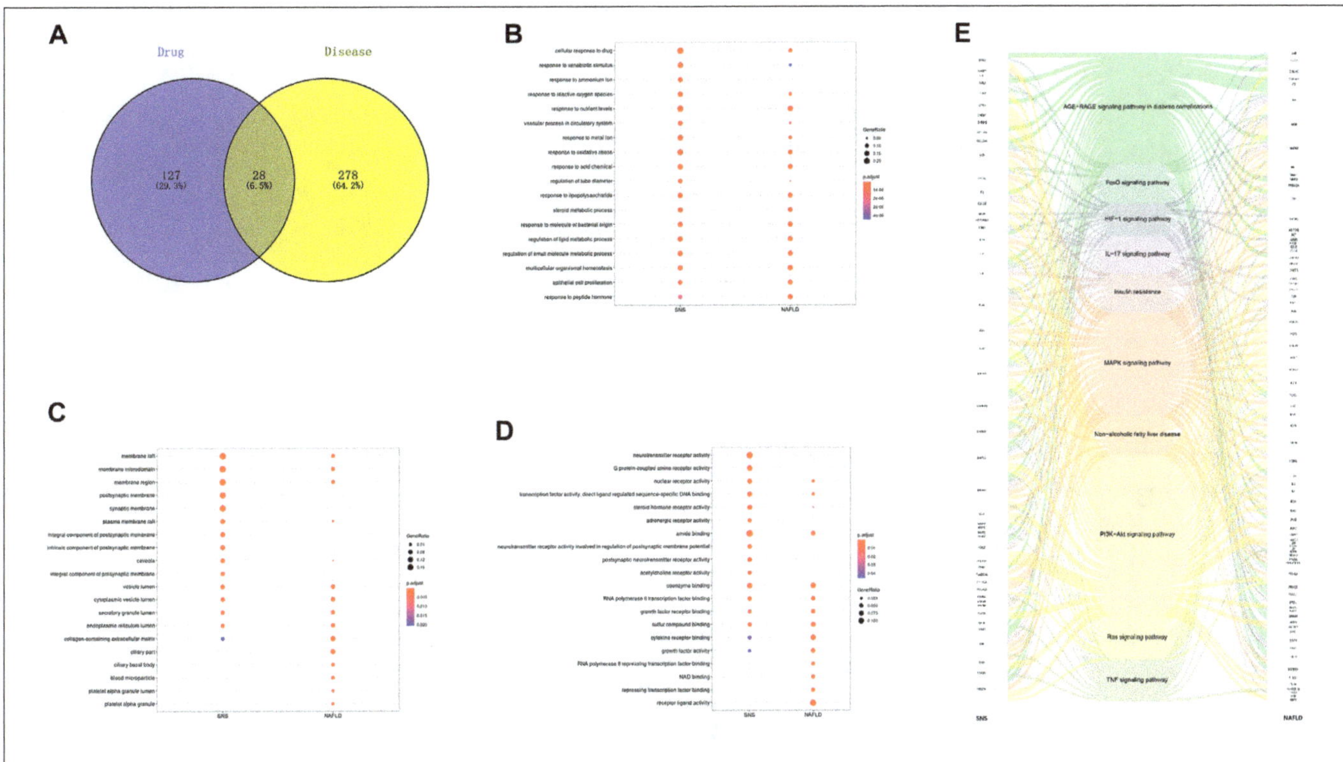

FIGURE 3 | Overlapped terms-based analysis. **(A)** Veen diagram of compound targets of SNS and NAFLD-related targets. Overlapped gene ontology (GO) and Kyoto Encyclopedia of Genes and Genomes (KEGG) terms of SNS and NAFLD: **(B)** biological processes (BPs), **(C)** cellular components (CCs), **(D)** molecular functions (MFs), and **(E)** KEGG pathways.

electro-transferred to PVDF membranes (Millipore, MA, United States). After blocking with 5% BSA, the membranes were incubated overnight at 4°C with specific primary antibodies against Phospho-JAK2 (Cell Signaling Technology, Danvers, MA, United States), Phospho-STAT3 (Cell Signaling Technology, Danvers, MA, United States), and β-actin (Cell Signaling Technology, Danvers, MA, United States) separately. Following four washes with Tris-buffered saline tween-20 (TBST), the membranes were incubated with the corresponding secondary antibodies as Goat Anti-Rabbit IgG (Lablead, China) and for 1 h at room temperature. Membranes were then washed four times with TBST, and the detection was carried out with an electrochemiluminescence (ECL) reagent (Applygen, China). The blot was imaged using EvolutionCapt FX6 and subjected to quantification analysis using Image J software. The results are expressed as the ratio of the relative intensity of the target proteins to that of the internal standard. JAK2 and STAT3 blots were performed by stripping and re-probing the blots with corresponding antibodies, respectively (Cell Signaling Technology, Danvers, MA, United States).

Statistical Analysis

All statistical analyses were performed using one-way ANOVA followed by Dunnett's Multiple Comparison Test, and all the bar plots were generated by GraphPad Prism 9 software; the data were expressed in terms of mean ± standard division (SD). Statistical significance was set at $p < 0.05$.

RESULTS

Compounds and Targets of Sinisan

After ADME screening, 137 unduplicated compounds and 155 unduplicated targets were obtained, which included 2,670 compound-target relationships (**Figure 2A**). Among four botanical drugs of Chaihu, Baishao, Zhishi, and Gancao, 17, 13, 22, and 92 compounds, respectively, were obtained (**Figure 2B**), which corresponded to 95, 77, 104, and 139 targets (**Figure 2C**). We found a potential synergistic effect of these four botanical drugs in the target level without many overlaps in the compound level. Gancao was the botanical drug that contributed to the highest proportion of collected compounds and targets.

Relationship Between Sinisan Targets and Non-Alcoholic Fatty Liver Disease Genes

After screening all of the compounds and targets, we want to recognize the potential corresponding compounds and targets of SNS anti-NAFLD effect. And we gathered genes related to NAFLD by database mining and removed predicted ones. As shown in **Figure 3A**, only 28 genes were overlapped between SNS genes and NAFLD genes. GO enrichment indicated that SNS targets and NAFLD genes could be enriched in the same GO terms with statistically significant difference (**Figures 3B–D**). These overlapped terms may involve lipid metabolism, oxidative stress, inflammatory

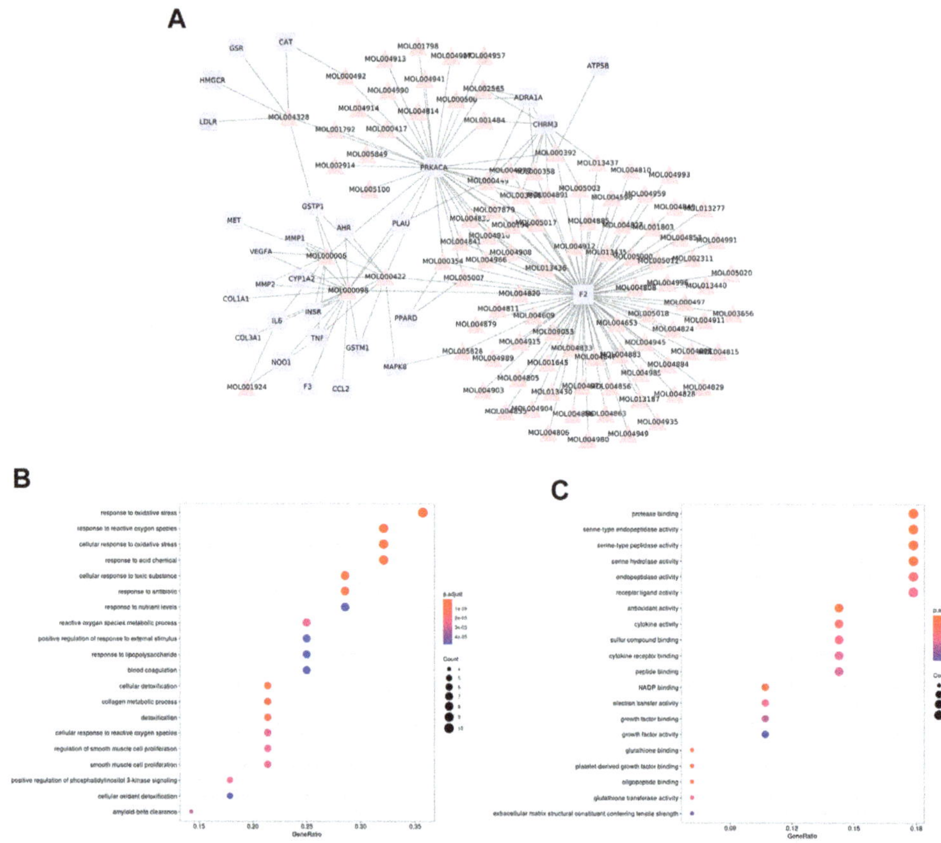

FIGURE 4 | Overlapped genes-based analysis. **(A)** Compound-target network of SNS against NAFLD. Gene ontology (GO) enrichment analysis of overlapped genes: **(B)** biological processes (BPs) and **(C)** molecular functions (MFs).

progress, and transcription. After KEGG enrichment of each gene set, 83 KEGG signals were overlapped. **Figure 3E** exhibited a complex relationship among SNS targets, NAFLD genes, and representative KEGG signals. These results showed similar terms enriched with SNS targets and NAFLD genes, indicating potential therapeutic effects of SNS against NAFLD.

Overlapped Gene-Based Enrichment Analysis

We firstly constructed a compound-target network based on overlapped genes between SNS targets and NAFLD genes (**Figure 4A**). GO enrichment of these overlapped genes indicated the potential mechanisms of SNS against NAFLD related to response to oxidative stress, response to lipopolysaccharide (LPS), phosphatidylinositol 3-kinase (PI3K) signaling, cytokine activity, and antioxidant activity (**Figures 4B,C**).

Protein-Protein Interaction Network-Based Proximity Analysis

According to previously published articles, disease genes tended to form a neighborhood in the human protein interactome, rather than being separate randomly (Cheng et al., 2019). And if a drug was effective for a disease, corresponding targets should be within or in the immediate vicinity of the corresponding disease module in the human protein interactome, indicating the role of neighborhood genes of disease genes in drug discovery. Our data showed the mean shortest path length between genes of SNS and NAFLD was 1.05, and the Z score was −9.51, indicating a significant difference between the mean shortest path lengths of SNS-NAFLD and random ones.

Protein-Protein Interaction Network-Based Cluster Analysis

The above results indicated a close relationship between SNS targets and NAFLD genes. Therefore, we hypothesized that SNS targets and NAFLD genes could form a network in the human protein interactome. To obtain data of high quality, a sub-PPI network with 1425 PPI relationships was grabbed from Snet. Further, **Figure 5** A-F showed six PPI clusters identified, containing both SNS targets (pink) and NAFLD genes (blue). Cluster 1 is related to the MAPK signaling pathway and FoxO signaling pathway, cluster 2 is related to the PI3K-Akt signaling pathway and HIF-1 signaling pathway, cluster 3 is related to TNF signaling pathway and AGE-RAGE signaling pathway, cluster 4 is related to Fatty acid degradation, cluster 5 is related to

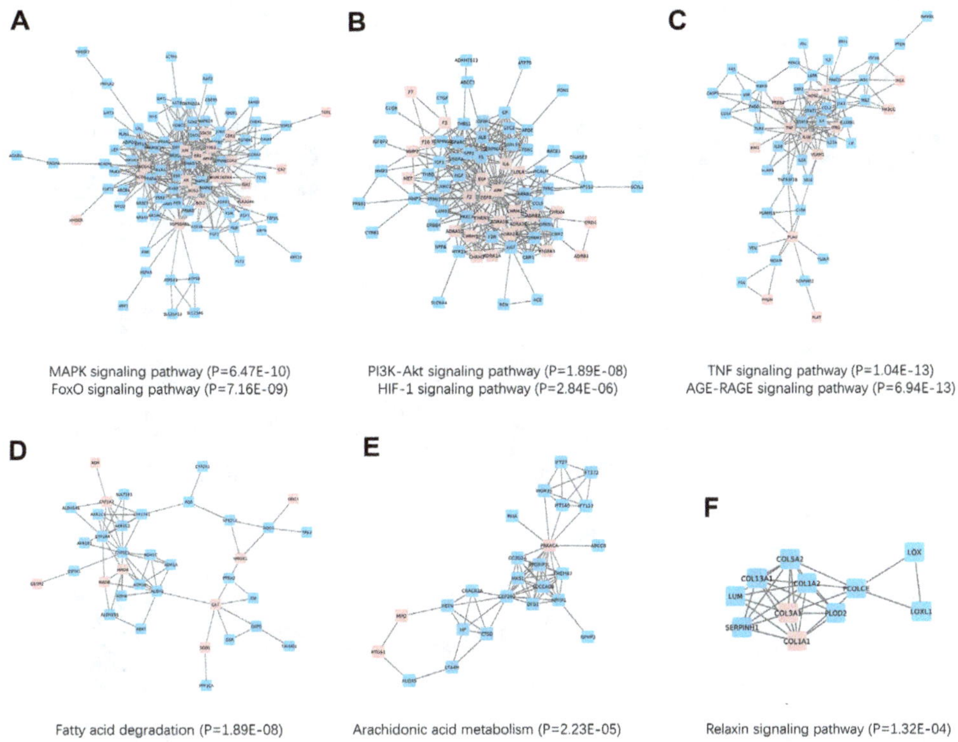

FIGURE 5 | Network-based clusters identification and Kyoto Encyclopedia of Genes and Genomes (KEGG) enrichment. **(A)** Cluster 1 was related to MAPK and FoxO pathways. **(B)** Cluster 2 was related to PI3K-Akt and HIF-1 pathways. **(C)** Cluster 3 was related to TNF and AGE-RAGE pathways. **(D)** Cluster 4 was related to the fatty acid degradation pathway. **(E)** Cluster 5 was related to the arachidonic acid metabolism pathway. **(F)** Cluster 6 was related to the relaxin pathway.

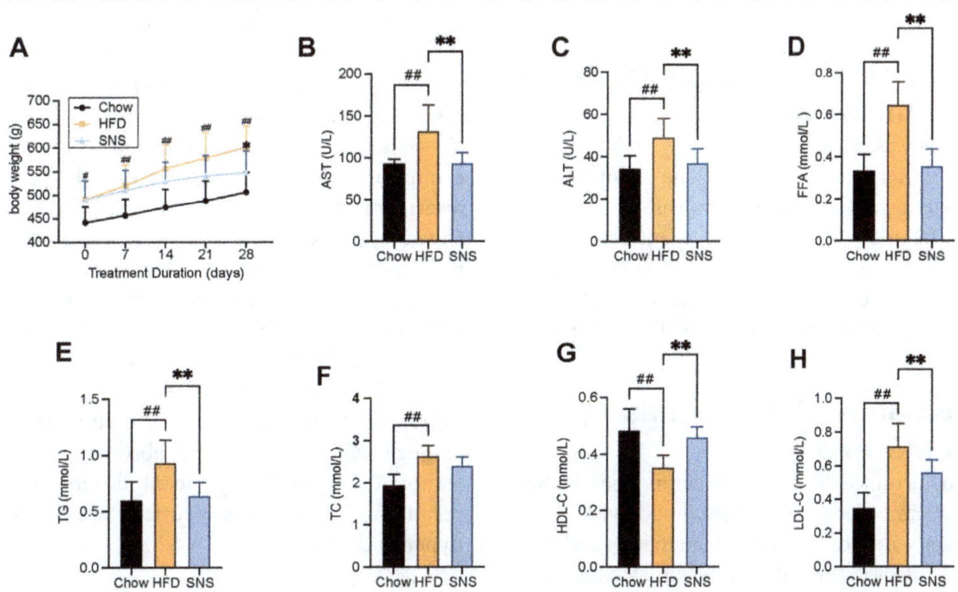

FIGURE 6 | Body weight and biochemical assays results after SNS treatment for rat NAFLD model. **(A)** Body weight measurement. **(B)** Serum aspartate aminotransferase (AST) levels. **(C)** Serum alanine aminotransferase (ALT) levels. **(D)** Serum free fatty acid (FFA) levels. **(E)** Serum total triglyceride (TG) levels. **(F)** Serum total cholesterol (TC) levels. **(G)** Serum high-density lipoprotein cholesterol (HDL-C) levels. **(H)** Serum low-density lipoprotein cholesterol (LDL-C) levels. Data are shown as mean ± SD (n = 9). $^{\#}p < 0.05$, $^{\#\#}p < 0.01$, $^{\#\#\#}p < 0.001$ when compared with chow group. $^{*}p < 0.05$, $^{**}p < 0.01$, $^{***}p < 0.001$ when compared with HFD group.

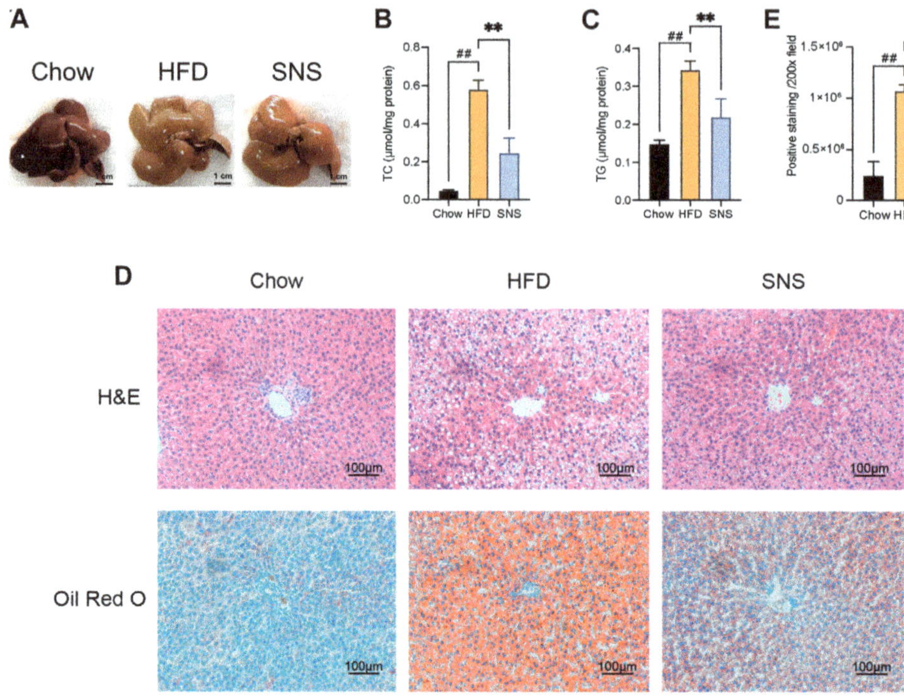

FIGURE 7 | Sinisan reduced liver lipid accumulation. **(A)** Morphology of the liver in each group. **(B)** Liver total cholesterol (TC) levels normalized by total protein. **(C)** Liver total triglyceride (TG) levels normalized by total protein. **(D)**. HE-stained and Oil Red O-stained liver tissue. **(E)** Relative evaluation of Oil Red O-staining. Three biological replicates were performed for each study. $^{\#}p < 0.05$, $^{\#\#}p < 0.01$, $^{\#\#\#}p < 0.001$ when compared with the Chow group, $^{*}p < 0.05$, $^{**}p < 0.01$, $^{***}p < 0.001$ when compared with HFD group.

Arachidonic acid metabolism, and cluster 6 is related to relaxin signaling pathway.

Protein-Protein Interaction Network-Based Hub Genes Identification

Although proximity analysis evaluated the efficacy of drug targets on disease genes, it was no help in hub gene identification. Therefore, we needed a ranking algorithm called RWR. As shown in **Table 1**, the top 10 genes were identified as hub genes by executing the RWR algorithm on the above sub-PPI network, including STAT3, CTNNB1, MAPK1, MAPK3, AGT, NQO1, TOP2A, FDFT1, ALDH4A1, and KCNH2 (**Table 1**).

Screening of Bioactive Compounds by UPLC-ESI-MS/MS Analysis

The present approach identified 58 bioactive compounds in SNS (**Table 2**), and some important bioactive compounds in the SNS compound-target network were identified, such as quercetin, kaempferol, medicarpin, luteolin, tetramethoxyluteolin, formononetin, isorhamnetin, naringenin, vestitol, and licochalcone A.

Sinisan Attenuated High Fat Diet-Induced Hyperlipidemia

To evaluate the therapeutic effect of SNS, a high fat diet- (HFD-) induced NAFLD rat model was used. As expected in the NAFLD model, HFD-treated rats exhibited an increased body weight. Compared with the HFD group, SNS treated rats showed significantly lowered body weights after a 4-week treatment (**Figure 6A**). The transaminase levels were assessed to evaluate whether SNS made improvements on liver function of NAFLD rats. The serum levels of AST and ALT were increased significantly in the HFD group compared with the Chow group, and these rises were reduced significantly by the SNS treatment compared with the HFD group (**Figures 6B,C**). It showed that levels of FFA were elevated in HFD rats, which manifests as metabolic disorders; however, it could be significantly alleviated after SNS intervention (**Figure 6D**). In addition, compared to the HFD group, SNS treatment influenced body lipid metabolism, including significantly decreasing the levels of serum TG and LDL-C (**Figures 6E,H**) and significantly increasing the levels of HDL-C (**Figure 6G**). SNS was also observed to decrease the levels of serum TC without significant difference (**Figure 6F**). These results indicated a therapeutic effect of SNS on HFD-induced hyperlipidemia.

Sinisan Reduced High Fat Diet-Induced Hepatic Steatosis

As shown in **Figure 7A**, in contrast to normal diet rats, HFD-fed rats developed a liver enlargement and discoloration, which were partially recovered with SNS treatment. Markedly, HFD-induced accumulation of lipid droplets in

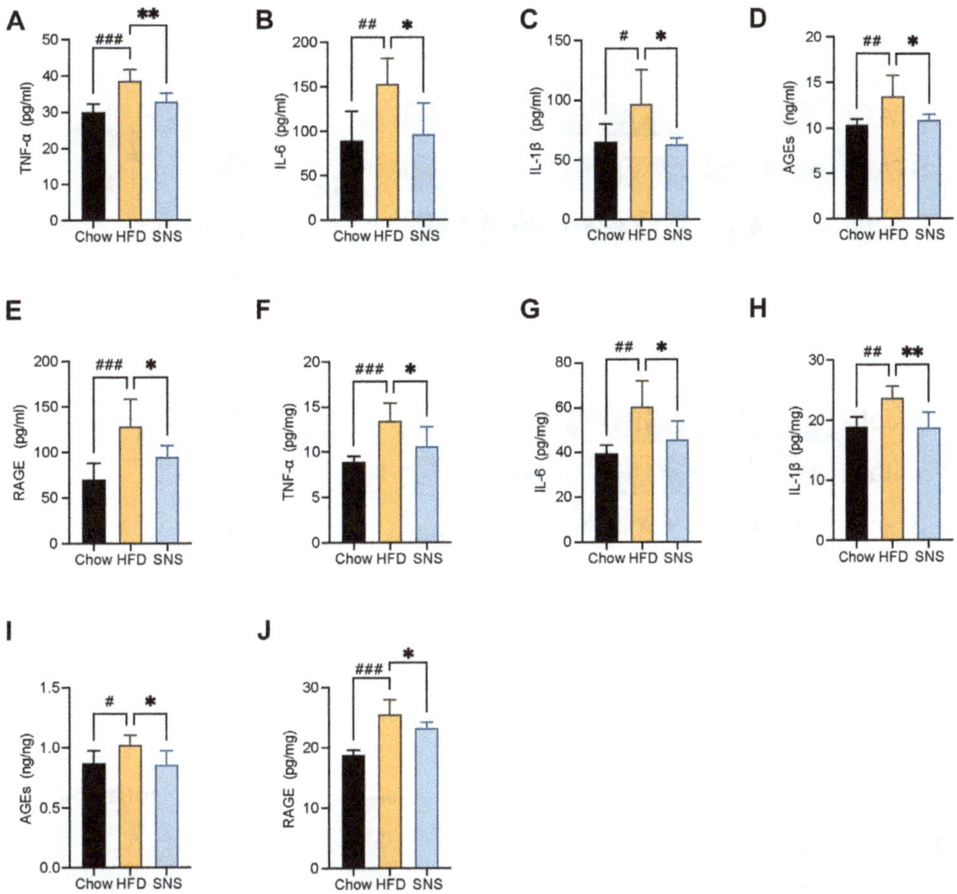

FIGURE 8 | SNS reduced liver pro-inflammatory cytokines, advanced glycation end-products (AGEs), and its receptor. **(A)** Serum levels of tumor necrosis factor alpha (TNFα). **(B)** Serum levels of interleukin 6 (IL6). **(C)** Serum levels of interleukin 1β (IL1β). **(D)** Serum levels of AGEs. **(E)** Serum levels of receptor for advanced glycation end-products (RAGE). **(F)** Liver levels of TNFα. **(G)** Liver levels of IL6. **(H)** Liver levels of IL1β. **(I)** Liver levels of AGEs. **(J)** Liver levels of receptor for RAGE. Data are shown as mean ± SD (n = 6). $^{\#}p < 0.05$, $^{\#\#}p < 0.01$, $^{\#\#\#}p < 0.001$ when compared with the Chow group, $^{*}p < 0.05$, $^{**}p < 0.01$, $^{***}p < 0.001$ when compared with the HFD group.

the liver was reduced by SNS, as evidenced by hepatic concentration of TC, TG (**Figures 7B,C**) and pathological staining (**Figure 7D**, representative histological liver H&E and Oil Red O staining). H&E staining revealed inflammatory cells and numerous lipid droplets in the livers of NAFLD rats, indicating inflammation and hepatocyte steatosis in the liver. SNS treatments showed less inflammation and hepatocyte steatosis than those of the NAFLD group. Oil Red O staining showed that there were many deposited lipid droplets in the HFD group. Compared with the HFD group, the lipid droplet quantity was lower in the SNS group (**Figure 7E**).

Sinisan Ameliorated High Fat Diet-Induced Hepatic Inflammation

To assess the extent of inflammatory, several inflammatory cytokines, AGEs, and RAGE in serum and liver were measured (**Figures 8A–J**). As a result, the HFD group displayed markedly higher expressions of IL6, IL1β, TNFα, AGEs, and RAGE compared with the Chow group. However, they were decreased in SNS-intervened rats compared with those in the HFD group, suggesting that SNS had an inhibitory effect on hepatic inflammation in NAFLD rats.

Sinisan Inhibited JAK2/Signal Transducer and Activator of Transcription 3 Phosphorylation

To investigate the potential of SNS's effect on the STAT3 signal in the NAFLD rat model, immunoblot analysis was performed for JAK2 and STAT3 phosphorylation (**Figures 9A–D**). It was demonstrated that expression of JAK2 and STAT3 phosphorylation was enhanced in NAFLD rats, while SNS reversed this activation to some extent. Therefore, we suggested that the inhibition of the JAK2/STAT3 signal may be the potential mechanism of SNS treating NAFLD (**Figure 9E**).

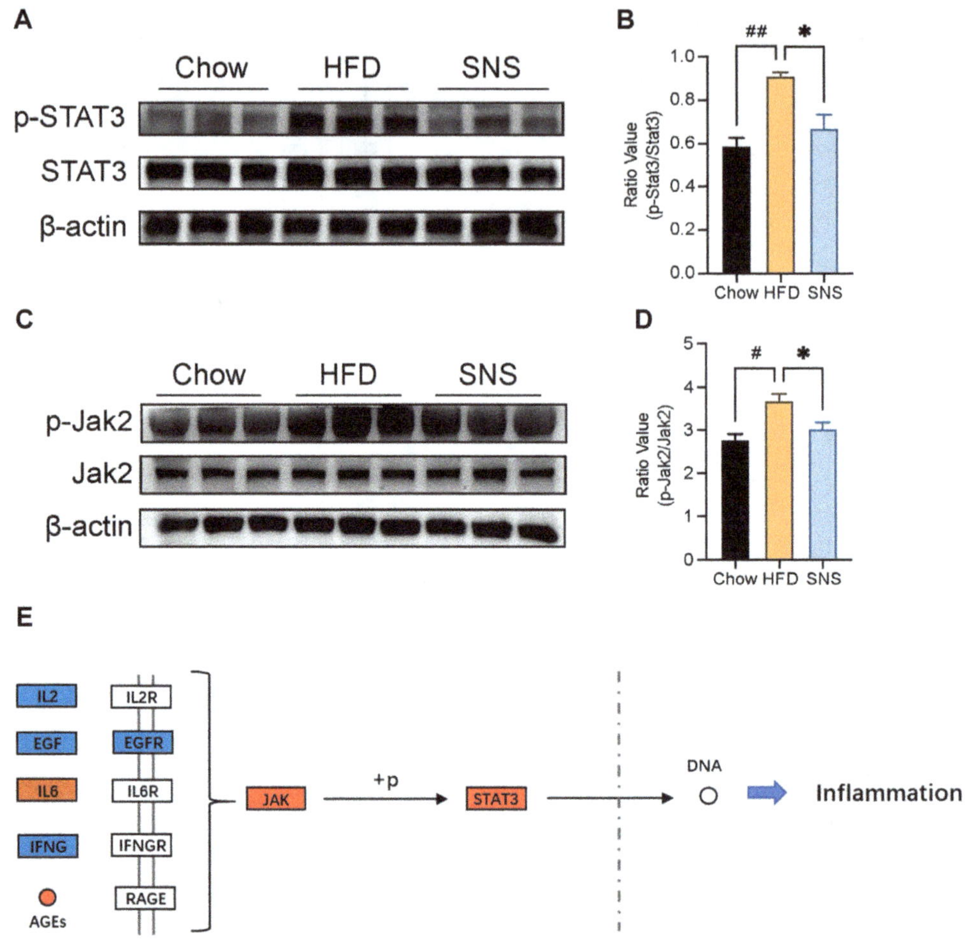

FIGURE 9 | SNS inhibited JAK2/STAT3 signal against NAFLD. **(A)** Expressions of signal transducer and activator of transcription (STAT3) and phosphorylated STAT3 (p-STAT3) were determined by Western blotting. **(B)** Quantitative analysis of p-STAT3:STAT3 expression ratio. **(C)** Expressions of Janus Kinase 2 (JAK2) and phosphorylated JAK2 (*p*-JAK2) were determined by Western blotting. **(D)** Quantitative analysis of *p*-JAK2:JAK2 expression ratio. Data are shown as mean ± SD (n = 3). $^{\#}p < 0.05$, $^{\#\#}p < 0.01$, $^{\#\#\#}p < 0.001$ when compared with the Chow group, $^{*}p < 0.05$, $^{**}p < 0.01$, $^{***}p < 0.001$ when compared with HFD group.

DISCUSSION

SNS has been widely applied in the treatment of chronic liver diseases in the clinic. As we previously mentioned, previous studies reported that SNS induced a decreased body weight and liver triglyceride accumulation in animal models (Cheng et al., 2017; Zhu et al., 2019). However, the underlying mechanisms of SNS against NAFLD are still difficult to understand, for it includes multiple compounds and multiple targets. In the present study, we modified our previously published network pharmacology approach (Ma et al., 2020) and used it to study the system-wide mechanism of SNS against NAFLD. This approach started from compounds screening, targets searching, and drug effect analyzing. Unlike previous studies, we hypothesized that SNS may influence NAFLD not only directly acting on the targets related to NAFLD, but also acting on the neighbors of NAFLD targets. Therefore, to evaluate the relationship between SNS targets and NAFLD targets, we used a well-performed network-based drug-disease proximity algorithm on the human interactome, which had an area under the receiver operating characteristic curve (AUC) of over 70% in a previous study (Cheng et al., 2018). After comparing with the reference distance distribution corresponding to the expected network topological distance between two randomly selected groups of proteins matched to size and degree as the NAFLD targets and SNS targets, the distance between the NAFLD targets and SNS targets was more close than the reference distance. These results indicated a therapeutic effect of SNS against NAFLD. To evaluate the importance of different targets, we used the RWR algorithm to sort the targets in a sub-PPI network only consisting of SNS targets and NAFLD targets. According to the RWR score, STAT3 was the most important target related to SNS targets. And most importantly, STAT3 played a core role in enriched KEGG pathways, including AGE-RAGE signal, FoxO signal, HIF-1 signal, and insulin resistance.

Our experimental data indicated that SNS treatment decreased Jak2/STAT3 activation, which could be activated by IL6 and

AGEs. Previous studies showed that STAT3 played important roles in liver inflammation and interacted with multiple signals. GWAS study validated the genetic associations of STAT3 with the susceptibility to NAFLD and disease progression in the Asian population (Sookoian et al., 2008; Kumar et al., 2019). *In vivo* study indicated that STAT3 was related to lipid synthesis by modulating the expression of SREBP1 in a high-fat diet model (Zeng et al., 2017). *In vitro* obesity model showed that STAT3 knockdown significantly attenuated TG content and expression of SREBP1 in LO2 cells (Chen et al., 2018). Another function of the STAT3 signal was activating liver inflammation. It has been reported that hepatocyte-specific STAT3 knockout markedly inhibited liver inflammation compared with wild-type mice (Miller et al., 2011). STAT3 was considered highly interconnected with NFκB signal, a core transcription factor in diverse immune responses. Many inflammatory factors transcribed by NFκB, such as IL6, are important STAT3 activators. In some conditions, STAT3 could directly interact with NFκB and lead to constitutive NFκB activation and numerous inflammatory genes transcription (Yu et al., 2009). According to previous reports, IL6, IL1b, and CCL2 were upregulated by STAT3 activation (Yu et al., 2009). And these pro-inflammatory factors played important roles in the progression of NAFLD (Kazankov et al., 2019). Recent data showed that STAT3-related lysosomal membrane permeabilization promoted ferroptosis via CTSB (cathepsin B) (Zhou et al., 2020). These data supported the therapeutic effect of SNS against NAFLD.

Our network pharmacology identified three compounds in SNS related to STAT3 inhibition, including quercetin, paeoniflorin, and luteolin. Recent studies reported that quercetin interrupted the positive feedback loop between STAT3 and IL-6 and exhibited an anti-inflammatory phenotype (Granato et al., 2019). Luteolin was also found to decrease STAT-binding activity and markedly suppress STAT3 phosphorylation in a dose-dependent manner (Aziz et al., 2018). Except for these two flavonoids, paeoniflorin, a monoterpene glucoside, was proved to markedly decrease STAT3 activation in immune cells (Zhang and Wei, 2020). Future studies should test the relationship between STAT3 and these compounds' treatment in NAFLD models.

CONCLUSION

In conclusion, in this study, we combined a PPI-network-based pharmacology analysis with biological validation to study the mechanism of the actions of SNS against NAFLD at the systemic level. We confirmed the anti-NAFLD effect of SNS was involved in multiple targets on Jak2/STAT3 signal pathway. In the future, other pathways or mechanisms predicted in this study should be further investigated.

AUTHOR CONTRIBUTIONS

CM, QZ, FC and XQW contributed to the study design, practical work, manuscript writing, and revision. XYW participated in research design and manuscript writing. JL, WH, DB, JS, ZW, QW, TX and PF participated in the implementation of some experiments and data analysis. All authors contributed to the article and approved the submitted version.

FUNDING

The present study was supported by grants from the National Natural Science Foundation of China (82004327, 81774122) and the Major Science and Technology Project for "Significant New Drugs Creation" New Drugs Creation (Grant No. 2019ZX09301-173).

ACKNOWLEDGMENTS

The authors thank Elsevier Language Services for providing language assistance and for proofreading the manuscript.

REFERENCES

Allen, A. M., Hicks, S. B., Mara, K. C., Larson, J. J., and Therneau, T. M. (2019). The Risk of Incident Extrahepatic Cancers Is Higher in Non-alcoholic Fatty Liver Disease Than Obesity - A Longitudinal Cohort Study. *J. Hepatol.* 71 (6), 1229–1236. doi:10.1016/j.jhep.2019.08.018

Aziz, N., Kim, M.-Y., and Cho, J. Y. (2018). Anti-inflammatory Effects of Luteolin: A Review of *In Vitro*, *In Vivo*, and In Silico Studies. *J. Ethnopharmacology* 225, 342–358. doi:10.1016/j.jep.2018.05.019

Chen, J., Yue, J., Liu, Y., Liu, J., Jiao, K., Teng, M., et al. (2018). Blocking of STAT-3/srebp1-Mediated Glucose-Lipid Metabolism Is Involved in Dietary Phytoestrogen-Inhibited Ovariectomized-Induced Body Weight Gain in Rats. *J. Nutr. Biochem.* 61, 17–23. doi:10.1016/j.jnutbio.2018.06.009

Cheng, F., Desai, R. J., Handy, D. E., Wang, R., Schneeweiss, S., Barabasi, A.-L., et al. (2018). Network-based Approach to Prediction and Population-Based Validation of In Silico Drug Repurposing. *Nat. Commun.* 9 (1), 2691. doi:10.1038/s41467-018-05116-5

Cheng, F., Kovacs, I. A., and Barabasi, A.-L. (2019). Network-based Prediction of Drug Combinations. *Nat. Commun.* 10 (1), 1197. doi:10.1038/s41467-019-09186-x

Cheng, F., Ma, C., Wang, X., Zhai, C., Wang, G., Xu, X., et al. (2017). Effect of Traditional Chinese Medicine Formula Sinisan on Chronic Restraint Stress-Induced Nonalcoholic Fatty Liver Disease: a Rat Study. *BMC Complement Altern. Med.* 17 (1), 203. doi:10.1186/s12906-017-1707-2

Cotter, T. G., and Rinella, M. (2020). Nonalcoholic Fatty Liver Disease 2020: The State of the Disease. *Gastroenterology* 158 (7), 1851–1864. doi:10.1053/j.gastro.2020.01.052

Granato, M., Gilardini Montani, M. S., Zompetta, C., Santarelli, R., Gonnella, R., Romeo, M. A., et al. (2019). Quercetin Interrupts the Positive Feedback Loop between STAT3 and IL-6, Promotes Autophagy, and Reduces ROS, Preventing EBV-Driven B Cell Immortalization. *Biomolecules* 9 (9), 482. doi:10.3390/biom9090482

Kanehisa, M., and Sato, Y. (2020). KEGG Mapper for Inferring Cellular Functions from Protein Sequences. *Protein Sci.* 29 (1), 28–35. doi:10.1002/pro.3711

Kazankov, K., Jørgensen, S. M. D., Thomsen, K. L., Møller, H. J., Vilstrup, H., George, J., et al. (2019). The Role of Macrophages in Nonalcoholic Fatty Liver Disease and Nonalcoholic Steatohepatitis. *Nat. Rev. Gastroenterol. Hepatol.* 16 (3), 145–159. doi:10.1038/s41575-018-0082-x

Kumar, A., Shalimar, D., Walia, G. K., Gupta, V., and Sachdeva, M. P. (2019). Genetics of Nonalcoholic Fatty Liver Disease in Asian Populations. *J. Genet.* 98. doi:10.1007/s12041-019-1071-8

Li, H., Zhao, L., Zhang, B., Jiang, Y., Wang, X., Guo, Y., et al. (2014). A Network Pharmacology Approach to Determine Active Compounds and Action Mechanisms of Ge-Gen-Qin-Lian Decoction for Treatment of Type 2 Diabetes. *Evidence-Based Complement. Altern. Med.* 2014, 1–12. doi:10.1155/2014/495840

Li, S., and Zhang, B. (2013). Traditional Chinese Medicine Network Pharmacology: Theory, Methodology and Application. *Chin. J. Nat. Medicines* 11 (2), 110–120. doi:10.1016/s1875-5364(13)60037-0

Ma, C., Wang, X., Xu, T., Zhang, S., Liu, S., Zhai, C., et al. (2020). An Integrative Pharmacology-Based Analysis of Refined Qingkailing Injection against Cerebral Ischemic Stroke: A Novel Combination of Baicalin, Geniposide, Cholic Acid, and Hyodeoxycholic Acid. *Front. Pharmacol.* 11, 519. doi:10.3389/fphar.2020.00519

Miller, A. M., Horiguchi, N., Jeong, W.-I., Radaeva, S., and Gao, B. (2011). Molecular Mechanisms of Alcoholic Liver Disease: Innate Immunity and Cytokines. *Alcohol. Clin. Exp. Res.* 35 (5), 787–793. doi:10.1111/j.1530-0277.2010.01399.x

Morris, J. H., Apeltsin, L., Newman, A. M., Baumbach, J., Wittkop, T., Su, G., et al. (2011). clusterMaker: a Multi-Algorithm Clustering Plugin for Cytoscape. *BMC Bioinformatics* 12, 436. doi:10.1186/1471-2105-12-436

Mu, J., Cheng, F., Wang, Q., Wang, X., Zhu, W., Ma, C., et al. (2020). Sini Powder Ameliorates the Inflammatory Response in Rats with Stress-Induced Non-alcoholic Fatty Liver Disease by Inhibiting the Nuclear Factor Kappa-B/Pyrin Domain-Containing Protein 3 Pathway. *J. Tradit Chin Med.* 40 (2), 253–266.

Nair, A., Morsy, M. A., and Jacob, S. (2018). Dose Translation between Laboratory Animals and Human in Preclinical and Clinical Phases of Drug Development. *Drug Dev. Res.* 79 (8), 373–382. doi:10.1002/ddr.21461

Piñero, J., Ramírez-Anguita, J. M., Saüch-Pitarch, J., Ronzano, F., Centeno, E., Sanz, F., et al. (2020). The DisGeNET Knowledge Platform for Disease Genomics: 2019 Update. *Nucleic Acids Res.* 48 (D1), D845–d855. doi:10.1093/nar/gkz1021

Sookoian, S., Castaño, G., Gianotti, T. F., Gemma, C., Rosselli, M. S., and Pirola, C. J. (2008). Genetic Variants in STAT3 Are Associated with Nonalcoholic Fatty Liver Disease. *Cytokine* 44 (1), 201–206. doi:10.1016/j.cyto.2008.08.001

Szklarczyk, D., Gable, A. L., Lyon, D., Junge, A., Wyder, S., Huerta-Cepas, J., et al. (2019). STRING V11: Protein-Protein Association Networks with Increased Coverage, Supporting Functional Discovery in Genome-wide Experimental Datasets. *Nucleic Acids Res.* 47 (D1), D607–d613. doi:10.1093/nar/gky1131

Targher, G., Byrne, C. D., and Tilg, H. (2020). NAFLD and Increased Risk of Cardiovascular Disease: Clinical Associations, Pathophysiological Mechanisms and Pharmacological Implications. *Gut* 69 (9), 1691–1705. doi:10.1136/gutjnl-2020-320622

Tilg, H., and Targher, G. (2020). NAFLD-related Mortality: Simple Hepatic Steatosis Is Not as 'benign' as Thought. *Gut* 70, 1212–1213. doi:10.1136/gutjnl-2020-323188

Valdeolivas, A., Tichit, L., Navarro, C., Perrin, S., Odelin, G., Levy, N., et al. (2019). Random Walk with Restart on Multiplex and Heterogeneous Biological Networks. *Bioinformatics* 35 (3), 497–505. doi:10.1093/bioinformatics/bty637

Wei, S.-S., Yang, H.-J., Huang, J.-W., Lu, X.-P., Peng, L.-F., and Wang, Q.-G. (2016). Traditional Herbal Formula Sini Powder Extract Produces Antidepressant-like Effects through Stress-Related Mechanisms in Rats. *Chin. J. Nat. Medicines* 14 (8), 590–598. doi:10.1016/s1875-5364(16)30069-3

Yang, J., Tian, S., Zhao, J., and Zhang, W. (2020). Exploring the Mechanism of TCM Formulae in the Treatment of Different Types of Coronary Heart Disease by Network Pharmacology and Machining Learning. *Pharmacol. Res.* 159, 105034. doi:10.1016/j.phrs.2020.105034

Yu, G., Wang, L.-G., Han, Y., and He, Q.-Y. (2012). clusterProfiler: an R Package for Comparing Biological Themes Among Gene Clusters. *OMICS: A J. Integr. Biol.* 16 (5), 284–287. doi:10.1089/omi.2011.0118

Yu, H., Pardoll, D., and Jove, R. (2009). STATs in Cancer Inflammation and Immunity: a Leading Role for STAT3. *Nat. Rev. Cancer* 9 (11), 798–809. doi:10.1038/nrc2734

Zeng, Z., He, W., Jia, Z., and Hao, S. (2017). Lycopene Improves Insulin Sensitivity through Inhibition of STAT3/Srebp-1c-Mediated Lipid Accumulation and Inflammation in Mice Fed a High-Fat Diet. *Exp. Clin. Endocrinol. Diabetes* 125 (9), 610–617. doi:10.1055/s-0043-101919

Zhang, L., and Wei, W. (2020). Anti-inflammatory and Immunoregulatory Effects of Paeoniflorin and Total Glucosides of Paeony. *Pharmacol. Ther.* 207, 107452. doi:10.1016/j.pharmthera.2019.107452

Zhou, B., Liu, J., Kang, R., Klionsky, D. J., Kroemer, G., and Tang, D. (2020). Ferroptosis Is a Type of Autophagy-dependent Cell Death. *Semin. Cancer Biol.* 66, 89–100. doi:10.1016/j.semcancer.2019.03.002

Zhu, F., Li, Y.-M., Feng, T.-T., Wu, Y., Zhang, H.-X., Jin, G.-Y., et al. (2019). Freeze-dried Si-Ni-San Powder Can Ameliorate High Fat Diet-Induced Non-alcoholic Fatty Liver Disease. *Wjg* 25 (24), 3056–3068. doi:10.3748/wjg.v25.i24.3056

4

A Computational Systems Pharmacology Approach to Investigate Molecular Mechanisms of Herbal Formula Tian-Ma-Gou-Teng-Yin for Treatment of Alzheimer's Disease

*Tianduanyi Wang, Zengrui Wu, Lixia Sun, Weihua Li, Guixia Liu and Yun Tang**

Shanghai Key Laboratory of New Drug Design, School of Pharmacy, East China University of Science and Technology, Shanghai, China

Correspondence:
Yun Tang
ytang234@ecust.edu.cn

Traditional Chinese medicine (TCM) is typically prescribed as formula to treat certain symptoms. A TCM formula contains hundreds of chemical components, which makes it complicated to elucidate the molecular mechanisms of TCM. Here, we proposed a computational systems pharmacology approach consisting of network link prediction, statistical analysis, and bioinformatics tools to investigate the molecular mechanisms of TCM formulae. Taking formula Tian-Ma-Gou-Teng-Yin as an example, which shows pharmacological effects on Alzheimer's disease (AD) and its mechanism is unclear, we first identified 494 formula components together with corresponding 178 known targets, and then predicted 364 potential targets for these components with our balanced substructure-drug–target network-based inference method. With Fisher's exact test and statistical analysis we identified 12 compounds to be most significantly related to AD. The target genes of these compounds were further enriched onto pathways involved in AD, such as neuroactive ligand–receptor interaction, serotonergic synapse, inflammatory mediator regulation of transient receptor potential channel and calcium signaling pathway. By regulating key target genes, such as ACHE, HTR2A, NOS2, and TRPA1, the formula could have neuroprotective and anti-neuroinflammatory effects against the progression of AD. Our approach provided a holistic perspective to study the relevance between TCM formulae and diseases, and implied possible pharmacological effects of TCM components.

Keywords: traditional Chinese medicine, compound–protein interactions, network-based inference, computational systems pharmacology, Alzheimer's disease

INTRODUCTION

With more than 5,000-year history, the traditional Chinese medicine (TCM) still plays key roles in the treatment of many diseases and disorders worldwide. However, TCM is usually prescribed as formulae, typically consisting of many herbs in different quantity, in which the composition theory "Monarch, Minister, Assistant and Guide" is observed (Jiang, 2005; Xiong et al., 2013; Zhang A. et al., 2013). Thus a TCM formula contains hundreds of chemical components, which makes it complicated and difficult to elucidate the molecular mechanisms of treatment.

In recent years, as the development of systems biology, network pharmacology has emerged as a new subject for us to understand the complex biological systems from an integrated multi-component network view (Hopkins, 2007, 2008). Network pharmacology is especially advantageous in analyzing 'multi-compound, multi-target, and multi-effect' scenario to reveal the molecular relationships among compounds and complex diseases from multiple scales (Zhao et al., 2010; Li et al., 2012). Therefore, it is very helpful for illustrating molecular mechanisms of TCM formulae and finding active constituents from herbs (Hao and Xiao, 2014). There are many studies published to date, such as *Radix Curcumae* formula against cardiovascular diseases (Tao et al., 2013), Qing-Luo-Yin against Rheumatoid arthritis (Zhang B. et al., 2013) and Ge-Gen-Qin-Lian decoction against type 2 diabetes (Li J. et al., 2014).

In our previous study, we developed a network pharmacological method, named network-based inference (NBI), to predict potential drug–target interactions (DTIs) between drugs and targets (Cheng et al., 2012). Because NBI method only could predict potential DTIs within a known drug–target network, we then proposed a new method, entitled substructure-drug–target network-based inference (SDTNBI), to predict potential targets for novel compounds without known targets (Wu et al., 2017). SDTNBI utilizes chemical substructures to bridge the gap between known drug–target network and novel compounds. Recently, we further improved SDTNBI by introducing three parameters (α, β, and γ) into it, namely balanced substructure-drug–target network-based inference (bSDTNBI), to identify potential targets for both old drugs and new chemical entities (Wu et al., 2016). With these methods, we developed computational systems pharmacology/toxicology approaches to investigate the molecular mechanisms of therapeutic effects of known drugs or active compounds, and side effects of known drugs or environmental compounds (Cheng et al., 2013a,b; Li H. et al., 2014; Li et al., 2016; Lu et al., 2015; Wang et al., 2017).

In this study, we proposed a computational systems pharmacology approach (**Figure 1**) combining our bSDTNBI method and statistical analysis to find out the molecular mechanisms of TCM formulae, taking formula Tian-Ma-Gou-Teng-Yin (TMGTY) as an example. TMGTY consists of 11 Chinese herbs, such as *Rhizoma Gastrodiae* (*Tianma*), *Ramulus Uncariae Cum Uncis* (*Gouteng*), *Concha Haliotidis* (*Shijueming*), *Fructus Gardeniae Jasminoidis* (*Zhizi*), and *Radix Scutellariae Baicalensis* (*Huangqin*). TMGTY was prescribed to alleviate hypertension-related symptoms and also showed therapeutic effects against dementia and Alzheimer's disease (AD) (Liu et al., 2014; May et al., 2016; Zhang et al., 2016; Chen et al., 2017). TMGTY was one of the 10 most commonly used formulae for treating AD in Taiwan, according to a cohort study of one million patients (Lin et al., 2016). TMGTY was also reported to have neuroprotective effects (Chik et al., 2013; Xian et al., 2016) and could enhance the effect of memory acquisition (Ho et al., 2005, 2008). However, its molecular mechanisms remain elusive.

Alzheimer's disease is a complex neurodegenerative disease that deteriorates memory, cognition, behavior and leads to dementia (Reitz et al., 2011). Several hypotheses were proposed to understand the pathogenesis of AD, including amyloid cascade hypothesis, Tau hypothesis, cholinergic hypothesis and neuroinflammation (Ballard et al., 2011; De Strooper and Karran, 2016; Selkoe and Hardy, 2016). Huge efforts were devoted to the discovery of anti-AD therapies based on these hypotheses, but no curable treatment is available yet. Due to the complex pathology of AD, drugs targeting single protein or pathway may not fully exert expected therapeutic effects. TCM formulae, along with network pharmacology approaches, provide a powerful tool to investigate AD pathology, and they are also promising outsets for anti-AD drug development (Dey et al., 2017; Lai et al., 2017).

For that purpose, we first collected chemical components of TMGTY from related databases, and predicted potential targets for the principal components. Those components were subsequently enriched onto AD-related pathways to find the most disease-relevant component groups. Then we applied gene set enrichment analysis on the groups to examine involved pathways and potential mechanisms in treatment of AD. In order to explore shared mechanisms between diseases, we also mapped disease-related proteins to a protein–protein interaction network to find disease modules. Overlapping sub-modules was presumed as shared mechanisms of which compound targets may affect corresponding diseases. Thus our approach provided a holistic perspective to look into combinations of natural compounds and helped to illustrate their molecular mechanisms.

MATERIALS AND METHODS

The whole workflow was illustrated in **Figure 1**.

Data Collection and Preparation

The formula of TMGTY was ascertained through literature survey. For each herb medicine in the formula, its constituents were mapped from TCM Systems Pharmacology Database (TCMSP) (Ru et al., 2014), TCM Integrated Database (TCMID) (Xue et al., 2013) and TCM Database@Taiwan (Chen, 2011). Then two important pharmacokinetic properties: human intestinal absorption (HIA) and blood brain barrier (BBB) penetration were predicted for every ingredient by our widely used webserver admetSAR[1]. Ingredients with HIA and BBB penetration classified as negatives were considered poorly absorbed by intestine and can hardly penetrate the BBB, and hence excluded from further analysis.

Alzheimer's disease and hypertension related genes were collected from The Comparative Toxicogenomics Database (CTD) (Davis et al., 2017), Human Genome Epidemiology (HuGE) Navigator (Yu et al., 2008), Kyoto Encyclopedia of Genes and Genomes (KEGG) (Kanehisa and Goto, 2000; Kanehisa et al., 2017), Online Mendelian Inheritance in Man (OMIM) (Amberger et al., 2009), and Pharmacogenetics

[1] http://lmmd.ecust.edu.cn/admetsar1/

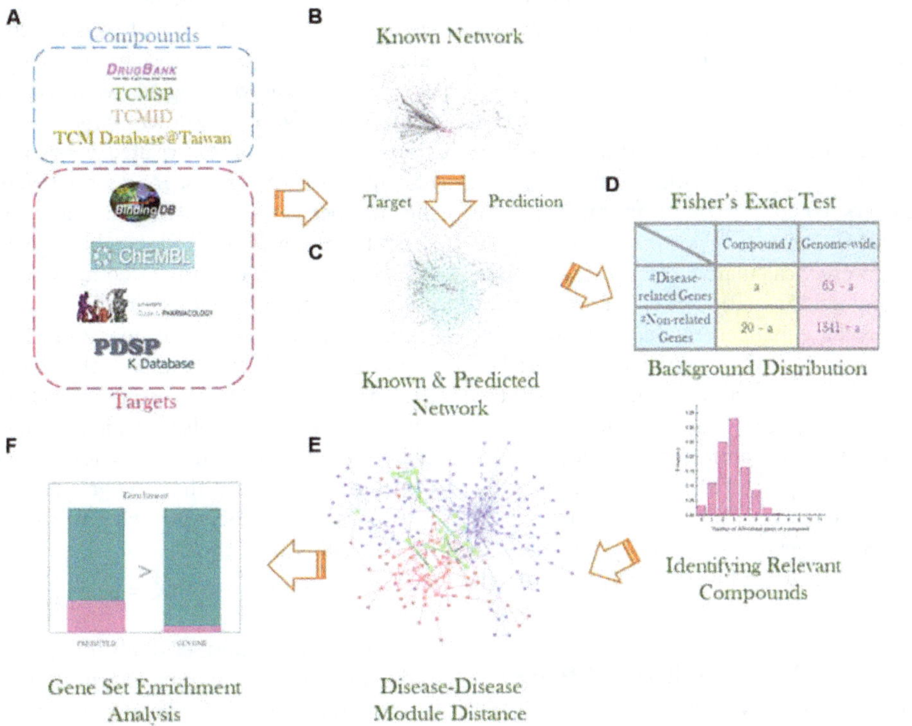

FIGURE 1 | Experiment workflow illustration: **(A)** compound and data collection from multiple databases; **(B)** construction of known compound–target network; **(C)** network link prediction via bSDTNBI method; **(D)** Fisher's exact test and background distribution to identify compounds significantly related to AD; **(E)** detection of AD and hypertension disease module and analysis of overlapping genes; **(F)** gene set enrichment analysis using DAVID v6.8 to investigate gene sets of interest.

and Pharmacogenomics Knowledge Base (PharmGKB) (Whirl-Carrillo et al., 2012). In CTD, only genes having a curated association to the disease were retained, i.e., genes marked as 'marker/mechanism' and/or 'therapeutic' in the 'direct evidence' column. In HuGE Navigator, genes with more than 20 publications were selected. In KEGG, 'KEGG Disease' was used to find disease genes of AD (KEGG Entry ID: H00056) and hypertension (KEGG Entry ID: H01633). In OMIM, associated genes of AD (Phenotype MIM number: 104300) and hypertension (Phenotype MIM number: 145500) were collected. AD (Accession ID: PA443319) and hypertension (Accession ID: PA444552) related genes in PharmGKB were downloaded. The collected genes were filtered using NCBI Gene database (Brown et al., 2015), and only protein-coding genes were retained.

To build network prediction models, a collection of TCM ingredients was made by combining molecules from above-mentioned TCM databases. Small molecules from DrugBank (Wishart et al., 2017) database were also collected.

For all ingredients, MacroModel 11.1 program (Schrödinger, LLC, New York, NY, United States, 2016) was applied to desalt and neutralize their structures. Then Epik 3.5 program (Schrödinger, LLC, New York, NY, United States, 2016) was used to generate tautomers. Only the most populated neutral tautomers were retained. The processed compounds were further converted to a canonical SMILES string by Open Babel toolkit (version 2.3.1) (O'Boyle et al., 2011). Duplicates were removed according to canonical SMILES string. Compounds without carbon atoms were also removed from the collection.

For each ingredient, the corresponding targets were matched from BindingDB (Gilson et al., 2016), ChEMBL (Gaulton et al., 2017), IUPHAR/BPS Guide to PHARMACOLOGY (Harding et al., 2017) and NIMH Psychoactive Drug Screening Program (PDSP) Ki Database (Roth et al., 2000) under criteria that: (1) target proteins are from *Homo sapiens* and have unique UniProt accession numbers; (2) K_i, K_d, IC_{50} or $EC_{50} \leq 10$ μM, or Potency ≤ 10 μM with "Activity Comment" marked as "Active." The Klekota-Roth (KR) fingerprint was used in this study and generated for every ingredient using PaDEL-Descriptor software (version 2.18) (Yap, 2011).

Construction of Compound–Target Networks

Three compound-target network models were built by our bSDTNBI method for new target prediction. The first was DrugBank network which contains only small molecules from DrugBank. The second was TCM network consisting of sole TCM ingredients from above collections. The last was a Global network merged by above two networks. The three models were evaluated independently to verify whether a combined model would outperform the others.

Ten-fold cross validation was applied to evaluate the performance of three models. In each fold, roughly 10% of DTIs were split from the network, serving as test set. Resources were redistributed among the remaining 90% of network (i.e., training set) to predict the 10% missing links. This process was repeated for ten times to reduce contingency. For three parameters α, β and γ used to tune the network performance, grid optimization was employed to search for the best set which maximizes the AUC of 10-fold cross validation. Detailed definition and description of these three parameters could be found in our previous publication (Wu et al., 2016).

Several indicators were calculated to assess model performance, such as precision (P), recall (R), precision enhancement (e_P), and recall enhancement (e_R). Furthermore, receiver operating characteristic (ROC) curves were plotted by true positive rate (TPR) against false positive rate (FPR). In this study, area under ROC curve (AUC) was calculated and used as an indicator to evaluate model performance since AUC is independent of the number of predicted targets. Basically, the higher the AUC value, the better the model performance. Above indicators were described in details and also widely used in previous studies (Cheng et al., 2012; Lü et al., 2012; Wu et al., 2016).

Target Prediction for TMGTY Ingredients

For all TMGTY ingredients, bSDTNBI was used to infer new targets. Most of the ingredients were not in the global network model, i.e., do not have known targets. They were represented by molecular fingerprints to link to the global network. The method redistributes known initial resources of drugs between different types of nodes to infer new targets. The resource diffusion number was set to 2 and the number of predicted targets was set to 20. The detailed description and evaluation of the method can be referred to our previous published papers (Wu et al., 2016, 2018).

Identification of AD-Related Components

Considering only a very small portion of natural products have known targets, the number of a compound's targets related to AD conforms approximately to hypergeometric distribution and its probability mass function is as following:

$$P(X = k) = \frac{\binom{K}{k}\binom{N-K}{n-k}}{\binom{N}{n}} \quad (1)$$

Where N is the total number of genes, K is the total number of AD-related genes, n is the number of predicted genes, k is the number of AD-related genes in predicted genes and $P(X = k)$ is the probability of k AD-related genes occurring in predicted genes for a compound.

However, the constructed network could not cover all protein-coding genes, so in a certain network, N was the number of protein-coding genes it covered, K was the number of all AD-related genes in the network and n was the number of predicted genes.

Fisher's exact test method was implemented to assess the significance of enrichment of AD-related genes in 20 predicted and known genes for each compound. Compounds with or without known targets were calculated separately. For compounds without known targets, n was set to 20 and k was the number of AD-related genes in n. As for compounds having s known targets, n was set to 20+s, and k was s plus the number of AD-related genes in n. P-value was calculated and adjusted by Benjamini–Hochberg method, and used to rank all compounds. Top-ranked compounds were presumed to be critical components of this formula in treating AD.

In order to take into consideration the properties of chemical components, all compounds collected from the three TCM databases were used to create a background component set. Twenty targets were also predicted for each compound. Then every compound had k AD-related genes. The frequency distribution of k in the background set was calculated and approximated roughly to the probability distribution of the background set:

$$P(X = k) = \frac{NP_k}{NP} \quad (2)$$

Where NP is the number of all collectable compounds and NP_k is the number of compounds having k AD-related genes. Then, if a compound has k AD-related genes where $P(X \geq k) < 0.01$, the compound is probably enriched onto AD. This was considered as a calibration and corroboration to Fisher's exact test.

Disease Module Analysis

Due to the complexity of biological network, common proteins may be shared among different diseases. Thus a drug acts on a single protein may produce effect on multiple diseases. The overlap of AD and hypertension disease modules was thus investigated to find common proteins. The collected AD-related proteins and hypertension related proteins were mapped onto a protein–protein interaction network which consisted of 13,460 proteins and 141,296 physical interactions. A disease module was calculated as the largest connected component (LCC) of the disease-related proteins in the protein–protein interaction network. Then the sizes of LCCs of 100,000 randomized protein sets in the network as large as the disease-related protein set were calculated and the distribution yielded. The statistical significance of the disease module was calculated as a z-score:

$$z - score = \frac{S - \overline{S^{rand}}}{\sigma(S^{\mathrm{rand}})} \quad (3)$$

Where S, $\overline{S^{rand}}$, and $\sigma(S^{\mathrm{rand}})$ denote the size of LCC of the disease-related protein set, the average value and standard deviation of the LCC size random distribution, respectively. A z-score greater than 1.96 indicates a significance p-value < 0.05, which suggests the disease module is larger than random observation. The above used protein–protein interaction network and algorithms were retrieved from the work of Menche et al. (2015).

Then the overlapping proteins of these two modules were extracted and gene set enrichment analysis was conducted to find enriched Gene Ontology biological processes with a cut-off adjusted p-value < 0.05.

Gene Set Enrichment Analysis

Predicted genes and overlapping genes of AD and hypertension modules were enriched onto KEGG Pathway and Gene Ontology (GO) biological process to detect key targets and pathways using the Database for Annotation, Visualization and Integrated Discovery (DAVID) v6.8 (Sherman et al., 2007; Jiao et al., 2012).

RESULTS

Formula Ingredients and Known Targets

A total of 731 compounds were collected from the above-mentioned three TCM databases for the formula TMGTY. In order to evaluate the pharmacokinetic properties of this oral administrated formula, HIA and BBB penetrations were predicted using our *in silico* system admetSAR. Only compounds that have both HIA and BBB penetrations predicted as positives were retained. After the screening, 494 herbal compounds were left for further study. 178 different known targets were matched for them from above described databases. Only 68 of 494 compounds had known targets. There were 394 known compound–target interaction pairs. All compounds and known targets information can be found in Supplementary Table S1.

AD and Hypertension Related Genes

From a series of gene databases, a total of 195 genes were collected and identified as AD-related genes, among which 10 are cytochrome P450 (CYPs). Two hundred and ninety-eight genes were collected as hypertension-related genes, within which nine were CYPs. CYPs are major catalysts contributing to the metabolism of a broad spectrum of endogenous compounds, xenobiotics, and nearly 90% marketing drugs (Guengerich et al., 2016). Due to the substrate promiscuity and wide existence, CYPs were thus excluded from this gene set. Then 185 AD-related genes and 289 hypertension-related genes were used for further experiment. The collected disease associated genes were listed in Supplementary Table S2. Gene set enrichment analyses of these gene groups were also shown in Supplementary Tables S3–S6.

Compound–Target Networks

Three compound–target interaction networks were constructed, namely DrugBank, TCM, and Global networks. Their details were shown in **Table 1**. The TCM network collected 1,495 compounds from TCM databases with 899 known targets, among which 287 compounds were also found in DrugBank network. The DrugBank network contains 2,672 small molecules and 1,326 protein targets. Only one hundred targets in TCM network were different from those in DrugBank network. It was thus combined with DrugBank network to form the Global network in order to introduce more targets and expand known network. In Global network, 45.1% targets were enzymes, 10.7% were GPCRs and about 6.7% were ion channels, while 23.7% fell into unknown category, according to IUPHAR classification (**Figure 2A**). As for compounds in Global network, their chemical space was described using three physicochemical descriptors, i.e., molecular weight, ALogP and topological polar surface area (TPSA), depicted in Figure. 2C. About 95% of all compounds have a molecular weight less than 600, TPSA value less than 200Å^2 and ALogP value lying in (−3, 3). Only a few TCM compounds have vast values, whose TPSA, for example, could be up to 800 Å^2. Similarities between all compounds were assessed by calculating Tanimoto coefficient on FCFP4 (**Figure 2D**). Compounds in **Figure 2D** were ordered as two groups: DrugBank small molecules and TCM compounds. Within each group, compounds were randomly distributed. An average Tanimoto coefficient of 0.13 was yielded, indicating a structural diversity among the compounds. The degree distributions of compound nodes and target nodes were calculated, as shown in **Figure 2B**, which succumb to power law distribution. This demonstrated that these networks are scale-free networks.

Our previously developed method bSDTNBI was applied to these three networks. Ten-fold cross validation was then conducted to assess model performance. Parameters α, β, and γ were determined as 0.32, 0.14, and -0.48, respectively. The performance is usually evaluated by several indicators such as AUC, precision and recall. The higher the values of indicators are, the better the performance is. Those indicators were listed in **Table 2** and corresponding ROC curves were plotted in Supplementary Figure S1. All three models performed well. The average recall values of DrugBank, TCM and Global network models were 0.729 ± 0.014, 0.694 ± 0.020, and 0.724 ± 0.012, respectively. A recall value around 70% indicated that, on average, approximately 70% of a drug's missing links were recovered correctly during 10 rounds of 10-fold cross validation. The value of AUC lies in [0, 1]. AUC value equals to 0.5 means the model gives a random prediction; it equals 1 means an ideal prediction. The AUC values of three above network models were 0.966 ± 0.002, 0.948 ± 0.005, and 0.968 ± 0.002, respectively, all larger than 95%, exhibiting high prediction accuracy. The Global network model outstripped the other two with greater indicator values. The Global network model was thus selected to predict targets for the TCM formula.

Target Prediction for Formula TMGTY

Based on the Global network, a total of 9,880 new compound–target interaction pairs were predicted via bSDTNBI method, which introduced 364 new targets for the 494 components of TMGTY. Together with the 178 known targets, a total of 542 targets formed 10,274 interactions with the 494 compounds. Compound–target pairs were hugely complemented from previous 394 interactions between 68 compounds and 178 targets. Among most predicted targets for novel compounds,

TABLE 1 | Overview of the three compound–target interaction (CTI) networks.

Network	N_C	N_T	N_{CTI}	Sparsity (%)
DrugBank	2,672	1,326	16,243	0.46
TCM	1,495	899	5,811	0.43
Global	3,880	1,426	19,800	0.36

N_C, the number of compounds; N_T, the number of targets; N_{CTI}, the number of CTIs; Sparsity: $N_{CTI}/(N_C \times N_T)$.

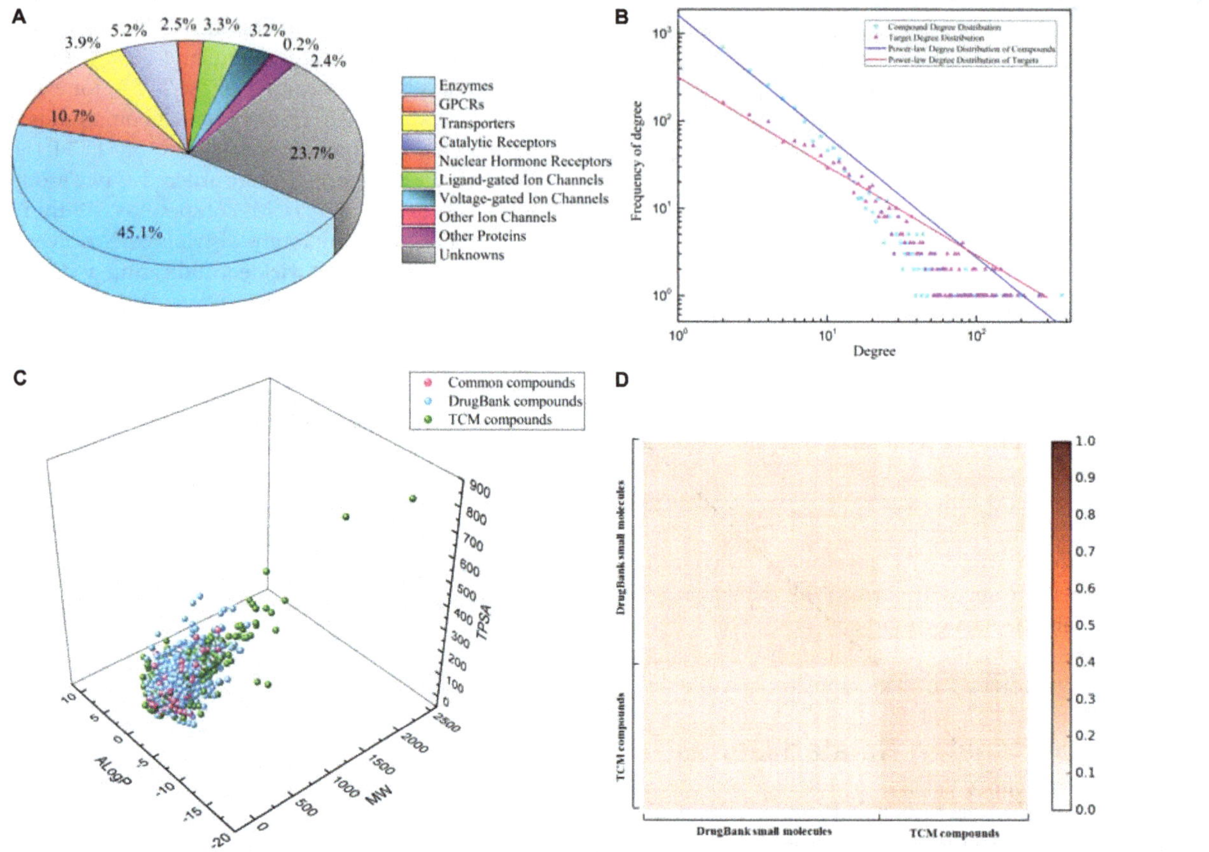

FIGURE 2 | Property analysis of Global network: **(A)** percentage of different kinds of predicted targets, according to IUPHAR classification; **(B)** power-law degree distribution of two kinds of nodes: compounds (blue), targets (red); **(C)** chemical space of all compounds in Global network, depicted by three descriptors: MW, ALogP, and TPSA, consisting of compounds form TCM database (blue), DrugBank database (green), and intersection (red); **(D)** chemical similarity of all compounds on FCFP4 fingerprints.

many were related to AD, such as ACHE, BCHE, BACE1, and MAOA (represented by official gene symbol). A complete list of known and predicted targets for all ingredients can be found in Supplementary Table S7.

Identification of AD-Related Components

In the Global network, only 1426 proteins were included, among which 65 proteins were AD-related. Thus, in the case of Global network, the probability of a compound having k AD-related targets conformed to an approximated hypergeometric distribution which had $K = 65$ and $N = 1{,}426$.

Then the adjusted p-value was proposed as an indicator: the lower is the adjusted p-value; the higher is the relevance to AD. A stringent p-value (less than 0.01) was used to identify compounds highly related to AD. Based on $P(X \geq k) = 0.007 < 0.01$, a compound having $k = 6$ or more predicted targets were considered significantly related to AD. For compounds having known targets, Fisher's exact test was applied separately. Compounds having p-values less than 0.01 were also considered enriched onto AD, regardless the number of AD-related targets they have.

Then a real distribution was investigated. A total of 57,741 compounds were collected and processed from TCMSP, TCMID, and TCM Database@Taiwan to serve as a background set. Twenty

TABLE 2 | Ten-fold cross validation performance of the three network models.

Network	AUC	Precision	Recall	e_P	e_R
DrugBank	0.966 ± 0.002	0.065 ± 0.001	0.729 ± 0.014	42.45 ± 0.81	47.20 ± 0.96
TCM	0.948 ± 0.005	0.049 ± 0.002	0.694 ± 0.020	28.81 ± 0.77	29.94 ± 0.83
Global	0.968 ± 0.002	0.061 ± 0.001	0.724 ± 0.012	46.41 ± 0.75	50.45 ± 0.83

AUC, area under receiver operating characteristic (ROC) curves; e_P, precision enhancement; e_R, recall enhancement.

novel targets were predicted for each compound and the number of AD-related genes was matched using previously collected AD-related genes. The number of AD-related targets of a compound ranged from 0 to 11.

In the background set, the probability of a natural product having k AD-related targets was approximated to the real frequency distribution. Only 3.0% natural products of all had 6 or more AD-related targets and 11.4% had 5 or more, in the real distribution (Supplementary Figure S2). Thus, $P(X \geq 6) = 0.030 < 0.05$ and it further corroborated that a compound having 6 or more AD-related targets was significantly enriched onto AD.

All compounds in the formula were assessed by above two methods. Twelve compounds met the criteria and thus were considered significantly related to AD (**Table 3**). Detailed information on these 12 compounds was listed in Supplementary Table S8.

Pathways Related to TMGTY

All known and predicted genes of these 12 compounds were enriched onto the KEGG pathways. 121 genes were significantly enriched onto 20 pathways with the adjusted p-value < 0.05 (Supplementary Figure S3). Many target genes were enriched onto pathways related to neurotransmitters. For example, there were 20 targets enriched onto serotonergic synapse pathway (adjusted p-value $= 3.5 \times 10^{-13}$) and 21 targets enriched onto neuroactive ligand–receptor interaction pathway (adjusted p-value $= 3.7 \times 10^{-7}$), while 10 targets were enriched onto dopaminergic synapse pathway (adjusted p-value $= 2.3 \times 10^{-3}$). There were also 15 targets enriched onto calcium signaling pathway (adjusted p-value $= 3.7 \times 10^{-7}$), eight onto arachidonic acid metabolism (adjusted p-value $= 3.7 \times 10^{-7}$) and seven onto inflammatory mediator regulation of TRP channels (adjusted p-value $= 3.7 \times 10^{-7}$). These pathways may involve in Ca^{2+} regulation and inflammation. Then a compound–target–pathway subnetwork was built according to target prediction and gene enrichment results, as shown in **Figure 3**. In the network, 11 genes had node degrees larger than 5, which indicated that they were potential targets to half or more than half of those 12 representative compounds. These genes were CYP3A4, ACHE, ABCG2, BACE1, CYP2D6, MAPT, MAOA, PTPN1, EHMT2, PTGS1, and CYP19A1.

Overlap of AD and Hypertension Disease Modules

A total of 172 AD-related proteins and 264 hypertension-related proteins were mapped onto the protein–protein interaction network. AD disease module and hypertension disease module were identified as the LCCs consisting of 86 and 166 proteins, respectively. The z-scores of AD and hypertension modules were 14.2 and 11.7, suggesting that the calculated modules were significantly larger than random expectations. Nineteen genes were shared by AD and hypertension, namely ABCB1, AHR, APOE, BCL2, CAT, CRP, ESR1, F2, GPX1, GSK3B, IL1B, LEP, MME, MTOR, NOS2, NOS3, PON1, SOD1, and SOD2. The disease relationship network was shown in Supplementary Figure S4. Then 26 key GO biological processes with p-values < 0.05 were identified by conducting gene set enrichment analysis on these 19 genes (Supplementary Figure S5). Biological processes such as response to reactive oxygen species, response to hydrogen peroxide, positive regulation of nitric oxide (NO) biosynthetic process, regulation of blood pressure, removal of superoxide radicals, and NO mediated signal transduction all together indicate that these overlapping genes are related to the progression of hypertension and inflammation.

DISCUSSION

The Computational Systems Pharmacology Approach Is Valuable for TCM Study

In this study, a computational systems pharmacology approach consisting of network link prediction, statistical analysis and bioinformatics tools was proposed to study TCM formula TMGTY, which has demonstrated a great advantage in investigation of molecular mechanisms of TCM formulae.

The network link prediction was performed with our bSDTNBI method, which was specifically developed for target prediction of new compounds outside of the compound–target network. Due to the scarcity of TCM ingredient–target interaction information, TCM ingredient–target network was highly incomplete and only covered a small range of targets, i.e., 899 targets, which limited its adaptability and impaired its prediction ability. Since an overlap of 287 compounds was found between collected TCM ingredients and DrugBank small molecules, a combined Global network was then used in order to cover more targets. The combined Global model also outperformed the other two. Comparing to other network prediction models for natural products (Fang et al., 2017a,b) which had approximately 750 drug targets in their global models, our global model covered a much wider range of targets, i.e., 1,426 drug targets, which empowered our model a greater potential to predict more diverse and credible targets for natural products with higher accuracy (using AUC value as an evaluation indicator).

The statistical analysis was conducted by Fisher's exact test. Comparing to gene set enrichment analysis methods (Huang et al., 2009), hypergeometric distribution was used to enrich AD-related genes on compounds. Natural products were enriched onto AD through AD-related genes using Fisher's exact test. For each compounds in the formula TMGTY, its known and predicted targets were identified as whether AD related or non-related. From the perspective of our bSDTNBI method, this resource diffusion method can in a way be envisaged as a distance-based similarity method. In the network, the more and the shorter the paths between a compound node and AD-related target nodes, the more resource it would be portioned from AD-related target nodes, i.e., more AD-related targets would be predicted for this compound. This implied certain intrinsic similarities between compounds represented by network topologies. Since the prediction cannot be perfectly accurate,

TABLE 3 | The 12 compounds were identified highly related to AD, using a cut-off p-value < 0.01.

ID	Structure	Number of AD-related genes	Source	Adjusted p-value
TMGTY067	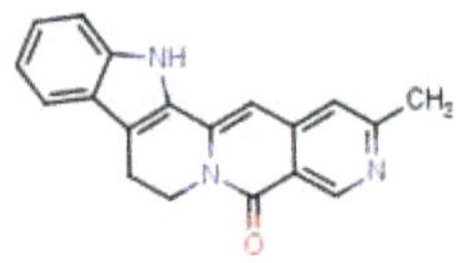	7	*Gouteng*	0.003503
TMGTY332	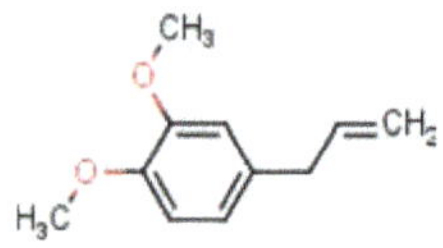	6	*Sangjisheng*	0.007194
TMGTY215	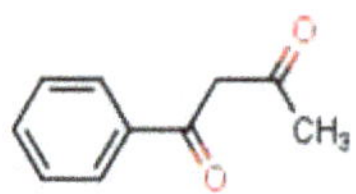	6	*Huangqin*	0.007194
TMGTY408	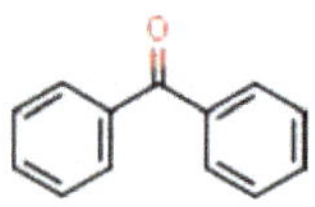	6	*Huangqin*	0.007194
TMGTY405	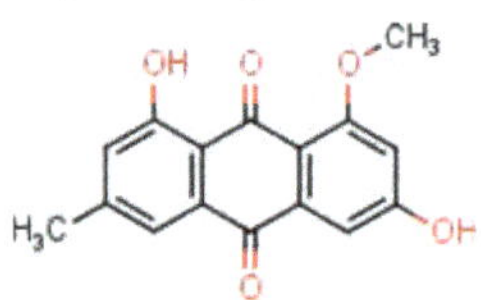	6	*Yejiaoteng*	0.007194
TMGTY404	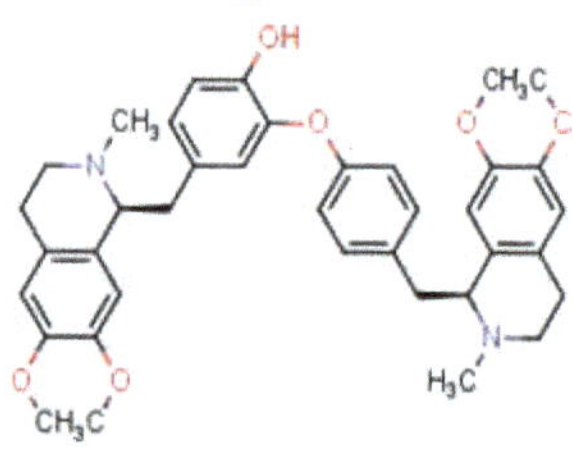	6	*Tianma*	0.007194
TMGTY293	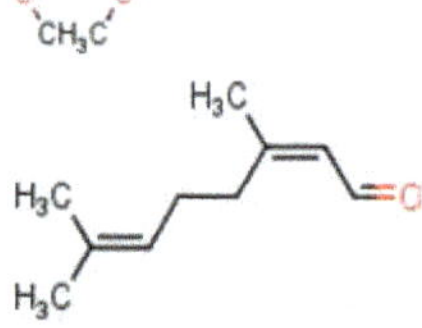	6	*Sangjisheng*	0.007194
TMGTY291	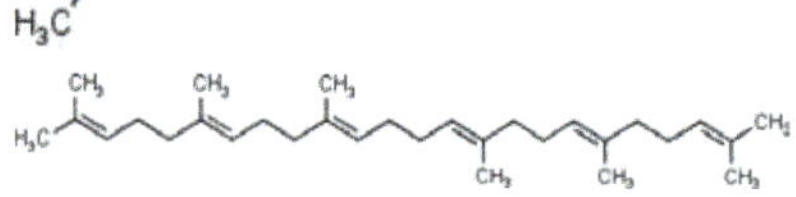	6	*Huangqin Zhizi*	0.007194
TMGTY114	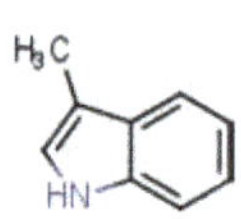	6	*Zhizi*	0.007194
TMGTY115	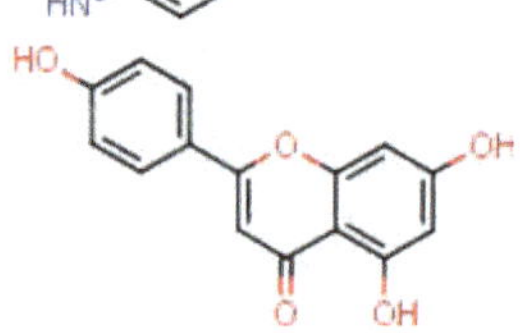	11	*Yimucao Zhizi Huangqin*	0.007194
TMGTY441	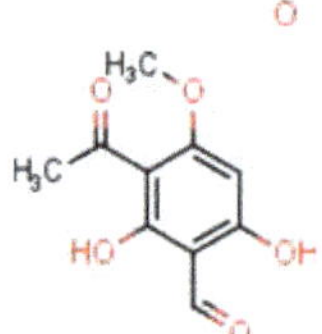	6	*Zhizi*	0.007194
TMGTY387	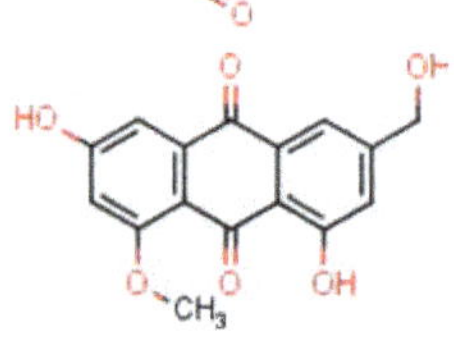	6	*Yejiaoteng*	0.007194

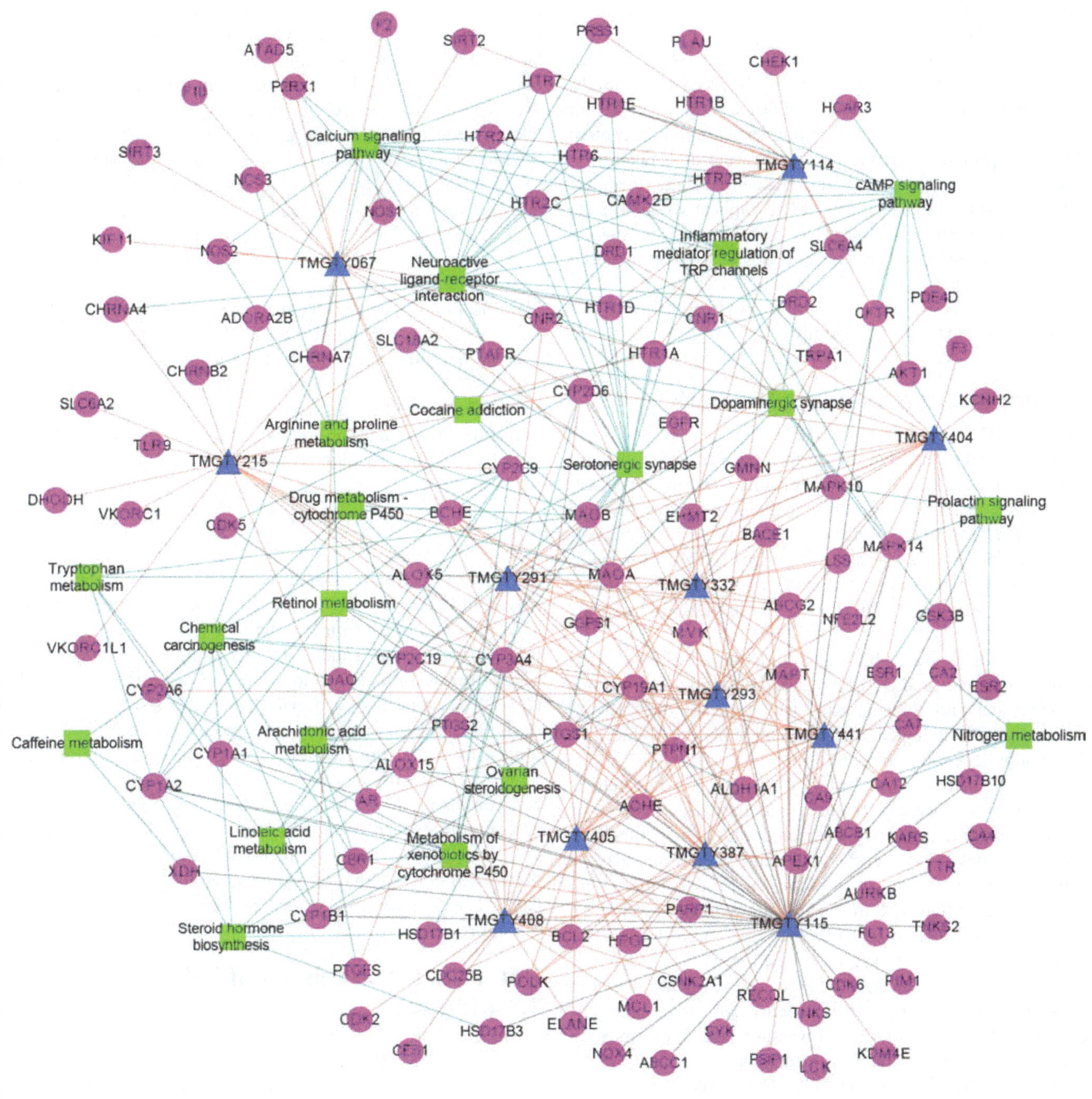

FIGURE 3 | The compound–target–pathway subnetwork of 12 compounds relating to AD. Compound was denoted by blue triangle, target by magenta circle and pathway by green rectangular. Known compound–target interaction was represented as gray line, predicted compound–target interaction as salmon line and target–pathway association as blue line. This figure was plotted using Cytoscape 3.3.0.

it was reasonable to consider that a compound having more predicted AD-related targets compared to non-related targets was more topologically similar to compounds having known AD-related targets, and thus more relevant to AD. Then Fisher's exact test was a good statistical tool to assess the relevance.

The cut-off p-value for compound selection and further analysis was set to 0.01. Twelve compounds were selected and a total of 121 targets were predicted for them. If the cut-off p-value were set to be 0.05, then 108 compounds would meet the criterion and 256 targets predicted. Compounds with a p-value between 0.01 and 0.05 were also considered relating to AD. However, 24 out of 121 targets for 12 compounds were AD-related while only 30 out of 256 targets for 108 compounds were AD-related. This suggested that many targets, especially AD-related targets, were shared among compounds with p-value less than 0.05. So the compounds with p-value less than 0.01 and their corresponding targets were representatives of the molecular mechanisms of formula TMGTY against AD.

The gap between compounds and diseases were bridged by combining above methods. The link between compounds, target genes and diseases was established and analyzed in the context of network science. Complex compound–protein and protein–protein interaction networks were both taken into consideration to facilitate the apprehension of the formula's mechanisms. Since TCM formulae have complicated constituents and are intrinsically multi-targeted and effective to diverse symptoms, our computational systems pharmacology approach provides a more comprehensive perspective to understand their mechanisms on a systematic level, and is easy to apply to various formulae, thus valuable to TCM study.

Evaluation of the Systems Network Pharmacology Approach

In order to further validate the performance of our approach, another traditional Chinese herbal formula Kai-Xin-San (KXS) was analyzed using this approach. KXS is a famous formula used for the treatment of neurosis and AD, which consists of four herbs: *Panax ginseng (Renshen), Wolfiporia cocos (Fuling), Polygala tenuifolia (Yuanzhi),* and *Acorus tatarinowii (Shichangpu)* (Zhou et al., 2012; Wang et al., 2015; Chu et al., 2016).

Three hundred and eighty-eight compounds were collected and 369 new targets predicted, then 28 representative compounds were identified and their targets were enriched onto KEGG pathway and GO biological process (Supplementary Tables S9–S13 and Supplementary Figure S6).

Among enriched pathways, nitrogen metabolism, neuroprotective ligand–receptor interaction, serotonergic synapse, dopaminergic synapse, arachidonic acid metabolism, linoleic acid metabolism, and tryptophan metabolism may be involved in AD pathology. GO biological process enrichment analysis indicated that KXS may involve in oxidation–reduction process, steroid metabolic process, memory, heterocycle metabolic process, lipoxygenase pathway and synaptic transmission, dopaminergic. These enrichment analyses suggested that KXS may exert neuroprotective effect by regulating metabolism networks, reversing oxidative damage in brain, as well as targeting neurotransmitter pathways.

Chu et al. (2016) discovered that KXS could alleviate cognitive deficits in AD model rats and more nerve cells survived than that in the control group. KXS could also regulate metabolism network, such as linoleic acid metabolism and arachidonic acid metabolism, by affecting certain metabolites to show anti-AD effects (Chu et al., 2016). Qiong et al. (2016) found that in rat models KXS could reduce the level of 3-nitro tyrosine (3-NT), and increase the activity of choline acetyltransferase, indicating antioxidant effects of KXS. Zhu et al. (2016a,b) discovered that KXS could induce synaptic protein expression in hippocampus neuron in rats and neuronal differentiation in PC12 cells.

In 28 representative compounds, Apigenin, Paeonol were reported to be important anti-AD compounds (Su et al., 2014). Eudesmin could up-regulate the expression of GABAA and Bcl-2, and it has significant anticonvulsant and sedative effects (Liu et al., 2015). 2′-*O*-Methylisoliquiritigenin was reported to have antioxidant activity and it was also active against human neuroblastoma cells (Batovska and Todorova, 2010). Marmesin was reported to have AChE inhibitory effects (Tumiatti et al., 2008; Cabral et al., 2012). Bergapten was discovered to have anti-inflammatory effects by suppressing the ROS and NO generation (Yang et al., 2018). Myrcene and eugenol was reported to have anti-inflammatory and antioxidant activities (Irie, 2006; Rufino et al., 2015).

The analyses of KXS further validated and proved our approach would be useful in the analyses of TCM formulae and identification of key herbal constituents. Detailed description of KXS can be found in Supplementary Data.

The precision values of three network models were among 0.049–0.065. Different from machine learning methods, bSDTNBI is a network-based method, and its evaluation indicators are from recommender systems (Zhou et al., 2010; Lü et al., 2012). The precision is defined as:

$$P = \frac{1}{c} \cdot \sum_{i=1}^{c} \frac{TP_i(L)}{L} \tag{4}$$

Where C is the number of compounds, L is the number of predicted targets and $TP_i(L)$ is the number of recovered missing links of compound i from test set in L targets. Hence, the more targets predicted, the smaller the precision.

The precision value of approximately 0.06 is relatively high (L = 20), comparing to previous network-based studies. Fang et al. (2017b) constructed network models with precision values ranged from 0.010 to 0.049. Precision values were among 0.042 to 0.072 in the work of Wu et al. (2016). They tested 56 available compounds predicted to act on estrogen receptor α (ERα), and 27 compounds were identified as active agonists or antagonists (Wu et al., 2016). Wu et al. (2018) also constructed global network models with precision values ranging from 0.045 to 0.055. The comparison also further validated the performance of our approach.

Potential Mechanisms of TMGTY in Treating AD

In the compound–target–pathway subnetwork, many enriched pathways were related to AD. For example, among target genes enriched onto serotonergic synapse pathway, 5-hydroxytryptamine receptor 2A (5-HT_{2A}), 5-hydroxytryptamine receptor 2C (5-HT_{2c}), and 5-hydroxytryptamine receptor 6 (5-HT_6) were reported to be related to AD (Wilkinson et al., 2014). 5-HT_{2A} and 5-HT_{2c} can modulate processing of amyloid protein precursor (APP) (Nitsch et al., 1996). Antagonists of 5-HT_6 can improve cognitive performance involving stimulation of glutamate, acetylcholine, and catecholamine release in brain (Benhamú et al., 2014). 5-HT_6 antagonists may also stimulate neurite outgrowth and inhibit mTOR pathway (Claeysen et al., 2015). All 12 compounds were predicted to act on targets in the pathway, mostly 5-HT receptors. Oxidative stress also contributes to neurodegeneration in AD (Barnham et al., 2004). The excessive generation of reactive oxygen species

(ROS) leads to free radical-mediated processes harmful to brain cells (Balaban et al., 2005). Monoamine oxidase A (MAO-A) and monoamine oxidase B (MAO-B) are involved in ROS production while catalyzing various amines (Melo et al., 2011). Acetylcholinesterase (AChE) was predicted to potentially interact with 10 compounds, which was also a neurotransmitter receptor. Thus it may also play an important role. Inhibitors of AChE, such as U.S. Food and Drug Administration (FDA) approved drugs donepezil and galantamine can stabilize or slow decline in cognition (Hansen et al., 2008). Efforts are made to develop multi-target drugs to improve therapeutic efficacy. Ladostigil, for example, is a multi-target drug designed to have AChE, butyrylcholinesterase (BChE) and brain selective MAO-A and MAO-B inhibitory activities (Mangialasche et al., 2010). This design strategy suggests an indigenous advantage of TCM formula in treating complex diseases, such as AD in this case: its multi-targeting attribute. Furthermore, compound TMGTY404 (Dauricine), from the main herb *Rhizoma Gastrodiae*, may potentially act on dopamine receptors, which could also help to stabilize neurodegeneration and cognitive decline in AD (Martorana and Koch, 2014). Twenty-one targets enriched onto neuroactive ligand–receptor interaction pathway were mostly neurotransmitter receptors. All above pathways suggested that this formula may exert neuroprotective effect by targeting various neurotransmitter receptors to treat AD.

Moreover, there were other enriched pathways may be involved in AD pathology, such as calcium signaling pathway, inflammatory mediator regulation of TRP channels and arachidonic acid metabolism. Ca^{2+} plays an important role in neuronal development, synaptic transmission and regulation of many neuronal metabolic pathways (Missiaen et al., 2000). It was also reported that the perturbed cellular Ca^{2+} homeostasis correlates with amyloid plaques and neurofibrillary tangles in AD (Hölscher, 1998). Several studies further revealed that the neurotoxicity of Aβ was diminished if cells were incubated in Ca^{2+}-free medium (Mattson et al., 1993) and Ca^{2+} from endoplasmic reticulum (ER) and mitochondria is involved into the pathogenesis of neuronal degeneration (Pereira et al., 2004; Takuma et al., 2005). Compounds that target neurotransmitters such as cholinergic receptors and 5-HT receptors may regulate the Ca^{2+} homeostasis, since Ca^{2+} signaling is initiated by neurotransmitters (Putney, 2003). Transient receptor potential (TRP) channels are plasma membrane cation channels consisting of six subfamilies: TRPA (ankyrin), TRPC (canonical), TRPM (melastatin), TRPML (mucolipin), TRPP (polycystin), and TRPV (vanilloid) (Moran, 2017). Aβ increases the production of ROS which further activates TRPC5, TRPM2, TRPM7, and TRPV1 and then triggers Ca^{2+} influx and induces NO production, finally leads to neurodegenerative and inflammatory processes (Yamamoto et al., 2007). In this case, TRPA1 was predicted as potential target for compounds TMGTY332, TMGTY293, and TMGTY291. TRPA1 is involved in the TRPA1-Ca^{2+}-PP2B signaling cascade which contributes to Aβ-triggered inflammation and AD pathogenesis. Aβ can trigger TRPA1-dependent Ca^{2+} influx and then enhance the activity of protein phosphatase 2B (PP2B), which then activates NF-κB and nuclear factor of activated T cells (NFAT), leading to produce pro-inflammatory cytokines. The inhibition of TRPA1 channel can slow down AD progression (Lee et al., 2016). The predicted target genes of these 12 compounds including TPRA1, PTGS1, PTGS2, HTR2A, CHRM1, NOS2, and ALOX5 are all important protein-coding genes in these pathways related to AD. Hence the speculation can be made that this TCM formula may exert its therapeutic effect against AD by targeting those proteins to regulate Ca^{2+} and NO level and mollify neuroinflammation.

In order to further corroborate the prediction, a literature review was conducted to check if any of these 12 compounds is already experimentally validated to have therapeutic effect against AD. TMGTY404 (Dauricine) was reported to have neuroprotective effect, which could reduce energy depletion and oxidative stress, thus attenuate neuronal apoptotic cell death (Li and Gong, 2007). Dauricine was predicted to have interactions with six AD-related targets: MAO-A, AChE, dopamine receptor D1 (D_1 receptor), $5\text{-}HT_{1A}$, MAO-B and beta-secretase 1 (BACE1). Targeting MAO-A and MAO-B could reduce the generation of ROS and targeting AChE, D_1 receptor and $5\text{-}HT_{1A}$ together could improve cognitive performance. Thus Dauricine may exert neuroprotective effect through predicted AD-related targets. TMGTY115 (Apigenin) was also reported to have antioxidant and anti-inflammatory properties. Similarly, Apigenin could reduce ROS, protect from Aβ-induced toxicity and suppress inflammatory mediators such as NO and prostaglandin in rat and mouse cell experiments (Venigalla et al., 2015).

Above all indicated the formula TMGTY may treat AD through complex mechanisms, showing both neuroprotective and anti-neuroinflammatory effects.

Overlapping Genes of AD and Hypertension Disease Modules

Nitric oxide plays a key role in the regulation of many physiological processes, such as vasodilation, inflammation, and neurodegeneration (Förstermann and Münzel, 2006; Brown, 2010). NO is generated by three NO synthase (NOS) isoforms: neuronal NOS (nNOS, encoded by NOS1), inducible NOS (iNOS, encoded by NOS2), and endothelial NOS (eNOS, encoded by NOS3). eNOS is constitutively expressed in the vascular endothelium where NO is continuously produced and involved in the regulation of vascular tone and blood pressure (Lundberg et al., 2015). In neurons, nNOS is activated by an influx of calcium to produce NO (Hall and Garthwaite, 2009). iNOS is highly expressed in inflammatory states and can produce high amounts of NO and other reactive nitrogen species such as peroxynitrite (Beckman et al., 1990). In diseased brain, iNOS is found mainly in microglia and astrocytes and may contribute to neuronal death and inflammatory neurodegeneration (Bal-Price and Brown, 2001; Brown and Bal-Price, 2003). So the overlapping genes may function in these enriched biological processes and involve in the regulation of blood pressure and NO levels in brain, thus contribute to the pathology of both AD and hypertension. Some other enriched biological processes such as positive regulation of neuron death and negative regulation of neuron apoptotic process suggested that

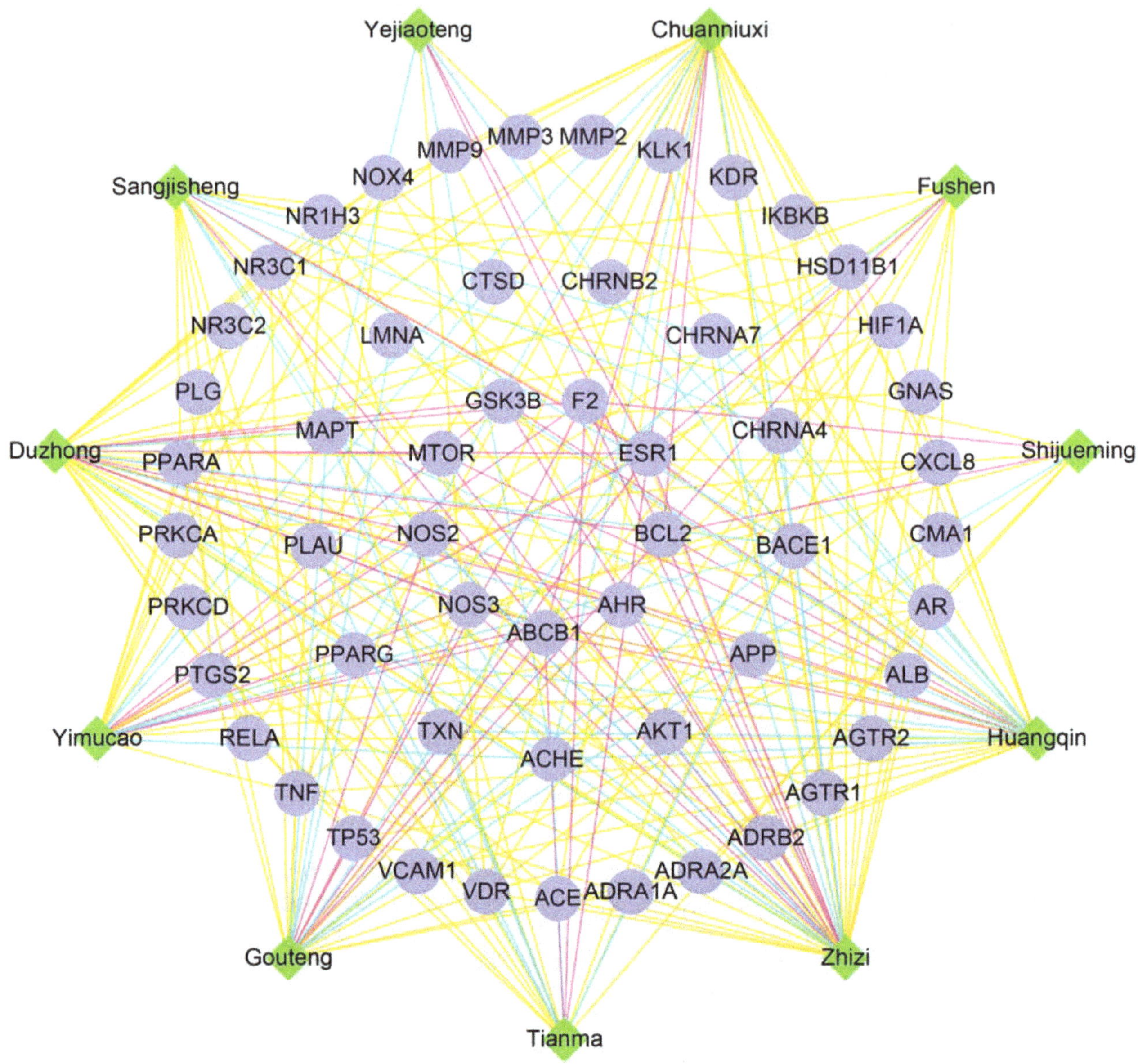

FIGURE 4 | The network of TMGTY herbs (green nodes) and AD, hypertension related genes (blue nodes) in detected disease modules. Herbal interactions with AD genes were noted as cyan edges, hypertension genes as yellow edges and common genes were red edges.

these genes may also engage in the physiology of neuron cells.

These enriched biological processes further suggested that common disease genes should be investigated from a more systematic view. Among common disease genes, several genes were connected in protein–protein interaction network, which suggested that these genes may together exert certain biological effects. The analyses of these genes may also help to understand the concept 'Syndrome' in TCM. Hence, a sub-module was defined as a group of genes containing more than two connected gene nodes in disease modules, which was involved in specific biological processes. Genes enriched onto those above-mentioned biological processes were APOE, BCL2, CAT, ESR1, GPX1, GSK3B, IL1B, LEP, MTOR, NOS2, NOS3, SOD1, and SOD2. Eleven out of these 13 genes were from two sub-modules of common genes, i.e., sub-module 1 (AHR, APOE, ESR1, GSK3B, MTOR, NOS2, NOS3) and sub-module 2 (BCL2, CAT, GPX1, SOD1, SOD2). Drugs acting on common genes, especially genes in sub-modules, may show therapeutic effect on both AD and hypertension. Several genes from sub-modules were potential targets to the 12 representative compounds. ESR1 was predicted to interact with TMGTY405, TMGTY404, TMGTY115, and TMGTY387; BCL2 was the possible target of TMGTY408, TMGTY405, and TMGTY387; NOS2, NOS3 may interact with TMGTY067, and GSK3B with TMGTY115. Taking compound TMGTY067 (Angustidine) as an example, it was predicted to interact with two protein-coding genes NOS2 and NOS3 in the sub-module 1. NOS2 and NOS3 were involved in the regulation of blood pressure, removal of superoxide radicals and NO mediated signal transduction. Thus Angustidine may potentially regulate both the blood pressure and neuro-inflammation and worth further investigation on its pharmacological effects through biological experiments.

The Synergistic Effect of TMGTY

Tian-Ma-Gou-Teng-Yin was prescribed for neurodegenerative diseases (Chik et al., 2013) such as AD (Liu et al., 2014; Lin et al., 2016) and Parkinson's disease (PD) (Pan et al., 2015), and also the prevention of hypertension (Zhang et al., 2016). Upon previously detected disease modules, a network illustration of potential interactions between herbs and AD, hypertension related gene targets was constructed to speculate the synergistic effect of herb formula (**Figure 4**). According to node degrees, AD-related genes were usually potential targets of multiple herbs, such as ACHE (of 10 herbs), BACE1 (9), MAPT (9), and PPARG (8). Thus TMGTY may have a synergistic effect on neurotransmitter-involved pathways to alleviate symptoms of AD. Nine common disease genes in the disease relationship network were predicted to be targets of herb components. Six of them were in sub-module 1, i.e., ESR1 (10), NOS2 (5), NOS3 (5), AHR (5), GSK3B (4), and MTOR (3). All herbs had potential effect on both AD and hypertension disease modules. *Tianma* and *Gouteng* were reported to have anti-AD effects on *in vitro* or *in vivo* models (Su et al., 2014). The water extract of *Tianma* and *Gouteng* showed antioxidant and antiapoptotic effects on neuronal differentiated PC12 cells (Xian et al., 2016). *Yejiaoteng* was a commonly prescribed herb for the treatment of AD and sleeping disorder, and a *Yejiaoteng* decoction was also reported to have sedative-hypnotic effect in an animal model (Chen et al., 2015). Studies have shown that *Huangqin* had antioxidant and anti-neuroinflammatory effects in PC12 cells and mice models (Shang et al., 2006; Jeong et al., 2011). *Yimucao* extract was tested to have cerebral protective effect by reducing neurological impairment, oxidative damage and apoptosis in cerebral occluded rats (Loh et al., 2009). The extract of *Zhizi* also had antioxidant activity (Debnath et al., 2011). Five herbs, *Gouteng, Tianma, Yimucao, Zhizi,* and *Duzhong*, were predicted to interact with genes in sub-module 1. Many of these herbs were involved in the production of ROS, and had antioxidant effects. Genes in the sub-module 1 were directly enriched onto GO biological processes such as positive regulation of neuron death and NO mediated signal transduction. Thus acting on sub-module 1 to regulate NO-related oxidative state may be attributed to the formula's common protective effects against both AD and hypertension.

A herb usually contains hundreds of compounds, and thus possesses a multi-target quality which results in multiple therapeutic effects. Subtly designed herb formulae consisting of several herbs may have synergistically enhanced therapeutic effects against certain symptoms. These symptoms may be a manifestation of functional gene groups. Thus a herb formula may possess complicated pharmacological activities.

CONCLUSION

In this study, we proposed a computational systems pharmacology approach to investigate the molecular mechanisms of TCM formula TMGTY. We first collected the principal components of this formula and predicted targets for them. Then using hypergeometric distribution and Fisher's exact test, those compounds were enriched onto AD through target proteins. The most representative compounds were selected and gene set enrichment analysis was conducted. Our approach revealed that formula TMGTY may have neuroprotective and anti-neuroinflammatory effects in treating AD. We further analyzed disease modules of AD and hypertension and found that some sub-modules of genes were shared between two diseases. Compounds (for example, Angustidine) targeting proteins in sub-modules (such as NOS2 and NOS3) may effect on both AD and hypertension.

Yet there are also limitations of our approach. To filter formula ingredients using predicted HIA and BBB properties may lead to an omission of some compounds. The incompleteness of herb ingredients, AD-related genes and PPI network would bring bias to the prediction and analysis. Furthermore our approach cannot discriminate whether a compound agonize or antagonize a target receptor, as well as the causal relationship between compounds and AD. For example, Isorhynchophylline and Gastrodin were not identified as top compounds since they were not predicted to have significant number of AD-related target genes. They had insufficient known target information and the prediction may be biased by above reasons. Thus the performance of our approach needs to be further improved, for example, by integrating drug-phenotype data. However, our approach is from a holistic perspective and easy to integrate new data to increase performance. At last but not least, our approach did not consider the quantity of each component in the formula, which is difficult currently and should be taken into account in future.

AUTHOR CONTRIBUTIONS

YT, GL, WL, and TW contributed to conception and design of the study. TW performed the experiments and wrote the manuscript. YT wrote sections of the manuscript. All authors contributed to manuscript revision, read and approved the submitted version.

FUNDING

This work was supported by the National Key Research and Development Program (Grant 2016YFA0502304), the National Natural Science Foundation of China (Grants 81673356 and U1603122) and the 111 Project (Grant B07023).

REFERENCES

Amberger, J., Bocchini, C. A., Scott, A. F., and Hamosh, A. (2009). McKusick's online mendelian inheritance in man (OMIM). *Nucleic Acids Res.* 37(Suppl. 1), D793–D796. doi: 10.1093/nar/gkn665

Balaban, R. S., Nemoto, S., and Finkel, T. (2005). Mitochondria, oxidants, and aging. *Cell* 120, 483–495. doi: 10.1016/j.cell.2005.02.001

Ballard, C., Gauthier, S., Corbett, A., Brayne, C., Aarsland, D., and Jones, E. (2011). Alzheimer's disease. *Lancet* 377, 1019–1031. doi: 10.1016/S0140-6736(10) 61349-9

Bal-Price, A., and Brown, G. C. (2001). Inflammatory neurodegeneration mediated by nitric oxide from activated glia-inhibiting neuronal respiration, causing glutamate release and excitotoxicity. *J. Neurosci.* 21, 6480–6491. doi: 10.1523/ JNEUROSCI.21-17-06480.2001

Barnham, K. J., Masters, C. L., and Bush, A. I. (2004). Neurodegenerative diseases and oxidative stress. *Nat. Rev. Drug Discov.* 3, 205–214. doi: 10.1038/nrd1330

Batovska, D. I., and Todorova, I. T. (2010). Trends in utilization of the pharmacological potential of chalcones. *Curr. Clin. Pharmacol.* 5, 1–29. doi: 10.2174/157488410790410579

Beckman, J. S., Beckman, T. W., Chen, J., Marshall, P. A., and Freeman, B. A. (1990). Apparent hydroxyl radical production by peroxynitrite: implications for endothelial injury from nitric oxide and superoxide. *Proc. Natl. Acad. Sci. U.S.A.* 87, 1620–1624. doi: 10.1073/pnas.87.4.1620

Benhamú, B., Martín-Fontecha, M., Vázquez-Villa, H., Pardo, L., and López-Rodríguez, M. L. (2014). Serotonin 5-HT6 receptor antagonists for the treatment of cognitive deficiency in Alzheimer's disease. *J. Med. Chem.* 57, 7160–7181. doi: 10.1021/jm5003952

Brown, G. C. (2010). Nitric oxide and neuronal death. *Nitric Oxide* 23, 153–165. doi: 10.1016/j.niox.2010.06.001

Brown, G. C., and Bal-Price, A. (2003). Inflammatory neurodegeneration mediated by nitric oxide, glutamate, and mitochondria. *Mol. Neurobiol.* 27, 325–355. doi: 10.1385/MN:27:3:325

Brown, G. R., Hem, V., Katz, K. S., Ovetsky, M., Wallin, C., Ermolaeva, O., et al. (2015). Gene: a gene-centered information resource at NCBI. *Nucleic Acids Res.* 43, D36–D42. doi: 10.1093/nar/gku1055

Cabral, R. S., Sartori, M. C., Cordeiro, I., Queiroga, C. L., Eberlin, M. N., Lago, J. H. G., et al. (2012). Anticholinesterase activity evaluation of alkaloids and coumarin from stems of *Conchocarpus fontanesianus*. *Rev. Bras. Farmacogn.* 22, 374–380. doi: 10.1590/S0102-695X2011005000219

Chen, C. Y.-C. (2011). TCM Database@Taiwan: the world's largest traditional Chinese medicine database for drug screening in silico. *PLoS One* 6:e15939. doi: 10.1371/journal.pone.0015939

Chen, K.-H., Yeh, M.-H., Livneh, H., Chen, B.-C., Lin, I. H., Lu, M.-C., et al. (2017). Association of traditional Chinese medicine therapy and the risk of dementia in patients with hypertension: a nationwide population-based cohort study. *BMC Complement. Altern. Med.* 17:178. doi: 10.1186/s12906-017-1677-4

Chen, Y.-L., Lee, C.-Y., Huang, K.-H., Kuan, Y.-H., and Chen, M. (2015). Prescription patterns of Chinese herbal products for patients with sleep disorder and major depressive disorder in Taiwan. *J. Ethnopharmacol.* 171, 307–316. doi: 10.1016/j.jep.2015.05.045

Cheng, F., Li, W., Wang, X., Zhou, Y., Wu, Z., Shen, J., et al. (2013a). Adverse drug events: database construction and in silico prediction. *J. Chem. Inform. Model.* 53, 744–752. doi: 10.1021/ci4000079

Cheng, F., Li, W., Wu, Z., Wang, X., Zhang, C., Li, J., et al. (2013b). Prediction of polypharmacological profiles of drugs by the integration of chemical, side effect, and therapeutic space. *J. Chem. Inform. Model.* 53, 753–762. doi: 10.1021/ ci400010x

Cheng, F., Liu, C., Jiang, J., Lu, W., Li, W., Liu, G., et al. (2012). Prediction of drug-target interactions and drug repositioning via network-based inference. *PLoS Comput. Biol.* 8:e1002503. doi: 10.1371/journal.pcbi.1002503

Chik, S. C. C., Or, T. C. T., Luo, D., Yang, C. L. H., and Lau, A. S. Y. (2013). Pharmacological effects of active compounds on neurodegenerative disease with Gastrodia and Uncaria decoction, a commonly used poststroke decoction. *Sci. World J.* 2013:896873. doi: 10.1155/2013/896873

Chu, H., Zhang, A., Han, Y., Lu, S., Kong, L., Han, J., et al. (2016). Metabolomics approach to explore the effects of Kai-Xin-San on Alzheimer's disease using UPLC/ESI-Q-TOF mass spectrometry. *J. Chromatogr. B* 101, 50–61. doi: 10.1016/j.jchromb.2016.02.007

Claeysen, S., Bockaert, J., and Giannoni, P. (2015). Serotonin: a new hope in Alzheimer's disease? *ACS Chem. Neurosci.* 6, 940–943. doi: 10.1021/ acschemneuro.5b00135

Davis, A. P., Grondin, C. J., Johnson, R. J., Sciaky, D., King, B. L., McMorran, R., et al. (2017). The comparative toxicogenomics database: update 2017. *Nucleic Acids Res.* 45, D972–D978. doi: 10.1093/nar/gkw838

De Strooper, B., and Karran, E. (2016). The cellular phase of Alzheimer's disease. *Cell* 164, 603–615. doi: 10.1016/j.cell.2015.12.056

Debnath, T., Park, P.-J., Deb Nath, N. C., Samad, N. B., Park, H. W., and Lim, B. O. (2011). Antioxidant activity of *Gardenia jasminoides* Ellis fruit extracts. *Food Chem.* 128, 697–703. doi: 10.1016/j.foodchem.2011.03.090

Dey, A., Bhattacharya, R., Mukherjee, A., and Pandey, D. K. (2017). Natural products against Alzheimer's disease: pharmaco-therapeutics and biotechnological interventions. *Biotechnol. Adv.* 35, 178–216. doi: 10.1016/j.biotechadv.2016.12.005

Fang, J., Gao, L., Ma, H., Wu, Q., Wu, T., Wu, J., et al. (2017a). Quantitative and systems pharmacology 3. Network-based identification of new targets for natural products enables potential uses in aging-associated disorders. *Front. Pharmacol.* 8:747. doi: 10.3389/fphar.2017.00747

Fang, J., Wu, Z., Cai, C., Wang, Q., Tang, Y., and Cheng, F. (2017b). Quantitative and systems pharmacology. 1. In silico prediction of drug–target interactions of natural products enables new targeted cancer therapy. *J. Chem. Inform. Model.* 57, 2657–2671. doi: 10.1021/acs.jcim.7b00216

Förstermann, U., and Münzel, T. (2006). Endothelial nitric oxide synthase in vascular disease: from marvel to menace. *Circulation* 113, 1708–1714. doi: 10.1161/circulationaha.105.602532

Gaulton, A., Hersey, A., Nowotka, M., Bento, A. P., Chambers, J., Mendez, D., et al. (2017). The ChEMBL database in 2017. *Nucleic Acids Res.* 45, D945–D954. doi: 10.1093/nar/gkw1074

Gilson, M. K., Liu, T., Baitaluk, M., Nicola, G., Hwang, L., and Chong, J. (2016). BindingDB in 2015: a public database for medicinal chemistry, computational chemistry and systems pharmacology. *Nucleic Acids Res.* 44, D1045–D1053. doi: 10.1093/nar/gkv1072

Guengerich, F. P., Waterman, M. R., and Egli, M. (2016). Recent structural insights into cytochrome P450 function. *Trends Pharmacol. Sci.* 37, 625–640. doi: 10.1016/j.tips.2016.05.006

Hall, C. N., and Garthwaite, J. (2009). What is the real physiological NO concentration in vivo? *Nitric Oxide* 21, 92–103. doi: 10.1016/j.niox.2009. 07.002

Hansen, R. A., Gartlehner, G., Webb, A. P., Morgan, L. C., Moore, C. G., and Jonas, D. E. (2008). Efficacy and safety of donepezil, galantamine, and rivastigmine for the treatment of Alzheimer's disease: a systematic review and meta-analysis. *Clin. Interv. Aging* 3, 211–225.

Hao, D. C., and Xiao, P. G. (2014). Network pharmacology: a rosetta stone for traditional Chinese medicine. *Drug Dev. Res.* 75, 299–312. doi: 10.1002/ddr. 21214

Harding, S. D., Sharman, J. L., Faccenda, E., Southan, C., Pawson, A. J., Ireland, S., et al. (2017). The IUPHAR/BPS guide to PHARMACOLOGY in 2018: updates and expansion to encompass the new guide to IMMUNOPHARMACOLOGY. *Nucleic Acids Res.* 46, D1091–D1106. doi: 10.1093/nar/gkx1121

Ho, S.-C., Ho, Y.-F., Lai, T.-H., Liu, T.-H., Su, S.-Y., and Wu, R.-Y. (2008). Effect of Tianma Gouteng Decoction with subtractive ingredients and its active constituents on memory acquisition. *Am. J. Chin. Med.* 36, 593–602. doi: 10.1142/S0192415X08006004

Ho, S.-C., Ho, Y.-F., Lai, T.-H., Liu, T.-H., and Wu, R.-Y. (2005). Traditional Chinese herbs against hypertension enhance the effect of memory acquisition. *Am. J. Chin. Med.* 33, 787–795. doi: 10.1142/S0192415X0500 3326

Hölscher, C. (1998). Possible causes of Alzheimer's disease: amyloid fragments, free radicals, and calcium homeostasis. *Neurobiol. Dis.* 5, 129–141. doi: 10.1006/ nbdi.1998.0193

Hopkins, A. L. (2007). Network pharmacology. *Nat. Biotechnol.* 25, 1110–1111. doi: 10.1038/nbt1007-1110

Hopkins, A. L. (2008). Network pharmacology: the next paradigm in drug discovery. *Nat. Chem. Biol.* 4, 682–690. doi: 10.1038/nchembio.118

Huang, D. W., Sherman, B. T., and Lempicki, R. A. (2009). Bioinformatics enrichment tools: paths toward the comprehensive functional analysis of large gene lists. *Nucleic Acids Res.* 37, 1–13. doi: 10.1093/nar/gkn923

Irie, Y. (2006). Effects of eugenol on the central nervous system: its possible application to treatment of Alzheimer's disease, depression, and Parkinson's disease. *Curr. Bioact. Compd.* 2, 57–66. doi: 10.2174/157340721060201005 7

Jeong, K., Shin, Y.-C., Park, S., Park, J.-S., Kim, N., Um, J.-Y., et al. (2011). Ethanol extract of *Scutellaria baicalensis* Georgi prevents oxidative damage and neuroinflammation and memorial impairments in artificial senescense mice. *J. Biomed. Sci.* 18:14. doi: 10.1186/1423-0127-18-14

Jiang, W.-Y. (2005). Therapeutic wisdom in traditional Chinese medicine: a perspective from modern science. *Trends Pharmacol. Sci.* 26, 558–563. doi: 10.1016/j.tips.2005.09.006

Jiao, X., Sherman, B. T., Huang, D. W., Stephens, R., Baseler, M. W., Lane, H. C., et al. (2012). DAVID-WS: a stateful web service to facilitate gene/protein list analysis. *Bioinformatics* 28, 1805–1806. doi: 10.1093/bioinformatics/bts251

Kanehisa, M., Furumichi, M., Tanabe, M., Sato, Y., and Morishima, K. (2017). KEGG: new perspectives on genomes, pathways, diseases and drugs. *Nucleic Acids Res.* 45, D353–D361. doi: 10.1093/nar/gkw1092

Kanehisa, M., and Goto, S. (2000). KEGG: Kyoto encyclopedia of genes and genomes. *Nucleic Acids Res.* 28, 27–30. doi: 10.1093/nar/28.1.27

Lai, C. Y., Wu, M. Y., Chiang, J. H., Sun, M. F., Chen, Y. H., Chang, C. T., et al. (2017). Utilization of Western medicine and traditional Chinese medicine among patients with Alzheimer's disease in Taiwan: a nationwide population-based study. *Eur. J. Neurol.* 24, 1166–1172. doi: 10.1111/ene.13361

Lee, K.-I., Lee, H.-T., Lin, H.-C., Tsay, H.-J., Tsai, F.-C., Shyue, S.-K., et al. (2016). Role of transient receptor potential ankyrin 1 channels in Alzheimer's disease. *J. Neuroinflammation* 13:92. doi: 10.1186/s12974-016-0557-z

Li, H., Zhao, L., Zhang, B., Jiang, Y., Wang, X., Guo, Y., et al. (2014). A network pharmacology approach to determine active compounds and action mechanisms of ge-gen-qin-lian decoction for treatment of type 2 Diabetes. *Evid. Based Complement. Altern. Med.* 2014:495840. doi: 10.1155/2014/495840

Li, J., Lei, K., Wu, Z., Li, W., Liu, G., Liu, J., et al. (2016). Network-based identification of microRNAs as potential pharmacogenomic biomarkers for anticancer drugs. *Oncotarget* 7, 45584–45596. doi: 10.18632/oncotarget.10052

Li, J., Lu, C., Jiang, M., Niu, X., Guo, H., Li, L., et al. (2012). Traditional Chinese medicine-based network pharmacology could lead to new multicompound drug discovery. *Evid. Based Complement. Altern. Med.* 2012:149762. doi: 10.1155/2012/149762

Li, J., Wu, Z., Cheng, F., Li, W., Liu, G., and Tang, Y. (2014). Computational prediction of microRNA networks incorporating environmental toxicity and disease etiology. *Sci. Rep.* 4:5576. doi: 10.1038/srep05576

Li, Y.-H., and Gong, P.-L. (2007). Neuroprotective effects of dauricine against apoptosis induced by transient focal cerebral ischaemia in rats via a mitochondrial pathway. *Clin. Exp. Pharmacol. Physiol.* 34, 177–184. doi: 10.1111/j.1440-1681.2007.04569.x

Lin, S.-K., Yan, S.-H., Lai, J.-N., and Tsai, T.-H. (2016). Patterns of Chinese medicine use in prescriptions for treating Alzheimer's disease in Taiwan. *Chin. Med.* 11:12. doi: 10.1186/s13020-016-0086-9

Liu, H., Song, Z., Liao, D. G., Zhang, T. Y., Liu, F., Zhuang, K., et al. (2015). Anticonvulsant and sedative effects of eudesmin isolated from *Acorus tatarinowii* on mice and rats. *Phytother. Res.* 29, 996–1003. doi: 10.1002/ptr.5337

Liu, P., Kong, M., Yuan, S., Liu, J., and Wang, P. (2014). History and experience: a survey of traditional Chinese medicine treatment for Alzheimer's disease. *Evid. Based Complement. Altern. Med.* 2014:642128. doi: 10.1155/2014/642128

Loh, K. P., Huang, S. H., Tan, B. K. H., and Zhu, Y. Z. (2009). Cerebral protection of purified Herba Leonuri extract on middle cerebral artery occluded rats. *J. Ethnopharmacol.* 125, 337–343. doi: 10.1016/j.jep.2009.05.025

Lü, L., Medo, M., Yeung, C. H., Zhang, Y.-C., Zhang, Z.-K., and Zhou, T. (2012). Recommender systems. *Phys. Rep.* 519, 1–49. doi: 10.1016/j.physrep.2012.02.006

Lu, W., Cheng, F., Jiang, J., Zhang, C., Deng, X., Xu, Z., et al. (2015). FXR antagonism of NSAIDs contributes to drug-induced liver injury identified by systems pharmacology approach. *Sci. Rep.* 5:8114. doi: 10.1038/srep08114

Lundberg, J. O., Gladwin, M. T., and Weitzberg, E. (2015). Strategies to increase nitric oxide signalling in cardiovascular disease. *Nat. Rev. Drug Discov.* 14:623. doi: 10.1038/nrd4623

Mangialasche, F., Solomon, A., Winblad, B., Mecocci, P., and Kivipelto, M. (2010). Alzheimer's disease: clinical trials and drug development. *Lancet Neurol.* 9, 702–716. doi: 10.1016/S1474-4422(10)70119-8

Martorana, A., and Koch, G. (2014). Is dopamine involved in Alzheimer's disease? *Front. Aging Neurosci.* 6:252. doi: 10.3389/fnagi.2014.00252

Mattson, M. P., Barger, S. W., Cheng, B., Lieberburg, I., Smith-Swintosky, V. L., and Rydel, R. E. (1993). β-Amyloid precursor protein metabolites and loss of neuronal Ca^{2+} homeostasis in Alzheimer's disease. *Trends Neurosci.* 16, 409–414. doi: 10.1016/0166-2236(93)90009-B

May, B. H., Feng, M., Zhou, I. W., Chang, S.-Y., Lu, S.-C., Zhang, A. L., et al. (2016). Memory impairment, dementia, and Alzheimer's disease in classical and contemporary traditional Chinese medicine. *J. Altern. Complement. Med.* 22, 695–705. doi: 10.1089/acm.2016.0070

Melo, A., Monteiro, L., Lima, R. M., Oliveira, D. M., Cerqueira, M. D., and El-Bachá, R. S. (2011). Oxidative stress in neurodegenerative diseases: mechanisms and therapeutic perspectives. *Oxid. Med. Cell. Longev.* 2011:467180. doi: 10.1155/2011/467180

Menche, J., Sharma, A., Kitsak, M., Ghiassian, S. D., Vidal, M., Loscalzo, J., et al. (2015). Uncovering disease-disease relationships through the incomplete interactome. *Science* 347:1257601. doi: 10.1126/science.1257601

Missiaen, L., Robberecht, W., Bosch, L. V. D., Callewaert, G., Parys, J. B., Wuytack, F., et al. (2000). Abnormal intracellular Ca^{2+} homeostasis and disease. *Cell Calcium* 28, 1–21. doi: 10.1054/ceca.2000.0131

Moran, M. M. (2017). TRP channels as potential drug targets. *Annu. Rev. Pharmacol. Toxicol.* 58, 309–330. doi: 10.1146/annurev-pharmtox-010617-052832

Nitsch, R. M., Deng, M., Growdon, J. H., and Wurtman, R. J. (1996). Serotonin 5-HT2a and 5-HT2c receptors stimulate amyloid precursor protein ectodomain secretion. *J. Biol. Chem.* 271, 4188–4194. doi: 10.1074/jbc.271.8.4188

O'Boyle, N. M., Banck, M., James, C. A., Morley, C., Vandermeersch, T., and Hutchison, G. R. (2011). Open Babel: an open chemical toolbox. *J. Cheminform.* 3:33. doi: 10.1186/1758-2946-3-33

Pan, W., Liu, J., Chen, X., Wang, Q., Wu, Y., Bai, Y., et al. (2015). A practical consensus guideline for the integrative treatment of Parkinson's disease in Shanghai, China. *Integr. Med. Int.* 2, 56–62. doi: 10.1159/000435813

Pereira, C., Ferreiro, E., Cardoso, S. M., and de Oliveira, C. R. (2004). Cell degeneration induced by amyloid-β peptides. *J. Mol. Neurosci.* 23, 97–104. doi: 10.1385/JMN:23:1-2:097

Putney, J. W. (2003). Capacitative calcium entry in the nervous system. *Cell Calcium* 34, 339–344. doi: 10.1016/S0143-4160(03)00143-X

Qiong, W., Yong-liang, Z., Ying-hui, L., Shan-guang, C., Jiang-hui, G., Yi-Xi, C., et al. (2016). The memory enhancement effect of Kai Xin San on cognitive deficit induced by simulated weightlessness in rats. *J. Ethnopharmacol.* 187, 9–16. doi: 10.1016/j.jep.2016.03.070

Reitz, C., Brayne, C., and Mayeux, R. (2011). Epidemiology of Alzheimer disease. *Nat. Rev. Neurol.* 7, 137–152. doi: 10.1038/nrneurol.2011.2

Roth, B. L., Lopez, E., Patel, S., and Kroeze, W. K. (2000). The multiplicity of serotonin receptors: uselessly diverse molecules or an embarrassment of riches? *Neuroscientist* 6, 252–262. doi: 10.1177/107385840000600408

Ru, J., Li, P., Wang, J., Zhou, W., Li, B., Huang, C., et al. (2014). TCMSP: a database of systems pharmacology for drug discovery from herbal medicines. *J. Cheminform.* 6:13. doi: 10.1186/1758-2946-6-13

Rufino, A. T., Ribeiro, M., Sousa, C., Judas, F., Salgueiro, L., Cavaleiro, C., et al. (2015). Evaluation of the anti-inflammatory, anti-catabolic and pro-anabolic effects of E-caryophyllene, myrcene and limonene in a cell model of osteoarthritis. *Eur. J. Pharmacol.* 750, 141–150. doi: 10.1016/j.ejphar.2015.01.018

Selkoe, D. J., and Hardy, J. (2016). The amyloid hypothesis of Alzheimer's disease at 25 years. *EMBO Mol. Med.* 8, 595–608. doi: 10.15252/emmm.201606210

Shang, Y.-Z., Qin, B.-W., Cheng, J.-J., and Miao, H. (2006). Prevention of oxidative injury by flavonoids from stems and leaves of Scutellaria *Baicalensis georgi* in PC12 cells. *Phytother. Res.* 20, 53–57. doi: 10.1002/ptr.1802

Sherman, B. T., Huang, D. W., Tan, Q., Guo, Y., Bour, S., Liu, D., et al. (2007). DAVID Knowledgebase: a gene-centered database integrating heterogeneous gene annotation resources to facilitate high-throughput gene functional analysis. *BMC Bioinformatics* 8:426. doi: 10.1186/1471-2105-8-426

Su, Y., Wang, Q., Wang, C., Chan, K., Sun, Y., and Kuang, H. (2014). The treatment of Alzheimer's disease using Chinese medicinal plants: from disease models to potential clinical applications. *J. Ethnopharmacol.* 152, 403–423. doi: 10.1016/j.jep.2013.12.053

Takuma, K., Yan, S. S., Stern, D. M., and Yamada, K. (2005). Mitochondrial dysfunction, endoplasmic reticulum stress, and apoptosis in Alzheimer's disease. *J. Pharmacol. Sci.* 97, 312–316. doi: 10.1254/jphs.CPJ04006X

Tao, W., Xu, X., Wang, X., Li, B., Wang, Y., Li, Y., et al. (2013). Network pharmacology-based prediction of the active ingredients and potential targets of Chinese herbal Radix Curcumae formula for application to cardiovascular disease. *J. Ethnopharmacol.* 145, 1–10. doi: 10.1016/j.jep.2012.09.051

Tumiatti, V., Bolognesi, M. L., Minarini, A., Rosini, M., Milelli, A., Matera, R., et al. (2008). Progress in acetylcholinesterase inhibitors for Alzheimer's disease: an update. *Expert Opin. Ther. Pat.* 18, 387–401. doi: 10.1517/13543776.18.4.387

Venigalla, M., Sonego, S., Gyengesi, E., and Münch, G. (2015). Curcumin and Apigenin - novel and promising therapeutics against chronic neuroinflammation in Alzheimer's disease. *Neural Regen. Res.* 10, 1181–1185. doi: 10.4103/1673-5374.162686

Wang, X., Han, Y., Zhang, A., and Sun, H. (2015). "Chapter 22 - Metabolic profiling provides a system for the understanding of Alzheimer's disease in rats post-treatment with Kaixin San," in *Chinmedomics*, eds X. Wang, H. Sun, and A. Zhang (Boston, MA: Academic Press), 347–362.

Wang, Y.-Y., Li, J., Wu, Z.-R., Zhang, B., Yang, H.-B., Wang, Q., et al. (2017). Insights into the molecular mechanisms of *Polygonum multiflorum* Thunb-induced liver injury: a computational systems toxicology approach. *Acta Pharmacol. Sin.* 38, 719–732. doi: 10.1038/aps.2016.147

Whirl-Carrillo, M., McDonagh, E. M., Hebert, J. M., Gong, L., Sangkuhl, K., Thorn, C. F., et al. (2012). Pharmacogenomics knowledge for personalized medicine. *Clin. Pharmacol. Ther.* 92, 414–417. doi: 10.1038/clpt.2012.96

Wilkinson, D., Windfeld, K., and Colding-Jørgensen, E. (2014). Safety and efficacy of idalopirdine, a 5-HT6 receptor antagonist, in patients with moderate Alzheimer's disease (LADDER): a randomised, double-blind, placebo-controlled phase 2 trial. *Lancet Neurol.* 13, 1092–1099. doi: 10.1016/S1474-4422(14)70198-X

Wishart, D. S., Feunang, Y. D., Guo, A. C., Lo, E. J., Marcu, A., Grant, J. R., et al. (2017). DrugBank 5.0: a major update to the DrugBank database for 2018. *Nucleic Acids Res.* 46, D1074–D1082. doi: 10.1093/nar/gkx1037

Wu, Z., Cheng, F., Li, J., Li, W., Liu, G., and Tang, Y. (2017). SDTNBI: an integrated network and chemoinformatics tool for systematic prediction of drug-target interactions and drug repositioning. *Brief. Bioinform.* 18, 333–347. doi: 10.1093/bib/bbw012

Wu, Z., Lu, W., Wu, D., Luo, A., Bian, H., Li, J., et al. (2016). In silico prediction of chemical mechanism of action via an improved network-based inference method. *Br. J. Pharmacol.* 173, 3372–3385. doi: 10.1111/bph.13629

Wu, Z., Lu, W., Yu, W., Wang, T., Li, W., Liu, G., et al. (2018). Quantitative and systems pharmacology 2. In silico polypharmacology of G protein-coupled receptor ligands via network-based approaches. *Pharmacol. Res.* 129, 400–413. doi: 10.1016/j.phrs.2017.11.005

Xian, J. W., Choi, A. Y.-T., Lau, C. B.-S., Leung, W. N., Ng, C. F., and Chan, C. W. (2016). *Gastrodia* and *Uncaria* (tianma gouteng) water extract exerts antioxidative and antiapoptotic effects against cerebral ischemia in vitro and in vivo. *Chin. Med.* 11:27. doi: 10.1186/s13020-016-0097-6

Xiong, X., Yang, X., Liu, Y., Zhang, Y., Wang, P., and Wang, J. (2013). Chinese herbal formulas for treating hypertension in traditional Chinese medicine: perspective of modern science. *Hypertens. Res.* 36, 570–579. doi: 10.1038/hr.2013.18

Xue, R., Fang, Z., Zhang, M., Yi, Z., Wen, C., and Shi, T. (2013). TCMID: traditional Chinese medicine integrative database for herb molecular mechanism analysis. *Nucleic Acids Res.* 41, D1089–D1095. doi: 10.1093/nar/gks1100

Yamamoto, S., Wajima, T., Hara, Y., Nishida, M., and Mori, Y. (2007). Transient receptor potential channels in Alzheimer's disease. *Biochim. Biophys. Acta* 1772, 958–967. doi: 10.1016/j.bbadis.2007.03.006

Yang, Y., Zheng, K., Mei, W., Wang, Y., Yu, C., Yu, B., et al. (2018). Anti-inflammatory and proresolution activities of bergapten isolated from the roots of *Ficus hirta* in an in vivo zebrafish model. *Biochem. Biophys. Res. Commun.* 496, 763–769. doi: 10.1016/j.bbrc.2018.01.071

Yap, C. W. (2011). PaDEL-descriptor: an open source software to calculate molecular descriptors and fingerprints. *J. Comput. Chem.* 32, 1466–1474. doi: 10.1002/jcc.21707

Yu, W., Gwinn, M., Clyne, M., Yesupriya, A., and Khoury, M. J. (2008). A navigator for human genome epidemiology. *Nat. Genet.* 40:124. doi: 10.1038/ng0208-124

Zhang, A., Sun, H., Qiu, S., and Wang, X. (2013). Advancing drug discovery and development from active constituents of Yinchenhao Tang, a famous traditional Chinese medicine formula. *Evid. Based Complement. Altern. Med.* 2013:257909. doi: 10.1155/2013/257909

Zhang, B., Wang, X., and Li, S. (2013). An integrative platform of TCM network pharmacology and its application on a herbal formula, Qing-Luo-Yin. *Evid. Based Complement. Altern. Med.* 2013:456747. doi: 10.1155/2013/456747

Zhang, G., Yang, G., Deng, Y., Zhao, X., Yang, Y., Rao, J., et al. (2016). Ameliorative effects of Xue-Fu-Zhu-Yu decoction, Tian-Ma-Gou-Teng-Yin and Wen-Dan decoction on myocardial fibrosis in a hypertensive rat mode. *BMC Complement. Altern. Med.* 16:56. doi: 10.1186/s12906-016-1030-3

Zhao, J., Jiang, P., and Zhang, W. (2010). Molecular networks for the study of TCM pharmacology. *Brief. Bioinform.* 11, 417–430. doi: 10.1093/bib/bbp063

Zhou, T., Kuscsik, Z., Liu, J.-G., Medo, M., Wakeling, J. R., and Zhang, Y.-C. (2010). Solving the apparent diversity-accuracy dilemma of recommender systems. *Proc. Natl. Acad. Sci. U.S.A.* 107, 4511–4515. doi: 10.1073/pnas.1000488107

Zhou, X.-J., Liu, M., Yan, J.-J., Cao, Y., and Liu, P. (2012). Antidepressant-like effect of the extracted of Kai Xin San, a traditional Chinese herbal prescription, is explained by modulation of the central monoaminergic neurotransmitter system in mouse. *J. Ethnopharmacol.* 139, 422–428. doi: 10.1016/j.jep.2011.11.027

Zhu, Y., Duan, X., Cheng, X., Cheng, X., Li, X., Zhang, L., et al. (2016a). Kai-Xin-San, a standardized traditional Chinese medicine formula, up-regulates the expressions of synaptic proteins on hippocampus of chronic mild stress induced depressive rats and primary cultured rat hippocampal neuron. *J. Ethnopharmacol.* 193, 423–432. doi: 10.1016/j.jep.2016.09.037

Zhu, Y., Duan, X., Huang, F., Cheng, X., Zhang, L., Liu, P., et al. (2016b). Kai-Xin-San, a traditional Chinese medicine formula, induces neuronal differentiation of cultured PC12 cells: modulating neurotransmitter regulation enzymes and potentiating NGF inducing neurite outgrowth. *J. Ethnopharmacol.* 193, 272–282. doi: 10.1016/j.jep.2016.08.013

5

Network Pharmacology and Experimental Assessment to Explore the Pharmacological Mechanism of Qimai Feiluoping Decoction Against Pulmonary Fibrosis

Yingying Yang[1,2†], Lu Ding[3†], Tingting Bao[1,2†], Yaxin Li[4], Jing Ma[5], Qingwei Li[2], Zezheng Gao[2], Siyu Song[4], Jing Wang[5], Jiachao Zhao[4], Ziyuan Wang[5], Daqing Zhao[3], Xiangyan Li[3], Zeyu Wang[6], Linhua Zhao[2*] and Xiaolin Tong[2*]*

[1]Graduate College, Beijing University of Chinese Medicine, Beijing, China, [2]Institute of Metabolic Diseases, Guang'anmen Hospital, China Academy of Chinese Medical Sciences, Beijing, China, [3]Jilin Ginseng Academy, Key Laboratory of Active Substances and Biological Mechanisms of Ginseng Efficacy, Ministry of Education, Jilin Provincial Key Laboratory of Bio-Macromolecules of Chinese Medicine, Changchun University of Chinese Medicine, Changchun, China, [4]College of Integrated Traditional Chinese and Western Medicine, Changchun University of Chinese Medicine, Changchun, China, [5]Affiliated Hospital of Changchun University of Chinese Medicine, Changchun, China, [6]Department of Scientific Research, Changchun University of Chinese Medicine, Changchun, China

***Correspondence:**
Zeyu Wang
zeyu781022@163.com
Linhua Zhao
melonzhao@163.com
Xiaolin Tong
tongxiaolin@vip.163.com*

†These authors have contributed equally to this work

Pulmonary fibrosis (PF) is one of the pathologic changes in COVID-19 patients in convalescence, and it is also a potential long-term sequela in severe COVID-19 patients. Qimai Feiluoping decoction (QM) is a traditional Chinese medicine formula recommended in the Chinese national medical program for COVID-19 convalescent patients, and PF is one of its indications. Through clinical observation, QM was found to improve the clinical symptoms and pulmonary function and reduce the degree of PF of COVID-19 convalescent patients. To further explore the pharmacological mechanisms and possible active components of QM in anti-PF effect, UHPLC/Q-TOF-MS was used to analyze the composition of the QM extract and the active components that can be absorbed into the blood, leading to the identification of 56 chemical compounds and 10 active components. Then, network pharmacology was used to predict the potential mechanisms and targets of QM; it predicted that QM exerts its anti-PF effects *via* the regulation of the epithelial–mesenchymal transition (EMT), extracellular matrix (ECM) degradation, and TGF-β signaling pathway. Finally, TGF-β1–induced A549 cells were used to verify and explore the pharmacological effects of QM and found that QM could inhibit the proliferation of TGF-β1–induced A549 cells, attenuate EMT, and promote ECM degradation by inhibiting the TGF-β/Smad3 pathway.

Keywords: COVID-19, pulmonary fibrosis, QM formula, network pharmacology, epithelial–mesenchymal transition, extracellular matrix accumulation, TGF-β1/Smad3 pathway

INTRODUCTION

Many interstitial lung diseases, such as idiopathic interstitial pneumonias and acute lung injury, can progress to pulmonary fibrosis (PF). Idiopathic PF (IPF) is a devastating, irreversible, and chronic progressive form of PF, and lung transplantation is the only treatment that can change the outcome of IPF patients (Richeldi et al., 2017). There are three million IPF patients around the world, and its incidence increases dramatically with age (Martinez et al., 2017). PF is also a pathological phenomenon in the development of various respiratory diseases, such as viral pneumonia and chronic obstructive pulmonary disease (COPD) (Meyer, 2017). The Coronavirus disease 2019 (COVID-19), which is caused by severe acute respiratory syndrome coronavirus 2 (SARS-CoV-2) (Asselah et al., 2021), has become a worldwide pandemic, infecting over 222 million people and killing more than 4.9 million people as of October 2021. However, the absence of SARS-CoV-2 nucleic acid in COVID-19 patients does not guarantee complete recovery, especially in severe and critical patients. A series of problems can occur during the COVID-19 recovery period, called post-acute COVID-19 syndrome, involving multiple disorders of the cardiovascular system, respiratory system, endocrine system, nervous system, urinary system, digestive system, and skin (Nalbandian et al., 2021). Several clinical studies have found that patients during the COVID-19 recovery period have imaging signs of PF, especially in critical patients. For example, a Chinese cohort study about post–COVID-19 indicated that in approximately 50% of 349 patients, at least one abnormal pattern was observed in high-resolution computed tomography (CT) scans of the chest at 6 months after discharge, with most abnormalities observed by CT being ground-glass opacities (Huang et al., 2021). Moreover, pathological studies of patients who died of COVID-19 revealed that PF was widespread in lung tissues (Bian, 2020). Consequently, PF could be a serious consequence of SARS-CoV-2 infection, according to the current information on COVID-19 and the data from severe acute respiratory syndrome (SARS) and Middle East respiratory syndrome (MERS) (George et al., 2020). Additionally, the major risk factors for severe COVID-19 are shared with that of IPF (George et al., 2020), including male sex, age, hypertension, diabetes, and other comorbidities. However, the treatment of IPF also remains supportive presently, with pirfenidone and nintedanib being among the few drugs that have anti-PF effects (King et al., 2014; Flaherty et al., 2019). Therefore, there is an urgent need to develop novel therapeutic strategies to delay the progressive stages of PF and deal with the possible arrival of post-COVID-19–related PF.

During the process of PF, epithelial cells can respond to microenvironmental cues and convert to mesenchymal cells, such as fibroblasts and myofibroblasts, which are direct effectors of organ fibrosis, *via* a process called the epithelial–mesenchymal transition (EMT) (King et al., 2011; Salton et al., 2019). Transforming growth factor beta (TGF-β) is an important fibrotic cytokine that can induce EMT and cause fibroblast differentiation into myofibroblast (Yan et al., 2014). Upon stimulation with cytokines such as TGF-β, angiotensin II, and interleukin-6 (IL-6), mesenchymal cells, especially myofibroblasts, could secrete large amounts of extracellular matrix (ECM), such as collagen I, laminin (LN), fibronectin (FN), and alpha-smooth muscle actin (α-SMA) (Meng et al., 2016; Forcina et al., 2019; Ji et al., 2019). Excessive deposition of ECM could result in scarring and destruction of the lung architecture (Bonnans et al., 2014). Thus, the inhibition of TGF-β–mediated EMT and ECM accumulation is a potential therapeutic strategy to prevent PF.

Based on the traditional Chinese medicine (TCM) theory, Qi-Yin deficiency and phlegm-stasis in channels are the key factors in the pathogenesis of PF; they are also observed in many COVID-19 convalescent patients, especially those with PF. Qimai Feiluoping decoction (QM), a TCM formula prescribed by Professor Tong Xiaolin, could nourish Qi-Yin, dissipate phlegm, invigorate blood circulation, and dredge collaterals. Therefore, QM is used to treat the convalescent patients of COVID-19 with the syndromes of phlegm-stasis in channels. QM consists of 18 Chinese medicines (**Table 1**). Through clinical observation, QM was found to be effective in improving fatigue, asthma, respiratory function, and abnormal lung CT manifestations (ground-glass shadow, fiber rope shadow, and mesh shadow) in COVID-19 convalescent patients. QM is also recommended in the Chinese rehabilitation guideline for major dysfunctions of COVID-19 discharged patients (http://www.nhc.gov.cn/xcs/zhengcwj/202005/b15d59b5228341129cc8c5126f663b10.shtml) to treat COVID-19 convalescent patients. In addition, a randomized controlled clinical trial (RCT) is being performed in the Hubei Provincial Hospital of Traditional Chinese Medicine (Wuhan, China) to further clarify i) the clinical effects of QM against COVID-19–related PF and ii) its stimulatory effects on lung function improvement in severe and critical COVID-19 convalescent patients (registration number: ChiCTR2000032165). The preliminary statistical results of the RCT have indicated the effectiveness of QM for preventing post-COVID-19–related PF.

Network pharmacology, as a systematic pharmacology research method, shares much with the key ideas of the holistic view of TCM. Based on network pharmacology, the mechanisms and possible active ingredients of many TCM formulas (Qing-Luo-Yin, Liu-Wei-Di-Huang pill, and Shen-Qi-Di-Huang decoction) against complex diseases, such as cancer, metabolic syndrome, and diabetic nephropathy, were revealed (Li et al., 2007; Li and Zhang, 2013; Di et al., 2018). A previous network pharmacological analysis had predicted the mechanism underlying the protective effects of QM against PF: VEGF, TNF-α, IL-6, MMP9, and TGF-β1 are potential targets, and the activation of VEGF, Toll-like receptor 4, MAPK, and TGF-β1 signaling pathways may protect patients against PF (Jin et al., 2021). However, the active components of QM were not identified, and these underlying mechanisms have not been further confirmed. Therefore, we used UHPLC/Q-TOF-MS analysis to identify the compounds of QM and combined network pharmacology to predict the potential mechanisms underlying the anti-PF effects of QM. TGF-β1–induced A549 cells were used to verify the hypothesis from the network pharmacological analysis. This study provides new insights

TABLE 1 | Compositions of QM.

Chinese name	Taxonomy name	Drug name	Abbr.	Family	Weight (g)	Part used	Voucher specimen
Huang-qi	*Astragalus mongholicus* Bunge	Astragali radix	HQ	Fabaceae	15	Root	202106-01
Dang-shen	*Codonopsis pilosula* (Franch.) Nannf.	Codonopsis radix	DGS	Campanulaceae	9	Root	202106-02
Bai-zhu	*Atractylodes macrocephala* Koidz.	Atractylodis macrocephalae rhizoma	BZ	Asteraceae	9	Rhizome	202106-03
Nan-sha-shen	*Adenophora triphylla* (Thunb.) ADC.	Adenophorae radix	NSS	Campanulaceae	9	Root	202106-04
Bei-sha-shen	*Glehnia littoralis* (A. Gray) F. Schmidt ex Miq.	Glehniae radix	BSS	Apiaceae	9	Root	202106-05
Mai-dong	*Ophiopogon japonicus* (Thunb.) Ker Gawl.	Ophiopogonis radix	MD	Asparagaceae	15	Rhizome	202106-06
Chen-pi	*Citrus x aurantium* L.	Citri reticulatae pericarpium	CP	Rutaceae	9	Rind	202106-07
Fu-ling	*Poria cocos* (Schw.) Wolf.	Poria	FL	Polyporaceae	15	Sclerotium	202106-08
Ban-xia	*Pinellia ternata* (Thunb.) Makino	Pinelliae rhizoma	BX	Araceae	6	Tuber	202106-09
Dan-shen	*Salvia miltiorrhiza* Bunge	Salviae miltiorrhizae radix et rhizoma	DS	Lamiaceae	9	Root	202106-10
Zhe-bei-mu	*Fritillaria thunbergii* Miq	Fritillariae thunbergii bulbus	ZBM	Liliaceae	3	Bulb	202106-11
Shui-zhi	*Whitmania pigra* Whitman	Hirudo	SZ	Hirudinidae	3	Whole animal	202106-12
Tu-bie-chong	*Eupolyphaga sinensis* Walker	Eupolyphaga steleophaga	TBC	Corydiidae	3	Whole animal	202106-13
Gan-cao	*Glycyrrhiza glabra* L.	Glycyrrhizae radix et rhizoma	GAC	Fabaceae	6	Rhizome	202106-14
Shan-zha	*Crataegus pinnatifida* Bunge	Crataegi fructus	SHZ	Rosaceae	3	Fruit	202106-15
Shen-qu		Massa medicata fermentata	SQ		3	Leavening	202106-16
Mai-ya	*Hordeum vulgare* L.	Hordei fructus germinatus	MY	Poaceae	3	Fruit	202106-17
Shan-yao	*Dioscorea oppositifolia* L.	Dioscoreae rhizoma	SY	Dioscoreaceae	9	Rhizome	202106-18

into the pharmacological mechanism and possible active components of QM, which could support its clinical application to prevent progressive fibrosis in patients with pulmonary diseases.

MATERIALS AND METHODS

Preparation of the QM Extract

The 18 Chinese medicines of QM (**Table 1**) were purchased from Beijing General Pharmaceutical Corporation (Beijing, China) and provided by the Department of Pharmacy, Affiliated Hospital of Changchun University of Traditional Chinese Medicine (Changchun, China). The voucher specimens were deposited at the Jilin Ginseng Academy, Changchun University of Chinese Medicine (Changchun, China). According to the standard procedure from Chinese Pharmacopoeia (2020 edition), all of the raw materials (138 g, clinical dosage) were decocted by distilled water twice (1 h each time) at a mass ratio of 1:10 to obtain the water extract of QM. The water extract was filtered and centrifuged to obtain the supernatant, which was dried in vacuum to obtain the powdery extract with a yield of 24.6% (34 g). The QM powdery extract was used for the UHPLC/Q-TOF-MS analysis and further experiments (Zhang et al., 2020).

UHPLC/Q-TOF-MS Analysis of the QM Extract

The following reference compounds were used for the UHPLC/Q-TOF-MS analysis: calycosin 7-O-glucoside (batch number: 5240), complanatuside (batch number: 3037), ononin (batch number: 3811), neoisoliquiritin (batch number: 6971), neoliquiritin (batch number: 7543), formononetin (batch number: 3523), quercetin (batch number: 1116), genistin (batch number: 9435), oleanolic acid (batch number: 1339), oroxylin A (batch number: 6180), isoquercitrin (batch number: 5650), atractylodin A (batch number: 7361), and methylnissolin-3-O-glucoside (batch number: 3816). All were bought from Shanghai Sidande Standard Technical Service Co., Ltd. Shanghai, China. Schaftoside (batch number: DST200524-006), calycosin (batch number: DST190915-012), isoliquiritigenin (batch number: DST190719-016), naringin (batch number: DST191011-099), naringenin (batch number: DST200109-100), peimine (batch number: DST200109-011), peiminine (batch number: DSTDB001201), hesperidin (batch number: DST190716-038), neohesperidin (batch number: DSTDX003901), nobiletin (batch number: DSTDC003701), lobetyolin (batch number: DATDD003501), caffeic acid (batch number: DST190517-013), 5-O-demethylnobiletin (batch number: DSTDQ009401), 3′-demethylnobiletin (batch number: DST210212-120), betulinic acid (batch number: DST190508-026), and isoastragaloside I (batch number: DST180315-022) were purchased from Chengdu Deste Biotechnology Co., Ltd. (Chengdu, China). Liquiritin (batch number: PS012028) was purchased from Chengdu Pusi Biotechnology Co., Ltd. (Chengdu, China). Rapid characterization of the multicomponent from the QM extract was performed using a Waters ACQUITY UPLC I-Class Plus/Xevo G2-XS QTOF system (Waters, Milford, United States). Chromatographic separation was performed on a Waters ACQUITY UPLC BEH C18 column (2.1 mm × 100 mm, 1.7 μm) maintained at 30°C. The mobile phase was composed of 0.1% formic acid in water (A) and

0.1% formic acid in acetonitrile (B) running at 0.3 ml/min consistent with the following optimal gradient elution program: 0–4 min, 2–8% B; 4–7 min, 8–15% B; 7–11 min, 15–21% B; 11–14 min, 21% B; 14–16 min, 21–32% B; 16–19 min, 32% B; 19–24 min, 32–50% B; 24–27 min, 50–80% B; and 27–30 min, 80–95% B. The injection volume was 1 μl. High-resolution MS data were recorded on a Xevo G2-XS QTOF mass spectrometer by MS^E in both the positive and negative ESI modes. The source parameters were as follows: capillary voltage, −2.0 kV in the negative ESI mode and 3.0 kV in the positive ESI mode; source temperature, 100°C; and cone voltage, 40 V. The mass analyzer scanned over the mass range of *m/z* 50–1,500 at a low collision energy of 6 V and a high collision energy of 40–60 V for the recording of MS^1 and MS^2 spectra by MS^E, respectively. Processing of the obtained MS^E data was conducted using UNIFI™ 1.9.3.0 software (Waters, Milford, United States).

Characterization of QM Components From Rat Plasma

Seven male Wistar rats (weighing 250 ± 20 g) were treated by oral gavage with the clinical equal dose of the QM powdery extract (3 g/kg/day, equal to 12.4 g raw materials/kg/day), and the blood samples were collected 10 days after oral administration of QM. Prior to analysis by UHPLC/IM-QTOF-MS, the plasma samples were processed as described below. An aliquot of 200 μl of the plasma sample was added with 600 μl of methanol. The mixed sample was then vortexed for 3 min and centrifuged at 13,000 rpm for 10 min, to precipitate the proteins. The resulting supernatant was evaporated to dryness under a stream of nitrogen at 40°C, and the dried residue was further dissolved in 200 μl of methanol–water (1:1, *v*/*v*) solution. After centrifugation at 13,000 rpm for 10 min, the supernatant was used as the test solution and injected for analysis. Characterization of the QM components from the rat plasma was performed using a Waters ACQUITY UPLC I-Class/Vion IMS-QTOF mass spectrometer (Waters, Manchester, United Kingdom) by MS^E in both positive and negative ESI modes, following the same chromatography and MS conditions as described above for characterizing the multiple components from the QM extract.

Collection of Components and Disease Targets

The PubChem database was used to obtain the molecular structure (SDF format) of each QM compound (Wang et al., 2012). Then, the molecular structural files of identified compounds were uploaded to the PharmaMapper database, the ChemMapper database, and the SwissTarget database to predict their potential targets (Gong et al., 2013; Gfeller et al., 2014; Wang et al., 2017). Meanwhile, PF-related targets were collected using the GeneCards database (Stelzer et al., 2016). The gene and UniProt IDs of these potential targets were obtained from the UniProt database. Finally, the overlapping targets between the potential therapeutic targets of QM and the disease targets in PF were obtained for further network analysis.

Network Construction and Analysis

Cytoscape 3.8.0 was used to visualize the relationship between components of QM and the potential targets of each compound. To explore the interaction among target proteins, overlapping targets were uploaded to STRING and the information about the protein-protein interaction (PPI) was obtained(Szklarczyk et al., 2015). Importantly, the significant Gene Ontology (GO), KEGG, and Reactome pathways were screened by the DAVID database (Huang et al., 2009).

Molecular Docking

The molecular structures of the compounds were searched from the PubChem database and reconstructed in the ChemBioDraw. Then, these structures were saved as "mol2" file with the energy minimized and saved as docking ligands as "pdbqt" files in AutoDock version 4.2, respectively. The PDB database (https://www.rcsb.org/) was used to retrieve the 3D structure of TGF-β1 (PDB ID: 1KLA) and TGF-β receptor 1 (TGF-βR1, PDB ID: 1PY5) with the files in the "pdb" format. Discovery Studio Client version 4.5 was used to hydrogenate proteins, remove water, and remove ligand molecules. AutoDock version 4.2 was used to add the nonpolar hydrogen, calculate Gasteiger charges for the protein, save it as "pdbqt" files, and finally, run Vina for molecular docking. The active site of molecular docking was determined by the ligand coordinates in the target protein complex. The ligand was set to be flexible, and the receptor was set to be rigid. Each receptor–ligand interaction generates 50 conformations, and the conformation with the best affinity was used as the final docking conformation. If the binding energy is less than 0, the compound (ligand) and protein (receptor) can bind spontaneously. If binding energy ≤ −1.2 kCal/mol, the ligand–receptor was considered stable (Gomez-Garcia et al., 2018).

Cell Culture and Model Establishment

Human adenocarcinomic A549 cells with type II alveolar epithelial cell features were bought from the cell bank of the Shanghai Institute of Cell Biology, Chinese Academy, and cultured in RPMI 1640 containing 10% fetal bovine serum (FBS, Clark Bioscience, Claymont, United States), 100 kU/L penicillin, and 100 mg/L streptomycin (Biosharp, Hefei, China) at 37°C in a 5% CO_2 humidified incubator. When the cells were in good condition, TGF-β1 (5 ng/ml) was added to induce A549 cell transformation into mesenchymal-like cells. After 24 h, the A549 cells were observed under the microscope (Olympus CKX53, Japan) to see whether their morphology had changed from hexagonal to a spindle shape after TGF-β1 treatment (Zhang et al., 2019).

Cell Viability Assay

A549 cells were seeded into 96-well plates at a density of 3,000, 6,000, or 8,000 cells/well. The effect of QM on cell viability was analyzed after treatment for 24, 48, or 72 h at a concentration of 7.8–1,000 μg/ml. Additionally, A549 cells were divided into the control group (dimethyl sulfoxide, DMSO alone), the model group (5 ng/ml TGF-β1), and the

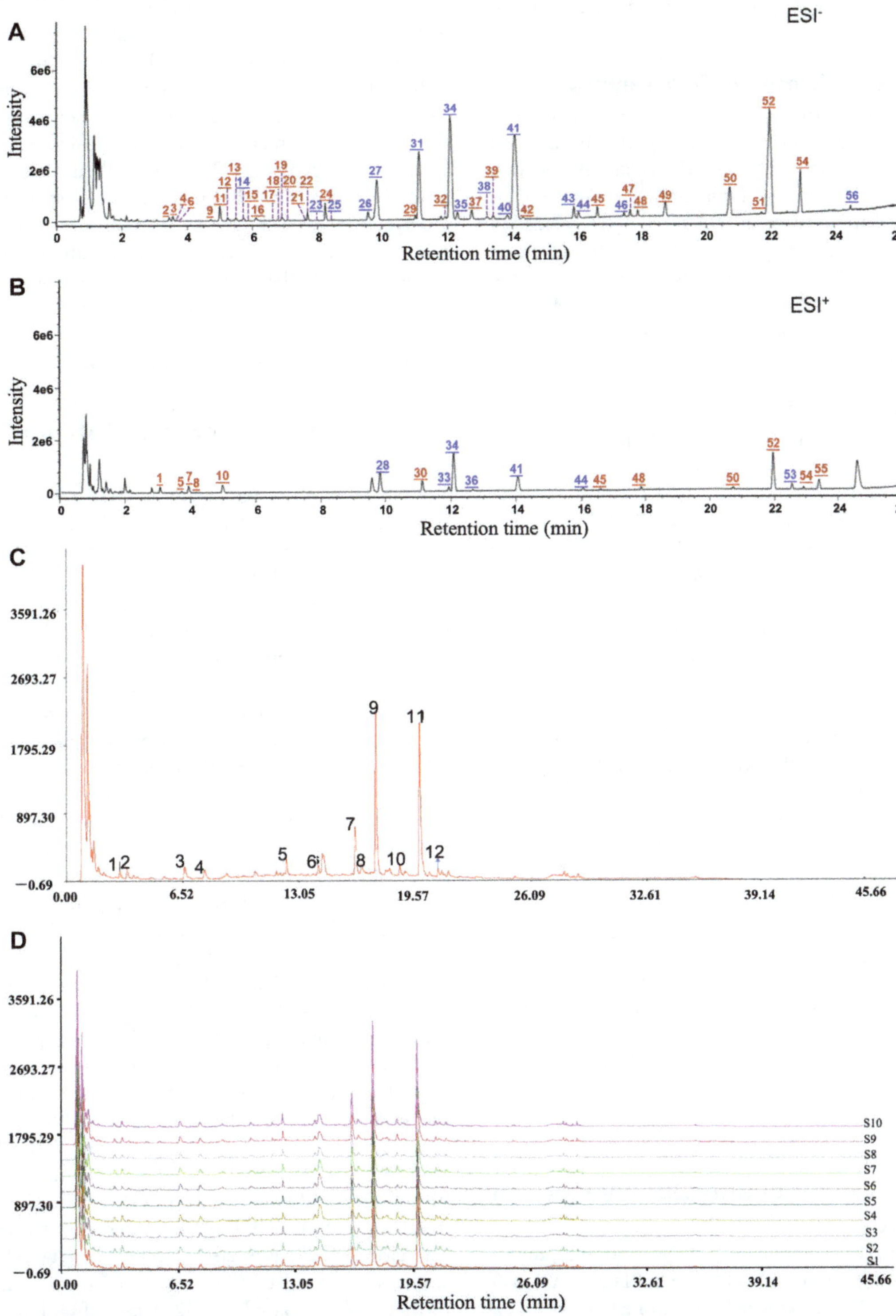

FIGURE 1 | Mass spectrum chromatograms of QM to screen for active components and analyze the reproducibility. **(A)** Negative ion mode. **(B)** Positive ion mode. Blue numbers represent those compounds that were identified through comparison with the reference standards. **(C,D)** The reproducible HPLC fingerprints of the mixture of 12 standard compounds and 10 batches of QM (S1–S10), using the Chinese Medicine Chromatographic Fingerprint Similarity Evaluation System (2012 Edition).

treatment group (5 ng/ml TGF-β1 + 7.8–1,000 μg/ml QM) to examine the effect of QM on the viability of TGF-β1-treated cells. After treatment for 24, 48, or 72 h, MTT (0.5 mg/ml) was added (Solibol, Beijing, China). DMSO (150 μl) was used to dissolve formazan crystals. Absorbance was measured at 490 nm using a microplate reader. The cell survival rate was calculated as the percentage of each group relative to the control group.

Quantitative Real-Time PCR Analysis

Total RNA was extracted from A549 cells using a total RNA extraction kit. Next, 1 μg of total RNA was reverse transcribed into cDNA with the iScript cDNA synthesis kit. A Bio-Rad CFX96 system was used to perform quantitative real-time PCR (qPCR) analysis, and the relative mRNA levels were calculated using the $2^{-\Delta\Delta Ct}$ method using GAPDH for normalization (Zhang et al., 2020). The primer sequences to amplify the genes encoding N-cadherin, E-cadherin, vimentin, α-SMA, LN, FN, collagen I, TGF-βR1, Smad7, and GAPDH are listed in **Supplementary Table S2**.

Western Blot Analysis

Antibodies against LN (ab11575), FN (ab2413), collagen I (ab34710), α-SMA (ab5694), E-cadherin (ab40772), N-cadherin (ab76011), vimentin (ab8978), TGF-βR1 (ab31013), Smad3 (ab40854), p-Smad3 (S423/S425 and ab52903), Smad7 (ab216428), and GAPDH (ab8245) were purchased from Abcam (Cambridge, MA, United States). After QM treatment, the total protein fraction was extracted from A549 cells by lysis in ice-cold RIPA buffer. Proteins were separated by SDS-PAGE and transferred onto PVDF membranes. After blocking for 1 h at room temperature with a blocking buffer containing 5% BSA, the membranes were incubated with the primary antibody overnight at 4°C. After washing, the membranes were incubated with the HRP-conjugated secondary antibody for 2 h. The protein bands were visualized using a chemiluminescent imaging system (ChemiDoc XRS+, Bio-Rad) and quantified by ImageJ software (Jiang et al., 2021).

Statistical Analysis

The data are expressed as mean ± standard deviation from three independent experiments. All of the data were statistically analyzed using GraphPad prism 9.0. Multiple groups were compared by one-way ANOVA (Tukey's *post hoc* test) to determine statistical significance. For all statistical analyses, $p < 0.05$ was considered to be statistically significant.

RESULTS

Chemical Components and Quality Control of QM Extract

To identify the chemical components of QM and analyze the consistency between various batches of QM, UHPLC/Q-TOF-MS analysis was conducted. The extracted ion chromatograms of all the compounds are shown in **Figures 1A,B**. A total of 56 components were characterized, among which 19 were accurately identified *via* comparison with the reference compounds. Information of these characterized components, including their assignments to the single drugs, is presented in **Supplementary Table S1**. These components were mainly from nine botanical drugs, that is, astragali radix (Huang-qi), citri reticulatae pericarpium (Chen-pi), salviae miltiorrhizae radix et rhizoma (Dan-shen), glycyrrhizae radix et rhizoma (Gan-cao), glehniae radix (Bei-sha-shen), atractylodis macrocephalae rhizoma (Bai-zhu), pinelliae rhizoma (Ban-xia), codonopsis radix (Dang-shen), and fritillariae thunbergii bulbus (Zhe-bei-mu). Nineteen compounds were identified by comparison with reference compounds, namely, atractyloside A, complanatuside, schaftoside, calycosin 7-O-glucoside, liquiritin, isoliquiritigenin, naringin, peimine, hesperidin, neohesperidin, peiminine, lobetyolin, neoisoliquiritin, ononin, methylnissolin-3-O-glucoside, calycosin, naringenin, nobiletin, and isoastragaloside I. Moreover, 10 batches of QM samples were analyzed, and similarity values of 0.983–0.999 were obtained by comparing with the reference spectrum, which indicated that the QM formula was reproducible (**Figures 1C,D**).

Network Establishment Between QM and PF

Combined with the PubChem database, 43 of the 56 chemical compounds from the UHPLC/Q-TOF-MS analysis had a well-defined molecular structure. Then, according to the "Network Pharmacology Evaluation Method Guidance" (Li, 2021), the 43 chemical compounds were used for the network pharmacological analysis. First, the PubChem database was used to obtain the molecular structure files of the 43 QM components. The potential therapeutic targets of the 43 ingredients were obtained from the PharmaMapper database, the ChemMapper database, the SwissTarget database, and the literature reports (Bunbupha et al., 2020; He et al., 2020a; Wang et al., 2021). These targets were screened according to many parameters, such as fit score ≥3.0 in the PharmaMapper database, score ≥0.4 in the ChemMapper database, and probability ≥0.4 in the SwissTarget database. After screening, we obtained the UniProt ID corresponding to each protein target and deleted reduplicated targets. Thus, a total of 452 potential therapeutic targets of QM were obtained (**Supplementary Table S4**). Second, the network of 43 active components and 452 potential targets of QM was constructed (**Supplementary Figure S1**). Furthermore, potential targets in PF were obtained from the GeneCards database, and 642 targets related to PF were obtained with the relevance score >11.63 (depending on the median to screen). Although the relevance score of angiotensin-converting enzyme 2 (ACE2) was lower than 11.63, ACE2 is an important target of COVID-19–related PF (Mourad and Levy, 2020), and QM is a TCM formula for the treatment of COVID-19 convalescent patients with PF. Therefore, ACE2 was also selected as a target of PF in this study, and a total of 643 targets of PF were screened out for further analysis. Based on 452 targets of QM and 643 targets in PF, 70 overlapping targets between QM and PF were obtained (**Supplementary Table S3**). Then, we established a network between the 43 QM components and 70 overlapping targets (**Figure 2A**). Through the network, we found that 2-succinyl-6-hydroxycyclohexa-2, 4-diene-1-carboxylic acid, and codonopsine were not connected with the overlapping targets. Then, the 70 overlapping targets were submitted to the STRING database to build the PPI network. As shown in

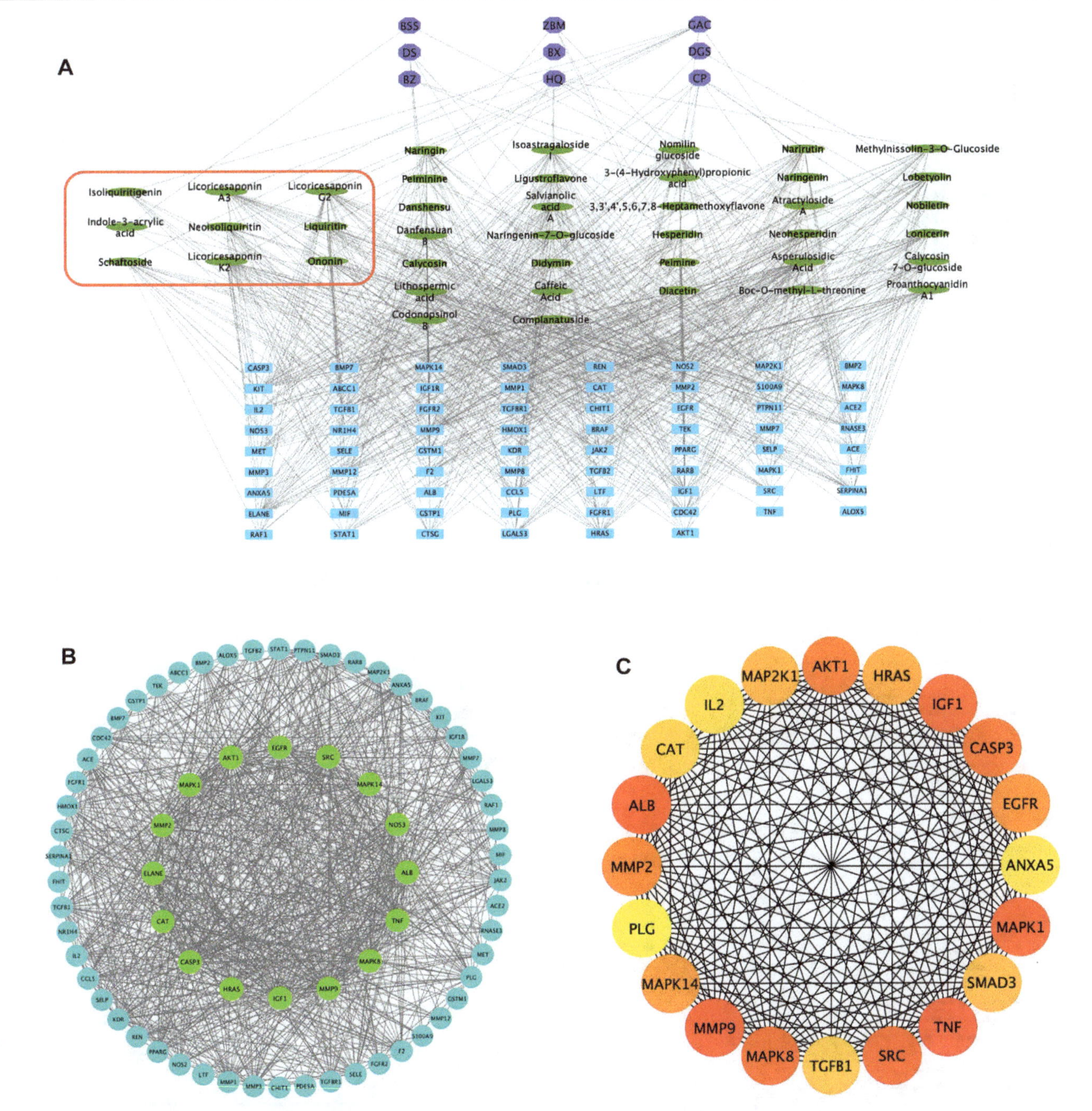

FIGURE 2 | Potential targets of QM components were predicted by network pharmacology analysis. **(A)** Construction of the network of 43 components–70 overlapping targets–nine botanical drugs. The green ovals represent the 43 active ingredients, the purple octagons represent the nine Chinese medicines, and the blue rectangles represent the 70 targets. The components circled by the red box are active ingredients isolated from rats' plasma. **(B)** Construction of the protein–protein network to identify potential targets of QM. The blue and green circles represent the overlapping targets. Topological analysis was used to screen more core targets of QM, according to degree ≥ 24, betweenness ≥ 0.01, and closeness ≥ 0.615, which are represented by the green circles. **(C)** The top 20 target networks are shown.

Figure 2B, the PPI network had 70 nodes and 866 edges. Subsequently, topological screening with degree ≥24, betweenness ≥0.01, and closeness ≥0.615 was used to screen key targets (**Figure 2B**). In addition, the top 20 targets of QM, such as TNF, MMP9, ALB, MAPK1, IGF1, SRC, MAPK8, CASP3, AKT1, MMP2, EGFR, MAPK14, HRAS, MAP2K1, SMAD3, TGFB1, CAT, IL2, ANXA5, and PLG, were selected and ranked with the maximal clique centrality (MCC) score (**Figure 2C**). Taken together, 70 potential targets of the 43 components of QM were obtained by network pharmacology.

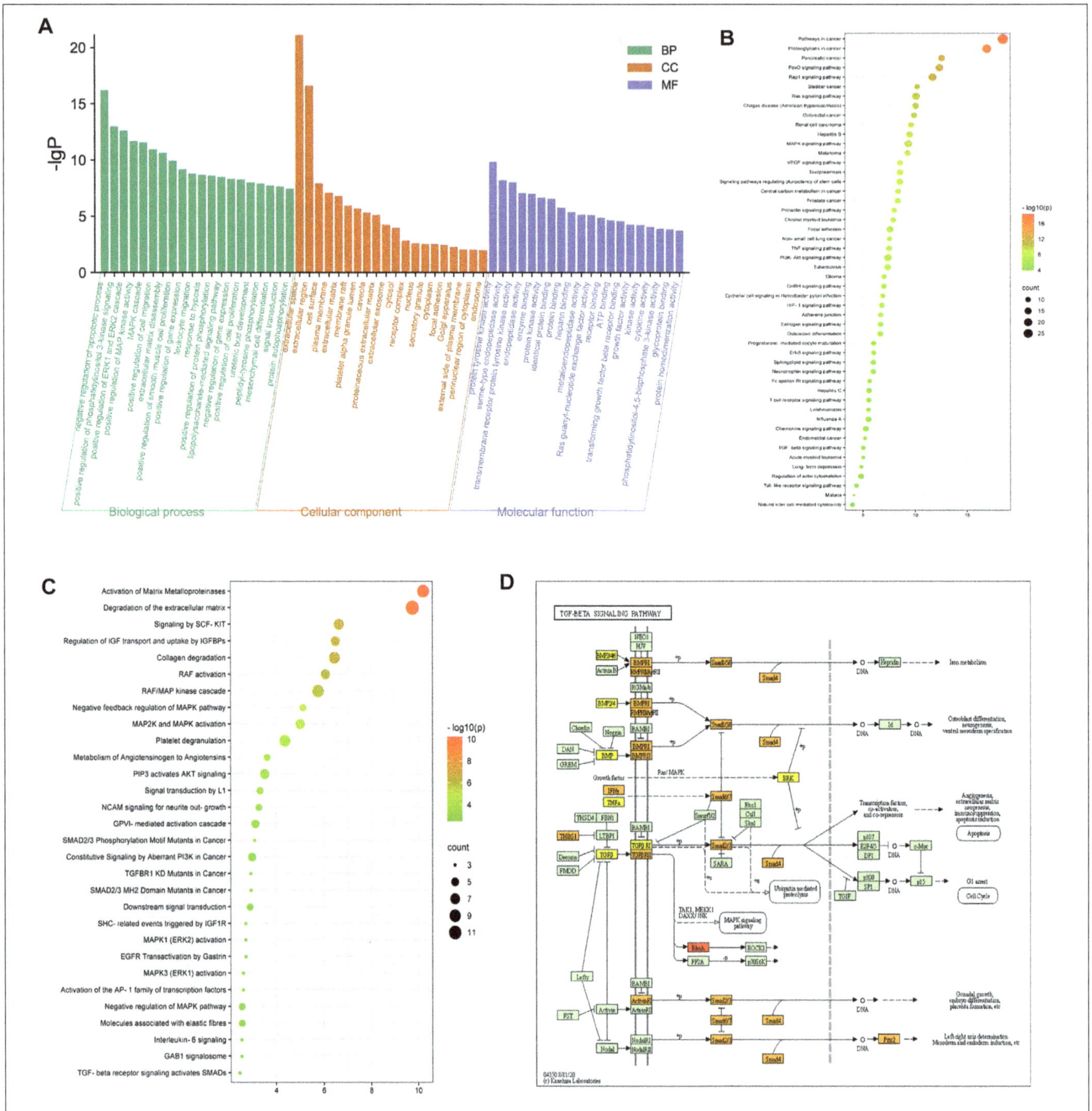

FIGURE 3 | Enrichment analysis of the potential targets of QM against PF was conducted based on the DAVID database. **(A)** Top 20 biological process (BP) terms, cellular component (CC) terms, and molecular function (MF) terms are shown as a bar diagram, according to the -lg p value. **(B,C)** The top 50 entries of KEGG pathway analysis and the top 30 entries of the Reactome pathway analysis were selected and ordered according to the -lg p value. **(D)** The TGF-β signaling pathway modified from hsa04350. Red represents targets of QM, orange represents key targets participated in PF, and yellow represents overlapping targets between QM and PF.

Enrichment Analysis

The 70 overlapping targets were submitted to the DAVID database to conduct GO enrichment analysis, from which we obtained 402 biological process (BP) terms (**Supplementary Table S5**), 36 cellular component (CC) terms (**Supplementary Table S6**), and 77 molecular function (MF) terms (**Supplementary Table S7**). The top 20 entries were respectively selected from BP, CC, and MF, in order of -lg p value (**Figure 3A**). In the BP category, ECM disassembly, mesenchymal cell differentiation, EMT, the collagen catabolic process, and proteolysis were directly related to PF. In the MF category, the targets were mainly involved in protein tyrosine

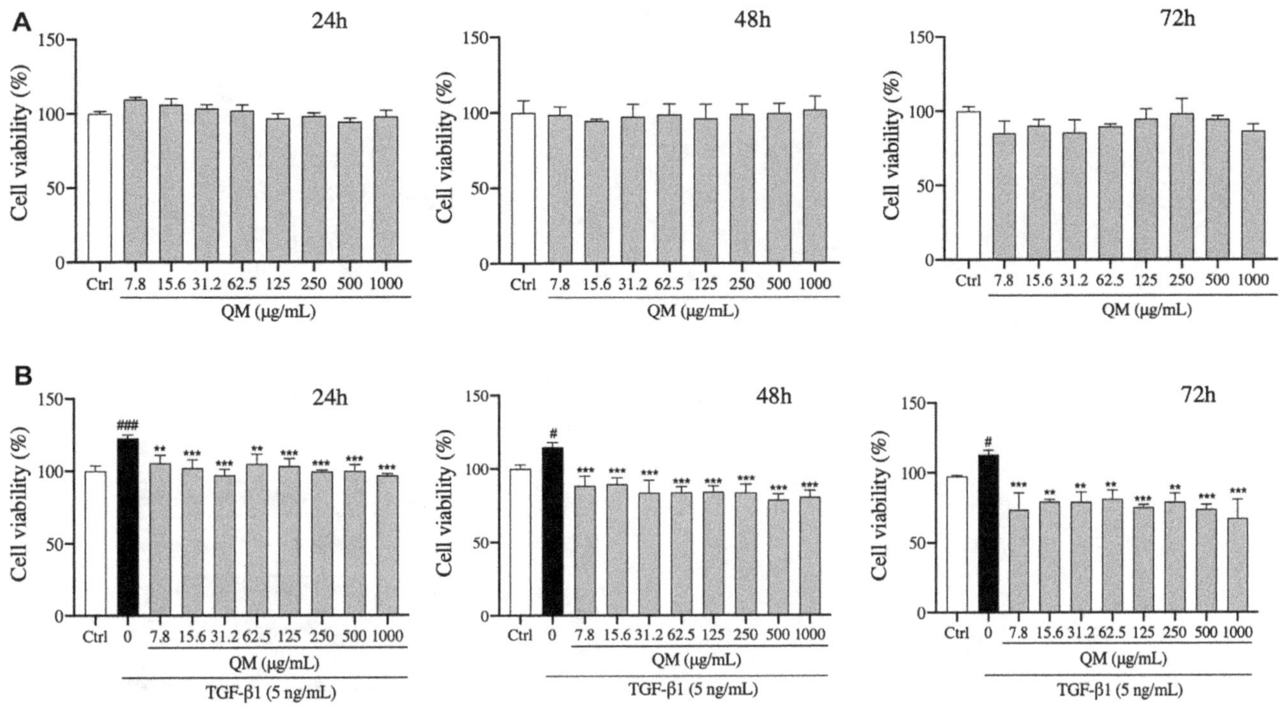

FIGURE 4 | QM inhibited the proliferation of TGF-β1–stimulated A549 cells. **(A)** After treatment with different doses of QM for 24, 48, and 72 h, the cytotoxicity of QM in A549 cells was evaluated by the MTT assay. **(B)** In TGF-β1–induced A549 cells, the effect of different doses of QM on cell viability after treatment for 24, 48, and 72 h was evaluated by the MTT assay. Data are shown as mean ± standard deviation from three independent experiments. $^{\#}p < 0.05$, $^{\#\#\#}p < 0.001$ versus the control group; $^{**}p < 0.01$ and $^{***}p < 0.001$ versus the model group (TGF-β1, 5 ng/ml).

kinase activity, protein kinase activity, TGF-β receptor binding, type II TGF-β receptor binding, protease binding, fibroblast growth factor–activated receptor activity, and fibroblast growth factor binding. The DAVID database was also used to obtain 71 Reactome pathway terms and 99 KEGG pathway terms (**Supplementary Tables S8, S9**). The top 50 entries of the KEGG database (**Figure 3B**) and the top 30 entries of the Reactome database (**Figure 3C**) were selected depending on the -lg p value. The KEGG pathways mainly included FoxO, Rap1, MAPK, VEGF, and TGF-β signaling pathways. The Reactome pathways mainly included activation of matrix metalloproteinases, degradation of the ECM, signaling by SCF-KIT, regulation of IGF transport and uptake by IGFBPs, collagen degradation, and activation of Smads by TGF-β receptor signaling. Collectively, the network pharmacological analysis indicated that QM may inhibit the TGF-β signaling pathway to mediate ECM accumulation, fibroblast activation, and EMT to prevent the progression of PF. The key targets of the TGF-β signaling pathway that participated in PF are shown in **Figure 3D**.

QM Inhibited TGF-β1–Induced A549 Cell Proliferation

The cytotoxicity of QM was tested. We found that QM at a concentration of 7.8–1,000 μg/ml was not cytotoxic for A549 cells after treatment for 24, 48, or 72 h (**Figure 4A**). Moreover, the viability of A549 cells was determined in the presence of TGF-β1 to mimic a pro-fibrotic environment. Compared with the control group, TGF-β1 significantly induced proliferation of A549 cells. After QM treatment at 7.8–1000 μg/ml for 24, 48, or 72 h, the proliferation of TGF-β1–induced A549 cells was decreased (**Figure 4B**). These data indicate that QM could inhibit the proliferation of TGF-β1–induced A549 cells.

QM Attenuated EMT in TGF-β1–Induced A549 Cells

TGF-β1 exerts strong pro-fibrotic effects and can induce EMT (Pezone et al., 2020), which is a phenomenon where inherent epithelial markers such as E-cadherin are lost and mesenchymal characteristics such as N-cadherin, vimentin, and α-SMA are gained (Cruz-Solbes and Youker, 2017). The morphology of A549 cells changes from hexagon to an elongated spindle-like shape when EMT occurs (Zhang et al., 2019). In the present study, after treatment with TGF-β1 (5 ng/ml) for 72 h, a spindle-like shape of A549 cells was observed (**Figure 5A**). When A549 cells were treated with QM at 125, 250, or 500 μg/ml, the mesenchymal-like morphology was attenuated compared with the TGF-β1–induced group (**Figure 5A**). To further verify the effects of QM in inhibiting EMT at the molecular level, qPCR and Western blot analyses were used to detect the EMT-related markers. After 72 h

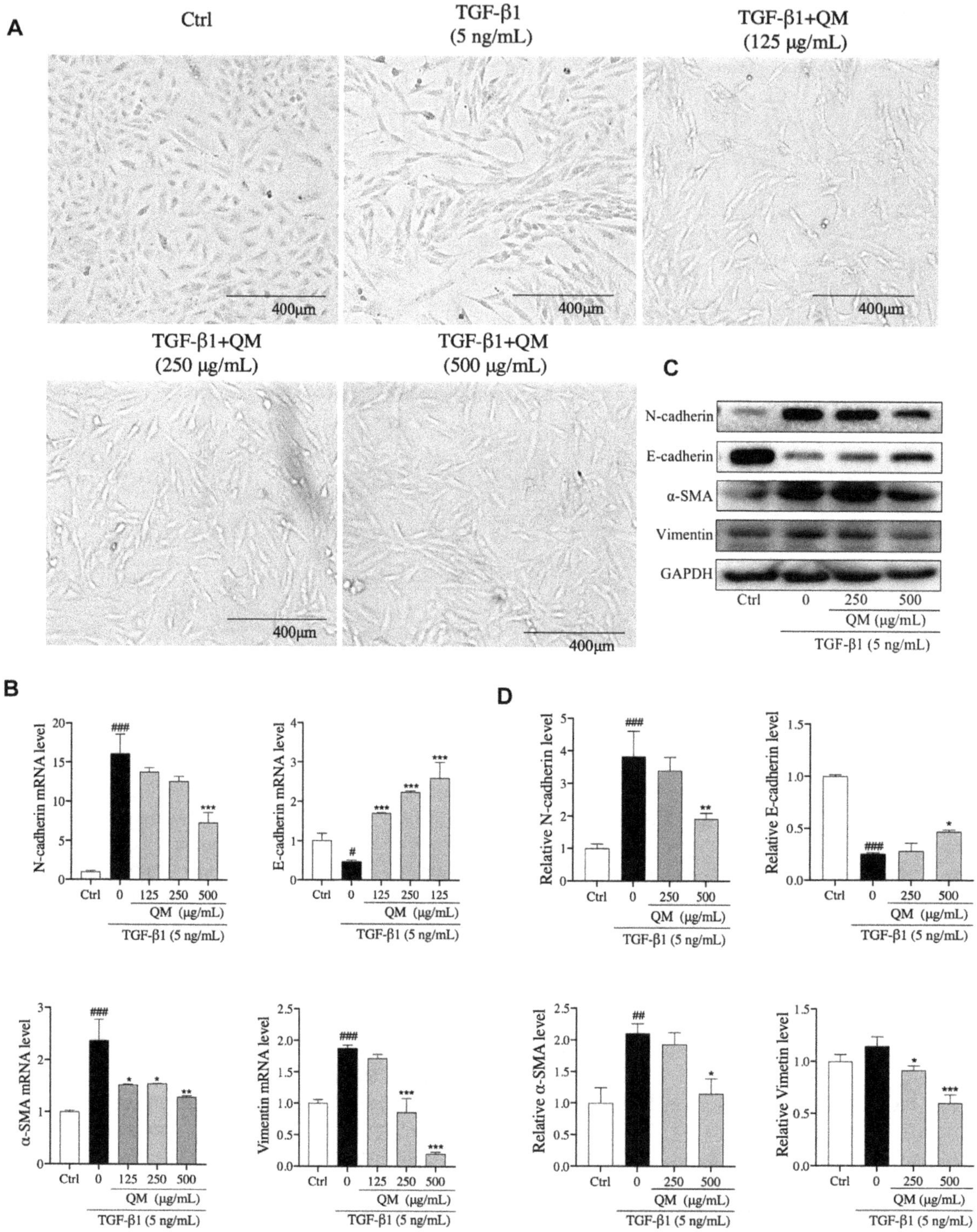

FIGURE 5 | QM-attenuated TGF-β1–induced EMT in A549 cells. **(A)** Representative light microscopic images of A549 cells treated with TGF-β1 and/or QM (125, 250, or 500 μg/ml). **(B)** After incubation with QM and TGF-β1 for 72 h, the mRNA levels of N-cadherin, E-cadherin, α-SMA, and vimentin in A549 cells were determined by qPCR analysis. GAPDH was used for normalization. **(C,D)** After treatment for 72 h, the protein levels of N-cadherin, E-cadherin, vimentin, and α-SMA in A549 cells from the control, TGF-β1, and TGF-β1 + QM groups were determined by Western blot analysis. GAPDH was used as the loading control. The relative levels of these proteins were calculated based on gray values from three independent experiments and normalized with GAPDH. $^{\#}p < 0.05$, $^{\#\#}p < 0.01$, $^{\#\#\#}p < 0.001$ versus the control group; $^{*}p < 0.05$, $^{**}p < 0.01$, and $^{***}p < 0.001$ versus the model group (TGF-β1, 5 ng/ml).

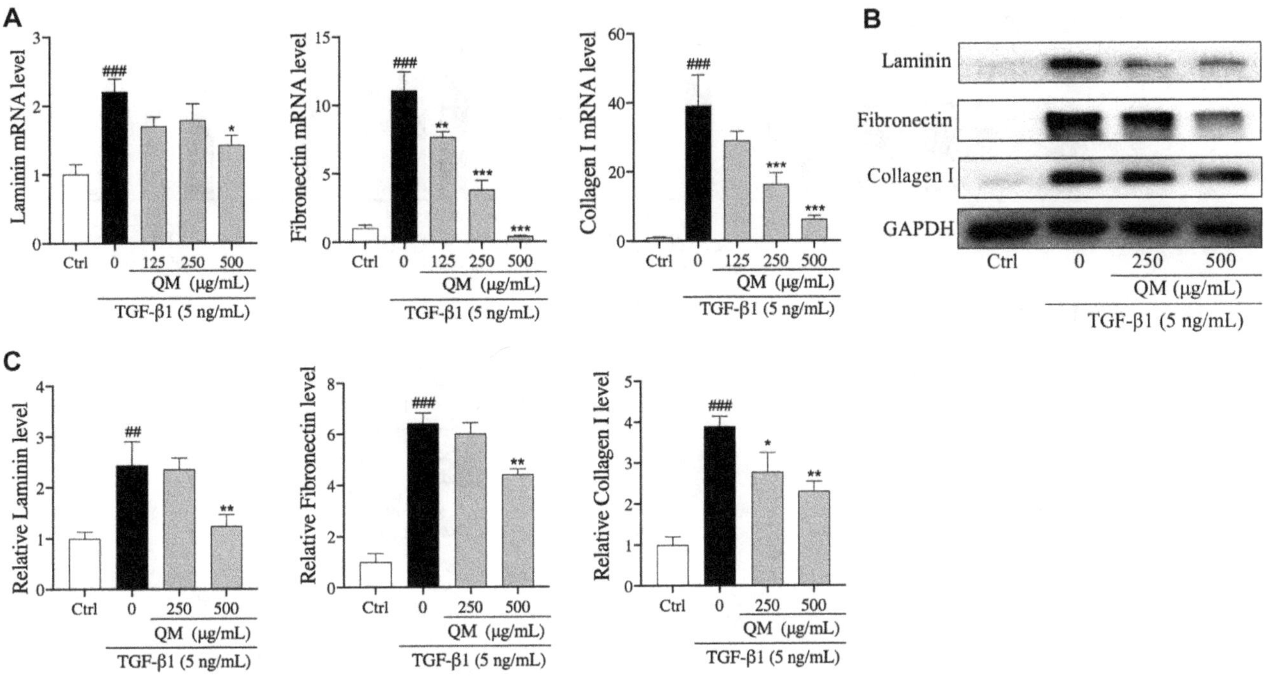

FIGURE 6 | QM promoted the degradation of ECM in TGF-β1–induced A549 cells. **(A)** After incubation with TGF-β1 and/or QM for 72 h, qPCR analysis was performed and the relative mRNA levels of laminin, fibronectin, and collagen I in A549 cells were calculated and normalized to GAPDH. **(B,C)** The protein levels of laminin, fibronectin, and collagen I in A549 cells treated with TGF-β1 and/or QM for 72 h were determined by Western blot analysis. GAPDH was used as the loading control. Data are from three independent experiments. $^{##}p < 0.01$, $^{###}p < 0.001$ versus the control group; $^{*}p < 0.05$, $^{**}p < 0.01$, and $^{***}p < 0.001$ versus the model group (TGF-β1, 5 ng/ml).

of incubation, qPCR results showed that the E-cadherin mRNA expression was decreased, whereas the mRNA levels of N-cadherin, α-SMA, and vimentin were upregulated in TGF-β1–induced A549 cells. Compared with the model group, the expression of E-cadherin was increased, and N-cadherin, α-SMA, and vimentin mRNA levels were downregulated after QM treatment at 125, 250, or 500 μg/ml (**Figure 5B**). Western blot analysis confirmed the qPCR results (**Figures 5C,D**). Together, these results demonstrated that QM inhibits EMT in TGF-β1–induced A549 cells.

QM Facilitated ECM Degradation in TGF-β1–Induced A549 Cells

The above findings revealed that EMT occurred in A549 cells after induction with TGF-β1. Cells with features of mesenchymal cells, such as fibroblasts and myofibroblasts, could secrete ECM proteins, such as collagen I, FN, and LN (Thiery et al., 2009). Excessive deposition of ECM is an important cause of organ fibrosis (Sun et al., 2013). In addition, the results of Reactome pathway enrichment from network pharmacology showed that QM could prevent PF *via* degrading ECM (**Figure 3**). To investigate the mechanisms by which QM stimulates ECM degradation, qPCR and Western blot analyses were conducted to investigate the protein and mRNA expression levels of key ECM markers, including LN, FN, and collagen I. The expression of collagen I, FN, and LN was significantly upregulated at the mRNA level in TGF-β1–induced A549 cells. QM treatment for 72 h decreased the level of collagen I, FN, and LN in a dose-dependent manner (**Figure 6A**). At the protein level, QM significantly reduced the TGF-β1–induced A549 cells which resulted in the increase in LN, FN, and collagen I levels. The inhibitory effects of QM on ECM accumulation were the strongest at a concentration of 500 μg/ml (**Figures 6B,C**). Together, these results suggested that QM stimulates ECM degradation in TGF-β1–induced A549 cells.

QM Inhibited the TGF-β/Smad3 Pathway

TGF-β/Smads signaling is a classical pathway in the occurrence and progression of organ fibrosis (He X. et al., 2020), giving rise to the occurrence of EMT and ECM deposition (Pardali et al., 2017). Moreover, the results of our network pharmacological analysis also showed that QM may exert its anti-PF effects through the TGF-β signaling pathway (**Figures 3B–D**). To further verify whether QM could regulate the TGF-β/Smads pathway, TGF-βR1, Smad7, and Smad3 and its phosphorylation, as downstream proteins of TGF-β1, were detected by western blot and/or qPCR. As shown in **Figure 7A**; **Supplementary Figure S2**, TGF-βR1 was significantly upregulated, and Smad3 phosphorylation was induced by TGF-β1 in the model group. After QM treatment for 72 h, these indicators were downregulated. Moreover, in TGF-β1–stimulated A549 cells, there was no change in the Smad3

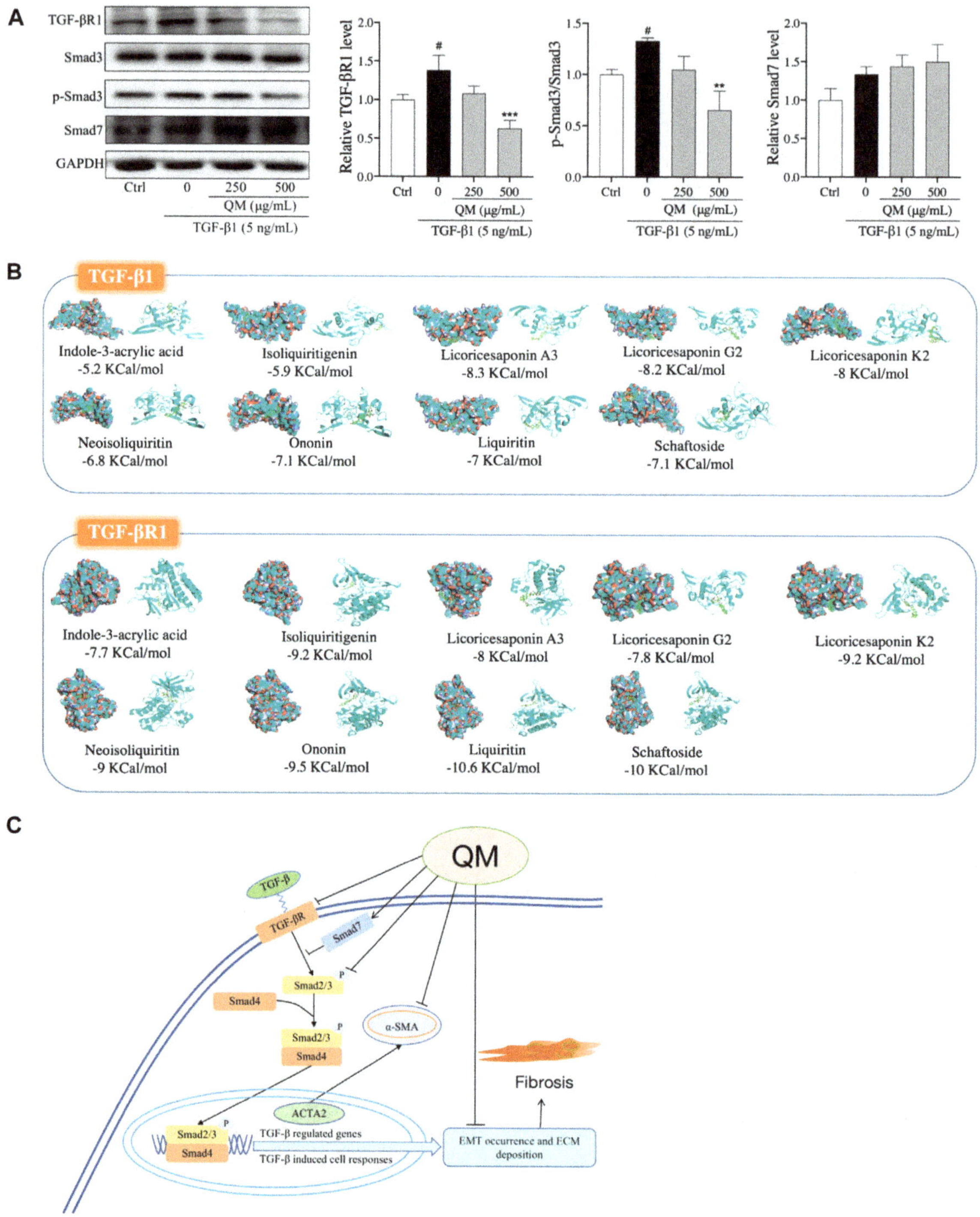

FIGURE 7 | QM inhibited the TGF-β1/Smad3 pathway to block PF progression. **(A)** After incubation with QM and TGF-β1 for 72 h, the protein levels of TGF-βR1, Smad3, *p*-Smad3 (S423/S425), and Smad7 in A549 cells were determined by Western blot analysis. GAPDH was used as the loading control. The ratio of *p*-Smad3/Smad3 was calculated from three independent experiments after normalization to GAPDH. $^{\#}p < 0.05$ versus the control group; $^{**}p < 0.01$ and $^{***}p < 0.001$ versus the model group (TGF-β1 5 ng/ml). **(B)** The molecular docking simulation results, including the compounds, the targets, and the lowest binding free energy. Green rectangles represent the compounds. The diagrams on the left are the surface appearances and those on the right are cartoon appearances of targets. **(C)** Scheme demonstrating the molecular mechanism underlying the effects of QM in preventing and treating PF.

protein level in the QM-treated group, which meant that QM inhibited the TGF-β1–induced increase in the p-Smad3/Smad3 ratio. In addition, as an inhibitor of the TGF-β/Smad3 pathway, TGF-β1 could increase the expression of Smad7 due to feedback action (Wang et al., 2014). But QM treatment had no effect on the increased Smad7 level induced by TGF-β1. Taken together, these results indicated that QM could inhibit the TGF-β1/Smad3 pathway in TGF-β1–induced A549 cells.

Analysis of Effective QM Components in the Rat Plasma

To identify the effective components of QM against PF, the QM components that could be absorbed into the bloodstream were characterized by UHPLC/IM-QTOF-MS. By comparing the MS data, the peaks that appeared in the corresponding positions of the QM-administered plasma and QM extract but did not appear in the blank rat plasma were considered as the prototype compounds absorbed into the plasma of rats. Accordingly, 10 prototype compounds were identified in the rat plasma: indole-3-acrylic acid from glehniae radix (Bei-sha-shen), schaftoside from pinelliae rhizoma (Ban-xia), and ononin from astragali radix (Huang-qi), and other seven components were from glycyrrhizae radix et rhizoma (Gan-cao), such as liquiritin, isoliquiritigenin, neoisoliquiritin, licoricesaponin A3, licoricesaponin G2, yunganoside G1, and licoricesaponin K2. The detailed information expressed by # is displayed in **Supplementary Table S1**. These results demonstrated that glycyrrhizae radix et rhizoma (Gan-cao) might be a key botanical drug of QM for preventing PF. However, the real and potential compounds responsible for the anti-PF effect of QM should be further identified in the mouse model with PF.

Molecular Docking

We further explored the relationship between i) the nine effective components that can be absorbed into the bloodstream and ii) the TGF-β signaling pathway. Molecular docking was used to analyze the binding energies of the nine compounds with TGF-β1 and TGF-βR1. As shown in **Figure 7B**, the nine compounds all had good binding affinities with TGF-β1 and TGF-βR1, especially the compounds from glycyrrhizae radix et rhizome (Gan-cao), such as liquiritin, isoliquiritigenin, neoisoliquiritin, licoricesaponin A3, licoricesaponin G2, and licoricesaponin K2. The molecular docking results indicated that the nine compounds from QM could all potentially regulate the TGF-β signaling pathway. However, the pharmacology action of these active components in inhibiting the TGF-β signaling pathway needs to further investigate in the cell or animal models.

DISCUSSION

In our study, UHPLC/Q-TOF-MS analysis was first used to analyze the composition of QM, leading to the identification of 56 components. Combined with the PubChem database and the literature studies, 43 compounds were identified or tentatively characterized. Based on these components, network pharmacology was used to predict the potential mechanisms of QM in preventing PF. First, 452 potential therapeutic targets of QM were obtained through several databases and the literature studies, and a network of 43 ingredients and 452 targets was established, from which the multicomponent and multi-target characteristics of the TCM formula were observed. Meanwhile, 643 genes related to PF were screened, and 70 overlapping targets between QM and PF were identified. Based on the STRING database and 70 overlapping targets, a PPI network was established and analyzed, from which the main targets of QM in anti-PF function were obtained, including TNF, MMPs, MAPKs, SRC, CASP3, AKT1, EGFR, IL2, SMAD3, TGFB1/2, and TGFBR1. These targets participate in many progresses involved in PF, such as the inflammatory response, ECM deposition, EMT, and fibroblast differentiation (Hou et al., 2018; Espindola et al., 2021). In addition, a previous study screening drugs by scoring viral fibrosis based on MAPK activity indicated EGFR is a main regulator of COVID-19–related fibrosis (Vagapova et al., 2021). Our GO functional enrichment results showed that QM mainly influences ECM degradation, mesenchymal cell differentiation, EMT, protein tyrosine and kinase activity, TGF-β and type II TGF-β receptor binding, fibroblast growth factor–activated receptor activity, and fibroblast growth factor binding, which are closely connected with the progression of PF. The KEGG and Reactome pathway enrichment analyses mainly revealed the involvement of the FoxO, Rap1, MAPK, VEGF, and TGF-β signaling pathways, activation of MMPs, and degradation of the ECM and collagen. Taken together, the results of network pharmacology indicated that EMT, fibroblast activation, ECM degradation, and the TGF-β/Smads signaling pathway are key mechanisms underlying the anti-PF effects of QM, among which the EMT and ECM accumulation are downstream actions of the TGF-β/Smads signaling pathway (Xu et al., 2009; Lederer and Martinez, 2018; Chen, 2020). However, except for the TGF-β pathway, the potential roles of other signaling pathways as targets of QM should be further investigated, based on our network pharmacology results.

To verify the effects of QM and the mechanism underlying TGF-β/Smads signaling pathway regulation, ECM degradation, and EMT inhibition, TGF-β1–induced A549 cells were used to conduct a series of experiments. The TGF-β/Smads signaling pathway was shown to mediate EMT (Pardali et al., 2017; Yao et al., 2019). Notably, lung cancer cells infected by SARS-CoV-2 could induce metabolic and transcriptional changes consistent with EMT (Stewart et al., 2021). In addition, TGF-β–induced fibroblast activation and myofibroblast differentiation is a central pathway of PF, which could increase ECM production and abnormal deposition. ECM deposition is a key factor in the development of tissue remodeling and may lead to impaired lung function and symptoms of diseases such as asthma, COPD, and IPF (Liu et al., 2021). Moreover, previous studies have shown that the level of TGF-β is elevated in COVID-19 patients' serum and upper airway samples (Montalvo Villalba et al., 2020; Ghazavi et al., 2021). Therefore, excessive ECM deposition is a main trigger for PF formation in COVID-19 convalescent patients (Habermann et al., 2020). In the present study, we first measured the markers related to EMT and ECM accumulation to evaluate the effects of QM in attenuating EMT and promoting ECM degradation. Then, the TGF-β1/Smad3 pathway was evaluated to confirm the mechanisms underlying the effects of QM. As shown in **Figure 7C**, our results demonstrate that QM can block the TGF-β1/Smad3 pathway to inhibit EMT and ECM deposition, which might be a critical functional mechanism of QM against PF.

To further analyze the possible active components of QM, the plasma of rats administrated with QM was analyzed by UHPLC/IM-QTOF-MS, and 10 active ingredients were obtained, among which the seven are originated from glycyrrhizae radix et rhizome (Gan-cao). Previous studies have shown that the components of glycyrrhizae radix et rhizome (Gan-cao) such as liquiritin, isoliquiritigenin, isoangustone A, and glycyrrhizin, could prevent organ fibrosis *via* many pathways, such as the TGF-β/Smad3, NF-κB, and MAPK signaling pathways (Li et al., 2010; Guan et al., 2012; Yan et al., 2018). Moreover, the ononin that originated from astragali radix (Huang-qi) was proven to inhibit cardiac fibrosis *via* the AMPK/mTOR signaling pathway (Pan et al., 2021). In addition, the binding energies were calculated based on molecular docking simulations, from which we found that the nine components potentially own the ability to bind to TGF-β1 and TGF-βR1 and, hence, regulate the TGF-β signaling pathway.

CONCLUSION

In summary, we identified 56 chemical compounds from the QM extract and 10 effective components from the plasma of QM-administrated rats, based on which, we conducted a network pharmacology analysis predicting that TGF-β–mediated EMT inhibition and ECM degradation are potential mechanisms underlying the anti-PF effects of QM. Furthermore, QM is proven to attenuate EMT and degrade ECM *via* the inhibition of the TGF-β1/Smad3 signaling pathway in TGF-β1–induced A549 cells. These findings shed light on the molecular mechanism and the possible active components of QM underlying its anti-PF effects, thus supporting the clinical application of QM for COVID-19 convalescent patients.

AUTHOR CONTRIBUTIONS

YY, LD, YL, JM, and SS performed the experiments. YY and TB performed the network pharmacology analysis. YY and LD analyzed data and drafted the manuscript. TB performed the molecular docking. ZG, QL, ZiW, JZ and JW assisted with experiments and revised the manuscript. XL and DZ supervised the experiments and the manuscript. ZeW, LZ and XT designed and revised the manuscript. All authors read and approved the final version of the manuscript.

FUNDING

This work was supported by the National Natural Science Foundation of China (No. 81804013), the Key Research and Development Program of Jilin Province (No. 20200404057YY), and the Special Project for Emergency of the Ministry of Science and Technology (No. 2020YFC0845000).

ACKNOWLEDGMENTS

We thank the kind support from Wenzhi Yang (State Key Laboratory of Component-based Chinese Medicine, Tianjin Key Laboratory of TCM Chemistry and Analysis, Tianjin University of Traditional Chinese Medicine, Tianjin, China) for detecting active components. We thank LetPub (www.letpub.com) for its linguistic assistance during the preparation of this manuscript.

REFERENCES

Asselah, T., Durantel, D., Pasmant, E., Lau, G., and Schinazi, R. F. (2021). COVID-19: Discovery, Diagnostics and Drug Development. *J. Hepatol.* 74, 168–184. doi:10.1016/j.jhep.2020.09.031

Bian, X. W. (2020). Autopsy of COVID-19 Patients in China. *Natl. Sci. Rev.* 7, 1414–1418. doi:10.1093/nsr/nwaa123

Bonnans, C., Chou, J., and Werb, Z. (2014). Remodelling the Extracellular Matrix in Development and Disease. *Nat. Rev. Mol. Cel Biol* 15, 786–801. doi:10.1038/nrm3904

Bunbupha, S., Apaijit, K., Maneesai, P., Prasarttong, P., and Pakdeechote, P. (2020). Nobiletin Ameliorates High-Fat Diet-Induced Vascular and Renal Changes by Reducing Inflammation with Modulating AdipoR1 and TGF-B1 Expression in Rats. *Life Sci.* 260, 118398. doi:10.1016/j.lfs.2020.118398

Chen, W. (2020). A Potential Treatment of COVID-19 with TGF-β Blockade. *Int. J. Biol. Sci.* 16, 1954–1955. doi:10.7150/ijbs.46891

Cruz-Solbes, A. S., and Youker, K. (2017). Epithelial to Mesenchymal Transition (EMT) and Endothelial to Mesenchymal Transition (EndMT): Role and Implications in Kidney Fibrosis. *Results Probl. Cel Differ* 60, 345–372. doi:10.1007/978-3-319-51436-9_13

Di, S., Han, L., Wang, Q., Liu, X., Yang, Y., Li, F., et al. (2018). A Network Pharmacology Approach to Uncover the Mechanisms of Shen-Qi-Di-Huang Decoction against Diabetic Nephropathy. *Evid. Based Complement. Alternat Med.* 2018, 7043402. doi:10.1155/2018/7043402

Espindola, M. S., Habiel, D. M., Coelho, A. L., Stripp, B., Parks, W. C., Oldham, J., et al. (2021). Differential Responses to Targeting Matrix Metalloproteinase 9 in Idiopathic Pulmonary Fibrosis. *Am. J. Respir. Crit. Care Med.* 203, 458–470. doi:10.1164/rccm.201910-1977OC

Flaherty, K. R., Wells, A. U., Cottin, V., Devaraj, A., Walsh, S. L. F., Inoue, Y., et al. (2019). Nintedanib in Progressive Fibrosing Interstitial Lung Diseases. *N. Engl. J. Med.* 381, 1718–1727. doi:10.1056/NEJMoa1908681

Forcina, L., Miano, C., Scicchitano, B. M., and Musarò, A. (2019). Signals from the Niche: Insights into the Role of IGF-1 and IL-6 in Modulating Skeletal Muscle Fibrosis. *Cells* 11, 232. doi:10.3390/cells8030232

George, P. M., Wells, A. U., and Jenkins, R. G. (2020). Pulmonary Fibrosis and COVID-19: the Potential Role for Antifibrotic Therapy. *Lancet Respir. Med.* 8, 807–815. doi:10.1016/S2213-2600(20)30225-3

Gfeller, D., Grosdidier, A., Wirth, M., Daina, A., Michielin, O., and Zoete, V. (2014). SwissTargetPrediction: a Web Server for Target Prediction of Bioactive Small Molecules. *Nucleic Acids Res.* 42, W32–W38. doi:10.1093/nar/gku293

Ghazavi, A., Ganji, A., Keshavarzian, N., Rabiemajd, S., and Mosayebi, G. (2021). Cytokine Profile and Disease Severity in Patients with COVID-19. *Cytokine* 137, 155323. doi:10.1016/j.cyto.2020.155323

Gomez-Garcia, O., Andrade-Pavon, D., Campos-Aldrete, E., Ballinas-Indili, R., Mendez-Tenorio, A., Villa-Tanaca, L., et al. (2018). Synthesis, Molecular Docking, and Antimycotic Evaluation of Some 3-Acyl Imidazo[1,2-A] pyrimidines. *Molecules* 23, 599. doi:10.3390/molecules23030599

Gong, J., Cai, C., Liu, X., Ku, X., Jiang, H., Gao, D., et al. (2013). ChemMapper: a Versatile Web Server for Exploring Pharmacology and Chemical Structure Association Based on Molecular 3D Similarity Method. *Bioinformatics* 29, 1827–1829. doi:10.1093/bioinformatics/btt270

Guan, Y., Li, F. F., Hong, L., Yan, X. F., Tan, G. L., He, J. S., et al. (2012). Protective Effects of Liquiritin Apioside on Cigarette Smoke-Induced Lung Epithelial Cell Injury. *Fundam. Clin. Pharmacol.* 26, 473–483. doi:10.1111/j.1472-8206.2011.00956.x

Habermann, A. C., Gutierrez, A. J., Bui, L. T., Yahn, S. L., Winters, N. I., Calvi, C. L., et al. (2020). Single-cell RNA Sequencing Reveals Profibrotic Roles of Distinct Epithelial and Mesenchymal Lineages in Pulmonary Fibrosis. *Sci. Adv.* 6, eaba1972. doi:10.1126/sciadv.aba1972

He, J., Peng, H., Wang, M., Liu, Y., Guo, X., Wang, B., et al. (2020a). Isoliquiritigenin Inhibits TGF-B1-Induced Fibrogenesis through Activating Autophagy via PI3K/AKT/mTOR Pathway in MRC-5 Cells. *Acta Biochim. Biophys. Sin (Shanghai)* 52, 810–820. doi:10.1093/abbs/gmaa067

He, X., Cheng, R., Huang, C., Takahashi, Y., Yang, Y., Benyajati, S., et al. (2020b). A Novel Role of LRP5 in Tubulointerstitial Fibrosis through Activating TGF-β/Smad Signaling. *Signal. Transduct Target. Ther.* 5, 45. doi:10.1038/s41392-020-0142-x

Hou, J., Ma, T., Cao, H., Chen, Y., Wang, C., Chen, X., et al. (2018). TNF-α-induced NF-Kb Activation Promotes Myofibroblast Differentiation of LR-MSCs and Exacerbates Bleomycin-Induced Pulmonary Fibrosis. *J. Cel Physiol* 233, 2409–2419. doi:10.1002/jcp.26112

Huang, C., Huang, L., Wang, Y., Li, X., Ren, L., Gu, X., et al. (2021). 6-month Consequences of COVID-19 in Patients Discharged from Hospital: a Cohort Study. *Lancet* 397, 220–232. doi:10.1016/S0140-6736(20)32656-8

Huang, D. W., Sherman, B. T., and Lempicki, R. A. (2009). Systematic and Integrative Analysis of Large Gene Lists Using DAVID Bioinformatics Resources. *Nat. Protoc.* 4, 44–57. doi:10.1038/nprot.2008.211

Ji, J., Tao, P., and He, L. (2019). Kangxianling Decoction Prevents Renal Fibrosis in Rats with 5/6 Nephrectomy and Inhibits Ang II-Induced ECM Production in Glomerular Mesangial Cells. *J. Pharmacol. Sci.* 139, 367–372. doi:10.1016/j.jphs.2019.03.003

Jiang, L., Yin, X., Chen, Y. H., Chen, Y., Jiang, W., Zheng, H., et al. (2021). Proteomic Analysis Reveals Ginsenoside Rb1 Attenuates Myocardial Ischemia/reperfusion Injury through Inhibiting ROS Production from Mitochondrial Complex I. *Theranostics* 11, 1703–1720. doi:10.7150/thno.43895

Jin, D., An, X., Zhang, Y., Zhao, S., Duan, L., Duan, Y., et al. (2021). Potential Mechanism Prediction of Herbal Medicine for Pulmonary Fibrosis Associated with SARS-CoV-2 Infection Based on Network Analysis and Molecular Docking. *Front. Pharmacol.* 12, 602218. doi:10.3389/fphar.2021.602218

King, T. E., Jr., Bradford, W. Z., Castro-Bernardini, S., Fagan, E. A., Glaspole, I., Glassberg, M. K., et al. (2014). A Phase 3 Trial of Pirfenidone in Patients with Idiopathic Pulmonary Fibrosis. *N. Engl. J. Med.* 370, 2083–2092. doi:10.1056/NEJMoa1402582

King, T. E., Jr., Pardo, A., and Selman, M. (2011). Idiopathic Pulmonary Fibrosis. *Lancet* 378, 1949–1961. doi:10.1016/S0140-6736(11)60052-4

Lederer, D. J., and Martinez, F. J. (2018). Idiopathic Pulmonary Fibrosis. *N. Engl. J. Med.* 378, 1811–1823. doi:10.1056/NEJMra1705751

Li, J., Kang, S. W., Kim, J. L., Sung, H. Y., Kwun, I. S., and Kang, Y. H. (2010). Isoliquiritigenin Entails Blockade of TGF-Beta1-SMAD Signaling for Retarding High Glucose-Induced Mesangial Matrix Accumulation. *J. Agric. Food Chem.* 58, 3205–3212. doi:10.1021/jf9040723

Li, S., and Zhang, B. (2013). Traditional Chinese Medicine Network Pharmacology: Theory, Methodology and Application. *Chin. J. Nat. Med.* 11, 110–120. doi:10.1016/S1875-5364(13)60037-0

Li, S., Zhang, Z. Q., Wu, L. J., Zhang, X. G., Li, Y. D., and Wang, Y. Y. (2007). Understanding ZHENG in Traditional Chinese Medicine in the Context of Neuro-Endocrine-Immune Network. *IET Syst. Biol.* 1, 51–60. doi:10.1049/iet-syb:20060032

Li, S. (2021). Network Pharmacology Evaluation Method Guidance-Draft. *World J. Traditional Chin. Med.* 7, 148. doi:10.4103/wjtcm.wjtcm_11_21

Liu, G., Philp, A. M., Corte, T., Travis, M. A., Schilter, H., Hansbro, N. G., et al. (2021). Therapeutic Targets in Lung Tissue Remodelling and Fibrosis. *Pharmacol. Ther.* 225, 107839. doi:10.1016/j.pharmthera.2021.107839

Martinez, F. J., Collard, H. R., Pardo, A., Raghu, G., Richeldi, L., Selman, M., et al. (2017). Idiopathic Pulmonary Fibrosis. *Nat. Rev. Dis. Primers* 3, 17074. doi:10.1038/nrdp.2017.74

Meng, X. M., Nikolic-Paterson, D. J., and Lan, H. Y. (2016). TGF-β: the Master Regulator of Fibrosis. *Nat. Rev. Nephrol.* 12, 325–338. doi:10.1038/nrneph.2016.48

Meyer, K. C. (2017). Pulmonary Fibrosis, Part I: Epidemiology, Pathogenesis, and Diagnosis. *Expert Rev. Respir. Med.* 11, 343–359. doi:10.1080/17476348.2017.1312346

Montalvo Villalba, M. C., Valdés Ramírez, O., Muné Jiménez, M., Arencibia Garcia, A., Martinez Alfonso, J., González Baéz, G., et al. (2020). Interferon Gamma, TGF-B1 and RANTES Expression in Upper Airway Samples from SARS-CoV-2 Infected Patients. *Clin. Immunol.* 220, 108576. doi:10.1016/j.clim.2020.108576

Mourad, J. J., and Levy, B. I. (2020). Interaction between RAAS Inhibitors and ACE2 in the Context of COVID-19. *Nat. Rev. Cardiol.* 17, 313. doi:10.1038/s41569-020-0368-x

Nalbandian, A., Sehgal, K., Gupta, A., Madhavan, M. V., Mcgroder, C., Stevens, J. S., et al. (2021). Post-acute COVID-19 Syndrome. *Nat. Med.* 27, 601–615. doi:10.1038/s41591-021-01283-z

Pan, R., Zhuang, Q., and Wang, J. (2021). Ononin Alleviates H2O2-Induced Cardiomyocyte Apoptosis and Improves Cardiac Function by Activating the AMPK/mTOR/autophagy Pathway. *Exp. Ther. Med.* 22, 1307. doi:10.3892/etm.2021.10742

Pardali, E., Sanchez-Duffhues, G., Gomez-Puerto, M. C., and Ten Dijke, P. (2017). TGF-β-Induced Endothelial-Mesenchymal Transition in Fibrotic Diseases. *Int. J. Mol. Sci.* 18, 2157. doi:10.3390/ijms18102157

Pezone, A., Taddei, M. L., Tramontano, A., Dolcini, J., Boffo, F. L., De Rosa, M., et al. (2020). Targeted DNA Oxidation by LSD1-Smad2/3 Primes TGF-B1/EMT Genes for Activation or Repression. *Nucleic Acids Res.* 48, 8943–8958. doi:10.1093/nar/gkaa599

Richeldi, L., Collard, H. R., and Jones, M. G. (2017). Idiopathic Pulmonary Fibrosis. *Lancet* 389, 1941–1952. doi:10.1016/S0140-6736(17)30866-8

Salton, F., Volpe, M. C., and Confalonieri, M. (2019). Epithelial⁻Mesenchymal Transition in the Pathogenesis of Idiopathic Pulmonary Fibrosis. *Medicina (Kaunas)* 55, 83. doi:10.3390/medicina55040083

Stelzer, G., Rosen, N., Plaschkes, I., Zimmerman, S., Twik, M., Fishilevich, S., et al. (2016). The GeneCards Suite: From Gene Data Mining to Disease Genome Sequence Analyses. *Curr. Protoc. Bioinformatics* 54, 1.30.1–1.30.33. doi:10.1002/cpbi.5

Stewart, C. A., Gay, C. M., Ramkumar, K., Cargill, K. R., Cardnell, R. J., Nilsson, M. B., et al. (2021). Lung Cancer Models Reveal SARS-CoV-2-Induced EMT Contributes to COVID-19 Pathophysiology. *bioRxiv.* doi:10.1101/2020.05.28.122291

Sun, K., Tordjman, J., Clément, K., and Scherer, P. E. (2013). Fibrosis and Adipose Tissue Dysfunction. *Cell Metab* 18, 470–477. doi:10.1016/j.cmet.2013.06.016

Szklarczyk, D., Franceschini, A., Wyder, S., Forslund, K., Heller, D., Huerta-Cepas, J., et al. (2015). STRING V10: Protein-Protein Interaction Networks, Integrated over the Tree of Life. *Nucleic Acids Res.* 43, D447–D452. doi:10.1093/nar/gku1003

Thiery, J. P., Acloque, H., Huang, R. Y., and Nieto, M. A. (2009). Epithelial-mesenchymal Transitions in Development and Disease. *Cell* 139, 871–890. doi:10.1016/j.cell.2009.11.007

Vagapova, E. R., Lebedev, T. D., and Prassolov, V. S. (2021). Viral Fibrotic Scoring and Drug Screen Based on MAPK Activity Uncovers EGFR as a Key Regulator of COVID-19 Fibrosis. *Sci. Rep.* 11, 11234. doi:10.1038/s41598-021-90701-w

Wang, C. M., Chen, J., Jiang, M., Xuan, X. P., and Li, H. X. (2014). Relationship between Artesunate Influence on the Process of TGF-Beta1 Induced Alveolar Epithelial Cells Transform into Mesenchymal Cells and on Idiopathic Pulmonary Fibrosis. *Yao Xue Xue Bao* 49, 142–147. doi:10.16438/j.0513-4870.2014.01.012

Wang, R., Wu, G., Dai, T., Lang, Y., Chi, Z., Yang, S., et al. (2021). Naringin Attenuates Renal Interstitial Fibrosis by Regulating the TGF-β/Smad Signaling Pathway and Inflammation. *Exp. Ther. Med.* 21, 66. doi:10.3892/etm.2020.9498

Wang, X., Shen, Y., Wang, S., Li, S., Zhang, W., Liu, X., et al. (2017). PharmMapper 2017 Update: a Web Server for Potential Drug Target Identification with a Comprehensive Target Pharmacophore Database. *Nucleic Acids Res.* 45, W356–w360. doi:10.1093/nar/gkx374

Wang, Y., Xiao, J., Suzek, T. O., Zhang, J., Wang, J., Zhou, Z., et al. (2012). PubChem's BioAssay Database. *Nucleic Acids Res.* 40, D400–D412. doi:10.1093/nar/gkr1132

Xu, J., Lamouille, S., and Derynck, R. (2009). TGF-beta-induced Epithelial to Mesenchymal Transition. *Cell Res* 19, 156–172. doi:10.1038/cr.2009.5

Yan, T., Wang, H., Cao, L., Wang, Q., Takahashi, S., Yagai, T., et al. (2018). Glycyrrhizin Alleviates Nonalcoholic Steatohepatitis via Modulating Bile Acids and Meta-Inflammation. *Drug Metab. Dispos* 46, 1310–1319. doi:10.1124/dmd.118.082008

Yan, Z., Kui, Z., and Ping, Z. (2014). Reviews and Prospectives of Signaling Pathway Analysis in Idiopathic Pulmonary Fibrosis. *Autoimmun. Rev.* 13, 1020–1025. doi:10.1016/j.autrev.2014.08.028

Yao, Y., Chen, R., Wang, G., Zhang, Y., and Liu, F. (2019). Exosomes Derived from Mesenchymal Stem Cells Reverse EMT via TGF-β1/Smad Pathway and Promote Repair of Damaged Endometrium. *Stem Cel Res Ther* 10, 225. doi:10.1186/s13287-019-1332-8

Zhang, C., Zhu, X., Hua, Y., Zhao, Q., Wang, K., Zhen, L., et al. (2019). YY1 Mediates TGF-B1-Induced EMT and Pro-fibrogenesis in Alveolar Epithelial Cells. *Respir. Res.* 20, 249. doi:10.1186/s12931-019-1223-7

Zhang, Z., Zhai, L., Lu, J., Sun, S., Wang, D., Zhao, D., et al. (2020). Shen-Hong-Tong-Luo Formula Attenuates Macrophage Inflammation and Lipid Accumulation through the Activation of the PPAR-Γ/lxr-A/abca1 Pathway. *Oxid Med. Cel Longev* 2020, 3426925. doi:10.1155/2020/3426925

6

Network Pharmacology Databases for Traditional Chinese Medicine

Runzhi Zhang, Xue Zhu, Hong Bai and Kang Ning**

School of Life Science and Technology, Huazhong University of Science and Technology, Wuhan, China

Correspondence:
Hong Bai
baihong@hust.edu.cn
Kang Ning
ningkang@hust.edu.cn

The research field of systems biology has greatly advanced and, as a result, the concept of network pharmacology has been developed. This advancement, in turn, has shifted the paradigm from a "one-target, one-drug" mode to a "network-target, multiple-component-therapeutics" mode. Network pharmacology is more effective for establishing a "compound-protein/gene-disease" network and revealing the regulation principles of small molecules in a high-throughput manner. This approach makes it very powerful for the analysis of drug combinations, especially Traditional Chinese Medicine (TCM) preparations. In this work, we first summarized the databases and tools currently used for TCM research. Second, we focused on several representative applications of network pharmacology for TCM research, including studies on TCM compatibility, TCM target prediction, and TCM network toxicology research. Third, we compared the general statistics of several current TCM databases and evaluated and compared the search results of these databases based on 10 famous herbs. In summary, network pharmacology is a rational approach for TCM studies, and with the development of TCM research, powerful and comprehensive TCM databases have emerged but need further improvements. Additionally, given that several diseases could be treated by TCMs, with the mediation of gut microbiota, future studies should focus on both the microbiome and TCMs to better understand and treat microbiome-related diseases.

Keywords: network pharmacology, Traditional Chinese Medicine, database, assessment and comparison, completeness

OPPORTUNITIES AND CHALLENGES FOR THE MODERNIZATION OF TRADITIONAL CHINESE MEDICINE

Traditional Chinese Medicine

Traditional Chinese Medicine (TCM) is one of the greatest treasures of Chinese culture, has a long history of use in East and Southeast Asia, and has been widely used since ancient civilization. Through continuous development and innovation, physicians have selected the essence and discarded the dross of TCM. As a result, TCM has become one of the main forms of alternative medicine in East Asia, North America, and Europe. TCMs use therapeutic herbs to treat diseases according to the combinatorial principle of "King, Vassal, Assistant, and Delivery servant" based on a patient's syndrome and to restore balance of life and body functions (Yi and Chang, 2004; Qiu, 2007). Each prescribed combination of these herbs is referred to as a TCM preparation, or TCM prescription, for example the LiuWeiDiHuangWan (LWDHW) pill. Traditionally, the discovery of most new drugs is focused on identifying or designing a pharmacologically effective agent that specifically interacts with a single target. During the past 30 years, such an approach has generated highly successful drugs. However, drugs acting on individual molecular targets usually exert unsatisfying therapeutic effects or have toxicity when used to treat certain diseases, such as diabetes, inflammation, and cancer (Kola and Landis, 2004). Given the major bottleneck in drug discovery, drug research, and development have gradually shifted from a "one-target, one-drug" mode to a "network-target, multiple-component-therapeutics" mode (Li, 2011; Li et al., 2011, 2014b). To treat disease, the holistic philosophy of TCM shares key concepts with the new mode of drug discovery. Therefore, making full use of TCM is of great importance for drug research. In recent years, TCM has gradually garnered interest thanks to its low toxicity and therapeutic effects (Chan, 1995; Corson and Crews, 2007; Qiu, 2007). For example, *Ganoderma lucidum,* termed "LingZhi" in China, has been used as a health-preserving and therapeutic agent. Previous studies have shown that it possesses medicinal properties, including anti-cancer, anti-diabetic, anti-hepatotoxic, and immunomodulatory effects (Paterson, 2006; Boh et al., 2007, Boh, 2013; Ma et al., 2015). *Panax ginseng* is another TCM that has been used therapeutically for more than 2,000 years to treat such diseases as cardiovascular disease, Alzheimer's disease, and diabetes (Lee et al., 2008; Kim, 2012; Yuan et al., 2012; Chan et al., 2013). Unlike modern drugs discovered by targeting a specific protein, however, the understanding of the molecular basis of TCM remains limited, and research into modern TCM theory has lagged, which has slowed down the development of novel TCMs (Corson and Crews, 2007). TCM studies must keep pace with the rapid development of modern science to remain relevant. Therefore, a scientific and effective assessment system needs to be established, which will be key for studying and making full use of TCMs.

Network Pharmacology: An Appropriate Approach for Modern TCM Research

Given the rapid progress in bioinformatics, systems biology, and polypharmacology, network-based drug discovery is considered to be a promising approach for cost-effective drug development. Systems biology examines biological systems by systematically perturbing them; monitoring the gene, protein, and informational pathway responses; integrating these data; and, ultimately, formulating mathematical models to describe the structure of the system and its response to individual perturbations (Ideker et al., 2001). Based on a systems biology approach, the concept of network pharmacology was first proposed by Li et al. (2014b). Because network pharmacology can provide a full or partial understanding of the principles of network theory and systems biology, it has been considered the next paradigm in drug discovery (Hopkins, 2008). Furthermore, the network pharmacology approach has been used to study "compound-proteins/genes-disease" pathways, which are capable of describing complexities among biological systems, drugs, and diseases from a network perspective, sharing a similar holistic philosophy as TCM. Applications of systems biology methods to determine the pharmacological action, mechanism of action, and safety of TCMs are invaluable for modern research and development of TCM. Thus, a new interdisciplinary method termed TCM network pharmacology has been proposed (Li and Zhang, 2013; Liang et al., 2014a; Li et al., 2014b), which has initiated a new research paradigm for transforming TCM from an experience-based to evidence-based medicine. In this work, we first summarized the currently widely used databases and tools for TCM network pharmacology research. Second, we concentrated on the different applications of network pharmacology to TCM research, including TCM recipes, target prediction, and network toxicology. Third, we compared different TCM databases based on their basic properties and search results (**Figure 1**).

TOOLS AND DATABASES FOR TCM NETWORK PHARMACOLOGY RESEARCH

With the rapid development of research, network pharmacology has become a new approach for drug mechanism research and drug development. In recent years, a variety of related databases and tools have provided crucial support for TCM network pharmacology research. Commonly used databases for TCM network pharmacology research include TCM databases [TCM database@Taiwan (Chen, 2011), HIT (Ye et al., 2011), TCMSP (Ru et al., 2014), and TCMID (Xue et al., 2013)), compound and drug information databases (Drugbank (Wishart et al., 2006), STITCH (Kuhn et al., 2014), ChEMBL (Gaulton et al., 2012), and PubChem (Wang et al., 2009)], target interaction databases [STRING (Szklarczyk et al., 2015), HPRD (Peri et al., 2003), MINT (Zanzoni et al., 2002), IntAct (Kerrien et al., 2012), Reactome (D'Eustachio, 2009), and HAPPI (Chen et al., 2009)], and gene-disease association databases [OMIM (Hamosh et al., 2002) and GAD (Becker et al., 2004; **Table 1**)]. Recently, we also proposed TCM-Mesh (Zhang et al., 2017), a more comprehensive TCM database that embodies the core idea of TCM network pharmacology. Based on these biological databases and clinical trial results, researchers can analyze the "herbs-compounds-proteins/genes-diseases" interaction network from the perspective of systems biology, which will provide an understanding of the effects of herbs on diseases. Furthermore, network pharmacology algorithms and tools are particularly vital in mining these databases for knowledge. For example, the Random Walk (Chen et al., 2012) algorithm is a commonly used network clustering algorithm, which starts from a random node (drug, target, or disease) and calculates the similarity of this node and its adjacent node to construct a "drug-target-disease" network. Moreover, the PRINCE (Vanunu et al., 2010) algorithm is used to prioritize disease genes and infer protein complex associations, based on formulating constraints on the prioritization function which is related with its smoothness over the network and usage of prior information. In addition to data acquisition and analysis, visualization is a key element of network pharmacology that makes the network more intuitive. Cytoscape (Shannon et al., 2003) is

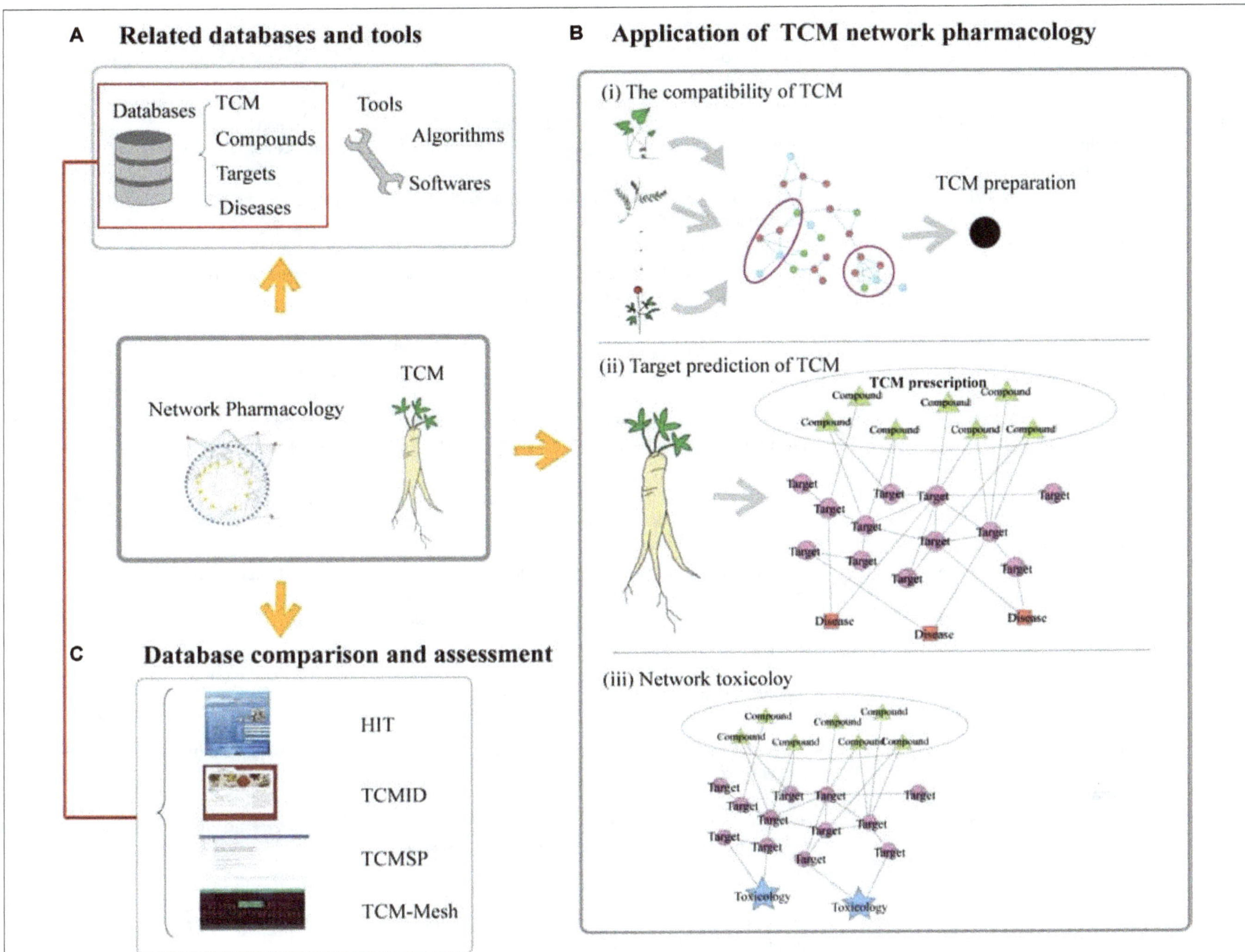

FIGURE 1 | Overall schema of the databases, tools, and applications of TCM network pharmacology analysis. **(A)** Related databases (TCM, compounds, targets, and disease databases) and tools (algorithms and software) used for TCM network pharmacology research. **(B)** The application of network pharmacology to TCM research: (i) the compatibility of TCM; (ii) target prediction of TCM; and (iii) network toxicology. **(C)** Comparison among several TCM databases based on the general statistics and search results.

an open-source platform suitable for visualizing molecular interaction networks and biological pathways and integrating these networks with annotations, gene expression profiles, and other state data. Pajek (Dohleman, 2006) is another powerful network analysis tool that is used to examine various complex non-linear networks.

NETWORK PHARMACOLOGY RESEARCH AND TCM

In recent years, an increasing number of studies have focused on the area of TCM network pharmacology. According to statistics in PubMed and the China National Knowledge Infrastructure (CNKI) databases, the number of published papers (**Figure 2**) has increased over time. These statistics demonstrate the increasing interest in the application of network pharmacology to TCM.

To date, network pharmacology has been applied to studies of many traditional Chinese herbs and herbal prescriptions. As listed in **Table 2**, researchers have conducted many network-based computational and experimental studies to detect effective substances and determine the mechanisms of herbal formulas against many diseases.

Compatibility of TCM Ingredients

Traditional Chinese Medicine preparation (in other words, TCM prescription) is the main form of TCM, and it is produced under the guidance of TCM syndrome differentiation and treatment, which is highly scientific. The traditional "King, Vassal, Assistant, and Delivery servant" combination rule of TCM herbal formulas contains the rich and profound scientific connotation of TCM theory. Thus, the ability to explain the compatibility of TCM is one of the most challenging tasks for TCM research. Li et al. (2010) proposed a method named the

TABLE 1 | Public databases, algorithms, and software related to TCM network pharmacology.

Type		Name	Description	Website for database or tool	Reference
Databases	**TCM-related databases**	TCM-Mesh	An integration of database and a data-mining system for network pharmacology analysis of TCM preparations	http://mesh.tcm.microbioinformatics.org	Zhang et al., 2017
		TCM database@Taiwan	The world's largest and most comprehensive free small molecular database on TCM for virtual screening	http://tcm.cmu.edu.tw	Chen, 2011
		HIT	A comprehensive and fully curated database to complement available resources on protein targets for FDA-approved drugs as well as the promising precursor compounds	http: //lifecenter.sgst.cn/hit	Ye et al., 2011
		TCMSP	A unique systems pharmacology platform of TCMs that captures the relationships among drugs, targets, and diseases	http://lsp.nwu.edu.cn/tcmsp.php	Ru et al., 2014
		TCMID	A comprehensive database that provides information and bridges the gap between TCM and modern life sciences	http://www.megabionet.org/tcmid	Xue et al., 2013
	Drug-related databases		A unique bioinformatics and cheminformatics resource that combines detailed drug data with comprehensive drug target information	https: //www.drugbank.ca	Wishart et al., 2006
		STITCH	A database of known and predicted interactions between chemicals and proteins	http://stitch.embl.de	Kuhn et al., 2014
		ChEMBL	An Open Data database containing binding, functional, and ADMET information for a large number of drug-like bioactive compounds	https://www.ebi.ac.uk/chembl	Gaulton et al., 2012
		PubChem	A public information system for analyzing the bioactivities of small molecules	https://pubchem.ncbi.nlm.nih.gov	Wang et al., 2009
	Target-related databases	STRING	A database of known and predicted protein-protein interactions	https://string-db.org	Szklarczyk et al., 2015
		HPRD	An object database that integrates a wealth of information relevant to the function of human proteins in health and disease	http://www.hprd.org	Peri et al., 2003
		MINT	A database that focuses on experimentally verified protein-protein interactions mined from the scientific literature by expert curators	https: //mint.bio.uniroma2.it	Zanzoni et al., 2002
		IntAct	A freely available, open-source database system and analysis tool for molecular interaction data	https: //www.ebi.ac.uk/intact	Kerrien et al., 2012
		Reactome	A free, open-source, curated, and peer-reviewed pathway database	https://reactome.org	D'Eustachio, 2009
		HAPPI	An online database of comprehensive human annotated and predicted protein interactions	http: //discovery.informatics.uab.edu/HAPPI	Chen et al., 2009
	Disease-related databases	OMIM	A comprehensive, authoritative compendium of human genes and genetic phenotypes that is freely available and updated daily	https://www.omim.org	Hamosh et al., 2002
		GAD	A database of genetic association data from complex diseases and disorders	https: //geneticassociationdb.nih.gov	Becker et al., 2004
Algorithms		Random walk	An algorithm that predicts potential drug-target interactions on a large scale under the hypothesis that similar drugs often target similar target proteins and the framework of Random Walk	https: //www.rdocumentation.org/packages/diffusr/versions/0.1.4/topics/random.walk	Chen et al., 2012
		PRINCE	A global, network-based method for prioritizing disease genes and inferring protein complex associations	https://github.com/fosterlab/PrInCE	Vanunu et al., 2010
Software		Cytoscape	A software environment for integrated models of biomolecular interaction networks	https://cytoscape.org	Shannon et al., 2003
		Pajek	A tool for complex network analysis	http://mrvar.fdv.uni-lj.si/pajek	Dohleman, 2006

These public databases are categorized into four types: TCM-related, drug-related, target-related, and disease-related. Publicly available tools and visualization software use data from these databases. Websites and references are provided for all of these resources.

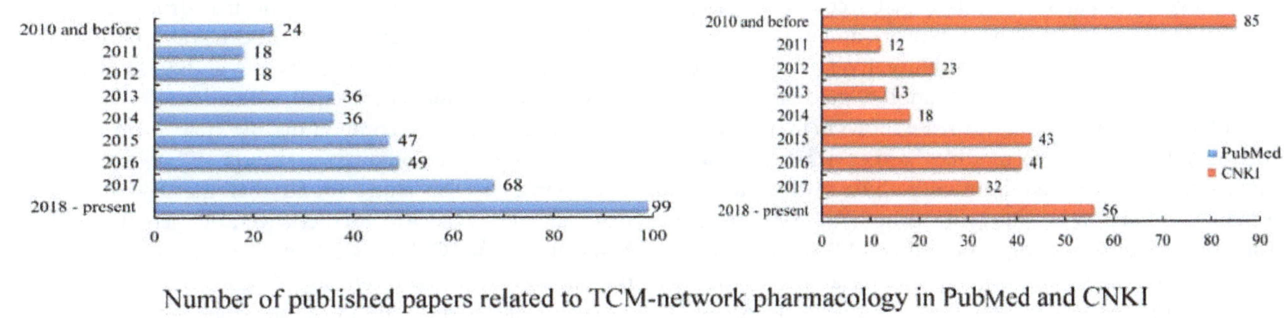

FIGURE 2 | Published papers identified from PubMed and CNKI databases. Papers in PubMed were searched by Title/Abstract containing the following keywords: "network pharmacology," "Chinese," and "medicine." Papers in CNKI were searched with the following key words: "network pharmacology" and "Chinese herb," excluding all conference papers. The analysis time was from 2010 and before, to the end of 2018.

TABLE 2 | TCM network pharmacology studies in international journals from 2011 to 2017.

Herb/Herbal prescription[a]	Related disease/effect	Year	Reference
Aconiti Lateralis Radix	Multi-targets	2011	Wu et al., 2011
Compound DanShen formula	Cardiovascular disease	2012	Li et al., 2012
Chinese herbal Radix Curcumae formula	Cardiovascular disease	2013	Tao et al., 2013
QingLuoYin	Rheumatoid arthritis	2013	Zhang et al., 2013
TaoHongSiWu decoction	Osteoarthritis	2013	Zheng et al., 2013
Eucommia ulmoides Oliv.	Hypertension	2014	Li et al., 2014d
GeGenQinLian decoction	Type 2 diabetes	2014	Li et al., 2014a
BuShenHuoXue formula	Chronic kidney disease	2014	Shi et al., 2014
LiuWeiDiHuang pill	Colon cancer and esophagitis	2014	Li et al., 2014b
QiShenYiQi formula	Myocardial infarction	2014	Li et al., 2014c
QiShenYiQi formula	Acute myocardial ischemia	2014	Wu et al., 2014
Dragon's blood tablet	Colitis	2014	Xu et al., 2014
ZhiZiDaHuang decoction	Alcoholic liver disease	2015	An and Feng, 2015
Rhubarb	Renal interstitial fibrosis	2015	Xiang et al., 2015
SiMiaoWan	Gout	2015	Zhao et al., 2015
ErXian decoction	Menopause-related symptoms	2015	Wang S. et al., 2015
QiGuiTongFeng tablet	Gout	2015	Ke et al., 2015
Salvia miltiorrhiza	Cardiovascular disease	2015	He et al., 2015
SiNiSan	Depression	2015	Wang H.H. et al., 2015
ShengMai preparations	Cardio-cerebral ischemic diseases	2015	Li F. et al., 2015
Dendrobium nobile	Type 2 diabetes	2015	Li M.M. et al., 2015
MaHuangFuZiXiXin decoction	Allergic rhinitis	2015	Tang et al., 2015
XiaoYaoSan	Depression	2015	Gao et al., 2015
Eriobotrya japonica - Fritillaria usuriensis dropping pills	Pulmonary diseases	2016	Tao et al., 2016
XiaoYao powder	Anovulatory infertility	2016	Liu et al., 2016
Euphorbia kansui and *Glycyrrhiza*	Hepatocellular carcinoma ascites	2016	Zhang et al., 2016
QingFeiXiaoYanWan	Acute lung inflammation	2016	Hou et al., 2016
YinChenHaoTang	Severe acute pancreatitis	2016	Xiang et al., 2016
YinHuangQingFei capsule	Chronic bronchitis	2016	Yu et al., 2017
YangHe decoction	Breast cancer	2017	Zeng and Yang, 2017
Fructus Aurantii Immaturus	Anti-coagulationGastrointestinalmotility regulation activities	2017	Tan et al., 2017
SheXiangBaoXin pill	Cardiovascular disease	2017	Fang et al., 2017
Radix *salviae miltiorrhizae*	Hepatoprotective effect	2017	Hong et al., 2017

[a] *The biological ingredients of herbal prescription were listed in* ***Supplementary Table S1****.*

Distance-Based Mutual Information Model (DMIM) to identify useful relationships that exist among herbs in numerous herbal formulas. DMIM combines mutual information entropy and "between-herb-distance" to score herb interactions and construct an herb network. It achieves a good balance among the herb's frequency, independence, and distance in herbal formulas when used to retrieve herb pairs. They used 3,865 collateral-related herbal formulas to construct an herb network and illustrated the traditional herbal pairing and compatibility. LWDHW was used as an example to identify possible compatibility mechanisms, and it was found that LWDHW-treated disease shows high phenotype similarity and that certain "co-modules" are enriched in cancer pathways and neuro-endocrine-immune pathways, which may be the mechanism of action by which the same LWDHW formula treats different diseases. Zhang et al. (2008, 2017) focused on the five flavors of Chinese medicinal properties and constructed Bayesian network models of bitterness, pungent flavor, and sugariness. The five flavors of some TCMs were predicted by these established models, providing crucial support for research on TCM compatibility.

Target Prediction of TCM

Understanding the molecular basis of TCM is crucial for the modernization of TCM, which not only would provide full theoretical support for TCM research but also would increase acceptance of TCM worldwide. In recent years, researchers have done a lot of work to study the molecular mechanisms of TCMs. We proposed the TCM-Mesh system (Zhang et al., 2017), which was designed as an integration of a database and a data-mining system for network pharmacology analysis of TCM preparations. We used TCM-Mesh to identify candidate targets for ginseng and LWDHW based on existing clues (e.g., molecular structures, bioactivity) from curated databases along with a pharmacology approach. The results showed that dammarane-type tetracyclic triterpenoids from ginseng (i.e., ginsenoside Rg1, ginsenoside Re, and ginsenoside Rb1) might be used to treat Alzheimer's disease, hypertension, and atherosclerosis by targeting tumor necrosis factor (TNF), nitric oxide synthase 3 (NOS3), and AKT serine/threonine kinase 1 (AKT1). Chemical constituents from LWDHW (i.e., loganin, paeonol) can be used to treat diabetes, diabetic nephropathy, and diabetic retinopathy by targeting intercellular adhesion molecule 1 and connective tissue growth factor. Li et al. (Liang et al., 2014b) established a novel pharmacology approach based on a network pharmacology approach to analyze the traditional herbal formulas for LWDHW. The authors found that the compounds of LWDHW may play an important role in esophagitis and colon cancer by regulating the expression of C-C chemokine receptor 2 (CCR2), estrogen receptor 1 (ESR1), peroxisome proliferator-activated receptor gamma (PPARG), and retinoic acid receptor alpha (RARA). They also selected a XinAn medical family's anti-rheumatoid arthritis (RA) herbal formula "QingLuoYin" (QLY) as an example (Zhang et al., 2013), which consisted of four herbs: KuShen (*Sophora flavescens*), QingFengTeng (*Sinomenium acutum*), HuangBai (*Phellodendron chinensis*), and BiXie (*Dioscorea collettii*). Some anti-angiogenic and anti-inflammatory active ingredients, such as kurarinone, matrine, sinomenine, berberine, and diosgenin, were identified among the 235 ingredients of QLY. In addition, the synergistic effects of the major ingredients were identified in QLY, such as matrine and sinomenine, which may have been derived from the feedback loop and compensatory mechanisms by targeting TNF- and vascular endothelial growth factor-induced signaling pathways involved in RA. According to the molecular structures of proteins and the corresponding targets of 1,401 drugs approved by the U.S. Food and Drug Administration, Wu et al. (2011) constructed a target prediction model by using the "Random Forest" algorithm. The authors used the compounds of "fuzi" (*Aconiti Lateralis Radix Praeparata*) to predict the targets and construct a multi-target network. The study found that the 22 compounds of "fuzi" have been used to predict several targets that reflect the characteristics of TCM. In addition, Li et al. (An and Feng, 2015) studied the antioxidant effects of ZhiZiDaHuang Decoction (ZZDHT) based on a network pharmacology approach. The authors found that ZZDHT may exert antioxidant effects to regulate reactive oxygen species, thereby treating alcoholic liver disease by targeting cytochrome P450 2E1 (CYP2E1), xanthine dehydrogenase (XDH), nitric oxide synthase 2 (NOS2), and prostaglandin-endoperoxide synthase 2 (PTGS2).

Network Toxicology

Network toxicology is based on an understanding of the "toxicity-(side effect)-gene-target-drug" interaction network, which utilizes network analysis to speculate and estimate the toxicity and side effects of drugs. Liu et al. (2012) proposed that technologies that feature rapid preparation, high-throughput screening, toxic components exclusion, and biochip along with the drug-target network are of great importance to TCM research on active ingredient screening, toxic components exclusion, and molecular mechanism, which could increase the safety of TCMs. Fan et al. (2011) proposed the concept and framework of network toxicology of TCM. The related tools and technologies were briefly introduced, and the prospects for network toxicology of TCM were forecasted. In their work, they used network pharmacology methods to reconstruct the network of "compound-protein/gene-toxicity" to identify toxic substances and predict the toxic side effects of known compounds, which provides valuable information for understanding the toxic mechanisms. Currently, the related databases for the study of network toxicology includes CTD (Davis et al., 2011), TOXNET (Wexler, 2001), and the National Toxicology Program. Furthermore, additional foresting toxicity software, such as TOPKAT, HazardExpert, and DEREK (Wolfgang and Johnson, 2002), are available for TCM network toxicology studies.

PROS AND CONS OF CURRENT TCM DATABASES: BENCHMARKING

Comparisons Among TCM Databases

As discussed, various databases are used for TCM analysis. However, network analysis of TCM is limited by several aspects of the currently available databases (**Figure 3**, current statistics on various databases can be obtained from the homepage of each database).

For example, HIT is a comprehensive TCM database that supports many different input formats. It is limited, however, in that the total information from HIT for TCM analysis is not sufficient, as it only contains about 586 compounds and 1,301 targets. Thus, the data that can be collected from the

		HIT	TCMID	TCMSP	TCM-Mesh
		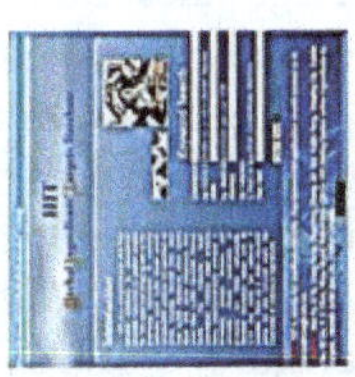	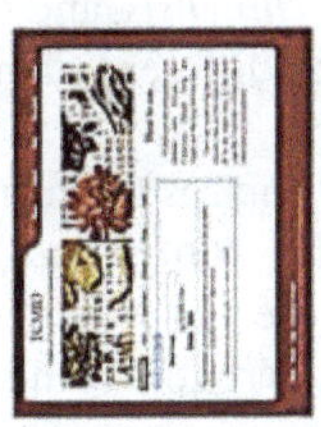	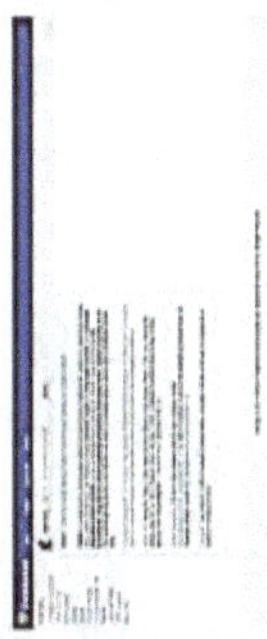	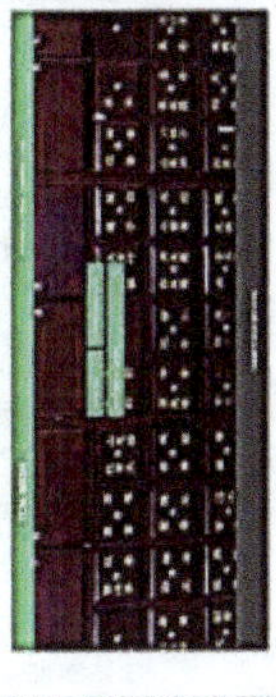
Paper	Reference	[21]	[23]	[22]	[36]
	Publisher	Nucleic Acids Research	Nucleic Acids Research	Journal of Cheminformatics	Scientific Reports
	Year of publication	2011	2013	2014	2017
Input types	Prescription	/	Pinyin name	/	/
	Herb	Latin name/Pinyin name/Chinese name	Pinyin name/English name	Latin name/Pinyin name/Chinese name	Pinyin name/English name
	Compound	English name/Abbreviation/CAS number/CID number	English name/STITCH ID/CAS number	English name/InChIKey/CAS number	English name/CAN string
	Target	Protein name	Protein name/gene symbol/Uniprot ID	Protein name	gene symbol
	Disease	/	Disease name/OMIM ID	Disease name	Disease name
General Statistics	Prescription	/	46,929	/	/
	Herb	1,305	8,159	499	6,235
	Compound	586	43,413	12,144	383,240
	Target	1,301	12,419	3,311	14,298
	Disease	/	3,854	837	6,204
	Side effect	/	/	/	163,221
	Toxicity	/	/	/	71
Limitations		· No prescirption, disease, side effect, toxicity related data · Recorded herbs, compounds and targets are limited	· No side effect, toxicity related data	· No prescription, side effect and disease retaled data · Recorded herbs and diseases are limited · A large amount of redundancies in the database when searched for herbs	· Limited inputs · Detailed descriptions about compounds, genes and diseases are lacked · No prescription related data

FIGURE 3 | Comparisons among the four TCM databases. The comparison contains the paper information, different input types, general statistics, and limitations of several TCM databases.

HIT are limited. TCMSP is a TCM database that captures the relationships among drugs, targets, and diseases. It allows users to use many input formats; however, TCMSP should be more concise as the database has a large amount of redundancies when searching for herbs, which must be trimmed to be improved. TCMID is another comprehensive database that provides information and bridges the gap between TCM and modern life science. It collects TCM-related information from the TCM@Taiwan database and the literature, including prescription of TCM, and also offers a module for network visualization. Although TCMID is available for multiple inputs, including compound name, STITCH database ID, and CAS number, when searching for ingredients, it is not sufficiently comprehensive, and many compounds are searched without a related network in TCMID. The newly launched TCM-Mesh is a more comprehensive database that not only contains the data on network pharmacology, including the "herb-compound-target-disease" network, but also includes data on TCM side effects and toxicity. As a result, TCM-Mesh offers a more holistic perspective for those conducting TCM research. Problems in TCM-Mesh remain to be resolved, however; for example, the web service is limited and many functions need to be improved, as the CAS number query is not supported. In addition, detailed descriptions about the compounds, genes, and diseases are lacking.

Detailed Information on Herbs and Prescriptions for Assessment

We used prescriptions for LWDHW and ZZDHT to assess TCM-Mesh and randomly selected 10 well-known herbs to test different TCM databases for systematic assessment (**Table 3**).

TABLE 3 | Detailed information on the data sets of herbs and prescriptions.

Herb or prescription	Index of assessment	Source
LWDHW	Targets	Liang et al., 2014b
ZZDHT		An and Feng, 2015
Ganoderma lucidum	(i) Number of ingredients of herbs found in the database	
Ginseng	(ii) Number of ingredient-target found in the database	Famous Chinese herbs
Codonopsis pilosula	(iii) Number of target-disease association found in the database	
Astragalus membranaceus		
Chinese yam		
Pseudo-ginseng		
Polygonum multiflorum		
Radix Angelicae dahuricae		
Coptis chinensis		
Cordyceps sinensis		

Assessment Using LWDHW as an Example

As mentioned earlier, Li et al. (2010) found that the compounds of LWDHW may play an indispensable role in esophagitis and colon cancer by regulating the expression of CCR2, ESR1, PPARG, and RARA. To validate the effects of LWDHW on esophagitis and colon cancer, we used TCM-Mesh. We found 11 candidate targets (including PPARG) for colon cancer and four potential targets for esophagitis (**Table 4**), all of which were validated by the literature.

Assessment Using ZZDHT as an Example

As discussed in Section 3.2, "Target prediction of TCM," ZZDHT decoction has been applied to treat alcoholic liver disease by targeting CYP2E1, XDH, NOS2, and PTGS2. We used TCM-Mesh to validate the effects of ZZDHT, leading to the identification of 12 candidate targets (including CYP2E1) for alcoholic liver disease (**Table 5**), all of which were supported by the literature.

Comparison of Search Results Among the TCM Databases

To further compare the databases, we selected 10 well-known herbs to randomly evaluate the TCM databases: *G. lucidum*, ginseng, *Codonopsis pilosula*, *Astragalus membranaceus*, Chinese yam, pseudo-ginseng, *Polygonum multiflorum*, Radix *Angelicae dahuricae*, *Coptis chinensis*, and *Cordyceps sinensis*. We used each herb to search the different databases and compared the search results (**Table 6**).

We compared the results from different databases and found that although the compound data recorded in TCM-Mesh were abundant, the data on the ingredients of the herb were limited. For each herb, the number of ingredients obtained from TCM-Mesh was lower than the number obtained from TCMID and TCMSP. We also found that the number of ingredients collected from TCMSP was much higher than that collected from the other two databases, in accordance with the fact that the database had a large amount of redundancies when searching for herbs. Additionally, we discovered higher completeness of TCM-Mesh in the ingredient-target associations and target-disease associations. For many herbs, the search results produced more hits in ingredient-target associations and target-disease associations in TCM-Mesh, although fewer ingredients were collected. Furthermore, a search for *P. multiflorum* in TCMSP produced no hits, revealing the limited herb data in TCMSP. The TCM database must keep pace with the development of TCM research to support the modernization of TCM. Therefore, a more comprehensive and complete database with powerful web services is necessary.

DISCUSSION AND CONCLUSION

Research on TCM has a long history in China, illustrating the enormous potential and opportunities for new drug innovation. The inception of TCM network pharmacology offers researchers a new chance to gain systematic insights into TCM, as the

TABLE 4 | Candidate targets of LWDHW for colon cancer and esophagitis validated by TCM-Mesh.

Disease	Target	Related compounds (herbs)	Reference
Colon cancer	ACP1 (acid phosphatase 1)	Adenine (*Poria cocos*)	Spina et al., 2008
	EGFR (epidermal growth factor receptor)	Capsaicin (Poria cocos), Cholesterol (Chinese yam)	Press et al., 2008
	GSTM1 (glutathione S-transferase mu 1)	Methyleugenol (cornel)	Huang et al., 2006
	IL10 (interleukin 10)	Dopamine (Chinese yam)	Cacev et al., 2008
	IL1B (IL-10b protein precursor)	Capsaicin (Poria cocos)	Lurje et al., 2009
	IL1RN (interleukin 1 receptor antagonist)	Palmitate (Poria cocos, Chinese yam, cornel)	Lurje et al., 2009
	PIK3CA (phosphatidylinositol-4,5-bisphosphate 3-kinase catalytic subunit alpha)	Palmitate (Poria cocos, Chinese yam, cornel)	Ogino et al., 2009
	PIK3R1 (phosphoinositide-3-kinase regulatory subunit 1)	Palmitate (Poria cocos, Chinese yam, cornel)	Li et al., 2008
	PPARG (peroxisome proliferator activated receptor gamma)	Capsaicin (Poria cocos)	Slattery et al., 2006
	RXRA (retinoid X receptor alpha)	Palmitate (Poria cocos, Chinese yam, cornel)	Egan et al., 2010
	SLC22A3 (solute carrier family 22 member 3)	Choline (Poria cocos), dopamine (Chinese yam)	Cui et al., 2011
Esophagitis	CYP2C19 (cytochrome P450 family 2 subfamily C member 19)	Capsaicin (Poria cocos), dopamine (Chinese yam), ursolic acid (cornel)	Kawamura et al., 2007
	GSTP1 (glutathione S-transferase pi 1)	Methyleugenol (cornel)	Kala et al., 2007
	IL1B (interleukin 1 beta)	Capsaicin (Poria cocos)	Koivurova et al., 2003
	IL1RN (interleukin 1 receptor antagonist)	Palmitate (Poria cocos, Chinese yam, cornel)	Koivurova et al., 2003

research strategy of network pharmacology is in accordance with the holistic understanding of the effects of TCM on disease. This understanding may lead to a new direction for the research of pharmacological mechanisms and safety evaluation of TCM. In addition, related methods and studies must keep pace with the rapid developments in TCM research and must continue to be powerful.

Unification and Integration: A More Powerful Database System

In recent years, several databases have been proposed, many of which share similar functions although they have different data sources. For most databases, the patterns of input differ from database to database. For example, the herb "Dried Tangerine Peel" in TCMSP must be searched by "chenpi" or "*Citrus reticulata*," whereas in TCMID, it must be searched by "chen pi" or "*Citri reticulatae pericarpium*." In addition, many compounds and proteins have different aliases in different databases (e.g., compounds: chemical name, CID number, STITCH ID, CAS number, PubChem CID, EC number, UNII; proteins: protein name, gene symbol, node ID, target ID, target drugbank ID, uniprot ID). The uniform format of input and output not only would make the current databases more concise, but also would enable researchers to take full advantage of the database resources. Thus, a standard transforming platform is needed. Such a platform should fully understand the data structure and content of various databases. Furthermore, it should support the translation among different formats of herbs, compounds, or proteins to bridge the gap between current databases for TCM research. Currently, the output of previous databases can be directly used as the input for another database. Most databases have associated web services; thus, the transforming platform that could transfer data from one database to another, can be presented to users as web services that are linked to different databases or to a browser plug-in. In addition to the unification of databases, the integration of diverse databases is also of great importance. Currently, more than 10,000 herbs used in more than 100,000 herbal formulas have been recorded in TCM (Qiu, 2007), posing a huge challenge for researchers who want to better understand the efficacy and the safety of the TCM. It is difficult for a single database to resolve all these problems as a result of the incompleteness of data. Each database has its own advantages regarding the specificity of its data and its algorithm. Therefore, the full integration of available resources will facilitate the production of an even more powerful and comprehensive database system, which undoubtedly will more effectively promote the modernization of TCM.

The Content of Compounds: A Crucial Factor

TCM aims to restore whole-body balance in patients by using a herbal formula (Li et al., 2007), and herbal prescriptions are usually composed of two or more medical herbs in a certain proportion. For example, LWDHW consists of six herbs (Zhao et al., 2007; Xie et al., 2008): *Rehmannia glutinosa* libosch., *Cornus officinalis* Sieb., *Dioscorea oppositifolia* L., *Paeonia ostii*, *Alisma orientale* Juz, and *Poria cocos* (Schw.) *Wolf*, with a dose proportion of 8:4:4:3:3:3 (Wu et al., 2007; Wang et al., 2010). For current studies on TCM formulas, researchers focus on the chemical composition rather than on the proportion of each

TABLE 5 | Candidate targets of ZZDHT for alcoholic liver disease validated by TCM-Mesh.

Disease	Target	Related chemical composition (herbs)	References
Alcoholic liver disease	ADH1B (alcohol dehydrogenase 1B (class I), beta polypeptide)	Zinc (Cape jasmine)	Lorenzo et al., 2006
	ADH1C (alcohol dehydrogenase 1C (class I), gamma polypeptide)	Zinc (Cape jasmine)	Khan et al., 2010
	ALDH2 (aldehyde dehydrogenase 2 family member)	Manganese (Cape jasmine)	Yu et al., 2002
	CYP1A1 (cytochrome P450 family 1 subfamily A member 1)	Apigenin, genistein, quercetin (Cape jasmine), naringin, nobiletin, sinensetin, tangeretin, progesterone (rheum officinale)-	Burim et al., 2004
	CYP2E1 (cytochrome P450 family 2 subfamily E member 1)	Calcium (Cape jasmine), Geniposide (Cape jasmine)	Khan et al., 2009
	GSTM1 (glutathione S-transferase mu 1)	Zinc (Cape jasmine)	Ladero et al., 2005
	HFE (homeostatic iron regulator)	Calcium (Cape jasmine)	Ropero et al., 2001
	IL10 (interleukin 10)	Beryllium (Cape jasmine)	Gleeson et al., 2008
	IL2 (interleukin 2)	Beryllium (Cape jasmine)	Marcos et al., 2008
	IL6 (interleukin 6)	Chromium (Cape jasmine)	Gleeson et al., 2008
	PPARG (peroxisome proliferator activated receptor gamma)	Genistein (Cape jasmine)	Marcos et al., 2009
	XRCC1 (X-ray repair cross-complementing 1)	Chromium (Cape jasmine)	Rossit et al., 2002

TABLE 6 | Search results of 10 well-known TCMs from three TCM databases.

Databases / Herbs	TCMID			TCM-Mesh			TCMSP		
	I	I-T	T-D	I	I-T	T-D	I	I-T	T-D
Ganoderma lucidum	160	1,164	771	32	150	238	484	543	365
Ginseng	293	4,820	2,913	153	4,144	2,970	380	748	486
Codonopsis pilosula	187	2,531	1,631	104	2,493	2,211	268	911	556
Astragalus membranaceus	70	1,832	1,186	35	2,426	2,376	174	953	605
Chinese yam	42	1,004	655	20	959	1,307	142	851	451
Pseudo-ginseng	157	900	635	71	1,104	1,591	238	716	506
Polygonum multiflorum	73	618	599	24	513	888	/	/	/
Radix *Angelicae dahuricae*	135	406	289	80	362	477	446	1,408	454
Coptis chinensis	30	238	231	23	142	274	96	596	513
Cordyceps sinensis	37	1,010	519	21	919	944	76	369	483

I, Ingredients of herb; I-T, Ingredient-target associations; T-D, Target-disease associations.

compound of TCM. Therefore, the influence of the compound content on the effect of the TCM is often ignored. The weight of the content of each compound should be taken into consideration in future studies to better understand the pharmacological effects of the TCM.

TCM-Gut Microbiota Network Pharmacology: A New Frontier

The significant involvement of the gut microbiota in human health and disease suggests that manipulation of commensal microbial composition through combinations of probiotics, antibiotics, and prebiotics could be a novel therapeutic approach. Previous studies have shown that many TCMs can be used as agents to prevent gut dysbiosis (Chang et al., 2015; Zhou et al., 2016). Therefore, a more comprehensive database about TCM and gut microbiota is needed, which should not only include information on the interaction between the TCM and the gut microbiota but also integrate respective advantages of TCM databases and microbiome databases. This integration will be conducive to accelerating the internationalization of TCM and will allow researchers to fully understand the efficacy of TCM from a holistic perspective. Research in the area of TCM network pharmacology is still in its infancy and remains to be developed. However, with data accumulation on TCM and clinical research and interaction of various methods of analysis and experiment, researchers can obtain more substantive and authentic information. This information is conducive to the modernization and internationalization of TCM and may offer critical technological support for drug development, clinical diagnosis, and personalized medicine.

AUTHOR CONTRIBUTIONS

KN and HB conceived and proposed the idea. KN, HB, and RZ designed the work. KN, RZ, and XZ contributed to the interpretation of data for the work. KN, HB, and RZ drafted the work. KN, HB, XZ, and RZ revised it critically for important intellectual content. All authors read and approved the final manuscript to be published, and agree to be accountable for all aspects of the work in ensuring that questions related to the accuracy or integrity of any part of the work are appropriately investigated and resolved.

FUNDING

This work was partially supported by National Science Foundation of China grants 81573702, 81774008, 31871334, and 31671374, and the Ministry of Science and Technology (High-Tech) grant (No. 2018YFC0910502).

REFERENCES

An, L., and Feng, F. (2015). Network pharmacology-based antioxidant effect study of zhi-zi-da-huang decoction for alcoholic liver disease. *Evid. Based. Complement. Alternat. Med.* 2015:492470. doi: 10.1155/2015/492470

Becker, K. G., Barnes, K. C., Bright, T. J., and Wang, S. A. (2004). The genetic association database. *Nat. Genet.* 36, 431–432. doi: 10.1038/ng0504-431

Boh, B. (2013). Ganoderma lucidum: a potential for biotechnological production of anti-cancer and immunomodulatory drugs. *Recent Pat. Anticancer Drug Discov.* 8, 255–287. doi: 10.2174/1574891X113089990036

Boh, B., Berovic, M., Zhang, J., and Zhi-Bin, L. (2007). Ganoderma lucidum and its pharmaceutically active compounds. *Biotechnol. Annu. Rev.* 13, 265–301. doi: 10.1016/s1387-2656(07)13010-6

Burim, R. V., Canalle, R., Martinelli Ade, L., and Takahashi, C. S. (2004). Polymorphisms in glutathione S-transferases GSTM1, GSTT1 and GSTP1 and cytochromes P450 CYP2E1 and CYP1A1 and susceptibility to cirrhosis or pancreatitis in alcoholics. *Mutagenesis* 19, 291–298. doi: 10.1093/mutage/geh034

Cacev, T., Radosević, S., Krizanac, S., and Kapitanović, S. (2008). Influence of interleukin-8 and interleukin-10 on sporadic colon cancer development and progression. *Carcinogenesis* 29, 1572–1580. doi: 10.1093/carcin/bgn164

Chan, G. H., Law, B. Y., Chu, J. M., Yue, K. K., Jiang, Z. H., Lau, C. W., et al. (2013). Ginseng extracts restore high-glucose induced vascular dysfunctions by altering triglyceride metabolism and downregulation of atherosclerosis-related genes. *Evid. Based. Complement. Alternat. Med.* 2013:797310. doi: 10.1155/2013/797310

Chan, K. (1995). Progress in traditional Chinese medicine. *Trends Pharmacol. Sci.* 16, 182–187. doi: 10.1016/S0165-6147(00)89019-7

Chang, C. J., Lin, C. S., Lu, C. C., Martel, J., Ko, Y. F., Ojcius, D. M., et al. (2015). Ganoderma lucidum reduces obesity in mice by modulating the composition of the gut microbiota. *Nat. Commun.* 6:7489. doi: 10.1038/ncomms8489

Chen, C. Y. (2011). TCM Database@Taiwan: the world's largest traditional Chinese medicine database for drug screening in silico. *PLoS One* 6:e15939. doi: 10.1371/journal.pone.0015939

Chen, J. Y., Mamidipalli, S., and Huan, T. (2009). HAPPI: an online database of comprehensive human annotated and predicted protein interactions. *BMC Genomics* 10:S16. doi: 10.1186/1471-2164-10-S1-S16

Chen, X., Liu, M. X., and Yan, G. Y. (2012). Drug-target interaction prediction by random walk on the heterogeneous network. *Mol. Biosyst.* 8, 1970–1978. doi: 10.1039/c2mb00002d

Corson, T. W., and Crews, C. M. (2007). Molecular understanding and modern application of traditional medicines: triumphs and trials. *Cell* 130, 769–774. doi: 10.1016/j.cell.2007.08.021

Cui, R., Okada, Y., Jang, S. G., Ku, J. L., Park, J. G., Kamatani, Y., et al. (2011). Common variant in 6q26-q27 is associated with distal colon cancer in an Asian population. *Gut* 60, 799–805. doi: 10.1136/gut.2010.215947

Davis, A. P., Murphy, C. G., Johnson, R., Lay, J. M., Lennonhopkins, K., Saracenirichards, C., et al. (2011). The comparative toxicogenomics database: update 2013. *Nucleic Acids Res.* 39, 1067–1072. doi: 10.1093/nar/gkq813

D'Eustachio, P. (2009). Reactome knowledgebase of human biological pathways and processes. *Nucleic Acids Res.* 37, D619–D622. doi: 10.1093/nar/gkn863

Dohleman, B. S. (2006). Exploratory social network analysis with Pajek. *Psychometrika* 71, 605–606. doi: 10.1007/s11336-005-1410-y

Egan, J. B., Thompson, P. A., Ashbeck, E. L., Conti, D. V., Duggan, D., Hibler, E., et al. (2010). Genetic polymorphisms in vitamin D receptor VDR/RXRA influence the likelihood of colon adenoma recurrence. *Cancer Res.* 70, 1496–1504. doi: 10.1158/0008-5472.CAN-09-3264

Fan, X., Zhao, X., Jin, Y., Shen, X., and Liu, C. (2011). Network toxicology and its application to traditional Chinese medicine. *Zhongguo Zhong Yao Za Zhi* 36, 2920–2922.

Fang, H. Y., Zeng, H. W., Lin, L. M., Chen, X., Shen, X. N., Fu, P., et al. (2017). A network-based method for mechanistic investigation of Shexiang Baoxin Pill's treatment of cardiovascular diseases. *Sci. Rep.* 7:43632. doi: 10.1038/srep43632

Gao, Y., Gao, L., Gao, X. X., Zhou, Y. Z., Qin, X. M., and Tian, J. S. (2015). An exploration in the action targets for antidepressant bioactive components of Xiaoyaosan based on network pharmacology. *Yao Xue Xue Bao* 50, 1589–1595.

Gaulton, A., Bellis, L. J., Bento, A. P., Chambers, J., Davies, M., Hersey, A., et al. (2012). ChEMBL: a large-scale bioactivity database for drug discovery. *Nucleic Acids Res.* 40, D1100–D1107. doi: 10.1093/nar/gkr777

Gleeson, D., Bradley, M. P., Jones, J., Peck, R. J., Bond, S. K., Teare, M. D., et al. (2008). Cytokine gene polymorphisms in heavy drinkers with and without decompensated liver disease: a case-control study. *Am. J. Gastroenterol.* 103, 3039–3046. doi: 10.1111/j.1572-0241.2008.02150.x

Hamosh, A., Scott, A. F., Amberger, J., Bocchini, C., Valle, D., and McKusick, V. A. (2002). Online mendelian inheritance in man (OMIM), a knowledgebase of human genes and genetic disorders. *Nucleic Acids Res.* 30, 52–55. doi: 10.1093/nar/30.1.52

He, S. B., Zhang, B. X., Wang, H. H., Wang, Y., and Qiao, Y. J. (2015). Study on mechanism of *Salvia miltiorrhiza* treating cardiovascular disease through auxiliary mechanism elucidation system for Chinese medicine. *Zhongguo Zhong Yao Za Zhi* 40, 3713–3717.

Hong, M., Li, S., Wang, N., Tan, H. Y., Cheung, F., and Feng, Y. (2017). A biomedical investigation of the hepatoprotective effect of *Radix salviae miltiorrhizae* and network pharmacology-based prediction of the active compounds and molecular targets. *Int. J. Mol. Sci.* 18:E620. doi: 10.3390/ijms18030620

Hopkins, A. L. (2008). Network pharmacology: the next paradigm in drug discovery. *Nat. Chem. Biol.* 4, 682–690. doi: 10.1038/nchembio.118

Hou, Y., Nie, Y., Cheng, B., Tao, J., Ma, X., Jiang, M., et al. (2016). Qingfei Xiaoyan Wan, a traditional Chinese medicine formula, ameliorates *Pseudomonas aeruginosa*-induced acute lung inflammation by regulation of PI3K/AKT and Ras/MAPK pathways. *Acta Pharm. Sin B* 6, 212–221. doi: 10.1016/j.apsb.2016.03.002

Huang, K., Sandler, R. S., Millikan, R. C., Schroeder, J. C., North, K. E., and Hu, J. (2006). GSTM1 and GSTT1 polymorphisms, cigarette smoking, and risk of colon cancer: a population-based case-control study in North Carolina (United States). *Cancer Causes Control* 17, 385–394. doi: 10.1007/s10552-005-0424-1

Ideker, T., Galitski, T., and Hood, L. (2001). A new approach to decoding life: systems biology. *Annu. Rev. Genomics Hum. Genet.* 2, 343–372. doi: 10.1146/annurev.genom.2.1.343

Kala, Z., Dolina, J., Marek, F., and Izakovicova Holla, L. (2007). Polymorphisms of glutathione S-transferase M1, T1 and P1 in patients with reflux esophagitis and Barrett's esophagus. *J. Hum. Genet.* 52, 527–534. doi: 10.1007/s10038-007-0148-z

Kawamura, M., Ohara, S., Koike, T., Iijima, K., Suzuki, H., Kayaba, S., et al. (2007). Cytochrome P450 2C19 polymorphism influences the preventive effect of lansoprazole on the recurrence of erosive reflux esophagitis. *J. Gastroenterol. Hepatol.* 22, 222–226. doi: 10.1111/j.1440-1746.2006.04419.x

Ke, Z. P., Zhang, X. Z., Ding, Y., Cao, L., Li, N., Ding, G., et al. (2015). Study on effective substance basis and molecular mechanism of Qigui Tongfeng tablet using network pharmacology method. *Zhongguo Zhong Yao Za Zhi* 40, 2837–2842.

Kerrien, S., Aranda, B., Breuza, L., Bridge, A., Broackescarter, F., Chen, C., et al. (2012). The IntAct molecular interaction database in 2012. *Nucleic Acids Res.* 40, D841–D846. doi: 10.1093/nar/gkr1088

Khan, A. J., Husain, Q., Choudhuri, G., and Parmar, D. (2010). Association of polymorphism in alcohol dehydrogenase and interaction with other genetic risk factors with alcoholic liver cirrhosis. *Drug Alcohol Depend.* 109, 190–197. doi: 10.1016/j.drugalcdep.2010.01.010

Khan, A. J., Ruwali, M., Choudhuri, G., Mathur, N., Husain, Q., and Parmar, D. (2009). Polymorphism in cytochrome P450 2E1 and interaction with other genetic risk factors and susceptibility to alcoholic liver cirrhosis. *Mutat. Res.* 664, 55–63. doi: 10.1016/j.mrfmmm.2009.02.009

Kim, J. H. (2012). Cardiovascular diseases and *Panax* ginseng: a review on molecular mechanisms and medical applications. *J. Ginseng. Res.* 36, 16–26. doi: 10.5142/jgr.2012.36.1.16

Koivurova, O. P., Karhukorpi, J. M., Joensuu, E. T., Koistinen, P. O., Valtonen, J. M., Karttunen, T. J., et al. (2003). IL-1 RN 2/2 genotype and simultaneous carriage of genotypes IL-1 RN 2/2 and IL-1beta-511 T/T associated with oesophagitis in *Helicobacter* pylori-negative patients. *Scand. J. Gastroenterol.* 38, 1217–1222. doi: 10.1080/00365520310006504

Kola, I., and Landis, J. (2004). Can the pharmaceutical industry reduce attrition rates? *Nat. Rev. Drug Discov.* 3, 711–715. doi: 10.1038/nrd1470

Kuhn, M., Szklarczyk, D., Pletscher-Frankild, S., Blicher, T. H., von Mering, C., Jensen, L. J., et al. (2014). STITCH 4: integration of protein-chemical interactions with user data. *Nucleic Acids Res.* 42, D401–D407. doi: 10.1093/nar/gkt1207

Ladero, J. M., Martinez, C., Garcia-Martin, E., Fernandez-Arquero, M., Lopez-Alonso, G., de la Concha, E. G., et al. (2005). Polymorphisms of the glutathione S-transferases mu-1 (GSTM1) and theta-1 (GSTT1) and the risk of advanced alcoholic liver disease. *Scand. J. Gastroenterol.* 40, 348–353. doi: 10.1080/00365520510012109

Lee, S. T., Chu, K., Sim, J. Y., Heo, J. H., and Kim, M. (2008). Panax ginseng enhances cognitive performance in Alzheimer disease. *Alzheimer Dis. Assoc. Disord.* 22, 222–226. doi: 10.1097/WAD.0b013e31816c92e6

Li, F., Lv, Y. N., Tan, Y. S., Shen, K., Zhai, K. F., Chen, H. L., et al. (2015). An integrated pathway interaction network for the combination of four effective compounds from ShengMai preparations in the treatment of cardio-cerebral ischemic diseases. *Acta Pharmacol. Sin.* 36, 1337–1348. doi: 10.1038/aps.2015.70

Li, H., Zhao, L., Zhang, B., Jiang, Y., Wang, X., Guo, Y., et al. (2014a). A network pharmacology approach to determine active compounds and action mechanisms of ge-gen-qin-lian decoction for treatment of type 2 diabetes. *Evid. Based. Complement. Alternat. Med.* 2014:495840. doi: 10.1155/2014/495840

Li, L., Plummer, S. J., Thompson, C. L., Tucker, T. C., and Casey, G. (2008). Association between phosphatidylinositol 3-Kinase regulatory subunit p85α Met326Ile genetic polymorphism and colon cancer Risk. *Clin. Cancer Res.* 14, 633–637. doi: 10.1158/1078-0432.CCR-07-1211

Li, M. M., Zhang, B. X., He, S. B., Zheng, R., Zhang, Y. L., and Wang, Y. (2015). Elucidating hypoglycemic mechanism of *Dendrobium nobile* through auxiliary elucidation system for traditional Chinese medicine mechanism. *Zhongguo Zhong Yao Za Zhi* 40, 3709–3712.

Li, S. (2011). Network target: a starting point for traditional Chinese medicine network pharmacology. *Zhongguo Zhong Yao Za Zhi* 36, 2017–2020.

Li, S., Fan, T. P., Jia, W., Lu, A., and Zhang, W. (2014b). Network pharmacology in traditional Chinese medicine. *Evid. Based. Complement. Alternat. Med.* 2014:138460. doi: 10.1155/2014/138460

Li, S., and Zhang, B. (2013). Traditional Chinese medicine network pharmacology: theory, methodology and application. *Chin. J. Nat. Med.* 11, 110–120. doi: 10.1016/s1875-5364(13)60037-0

Li, S., Zhang, B., Jiang, D., Wei, Y., and Zhang, N. (2010). Herb network construction and co-module analysis for uncovering the combination rule of traditional Chinese herbal formulae. *BMC Bioinformatics* 11:S6. doi: 10.1186/1471-2105-11-S11-S

Li, S., Zhang, B., and Zhang, N. (2011). Network target for screening synergistic drug combinations with application to traditional Chinese medicine. *BMC Syst. Biol.* 5(Suppl. 1):S10. doi: 10.1186/1752-0509-5-s1-s10

Li, S., Zhang, Z. Q., Wu, L. J., Zhang, X. G., Li, Y. D., and Wang, Y. Y. (2007). Understanding ZHENG in traditional Chinese medicine in the context of neuro-endocrine-immune network. *IET Syst. Biol.* 1, 51–60. doi: 10.1049/iet-syb:20060032

Li, X., Wu, L., Liu, W., Jin, Y., Chen, Q., Wang, L., et al. (2014c). A network pharmacology study of Chinese medicine QiShenYiQi to reveal its underlying multi-compound, multi-target, multi-pathway mode of action. *PLoS One* 9:e95004. doi: 10.1371/journal.pone.0095004

Li, X., Xu, X., Wang, J., Yu, H., Wang, X., Yang, H., et al. (2012). A system-level investigation into the mechanisms of Chinese traditional medicine: compound Danshen formula for cardiovascular disease treatment. *PLoS One* 7:e43918. doi: 10.1371/journal.pone.0043918

Li, Y., Han, C., Wang, J., Xiao, W., Wang, Z., Zhang, J., et al. (2014d). Investigation into the mechanism of *Eucommia ulmoides Oliv.* based on a systems pharmacology approach. *J. Ethnopharmacol.* 151, 452–460. doi: 10.1016/j.jep.2013.10.067

Liang, X., Li, H., and Li, S. (2014a). A novel network pharmacology approach to analyse traditional herbal formulae: the Liu-Wei-Di-Huang pill as a case study. *Mol. Biosyst.* 10, 1014–1022. doi: 10.1039/C3MB70507B

Liang, X., Li, H., and Li, S. (2014b). A novel network pharmacology approach to analyse traditional herbal formulae: the Liu-Wei-Di-Huang pill as a case study. *Mol. Biosyst.* 10, 1014–1022. doi: 10.1039/c3mb70507b

Liu, H., Zeng, L., and Yang, K. (2016). A network pharmacology approach to explore the pharmacological mechanism of xiaoyao powder on anovulatory infertility. *Evid. Based. Complement. Alternat. Med.* 2016:2960372. doi: 10.1155/2016/2960372

Liu, Q., Zhang, Z., Fang, L., Jiang, Y., and Yin, X. (2012). Application of network pharmacology and high through-put technology on active compounds screening from traditional Chinese medicine. *Zhongguo Zhong Yao Za Zhi* 37, 134–137.

Lorenzo, A., Auguet, T., Vidal, F., Broch, M., Olona, M., Gutiérrez, C., et al. (2006). Polymorphisms of alcohol-metabolizing enzymes and the risk for alcoholism and alcoholic liver disease in Caucasian Spanish women. *Drug Alcohol Depend.* 84, 195–200. doi: 10.1016/j.drugalcdep.2006.03.002

Lurje, G., Hendifar, A. E., Schultheis, A. M., Pohl, A., Husain, H., Yang, D., et al. (2009). Polymorphisms in interleukin 1 beta and interleukin 1 receptor antagonist associated with tumor recurrence in stage II colon cancer. *Pharmacogenet. Genomics* 19, 95–102. doi: 10.1097/FPC.0b013e32831a9ad1

Ma, H. T., Hsieh, J. F., and Chen, S. T. (2015). Anti-diabetic effects of *Ganoderma lucidum*. *Phytochemistry* 114, 109–113. doi: 10.1016/j.phytochem.2015.02.017

Marcos, M., Pastor, I., Gonzalez-Sarmiento, R., and Laso, F. J. (2008). A new genetic variant involved in genetic susceptibility to alcoholic liver cirrhosis: -330T > G polymorphism of the interleukin-2 gene. *Eur. J. Gastroenterol. Hepatol.* 20, 855–859. doi: 10.1097/MEG.0b013e3282fd0db1

Marcos, M., Pastor, I., Gonzalez-Sarmiento, R., and Laso, F. J. (2009). A functional polymorphism of the NFKB1 gene increases the risk for alcoholic liver cirrhosis in patients with alcohol dependence. *Alcohol. Clin. Exp. Res.* 33, 1857–1862. doi: 10.1111/j.1530-0277.2009.01023.x

Ogino, S., Nosho, K., Kirkner, G. J., Shima, K., Irahara, N., Kure, S., et al. (2009). PIK3CA mutation is associated with poor prognosis among patients with curatively resected colon cancer. *J. Clin. Oncol.* 27, 1477–1484. doi: 10.1200/JCO.2008.18.6544

Paterson, R. R. (2006). Ganoderma - a therapeutic fungal biofactory. *Phytochemistry* 67, 1985–2001. doi: 10.1016/j.phytochem.2006.07.004

Peri, S., Navarro, J. D., Amanchy, R., Kristiansen, T. Z., Jonnalagadda, C. K., Surendranath, V., et al. (2003). Development of human protein reference database as an initial platform for approaching systems biology in humans. *Genome Res.* 13, 2363–2371. doi: 10.1101/gr.1680803

Press, O. A., Zhang, W., Gordon, M. A., Yang, D., Lurje, G., Iqbal, S., et al. (2008). Gender-related survival differences associated with EGFR polymorphisms in metastatic colon cancer. *Cancer Res.* 68, 3037–3042. doi: 10.1158/0008-5472.CAN-07-2718

Qiu, J. (2007). Traditional medicine: a culture in the balance. *Nature* 448, 126–128. doi: 10.1038/448126a

Ropero Gradilla, P., Villegas Martínez, A., Fernández Arquero, M., García-Agúndez, J. A., González Fernández, F. A., Benítez Rodríguez, J., et al. (2001).

C282Y and H63D mutations of HFE gene in patients with advanced alcoholic liver disease. *Rev. Esp. Enferm. Dig.* 93, 156–163.

Rossit, A. R., Cabral, I. R., Hackel, C., da Silva, R., Froes, N. D., and Abdel-Rahman, S. Z. (2002). Polymorphisms in the DNA repair gene XRCC1 and susceptibility to alcoholic liver cirrhosis in older Southeastern Brazilians. *Cancer Lett.* 180, 173–182. doi: 10.1016/S0304-3835(02)00029-0

Ru, J., Li, P., Wang, J., Zhou, W., Li, B., Huang, C., et al. (2014). TCMSP: a database of systems pharmacology for drug discovery from herbal medicines. *J. Cheminform.* 6:13. doi: 10.1186/1758-2946-6-13

Shannon, P., Markiel, A., Ozier, O., Baliga, N. S., Wang, J. T., Ramage, D., et al. (2003). Cytoscape: a software environment for integrated models of biomolecular interaction networks. *Genome Res.* 13, 2498–2504. doi: 10.1101/gr.1239303

Shi, S. H., Cai, Y. P., Cai, X. J., Zheng, X. Y., Cao, D. S., Ye, F. Q., et al. (2014). A network pharmacology approach to understanding the mechanisms of action of traditional medicine: bushenhuoxue formula for treatment of chronic kidney disease. *PLoS One* 9:e89123. doi: 10.1371/journal.pone.0089123

Slattery, M. L., Curtin, K., Wolff, R., Ma, K. N., Sweeney, C., Murtaugh, M., et al. (2006). PPARγ and colon and rectal cancer: associations with specific tumor mutations, aspirin, ibuprofen and insulin-related genes (United States). *Cancer Causes Control* 17, 239–249. doi: 10.1007/s10552-005-0411-6

Spina, C., Bottini, P. S., and Gloria-Bottini, F. (2008). ACP1 genetic polymorphism and colon cancer. *Cancer Genet. Cytogenet.* 186, 61–62. doi: 10.1016/j.cancergencyto.2008.06.006

Szklarczyk, D., Franceschini, A., Wyder, S., Forslund, K., Heller, D., Huerta-Cepas, J., et al. (2015). STRING v10: protein-protein interaction networks, integrated over the tree of life. *Nucleic Acids Res.* 43, D447–D452. doi: 10.1093/nar/gku1003

Tan, W., Li, Y., Wang, Y., Zhang, Z., Wang, T., Zhou, Q., et al. (2017). Anti-coagulative and gastrointestinal motility regulative activities of Fructus Aurantii immaturus and its effective fractions. *Biomed. Pharmacother.* 90, 244–252. doi: 10.1016/j.biopha.2017.03.060

Tang, F., Tang, Q., Tian, Y., Fan, Q., Huang, Y., and Tan, X. (2015). Network pharmacology-based prediction of the active ingredients and potential targets of Mahuang Fuzi Xixin decoction for application to allergic rhinitis. *J. Ethnopharmacol.* 176, 402–412. doi: 10.1016/j.jep.2015.10.040

Tao, J., Hou, Y., Ma, X., Liu, D., Tong, Y., Zhou, H., et al. (2016). An integrated global chemomics and system biology approach to analyze the mechanisms of the traditional Chinese medicinal preparation *Eriobotrya japonica - Fritillaria usuriensis* dropping pills for pulmonary diseases. *BMC Complement. Altern. Med.* 16:4. doi: 10.1186/s12906-015-0983-y

Tao, W., Xu, X., Wang, X., Li, B., Wang, Y., Li, Y., et al. (2013). Network pharmacology-based prediction of the active ingredients and potential targets of Chinese herbal Radix Curcumae formula for application to cardiovascular disease. *J. Ethnopharmacol.* 145, 1–10. doi: 10.1016/j.jep.2012.09.051

Vanunu, O., Magger, O., Ruppin, E., Shlomi, T., and Sharan, R. (2010). Associating genes and protein complexes with disease via network propagation. *PLoS Comput. Biol.* 6:e1000641. doi: 10.1371/journal.pcbi.1000641

Wang, H. H., Zhang, B. X., Ye, X. T., He, S. B., Zhang, Y. L., and Wang, Y. (2015). Study on mechanism for anti-depression efficacy of Sini San through auxiliary mechanism elucidation system for Chinese medicine. *Zhongguo Zhong Yao Za Zhi* 40, 3723–3728.

Wang, P., Sun, H., Lv, H., Sun, W., Yuan, Y., Han, Y., et al. (2010). Thyroxine and reserpine-induced changes in metabolic profiles of rat urine and the therapeutic effect of Liu Wei Di Huang Wan detected by UPLC-HDMS. *J. Pharm. Biomed. Anal.* 53, 631–645. doi: 10.1016/j.jpba.2010.04.032

Wang, S., Tong, Y., Ng, T. B., Lao, L., Lam, J. K., Zhang, K. Y., et al. (2015). Network pharmacological identification of active compounds and potential actions of Erxian decoction in alleviating menopause-related symptoms. *Chin. Med.* 10:19. doi: 10.1186/s13020-015-0051-z

Wang, Y., Xiao, J., Suzek, T. O., Jian, Z., Wang, J., and Bryant, S. H. (2009). PubChem: a public information system for analyzing bioactivities of small molecules. *Nucleic Acids Res.* 37, W623–W633. doi: 10.1093/nar/gkp456

Wexler, P. (2001). TOXNET: an evolving web resource for toxicology and environmental health information. *Toxicology* 157, 3–10. doi: 10.1016/S0300-483X(00)00337-1

Wishart, D. S., Knox, C., Guo, A. C., Shrivastava, S., Hassanali, M., Stothard, P., et al. (2006). DrugBank: a comprehensive resource for in silico drug discovery and exploration. *Nucleic Acids Res.* 34, D668–D672. doi: 10.1093/nar/gkj067

Wolfgang, G. H., and Johnson, D. E. (2002). Web resources for drug toxicity. *Toxicology* 173, 67–74. doi: 10.1016/S0300-483X(02)00022-7

Wu, C. R., Lin, L. W., Wang, W. H., and Hsieh, M. T. (2007). The ameliorating effects of LiuWei Dihuang Wang on cycloheximide-induced impairment of passive avoidance performance in rats. *J. Ethnopharmacol.* 113, 79–84. doi: 10.1016/j.jep.2007.05.003

Wu, L., Gao, X., Wang, L., Liu, Q., Fan, X., Wang, Y., et al. (2011). Prediction of multi-target of Aconiti Lateralis Radix Praeparata and its network pharmacology. *Zhongguo Zhong Yao Za Zhi* 36, 2907–2910.

Wu, L., Wang, Y., Li, Z., Zhang, B., Cheng, Y., and Fan, X. (2014). Identifying roles of "Jun-Chen-Zuo-Shi" component herbs of QiShenYiQi formula in treating acute myocardial ischemia by network pharmacology. *Chin. Med.* 9:24. doi: 10.1186/1749-8546-9-24

Xiang, H., Wang, G., Qu, J., Xia, S., Tao, X., Qi, B., et al. (2016). Yin-Chen-Hao tang attenuates severe acute pancreatitis in rat: an experimental verification of in silico network target prediction. *Front. Pharmacol.* 7:378. doi: 10.3389/fphar.2016.00378

Xiang, Z., Sun, H., Cai, X., Chen, D., and Zheng, X. (2015). The study on the material basis and the mechanism for anti-renal interstitial fibrosis efficacy of rhubarb through integration of metabonomics and network pharmacology. *Mol. Biosyst.* 11, 1067–1078. doi: 10.1039/c4mb00573b

Xie, B., Gong, T., Tang, M., Mi, D., Zhang, X., Liu, J., et al. (2008). An approach based on HPLC-fingerprint and chemometrics to quality consistency evaluation of Liuwei Dihuang Pills produced by different manufacturers. *J. Pharm. Biomed. Anal.* 48, 1261–1266. doi: 10.1016/j.jpba.2008.09.011

Xu, H., Zhang, Y., Lei, Y., Gao, X., Zhai, H., Lin, N., et al. (2014). A systems biology-based approach to uncovering the molecular mechanisms underlying the effects of dragon's blood tablet in colitis, involving the integration of chemical analysis, ADME prediction, and network pharmacology. *PLoS One* 9:e101432. doi: 10.1371/journal.pone.0101432

Xue, R., Fang, Z., Zhang, M., Yi, Z., Wen, C., and Shi, T. (2013). TCMID: traditional Chinese medicine integrative database for herb molecular mechanism analysis. *Nucleic Acids Res.* 41, D1089–D1095. doi: 10.1093/nar/gks1100

Ye, H., Ye, L., Kang, H., Zhang, D., Tao, L., Tang, K., et al. (2011). HIT: linking herbal active ingredients to targets. *Nucleic Acids Res.* 39, D1055–D1059. doi: 10.1093/nar/gkq1165

Yi, Y. D., and Chang, I. M. (2004). An overview of traditional Chinese herbal formulae and a proposal of a new code system for expressing the formula title. *Evid. Based. Complement. Alternat. Med.* 1, 125–132. doi: 10.1093/ecam/neh019

Yu, C., Li, Y., Chen, W., and Yue, M. (2002). Genotype of ethanol metabolizing enzyme genes by oligonucleotide microarray in alcoholic liver disease in Chinese people. *Chin. Med. J.* 115, 1085–1087.

Yu, G., Zhang, Y., Ren, W., Ling, D., Li, J., Geng, Y., et al. (2017). Network pharmacology-based identification of key pharmacological pathways of Yin–Huang–Qing–Fei capsule acting on chronic bronchitis. *Int. J. Chron. Obstruct. Pulmon. Dis.* 12, 85–94. doi: 10.2147/COPD.S121079

Yuan, H. D., Kim, J. T., Kim, S. H., and Chung, S. H. (2012). Ginseng and diabetes: the evidences from in vitro, animal and human studies. *J. Ginseng. Res.* 36, 27–39. doi: 10.5142/jgr.2012.36.1.27

Zanzoni, A., Montecchi-Palazzi, L., Quondam, M., Ausiello, G., Helmer-Citterich, M., and Cesareni, G. (2002). MINT: a Molecular INTeraction database. *FEBS Lett.* 513, 135–140. doi: 10.1016/S0014-5793(01)03293-8

Zeng, L., and Yang, K. (2017). Exploring the pharmacological mechanism of Yanghe Decoction on HER2-positive breast cancer by a network pharmacology approach. *J. Ethnopharmacol.* 199, 68–85. doi: 10.1016/j.jep.2017.01.045

Zhang, B., Wang, X., and Li, S. (2013). An integrative platform of TCM network pharmacology and its application on a herbal formula, Qing-Luo-Yin. *Evid. Based. Complement. Alternat. Med.* 2013:456747. doi: 10.1155/2013/456747

Zhang, P., Li, J., and Wang, Y. (2008). Bayesian belief network and its application in predicting the five flavors of Chinese medicinal components. *Mod. Tradit. Chin. Med. Mater. Mater. World Sci. Technol.* 10, 114–117. doi: 10.11842/wst.2008.5

Zhang, R. Z., Yu, S. J., Bai, H., and Ning, K. (2017). TCM-Mesh: the database and analytical system for network pharmacology analysis for TCM preparations. *Sci. Rep.* 7:2821. doi: 10.1038/s41598-017-03039-7

Zhang, Y., Lin, Y., Zhao, H., Guo, Q., Yan, C., and Lin, N. (2016). Revealing the effects of the herbal pair of euphorbia kansui and glycyrrhiza on hepatocellular carcinoma ascites with integrating network target analysis and experimental validation. *Int. J. Biol. Sci.* 12, 594–606. doi: 10.7150/ijbs.14151

Zhao, F., Guochun, L., Yang, Y., Shi, L., Xu, L., and Yin, L. (2015). A network pharmacology approach to determine active ingredients and rationality of herb combinations of Modified-Simiaowan for treatment of gout. *J. Ethnopharmacol.* 168, 1–16. doi: 10.1016/j.jep.2015.03.035

Zhao, X., Wang, Y., and Sun, Y. (2007). Quantitative and qualitative determination of Liuwei Dihuang tablets by HPLC-UV-MS-MS. *J. Chromatogr. Sci.* 45, 549–552. doi: 10.1093/chromsci/45.8.549

Zheng, C. S., Xu, X. J., Ye, H. Z., Wu, G. W., Li, X. H., Xu, H. F., et al. (2013). Network pharmacology-based prediction of the multi-target capabilities of the compounds in Taohong Siwu decoction, and their application in osteoarthritis. *Exp. Ther. Med.* 6, 125–132. doi: 10.3892/etm.2013.1106

Zhou, S. S., Xu, J., Zhu, H., Wu, J., Xu, J. D., Yan, R., et al. (2016). Gut microbiota-involved mechanisms in enhancing systemic exposure of ginsenosides by coexisting polysaccharides in ginseng decoction. *Sci. Rep.* 6:22474. doi: 10.1038/srep22474

7

The Key Target and Molecular Mechanism of the Volatile Component of *Scutellaria baicalensis* Georgi in Acute Lung Injury Based on Network Pharmacology

Guosong Zhu[1], Jiaqiang Zhang[1], Yali Yang[1], Haoran Zhang[1], Wenwen Jin[2], Fangchu Su[2], Junting Liang[3], Kaiwei Wang[1], Jianhua Zhang[2]* and Chuanliang Chen[3]**

[1]Department of Anesthesia and Perioperative Medicine, Henan Provincial People's Hospital, People's Hospital of Zhengzhou University, Zhengzhou, China, [2]Medical Engineering Technology and Data Mining Institute, Zhengzhou University, Zhengzhou, China, [3]Clinical Bioinformatics Experimental Center, Henan Provincial People's Hospital, People's Hospital of Zhengzhou University, Zhengzhou, China

***Correspondence:**
Kaiwei Wang
wangkw1975@163.com
Jianhua Zhang
petermail@zzu.edu.cn
Chuanliang Chen
henanccl@163.com

Ethnopharmacological relevance: *Scutellaria baicalensis* georgi is one of the most widely studied TCMs; its effects in ALI have been studied in a large number of experiments, and the efficacy of volatile oil from TCM remains to be studied.

Aim: The volatile component of *Scutellaria baicalensis* georgi was selected to act on the key target of acute lung injury and was preliminarily studied for its specific molecular mechanism.

Methods: The volatile active substances of *Scutellaria baicalensis* georgi were extracted by GC–MS, and the active ingredients related with the occurrence and development of acute lung injury were searched and matched by the TCMSP database. The pharmacologic data and analysis platform of TCM were used to retrieve and screen for the volatile active components and the possible therapeutic targets of *Scutellaria baicalensis* georgi. In addition, acute lung injury was searched in the disease target database to identify the corresponding disease target proteins, thereby establishing a protein–protein interaction network. Finally, the effects of wogonin on the apoptotic and inflammatory factors in the acute lung injury cell model were analyzed experimentally.

Results: We identified 100 candidate targets and successfully constructed a complex target network. The targets identified by the above gene enrichment analysis played important roles in the autoimmune disease cell cycle apoptosis and related signaling pathways. The KEGG pathway analysis showed that most of the target genes were involved in the inflammatory response regulation of the TRP, PI3K-Akt, and IL-17 signaling pathways. The participation of wogonin in the specific regulatory pathways of PI3K-Akt signaling and IL-17 signaling was verified through experiments. In the lung-injured cell model, the results showed that wogonin inhibited the apoptosis of injured lung cells by inhibiting the expression of *BAD* gene and the activation of cleaved *caspase-3* gene while increasing Bcl-2 expression. In addition, wogonin inhibited the expression of the abovementioned inflammatory factors and further inhibited the inflammatory response in the lung injury cells.

Conclusion: The results of pharmacological network analysis can predict and explain the regulation mechanism of multi-target and multi-pathway of TCM components. This study identified the potential target and important pathway of wogonin in regulating acute lung injury. At the same time, the accuracy of network pharmacological prediction is also preliminarily verified by molecular biology experiment.

Keywords: key target, signal pathway, acute lung injury, network pharmacology, wogonin

INTRODUCTION

The pathogenesis of acute lung injury (ALI) essentially includes uncontrolled inflammatory response in the body, with injury of alveolar epithelial and pulmonary capillary endothelial cells as the main pathologic manifestations (Gouda and Bhandary, 2019; Mokra et al., 2019). The most important treatment strategy for ALI is mechanical ventilation. Drug therapy mainly comprises statins which have rich pharmacologic activities, can inhibit the release of inflammatory mediators and platelet aggregation, act as anticoagulant and antioxidant, and can improve endothelial function (Xu et al., 2019). In addition to statins, keratinized cell growth factor and neutrophil elastase inhibitors may be given for ALI (Hiroshima et al., 2017; Patel et al., 2018). In China, traditional Chinese medicine (TCM) is mainly used to treat ALI by regulating inflammatory mediators. *Scutellaria baicalensis* georgi is one of the most widely studied TCMs that were shown to have significant effects in the treatment of ALI; its active ingredients include baicalin and flavonoids (Ding et al., 2016; Meng et al., 2019; Peng et al., 2019; Zhi et al., 2020). However, only few have studied the effects of the volatile components of *Scutellaria baicalensis* georgi on ALI.

Network pharmacology is based on large data on background fusion system biology, molecular biology, and pharmacology, and a variety of emerging macroscopic to microcosmic disciplines on network computer platform (Poornima et al., 2016; Jain et al., 2018). It screens and builds a multilevel network, using a variety of database platform and computer software and data visualization that are more directed to interpret the correlation of TCM compounds with disease (Li et al., 2017; Sidders et al., 2018). Based on these, the volatile components in *S. baicalensis* were extracted by GC–MS experiment. The active components related with the development and progression of ALI were searched and matched with the TCMSP database. Then, based on network pharmacology, the volatile components of Radix Scutellariae and the network relationship among the ALI-related targets were simulated to clarify the mechanisms in ALI. In addition, we carried out a large number of biological experiments to validate the volatile components of Radix Scutellariae and to investigate the mechanism of wogonin for the treatment of ALI.

MATERIALS AND METHODS

Extraction of Volatile Components From *Scutellaria baicalensis* by GC–MS

a) Sample preparation: 30 g of *Scutellaria* was crushed and sifted before being divided into three equal parts of 10 g each. Ethanol, methanol, and benzenol were respectively extracted using hot water for 4 h. After passing through a 0.22-μm ultrafiltration membrane, the filtrate was concentrated to 5 ml using a rotating evaporator, and again filtered through a 0.22-μm filter membrane to obtain samples in an injection bottle. The sample was set aside for GC–MS analysis (Agilent).
b) Gas chromatography conditions: the elastic quartz capillary column (RTX-5MS; 30 m × 0.25 mm, 0.25 μm) was heated by the program. The column temperature was successively increased to 210°C for 10 min, 220°C for 1 min, and 280°C for 10 min and was kept for 1 min; the determination time was 20 min in total. The shunting ratio was 20:1. The inlet temperature was 280°C and the column front pressure was 50 kPa. The injection volume was 1 μl, the carrier gas was high purity nitrogen (99.999%) and the flow rate was 1.1 ml/min.
c) Mass spectrum conditions: the EI ion source temperature was 200°C. The electron energy was 70 eV. The connector temperature was 250°C. The solvent delay was 3.5 min. The scanning range was 50–600 amu. The voltage of the electron multiplier was 1200 V.
d) Screening with the prior data: the corresponding compound ion flow chart was generated, according to the mass spectrum of each chromatographic peak fragments figure, literature report, and database data. The mass spectrum data was checked based on the peak mass-to-charge ratio and the relative abundance conditions, such as intuitive comparison. The chemical composition of the physical and chemical properties, as well as the pharmacologic action of the selected crude drug was determined.

Screening of Active Ingredients in TCM

The bioactive compounds of TCM were downloaded from the TCMSP database. According to the absorption, distribution, metabolism, and excretion model of the body, oral bioavailability (OB) and drug similarity (DL) were used to screen the candidate active ingredients. DL ≥ 0.18 and OB ≥ 30% were set as the thresholds for screening the active ingredients. Thereafter, the chemical structure formula of each active ingredient compound was downloaded to predict the target gene.

Prediction of the Action Targets of the Active Ingredients Contained in TCM

The compound structure of the active ingredient downloaded from the TCMSP database was uploaded to Baton-TCM and the SwissTargetPrediction database and its parameters were set as default values.

Screening of Target Genes Associated With ALI

The target information related with ALI was obtained from the OMIM, NCBI-gene, and GeneCards database. By entering the information of the relevant gene of ALI, the target information related with ALI was finally obtained.

Network Construction and Annotation Analysis Based on the Active Components of TCM and Targets of ALI

Cytoscape 3.6.1 software was used to establish the protein interaction network between the active components of TCM and the targets related with ALI, to integrate and extract the intersection network, and to perform topological structure analysis. The degree of topology eigenvalue in the network nodes was used as the index to screen the key targets. R language was used to extract the target gene information related with ALI. GO enrichment and KEGG pathway analyses were performed.

Experimental Verification

Cell Culture and Treatments

BEAS-2B cells were cultured in an incubator with 37.5% carbon dioxide. According to previous report (Wang and Cui, 2019), wogonin concentration gradients 0,5,10, 15, 20, 25, 30, and 50 µmol/l, CCK-8 were designed to detect the effect of wogonin on cell activity. The final choice of wogonin was 50 µmol/l. The cells were pretreated with 50 µmol/l of wogonin for 8 h, followed by treatment with 50 g/ml of LPS for 16 h. CCK-8 detection was performed after reaching the time point.

Cell Activity Detection

The cells of each group at a specific time were placed into a 100-µl normal medium for each well, mixed with 10 µl of CCK-8, and incubated at 37°C for 1 h. The OD value at 450 nm was measured on a microplate analyzer for data analysis.

Western Blot

The cells were lyzed, the cellular proteins were extracted, and the protein concentration of the samples was quantified by an assay kit (Wanleibio Co., Ltd. Shenyang, China). Proteins were separated from each group of lysates (20 µg) using polyacrylamide gel and were transferred to polyvinylidene difluoride membranes (Millipore, Bedford, MA, United States). The membranes were washed in Tris-buffered saline with 0.5% Tween 20 (TBST) for 5 min and blocked in 5% skim milk for 1 h. The membranes were incubated with antibodies against caspase-3/cleaved caspase-3, BAD, and Bcl-2 (Wanleibio Co., Ltd. Shenyang, China, 1:2000 dilution) overnight at 4°C. Successively thereafter, the membranes were washed three times with TBST for 5 min each, incubated for 1 h at 37°C with rabbit HRP–conjugated anti-mouse antibody (1:1000) (Wanleibio Co., Ltd. Shenyang, China), and washed three times with TBST for 5 min each. We detected protein bands using an electrochemiluminescence agent (Wanleibio Co., Ltd. Shenyang, China). β-actin was used to normalize the band densities.

ELISA

Biochemical estimations of TNF-α, IL-1β, and IL-6 were performed using ELISA kits (Wanleibio Co., Ltd.), according to the manufacturer's instructions.

Statistical Analyses

All experimental data were tested for homogeneity and normality and were expressed as mean ± S.D. Analyses were performed using SPSS23.0 software. Comparison of the same time points was performed by independent sample t-test or analysis of variance. One-way analysis of variance was used and the data between the two groups were compared using the LSD test. $p < 0.05$ denoted statistical significance.

RESULTS

Extraction of Volatile Components From *S. baicalensis* by GC–MS

The volatile active ingredients of *S. baicalensis* were fully extracted by GC–MS using methanol, ethanol, and benzenol, and the results of the ion flow diagram are shown in **Figure 1**. Thereafter, the substances related with the development of ALI were searched and matched by TCMSP database. Finally, the volatile active ingredients of Scutellaria wogonin were identified by GC–MS analysis.

The extract of *Scutellaria baicalensis* was analyzed by GC–MS, and the volatile components of *Scutellaria baicalensis* were obtained by chromatography-mass spectrometry. Subsequently, the TCMSP database was used to identify the volatile components. As shown in **Figure 1** and **Table 1**, a total of 31 volatile substances were obtained. Meanwhile, taking the peak area and peak area percentage as parameters and combining with 31 active components, the ratio of wogonin in the total 31 active volatile components was 49.38%. The phenylethanol extraction method had the highest volatile component content, which was 3.67 times and 3.95 times higher than that of ethanol extraction and

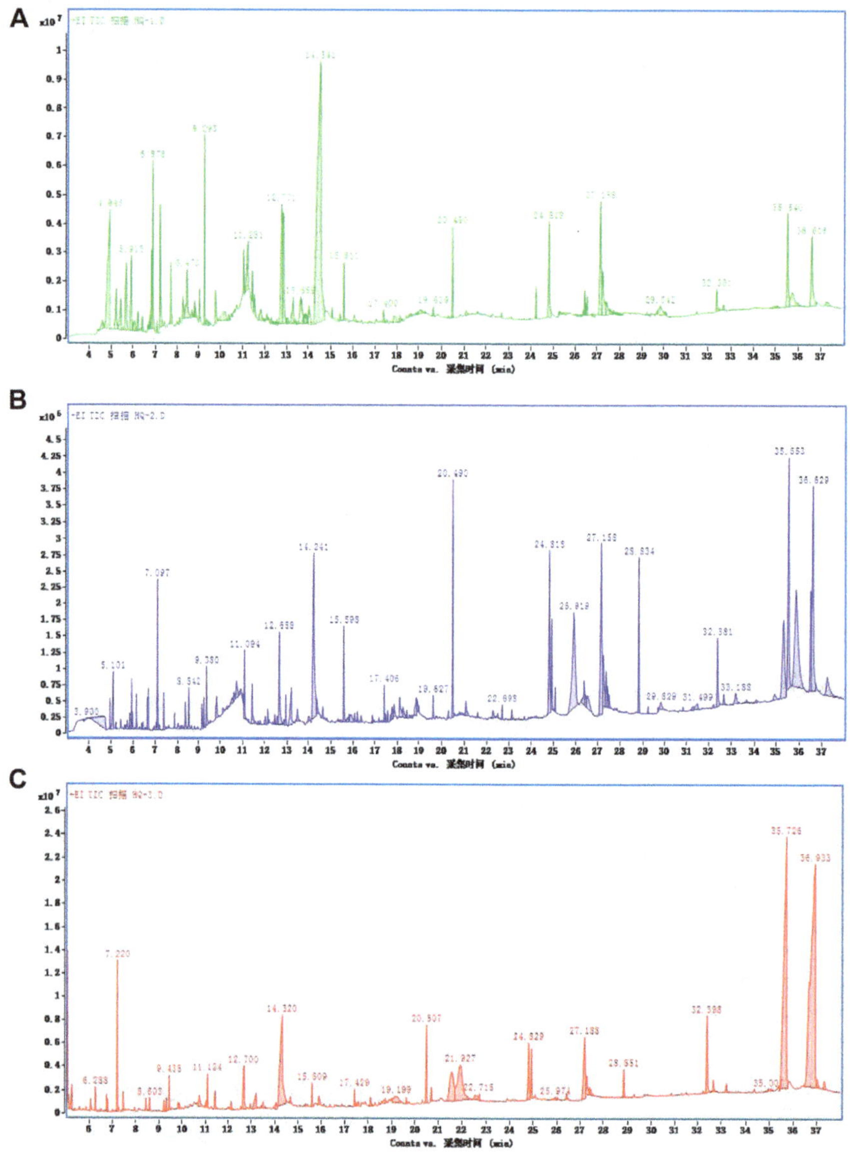

FIGURE 1 | Ion flow diagram of *Scutellaria baicalensis georgi* detected by GC–MS. GC–MS detection ion flow diagram for extraction of *S. baicalensis* by **(A)** ethanol, **(B)** methanol, and **(C)** benzenol.

methanol extraction, respectively. In the phenylethanol extraction method, the total amount of 43 compounds of wogonin accounted for 53.91%, the volatile components of wogonin were finally obtained.

Identification and Analysis of the Effects of the Volatile Components of Scutellaria on Human Targets

Using the Baton-TCM and SwissTargetPrediction database, which predicted the corresponding human target information of the compound, we obtained 117 targets of wogonin in the human body.

Identification and Analysis of Targets Related With ALI

We retrieved a list of genes associated with ALI: 106 genes were obtained from OMIM, 7966 genes were obtained from the GENECARDS tool, and 1265 genes were obtained from NCBI-GENE. Combination of the three databases obtained 7993 gene information related with ALI. After statistical analysis of the targets of the Scutellaria volatile components and the related targets of ALI, a combination of 100 targets were obtained (**Figure 2**). Using Cytoscape software, the network of the related targets of Scutellaria volatile components acting on ALI was analyzed to obtain the protein interaction network (**Figure 3**).

TABLE 1 | Volatile components of *Scutellaria baicalensis*.

Molecule name	CAS	OB (%)	DL
cis-5,8,11,14,17-Eicosapentaenoic acid	10417-94-4	45.66	0.21
1-Heptatriacotanol	105794-58-9	9.83	0.39
Hexadecanoic acid, methyl ester	112-39-0	18.09	0.12
delta-tocopherol	119-13-1	16.36	0.48
3-tert-butyl-4-hydroxyanisole	121-00-6	66.46	0.05
Ginsenoyne E	126146-63-2	36.53	0.13
Tributyl phosphate	126-73-8	27.76	0.06
1-Penten-3-one	1629-58-9	69.46	0
Dihydrooroxylin A	18956-18-8	38.72	0.23
Lactose	63-42-3	1.43	0.2
4-Mercaptophenol	637-89-8	60.34	0.01
5-Hydroxymethylfurfural	67-47-0	45.07	0.02
Panaxydol	72800-72-7	61.67	0.13
Cedrol	77-53-2	16.23	0.12
2-Methoxy-4-vinylphenol	7786-61-0	38.39	0.03
beta-Guaiene	88-84-6	19.91	0.07
4-Cyclopentene-1,3-dione	930-60-9	49.25	0.01
Benzoic acid, ethyl ester	93-89-0	27.58	0.03
Acetophenone	98-86-2	48.19	0.02
4H-Pyran-4-one, 2,3-dihydro-3,5-dihydroxy-6-methyl-	28564-83-2	37.8	0.03
1H-3a,7-Methanoazulene, 2,3,4,7,8,8a-hexahydro-3,6,8,8-tetramethyl-, [3 R-(3.alpha., 3a.beta., 7.beta., 8a.alpha.)]-	469-61-4	55.56	0.1
3-Furaldehyde	498-60-2	50.96	0.01
Orcinol	504-15-4	48.14	0.02
Di-epi-.alpha.-cedrene	50894-66-1	52.87	0.1
(1S,2S)-(+)-N-methylpseudoephedrine	51018-28-1	37.12	0.04
n-Hexadecanoic acid	57-10-3	19.3	0.1
2,5-Octadecadiynoic acid, methyl ester	57156-91-9	6.88	0.17
9,12-Octadecadienoic acid (Z,Z)-	60-33-3	41.9	0.14
2-Furancarboxaldehyde, 5-methyl-	620-02-0	43.92	0.01
Hexadecanoic acid, ethyl ester	628-97-7	18.99	0.14
Wogonin	632-85-9	30.68	0.23

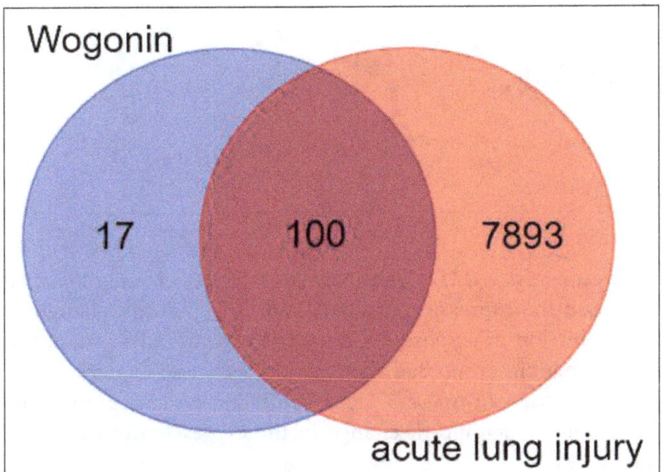

FIGURE 2 | Venn diagram of the volatile components of *Scutellaria* and the targets related with ALI.

Functional Enrichment Analysis of TCM Targets

The GO annotation analysis showed that the target of the Scutellaria volatile components on ALI was related with the regulation of fatty acid metabolism (**Figure 4**). The KEGG pathway analysis showed that most of the target genes were involved in the inflammatory response regulation of the TRP, PI3K-Akt, and IL-17 signaling pathways (**Figure 5**). ALI was mainly induced by LPS, resulting in a severe inflammatory response in the body. Our analysis showed relationship with the apoptotic signaling pathway of PI3K-Akt and the inflammatory factor signaling pathway of IL-17. According to KEGG results, the specific regulation paths of the two signaling pathways were further obtained and the results are shown in **Figure 6**.

Based on the results of the network pharmacology analysis, we used biological experiments to verify the molecular model of the Scutellaria volatile components acting on ALI.

Effects of Wogonin on the Key Targets in the Lung Injury Cell Model

The effect of wogonin on the activity of BEAS-2B cells was not significantly different under different concentration gradients, and the effect of wogonin on cell proliferation was not significantly different between all concentration gradients and without the addition of wogonin. In conclusion, different concentrations of wogonin (5, 10, 15, 20, 25, 30, and 50 μmol/l) had no effect on the activity of BEAS-2B cells (**Figure 7**). Finally, in order to increase the effect of wogonin on lung injury cells and facilitate the subsequent study of the mechanism, we

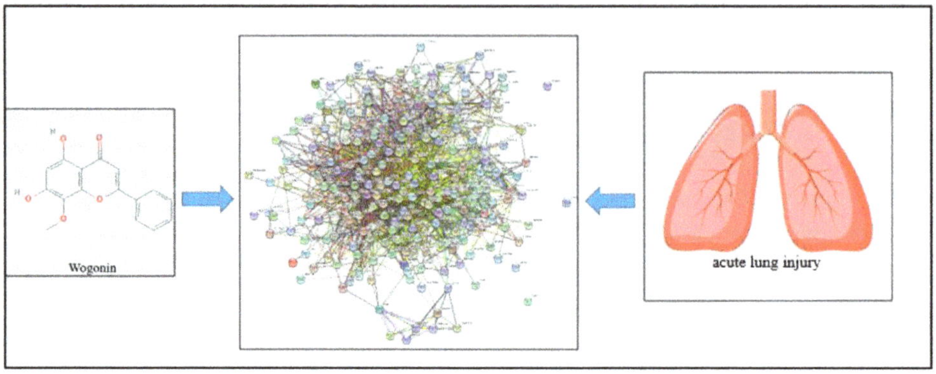

FIGURE 3 | Regulatory network model of the volatile components of *Scutellaria* acting on ALI.

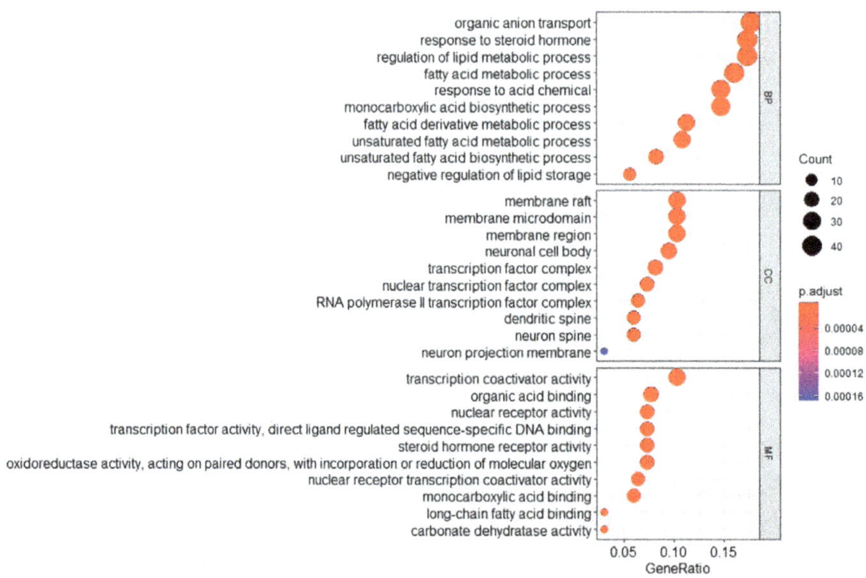

FIGURE 4 | GO annotation of *Scutellaria* volatile components acting on the target of ALI.

chose the maximum concentration of 50 µmol/l in the concentration gradient for subsequent experimental studies.

For the subsequent tests, the concentration of wogonin was selected as 50 µmol/l, as previously reported (Wang and Cui, 2019). In the lung injury cell model, the cell activity of the normal BEAS-2B cells decreased significantly after the addition of LPS; the model was successfully constructed. After the addition of wogonin, the activity of the BEAS-2B cells significantly increased (**Figure 8**).

In order to further verify the antiapoptotic mechanism of wogonin in lung injury, we analyzed the regulatory effect of wogonin on the PI3K-Akt apoptotic signaling pathway, according to the amplification analysis results of KEGG. On the Western blot analysis, we detected the expression of the apoptotic regulation genes, such as *caspase-3/cleaved caspase-3*, *BAD*, and *Bcl-2*. The results showed that compared with the blank control group, the LPS group had significantly increased expressions of *BAD* and *cleaved caspase-3*, significantly decreased the expression of *Bcl-2*, and no significant change in the expression of *caspase-3*. Compared with the LPS group, the LPS + wogonin group had significantly decreased expressions of *BAD* and *cleaved caspase-3*, significantly increased expression of *Bcl-2*, and no significant change in the expression of *caspase-3* (**Figure 9**).

In order to further verify the anti-inflammatory mechanism of wogonin in ALI, we analyzed the regulatory effect of wogonin on the IL-17 signaling pathway, according to the amplified analysis results of KEGG. TNF-α, IL-1, and IL-6 secretions were significantly increased in the LPS group, compared with those in the blank control group. Compared with the LPS group, the LPS + wogonin groups had significantly decreased secretion of inflammatory factors. As shown in **Figure 10** and **Table 2**, wogonin inhibited the expression of the inflammatory factors in the lung injury cell model.

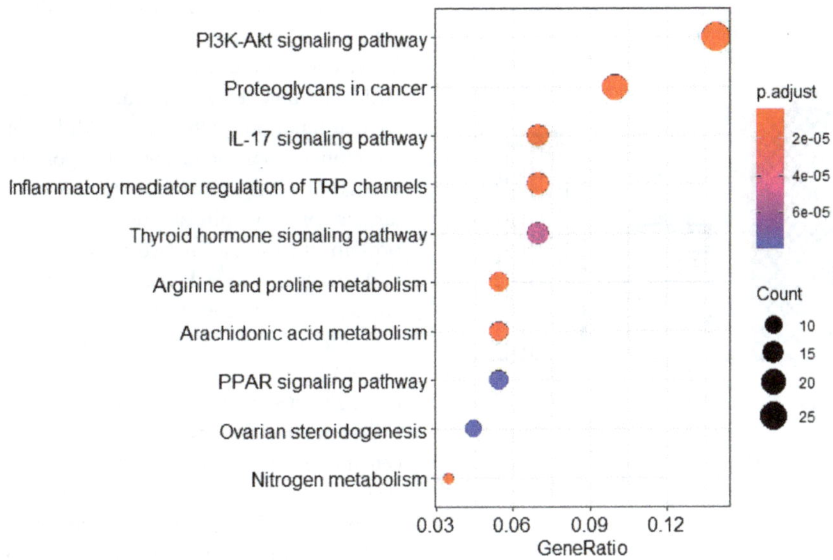

FIGURE 5 | KEGG pathway analysis of the *Scutellaria* volatile components acting on the targets of ALI.

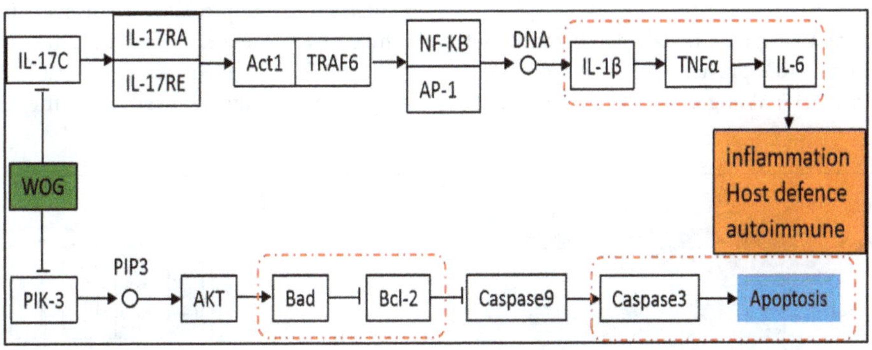

FIGURE 6 | Pathway diagram of the wogonin involved in the PI3K-Akt and IL-17 signaling pathways.

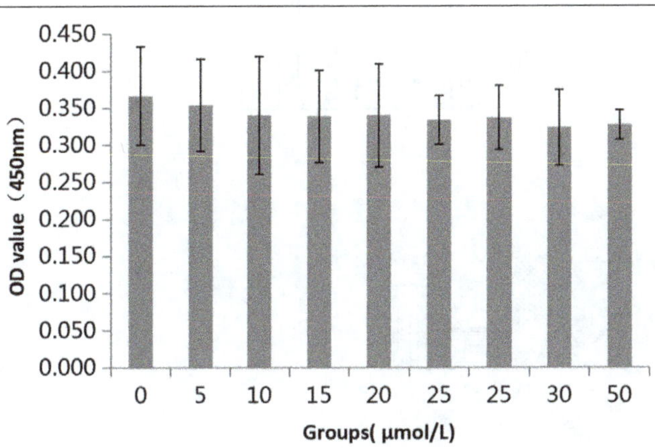

FIGURE 7 | Effect of wogonin on BEAS-2B cell viability.

DISCUSSION

At present, most conventional TCM use water-boiled processing to extract the hydrothermally soluble material components. In recent years, the pharmacologic effects of nonhydrothermally soluble substances contained in Chinese medicines have gradually gained the attention of researchers (Zorzetto et al., 2015). However, because of the pharmacologic effects of the volatile components in TCM, research and development of these volatile components have been limited by the prolonged period of animal experiments. Therefore, only few have studied the pharmacologic effects of the volatile oils in TCM. With the discovery of modern pharmacologic studies in recent years, more studies on the chemical properties and pharmacologic activities of the volatile substances in Chinese herbal medicines have been conducted. The volatile components of Chinese herbal medicines not only have analgesic, antibacterial,

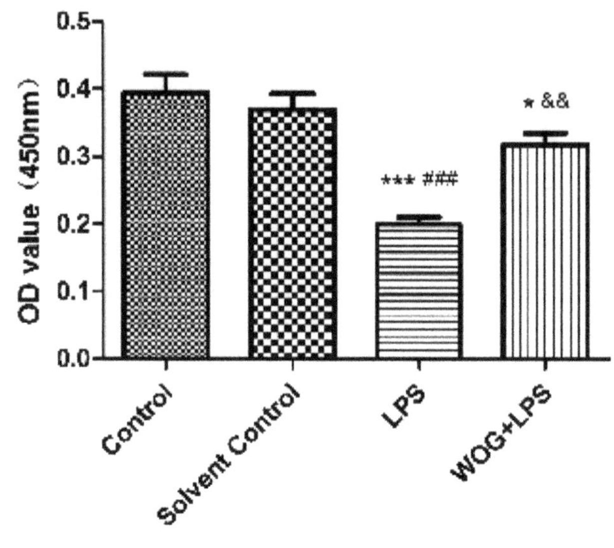

FIGURE 8 | Effect of wogonin on the activity of BEAS-2B cells with LPS. $^{*}p < 0.05$, $^{**}p < 0.01$, $^{***}p < 0.001$, compared with the control group. $^{\#}p < 0.05$, $^{\#\#}p < 0.01$, $^{\#\#\#}p < 0.001$, compared with the solvent control group. $^{\&}p < 0.05$, $^{\&\&}p < 0.01$, $^{\&\&\&}p < 0.001$, compared with the LPS group.

and anti-inflammatory effects to improve myocardial function but also have curative effects to prevent hypertension and hyperlipidemia (Singh et al., 2015; Wang et al., 2016; Zhou et al., 2016; Bui et al., 2017). In this study, the volatile components of *Scutellaria baicalensis* georgi were extracted by GC–MS, and the active components related with the development and progression of ALI were matched with the active components of Scutellaria baicalin in combination with the TCMSP database. The active volatile components of Scutellaria (wogonin) were screened for their effects on lung injury, the network analysis on the relevant targets of wogonin acting on ALI were conducted, and the protein interaction network was obtained. Further KEGG and GO analyses found that the role of wogonin was mainly concentrated in the apoptotic signaling pathway of PI3K-Akt and the inflammatory factor signaling pathway of IL-17. Therefore, we hypothesized that wogonin may exert therapeutic effects on ALI through negative regulation of apoptotic factors and pro-inflammatory factors. Furthermore, we established a lung injury cell model *in vitro* using LPS-induced BEAS-2B cells, verified the systematic pharmacologic prediction results, and discussed the mechanism of wogonin in treating ALI.

In the PI3K/AKT signaling pathway, *Bcl-2* is a gene that inhibits the apoptosis caused by a variety of cytotoxic factors and enhances the resistance of cells to most factors that cause DNA damage (Ashkenazi et al., 2017; Zhang et al., 2020). The downstream factor *BAD* is a target proapoptotic gene that regulates cell apoptosis and survival. In some studies on ALI induced by OA experiments, detecting the expression of VEGF, Bcl-2, BAD, and PI3K/AKT in serum of pulmonary bronchial lavage, the results showed that the increased Bcl-2 protein

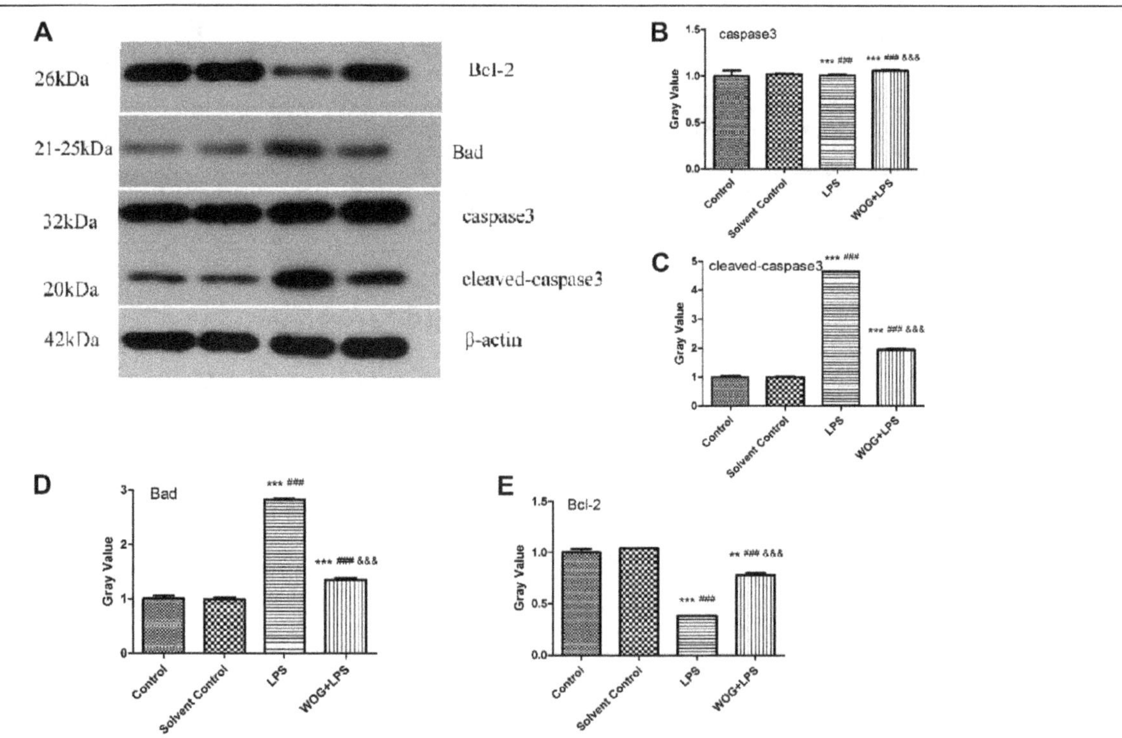

FIGURE 9 | Effect of wogonin on the BEAS-2B cells with LPS **(A)** Western blot analysis and **(B–E)** Gray analysis inhibited expressions of caspase-3/cleaved caspase-3, BAD, and Bcl-2 proteins. $^{*}p < 0.05$, $^{**}p < 0.01$, $^{***}p < 0.001$, compared with the control group. $^{\#}p < 0.05$, $^{\#\#}p < 0.01$, $^{\#\#\#}p < 0.001$, compared with the solvent control group. $^{\&}p < 0.05$, $^{\&\&}p < 0.01$, $^{\&\&\&}p < 0.001$, compared with the LPS group.

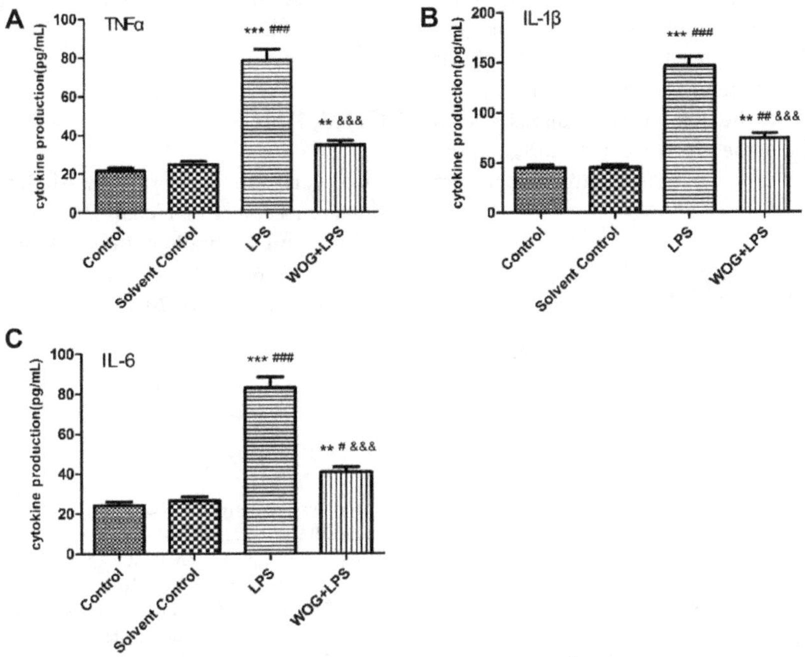

FIGURE 10 | Effect of wogonin on the BEAS-2B cells with LPS. The expressions of **(A)** TNF-α, **(B)** IL-1β, and **(C)** IL-6 are inhibited. $^{*}p < 0.05$, $^{**}p < 0.01$, $^{***}p < 0.001$, compared with the control group. $^{\#}p < 0.05$, $^{\#\#}p < 0.01$, $^{\#\#\#}p < 0.001$, compared with the solvent control group. $^{\&}p < 0.05$, $^{\&\&}p < 0.01$, $^{\&\&\&}p < 0.001$, compared with the LPS group.

TABLE 2 | Effects of wogonin on the BEAS-2B cells with LPS on the expressions of TNF-α, IL-1β, and IL-6.

Group	TNF-α	IL-1β	IL-6
Control	21.577 ± 2.712	44.776 ± 5.462	24.258 ± 2.936
Solvent control	24.738 ± 2.988	45.219 ± 4.889	26.484 ± 3.374
LPS	78.438 ± 10.109	146.657 ± 15.757	82.992 ± 9.485
LPS + wogonin	34.896 ± 3.910	74.352 ± 8.463	40.716 ± 4.324

expression was associated with the activation of AKT, the activation of AKT inhibited the expression of BAD factors, thereby, inhibiting lung cell apoptosis; this effect was achieved by the PI3K/AKT pathway. Caspase is the executor of apoptosis and other families regulate apoptosis by directly or indirectly inhibiting the activation of the members of the Caspase family (Bolívar et al., 2019). These proteases exist in the normal state as inactive progenases and are activated by apoptotic signals that stimulate the cleavage of their specific aspartic acid residues (Larsen and Sørensen, 2017). Caspase in the upstream can sequentially activate caspase downstream, forming a cascade reaction and transmitting apoptotic signals to apoptotic substrates. Both extracellular and intracellular apoptosis signals need to activate caspase-6 and caspase-7 through caspase-3 and activate various enzymes to directly lead to the characteristic apoptotic manifestations, such as DNA degradation cell wrinkling (Sergio et al., 2018). Therefore, caspase-3 is the central link in the apoptotic signal transduction process and the detection of activated caspase-3 level can reflect the apoptotic process (Messer et al., 2013). In our experiment, the cell expressions of Bcl-2, BAD, caspase-3, and cleaved caspase-3 were detected by Western blot. The results showed that, in the lung injury cell model, wogonin inhibited the expression of the *BAD* gene and activation of the *cleaved caspase-3* gene and increased the expression of *Bcl-2*, thereby, inhibiting the apoptosis of lung injury cells. In summary, these data indicated that wogonin effectively inhibited the apoptosis of lung injury cells and confirmed the results of functional enrichment analysis.

Multiple inflammatory cytokines are expressed in the lung tissue cells in ALI, and the IL-17 signaling pathway was involved in the secretion of TNF-α, IL-1β, and IL-6 (Ding et al., 2017). TNF-α is an important bioactive medium in the human body and can activate TNF-α to induce cell apoptosis and IL-6 expression and promote fibroblast proliferation (Lai et al., 2019). Il-1β, which is an endogenous source of heat, is a proinflammatory cytokine that triggers immune and inflammatory responses and can be synthesized and secreted by a variety of cells. Studies have shown that IL-1β was a promoter of inflammatory amplification and was involved in the development of inflammation (Jia et al., 2019). In this experiment, LPS was used to construct a lung injury cell model, and TNF-α, IL-6, and IL-1β were detected by ELISA. The results showed that wogonin inhibited the expression of TNF-α, IL-6, and IL-1β in lung injury cells. Therefore, these data indicated that wogonin effectively inhibited the inflammatory response of lung injury and confirmed the results of functional enrichment analysis.

In summary, this study preliminarily identified the key targets and important pathways of wogonin regulating acute lung injury through network pharmacology. At the same time, we carried out molecular biological verification on the key targets, and the experimental results also confirmed the accuracy of network pharmacological prediction. Using network pharmacological methods, this study provides an alternative strategy to help us understand the specific mechanism of traditional Chinese medicines such as wogonin in the treatment of diseases such as acute lung injury. At the same time, we will design more reasonable experiments to carry out in-depth mechanism research in the future.

AUTHOR CONTRIBUTIONS

GZ, KW, JZ, and CC participated in the research design. GZ, JZ, YY, and HZ carried out the experiment. GZ, JZ, WJ, JL, and FS performed the data analysis. GZ, JZ, YY, KW, and CC wrote the manuscript.

FUNDING

This work was supported by Medical Science and Technology Research Project of Henan Province (Grant no. SB201901098), Science and Technology Research in Henan Province (Grant no. 202102310463), the Natural Science Foundation of Henan Province (Grant no. 202300410447), and 23456 Talent Project.

REFERENCES

Ashkenazi, A., Fairbrother, W. J., Leverson, J. D., and Souers, A. J. (2017). From Basic Apoptosis Discoveries to Advanced Selective BCL-2 Family Inhibitors. *Nat. Rev. Drug Discov.* 16 (4), 273–284. doi:10.1038/nrd.2016.253

Bolívar, B. E., Vogel, T. P., and Bouchier-Hayes, L. (2019). Inflammatory Caspase Regulation: Maintaining Balance between Inflammation and Cell Death in Health and Disease. *FEBS J.* 286 (14), 2628–2644. doi:10.1111/febs.14926

Bui, T. T., Piao, C. H., Song, C. H., Lee, C.-H., Shin, H. S., and Chai, O. H. (2017). Baicalein, Wogonin, andScutellaria Baicalensisethanol Extract Alleviate Ovalbumin-Induced Allergic Airway Inflammation and Mast Cell-Mediated Anaphylactic Shock by Regulation of Th1/Th2 Imbalance and Histamine Release. *Anat. Cell Biol.* 50 (2), 124–134. doi:10.5115/acb.2017.50.2.124

Ding, Q., Liu, G.-Q., Zeng, Y.-Y., Zhu, J.-J., Liu, Z.-Y., HuangJA, X., et al. (2017). Role of IL-17 in LPS-Induced Acute Lung Injury: an In Vivo Study. *Oncotarget* 8 (55), 93704–93711. doi:10.18632/oncotarget.21474

Ding, X.-M., Pan, L., Wang, Y., and Xu, Q.-Z. (2016). Baicalin Exerts Protective Effects against Lipopolysaccharide-Induced Acute Lung Injury by Regulating the Crosstalk between the CX3CL1-Cx3cr1 axis and NF-Kb Pathway in CX3CL1-Knockout Mice. *Int. J. Mol. Med.* 37 (3), 703–715. doi:10.3892/ijmm.2016.2456

Gouda, M. M., and Bhandary, Y. P. (2019). Acute Lung Injury: IL-17A-Mediated Inflammatory Pathway and its Regulation by Curcumin. *Inflammation* 42 (4), 1160–1169. doi:10.1007/s10753-019-01010-4

Hiroshima, Y., Hsu, K., Tedla, N., Wong, S. W., Chow, S., Kawaguchi, N., et al. (2017). S100A8/A9 and S100A9 Reduce Acute Lung Injury. *Immunol. Cell Biol.* 95 (5), 461–472. doi:10.1038/icb.2017.2

Jain, B., Raj, U., and Varadwaj, P. K. (2018). Drug Target Interplay: A Network-Based Analysis of Human Diseases and the Drug Targets. *Curr. Top. Med. Chem.* 18 (13), 1053. doi:10.2174/1568026618666180719160922

Jia, X., Cao, B., An, Y., Zhang, X., and Wang, C. (2019). Rapamycin Ameliorates Lipopolysaccharide-Induced Acute Lung Injury by Inhibiting IL-1β and IL-18 Production. *Int. Immunopharmacol.* 67, 211–219. doi:10.1016/j.intimp.2018.12.017

Lai, W. Y., Wang, J. W., Huang, B. T., Lin, E. P., and Yang, P. C. (2019). A Novel TNF-α-Targeting Aptamer for TNF-α-Mediated Acute Lung Injury and Acute Liver Failure. *Theranostics* 9 (6), 1741–1751. doi:10.7150/thno.30972

Larsen, B. D., and Sørensen, C. S. (2017). The Caspase-activated DN Ase: Apoptosis and beyond. *FEBS J.* 284 (8), 1160–1170. doi:10.1111/febs.13970

Li, X., Xu, Y., Cui, H., Huang, T., Wang, D., Lian, B., et al. (2017). Prediction of Synergistic Anti-cancer Drug Combinations Based on Drug Target Network and Drug Induced Gene Expression Profiles. *Artif. Intelligence Med.* 83, 35–43. doi:10.1016/j.artmed.2017.05.008

Meng, X., Hu, L., and Li, W. (2019). Baicalin Ameliorates Lipopolysaccharide-Induced Acute Lung Injury in Mice by Suppressing Oxidative Stress and Inflammation via the Activation of the Nrf2-Mediated HO-1 Signaling Pathway. *Naunyn-schmiedeberg's Arch. Pharmacol.* 392 (11), 1421–1433. doi:10.1007/s00210-019-01680-9

Messer, M. P., Kellermann, P., Weber, S. J., Hohmann, C., Denk, S., Klohs, B., et al. (2013). Silencing of Fas, Fas-Associated via Death Domain, or Caspase 3 Differentially Affects Lung Inflammation, Apoptosis, and Development of Trauma-Induced Septic Acute Lung Injury. *Shock* 39 (1), 19–27. doi:10.1097/shk.0b013e318277d856

Mokra, D., Mikolka, P., Kosutova, P., and Mokry, J. (2019). Corticosteroids in Acute Lung Injury: The Dilemma Continues. *Ijms* 20 (19), 4765. doi:10.3390/ijms20194765

Patel, V. J., Biswas Roy, S., Mehta, H. J., Joo, M., and Sadikot, R. T. (2018). Alternative and Natural Therapies for Acute Lung Injury and Acute Respiratory Distress Syndrome. *Biomed. Res. Int.* 2018, 2476824. doi:10.1155/2018/2476824

Peng, L.-Y., Yuan, M., Song, K., Yu, J.-L., Li, J.-H., Huang, J.-N., et al. (2019). Baicalin Alleviated APEC-Induced Acute Lung Injury in Chicken by Inhibiting NF-Kb Pathway Activation. *Int. Immunopharmacol.* 72, 467–472. doi:10.1016/j.intimp.2019.04.046

Poornima, P., Kumar, J. D., Zhao, Q., Blunder, M., and Efferth, T. (2016). Network Pharmacology of Cancer: From Understanding of Complex Interactomes to the Design of Multi-Target Specific Therapeutics from Nature. *Pharmacol. Res.* 111 (111), 290–302. doi:10.1016/j.phrs.2016.06.018

Sergio, L. P. d. S., Thomé, A. M. C., Trajano, L. A. d. S. N., Mencalha, A. L., da Fonseca, A. d. S., and de Paoli, F. (2018). Photobiomodulation Prevents DNA Fragmentation of Alveolar Epithelial Cells and Alters the mRNA Levels of Caspase 3 and Bcl-2 Genes in Acute Lung Injury. *Photochem. Photobiol. Sci.* 17 (7), 975–983. doi:10.1039/c8pp00109j

Sidders, B., Karlsson, A., Kitching, L., Torella, R., Karila, P., and Phelan, A. (2018). Network-Based Drug Discovery: Coupling Network Pharmacology with Phenotypic Screening for Neuronal Excitability. *J. Mol. Biol.* 430 (18 Pt A), 3005–3015. doi:10.1016/j.jmb.2018.07.016

Singh, V., Rana, M., Jain, M., Singh, N., Naqvi, A., Malasoni, R., et al. (2015). Curcuma Oil Attenuates Accelerated Atherosclerosis and Macrophage Foam-Cell Formation by Modulating Genes Involved in Plaque Stability, Lipid Homeostasis and Inflammation. *Br. J. Nutr.* 113 (1), 100–113. doi:10.1017/s0007114514003195

Wang, C., and Cui, C. (2019). Inhibition of Lung *Cancer* Proliferation by Wogonin Is Associated with Activation of Apoptosis and Generation of Reactive Oxygen Species. *Balkan Med. J.* 37 (1), 29–33. doi:10.4274/balkanmedj.galenos.2019.2019.7.75

Wang, L., Jiang, Q., Hu, J., Zhang, Y., and Li, J. (2016). Research Progress on Chemical Constituents of Lonicerae Japonicae Flos. *Biomed. Res. Int.* 2016, 8968940. doi:10.1155/2016/8968940

Xu, W.-j., Wang, X.-x., Jin, J.-j., Zou, Q., Wu, L., Lv, T.-f., et al. (2019). Inhibition of GGPPS1 Attenuated LPS-Induced Acute Lung Injury and Was Associated with NLRP3 Inflammasome Suppression. *Am. J. Physiology-Lung Cell Mol. Physiol.* 316 (3), L567–L577. doi:10.1152/ajplung.00190.2018

Zhang, Z. H., Chen, Z. G., Liu, R. M., Liang, Q. C., Peng, Z. Y., Yin, S., et al. (2020). Bcl-2 Proteins Regulate Mitophagy in Lipopolysaccharide-Induced Acute Lung

Injury via PINK1/Parkin Signaling Pathway. *Oxid Med. Cel Longev.* 2020, 6579696. doi:10.1155/2020/6579696

Zhi, H., Jin, X., Zhu, H., Li, H., Zhang, Y., Lu, Y., et al. (2020). Exploring the Effective Materials of Flavonoids-Enriched Extract from Scutellaria Baicalensis Roots Based on the Metabolic Activation in Influenza A Virus Induced Acute Lung Injury. *J. Pharm. Biomed. Anal.* 177, 112876. doi:10.1016/j.jpba.2019.112876

Zhou, X., Choi, P. S., Yang, J. M., Or, P. M. Y., HoiPMLee, S. M. Y., et al. (2016). Chemical and Pharmacological Evaluations on the Extract of Scutellaria Baicalensis Georgi (Huang-Qin) Prepared by Various Extraction Methods. *Springerplus* 5 (1), 1438. doi:10.1186/s40064-016-3115-3

Zorzetto, C., Sanchez-Mateo, C. C., Rabanal, R. M., Lupidi, G., Bramucci, M., Quassinti, L., et al. (2015). Antioxidant Activity and Cytotoxicity on Tumour Cells of the Essential Oil from Cedronella Canariensis Var. Canariensis (L.) Webb & Berthel. (Lamiaceae)[J]. *Nat. Prod. Res.* 29 (17), 1641–1649. doi:10.1080/14786419.2014.994213

8

Systems Pharmacology for Investigation of the Mechanisms of Action of Traditional Chinese Medicine in Drug Discovery

Wenjuan Zhang[1,2,3], Ying Huai[1,2,3], Zhiping Miao[1,2,3], Airong Qian[1,2,3] and Yonghua Wang[4]**

[1] Lab for Bone Metabolism, Key Lab for Space Biosciences and Biotechnology, School of Life Sciences, Northwestern Polytechnical University, Xi'an, China, [2] Research Center for Special Medicine and Health Systems Engineering, School of Life Sciences, Northwestern Polytechnical University, Xi'an, China, [3] NPU-UAB Joint Laboratory for Bone Metabolism, School of Life Sciences, Northwestern Polytechnical University, Xi'an, China, [4] Lab of Systems Pharmacology, College of Life Sciences, Northwest University, Xi'an, China

Correspondence:
Airong Qian
qianair@nwpu.edu.cn
Yonghua Wang
yhwang@nwu.edu.cn

As a traditional medical intervention in Asia and a complementary and alternative medicine in western countries, traditional Chinese medicine (TCM) has attracted global attention in the life science field. TCM provides extensive natural resources for medicinal compounds, and these resources are generally regarded as effective and safe for use in drug discovery. However, owing to the complexity of compounds and their related multiple targets of TCM, it remains difficult to dissect the mechanisms of action of herbal medicines at a holistic level. To solve the issue, in the review, we proposed a novel approach of systems pharmacology to identify the bioactive compounds, predict their related targets, and illustrate the molecular mechanisms of action of TCM. With a predominant focus on the mechanisms of actions of TCM, we also highlighted the application of the systems pharmacology approach for the prediction of drug combination and dynamic analysis, the synergistic effects of TCMs, formula dissection, and theory analysis. In summary, the systems pharmacology method contributes to understand the complex interactions among biological systems, drugs, and complex diseases from a network perspective. Consequently, systems pharmacology provides a novel approach to promote drug discovery in a precise manner and a systems level, thus facilitating the modernization of TCM.

Keywords: bioactive compounds, target identification, systems pharmacology, synergistic effect, drug discovery

INTRODUCTION

Traditional Chinese medicine (TCM) plays important roles in the prevention and treatment of complex diseases, which has been developed in China for thousands of years (Tang et al., 2009). In recent decades, TCM has been widely used as the complementary and alternative medicine in Western countries. Generally, Chinese herbal prescriptions or formulae (also called "Fangji") are

Abbreviations: TCM, traditional Chinese medicine; ADME, absorption, distribution, metabolism, and excretion; SOD, superoxide dismutase; CK, creatine kinase; cAMP, cyclic adenosine monophosphate; cTnI, cardiac troponin I; ALOX5, arachidonate 5-lipoxygenase; TOP2A, topoisomerase 2-alpha; ADCY1, adenylate cyclase type 1; SCD, stearoyl-coenzyme A desaturase; BCHE, butyrylcholinesterase.

used in clinical practice, and they can exhibit coordinating roles through the rational combination of multiple herbs to achieve good efficacy and few side effects for various diseases' prevention and treatment (Li et al., 2009). Despite the widespread use of TCM in clinical practice, proving its effectiveness *via* scientific trials and dissecting the molecular mechanisms are still big challenges.

Indeed, TCM and Chinese medicine formulae are designed under the principle of "syndrome differentiation" according to the combination rule of medicinal properties in TCM with obvious multiple-compound characteristics (Li, 2009). In ancient times, ancestors usually tested poison to identify effective herbs; for example, Li Shizhen was a famous physician and pharmacologist in the Ming Dynasty, who tested drugs and tried poison in the spirit of dedication to science. There is no doubt that viewing humans as the testers would be risky, but knowledge on common herbs is the achievement of an Ancient Chinese medical scientist who tried poison. Nowadays, great efforts have been made to extract and isolate compounds in herbs and prescriptions, resulting in the emergence of numerous newly identified ingredients (Zhang et al., 2018). In addition, the absorption, distribution, metabolism, and excretion (ADME) properties are defined as the dynamic changes in drugs within an animal or the human body, such as oral bioavailability (OB), drug-likeness, and half-life, which are critical in drug discovery and development (Su et al., 2007). It has been reported that nearly 95% of lead compounds fail in the drug development in clinical trials each year, and approximately 50% of these failures are due to poor ADME properties (Kassel, 2004). Therefore, the optimization of the ADME properties of lead compounds may be a critical factor that determines whether the drug can be successfully developed (MacCoss and Baillie, 2004). Many clinical studies including randomized controlled trials (RCTs) of the herbs have been conducted, some demonstrating hepatotoxicity and toxicity (Hu et al., 2017). However, because the extraction and isolation of compounds derived from herbs are costly and time-consuming, as well as only a few of them have satisfactory ADME properties and less side effects, there is an urgent need to develop a fast and effective novel strategy for identifying potential active compounds.

Furthermore, the identification of compounds derived from TCM is also an important process for drug development and an essential factor for the dissection of the holistic mechanisms of action of TCM (Cao et al., 2012). Currently, the ligand-based virtual screening (LBVS), structured-based virtual screening (SBVS), and the text mining-based approach are widely used to predict the target–ligand interactions (Ballesteros and Palczewski, 2001; Byvatov et al., 2003; Krejsa et al., 2003). In addition, several chemical genomics approaches, such as the ligand-based, target-based, or target–ligand methods, are more effective to predict the compound–protein interactions (Balakin et al., 2003; Frimurer et al., 2005; Nagamine and Sakakibara, 2007; Rognan, 2007; Xia et al., 2009; He et al., 2010; Yamanishi et al., 2011). For example, Frimurer et al. have established a target-based approach to divide the receptors and the known ligands into clusters and further to discover each cluster with shared ligands (Frimurer et al., 2005). However, the target–ligand approach integrates the ligand chemical space, target space, and the available known drug–target network information to construct a complex predictive model to predict ligands or targets. For example, the *in silico* models integrated the amino acid sequences, two-dimensional chemical structures, and mass spectrometry data, as well as the chemical functional groups and biological features, for predicting the drug–target interactions (Nagamine and Sakakibara, 2007). However, all these approaches only focused on limited receptor space with certain protein families or the limited chemical space of US Food and Drug Administration (FDA)-approved drugs, and maybe they are not suitable for the unknown compounds of TCM. Therefore, novel approaches to identify the drug targets of TCM are valuable for understanding the mechanisms of TCM.

More importantly, TCM views the human body as a complex dynamical system and focuses on the balance of the human body, both internally and with its external environment (Ma et al., 2016). Previously, the researchers could only focus on the human body's reaction to herbal medicines, such as alleviating cough, reducing heat, and limiting bleeding. However, how these active molecules combine with each other to assemble as a whole to exert their therapeutic effects is still unclear, and it is of great significance to understand the molecular mechanisms of TCM. Therefore, efficient approaches to dissecting the mechanisms of drug combinations in TCM are of great significance to understand the underlying mechanisms of action of TCM.

Fortunately, the advent of systems pharmacology has provided the opportunity and methodologies for the development and modernization of TCM. In the recent year, systems pharmacology has been used to identify active natural products and investigate the mechanism of natural products (Li et al., 2015a, Li et al., 2012b; Zhang et al., 2016; Fang et al., 2017; Wang et al., 2017; Yang et al., 2017). Also, systems pharmacology provides new strategy for discovering novel drug combinations for the treatment of complex diseases. Integrated TCM for treatment of various diseases based on syndrome differentiations is one essential factor of the compatibility principles contributing to the drug efficacy (Zhang and Wang, 2015; Wang and Li, 2016a; Zhu et al., 2018). However, in contrast to Western medicine, TCM is overly dependent on the experiences of patients and practitioners and lacks systematic research methods. Therefore, there are many issues that need to be resolved in the development of TCM, for example: 1) TCM focused on the overall efficacy and clinical safety, but there is a lack of precise analysis and monitoring, including few studies on the pharmacodynamic and toxicological mechanisms; 2) the quality of herbs is one of the most important factors for the modernization of TCM, which has a major effect on the efficacy of TCM, but the quality is difficult to control; 3) the synergistic, additive, or antagonistic effects of TCM depend on the different properties of absorption, distribution, metabolism, excretion, and the toxicity of the pharmacodynamic components, which remain unclear; 4) the active ingredients and the mechanisms of action of TCM are unclear, which restrict the acceptance and development of TCM and seriously hinder the modernization processes. Owing to its complex composition and multiple systems, it is difficulty to dissect the underlying mechanisms of TCM at the systems level. Furthermore, the methodology often leads to controversy. Therefore, there is an urgent need to develop a new systematic and holistic research method.

In this review, we first introduced the concept and principle of systems pharmacology, and then we reviewed the computational methods of systems pharmacology for bioactive compound screening, target fishing, drug combination, and network analysis. In addition, we detailed the applications of systems pharmacology, including the elucidation of the mechanisms of action of herbal formulae, the design of multi-target drugs or drug combinations, and the theoretical analysis of Chinese medicine to guide the development of herbal medicine.

CONCEPT AND PRINCIPLE OF SYSTEMS PHARMACOLOGY

The exploration of the mechanism of action of the multiple compounds within a TCM prescription is the inevitable requirement for the modernization of TCM. In addition, to uncover the mechanism of actions of TCM, the modern scientific and technological methods need to propose for the foundation to promote the global development of TCM. Owing to its complexity, the holistic concept, and syndrome differentiation of TCM theory, the dissection of mechanisms of action of TCM is difficult. Therefore, we proposed the systematic research approach of systems pharmacology, based on the dynamic interaction of TCM with the human body from different levels, such as cellular, molecular, tissue, organ, and holistic levels (Wang and Yang, 2013) (**Figure 1**).

Systems pharmacology is an emerging discipline that focuses on the interaction between drugs and the body and the rules and mechanisms of drugs at a systems level. More specifically, the interactions between drugs and the body are illustrated from the microscopic levels (molecular and biochemical network levels) to the macroscopic levels (tissue, organ, and holistic levels). Systems pharmacology aims to investigate the changes in the functions and reactions in the human body induced by drugs, thus providing new strategies and tools to achieve precise control of the complex biological networks inside cells, thus altering disease pathophysiology, improving drug efficacy, and reducing adverse reactions (Wang and Yang, 2013; Zhang and Wang, 2015). To enhance the systems pharmacology platform, theoretic calculations and experimental methods were integrated into the models for the discovery of bioactive molecules, the identification of new drug targets, the prediction of adverse drug reactions, the exploration of therapeutic mechanisms, and the elucidation of the rules of drug combination (Huang et al., 2013a). This platform allows the large-scale analysis of simulation methodology and optimization algorithms, which can be applied to determine the molecular mechanisms of TCM and to assist the development of novel drugs.

METHODOLOGY OF SYSTEMS PHARMACOLOGY IN TCM

ADME Screening Methods of Bioactive Ingredients in TCM

The ADME properties consist of drug solubility, permeability, protein binding ability, oral bioavailability, drug-likeness, blood–brain barrier (BBB) permeability, small intestine absorption, and half-life. TCM is a multifaceted system consisting of numerous compounds, of which only a few exhibit favorable ADME properties. Therefore, the screening and analysis of bioactive components in TCM are extremely challenging. To solve this problem, in the following section, we have focused on the introduction of an *in silico* ADME system (SysADME) (**Figure 2**), which is a rapid, efficient, and cost-effective strategy to explore the potential bioactive compounds of herbal medicines.

First, from the structure of the compounds and the help of system theory and artificial intelligence, the SysADME system integrates more than 20 models, including P-glycoprotein substrate inhibitor (Pgp) recognition, small intestine absorption, BBB permeability, and a mathematical forecast of plasma protein binding (Ai et al., 2009; Wang et al., 2009; Ai et al., 2010). In addition, we have built a series of predictive toxicity analysis (toxicology) models through the integration of modern statistics, chemical informatics, and other techniques (Hao et al., 2011; Xu et al., 2011a; Xu et al., 2011b). In the following part, we will review three representative models in details.

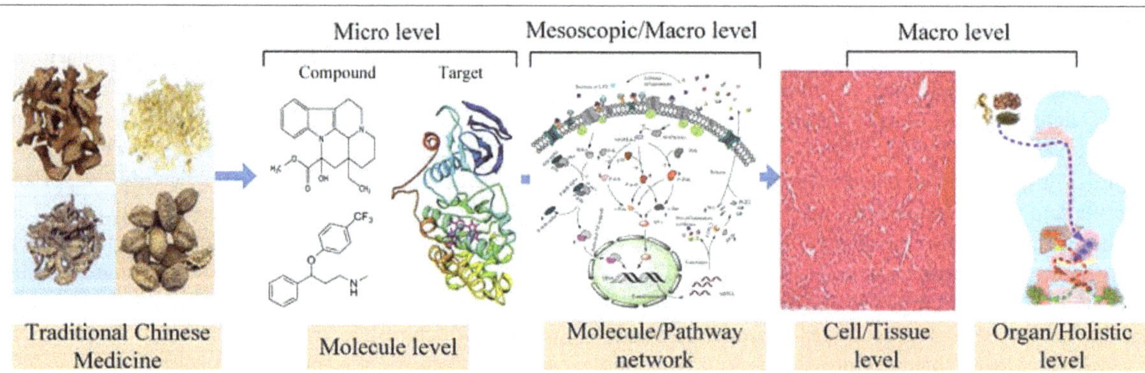

FIGURE 1 | Multi-scale models and approaches of systems pharmacology.

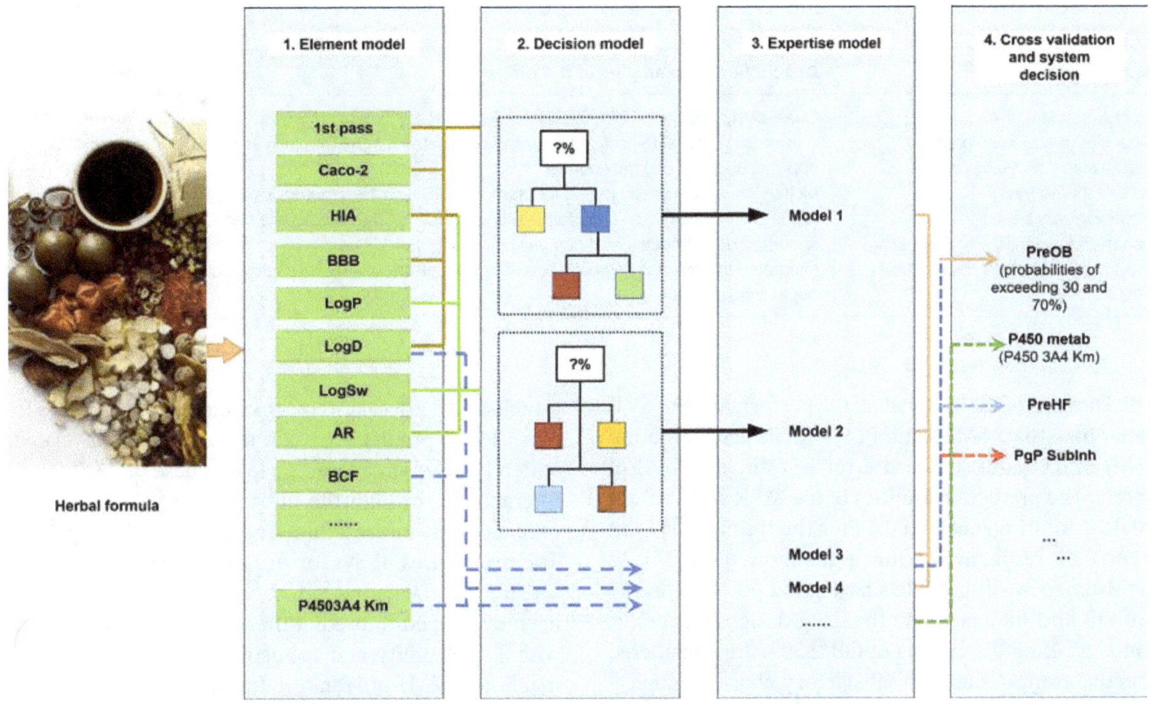

FIGURE 2 | SysADME/t system for the screening of bioactive ingredients of traditional Chinese medicines (TCMs).

The Prediction of Human Oral Bioavailability (OB)

Because the predominant and most convenient way to deliver drugs of TCM is the oral route, the good OB of a new drug candidate is one of the essential pharmacokinetic parameters of ADME properties. Recently, multiple large-scale experiments have been conducted to evaluate the OB values of drugs, but they are labor-intensive and time-consuming. At first, Lipinski's "rule of five" has been qualitatively used to predict the absorption and permeability of drugs to guide the prediction of OB (Lipinski et al., 2012). And then many *in silico* models have been established to predict OB of drug molecules in the early stages of drug discovery (Aller et al., 2009). Quantitative structure–property relationship (QSPR), rule of thumb (RoT), and physiologically based-pharmacokinetic (PBPK) approaches are promising alternatives to the OB prediction (Agoram et al., 2001; Cabrera-Pérez et al., 2018). Since 2000, numerous QSPR models have been developed to predict OB; for example, Andrews et al. constructed a regression model to predict OB based on a dataset of 591 molecules by applying 85 structural descriptors (Aller et al., 2009). Compared to Lipinski's "rule of five," the false-negative rate was reduced from 5% to 3%, and the false-positive rate decreased from 78% to 53%. In addition, Yoshida et al. used the multiple linear regression model for predicting OB with 15 structural descriptors (Yoshida and Topliss, 2000). However, the correct accuracy of this model can only achieve 60% for the test compounds. As for PBPK models, Yu and Amidon have established a compartmental model of absorption and transit (CAT) to predict the fraction of absorbed dose of different drugs (Yu, 1999). These integrated models were established based on seven transit compartments, which represent different anatomical regions of the small intestine. The limitation of the CAT model is that it ignored several properties that affect drug absorption, such as rate of dissolution, pH dependence on drug solubility, absorption in the stomach and/or colon, first-pass metabolism, and drug degradation in the intestine and liver, leading to the prediction of absorption with low solubility or permeability (Cabrera-Pérez et al., 2018). Up to now, there are no reliable and efficient models for prediction of OB based on simple descriptors.

In our previous work, given the multiple compounds, multiple targets, and synergetic effects of TCM, we have proposed a mathematical model called prediction of oral drug bioavailability (PreOB), which integrated the effects of Pgp efflux and P450 metabolism to ensure the accuracy of OB prediction of drugs (Xu et al., 2012). The PreOB was carried out by the following steps: first, 805 drug and drug-like molecules and their OB values were collected from the bioavailability database (Hou and Xu, 2002), and all the OB values were transformed into the common logarithm of log (oral bioavailability) (logB). Besides, a total of 1,536 dragon descriptors were calculated by Professional 5.4, 2006 (Talete, 2011). Then, all the 805 drugs were divided into several statistical subsets according to the geometry-based algorithm and iterative self-consistent approach (Jain, 2003). Next, by self-organizing map (SOM) (Vesanto, 2002), the compounds in each subset were split into training and independent validation sets based on their distribution in the chemical space. The two linear methods including multiple linear regression (MLR) and partial least squares regression (PLS), and the non-linear method support vector regression model (SVR) were available to perform prediction with five-fold cross-validation and independent

TABLE 1 | The comparisons between the tools of the prediction of oral bioavailability (OB) developed by the other groups and prediction of oral drug bioavailability (PreOB) model.

Number	Model name	Description or examples of the model	Reference
1	Lipinski's "rule of five"	Qualitatively used to predict the absorption and permeability of drugs	(Lipinski et al., 2012)
2	Quantitative structure–property relationship (QSPR) model	A regression model to predict OB based on a dataset of 591 molecules by applying 85 structural descriptors	(Aller et al., 2009)
3	Rule of thumb (RoT)	Multiple linear regression model for predicting OB with 15 structural descriptors	(Yoshida and Topliss, 2000)
4	Physiologically based-pharmacokinetic (PBPK) approach	A compartmental model of absorption and transit (CAT) to predict the fraction of absorbed dose of different drugs	(Yu, 1999)
5	Prediction of oral drug bioavailability (PreOB)	Integrated the effects of Pgp efflux and P450 metabolism to ensure the accuracy of OB prediction	(Xu et al., 2012)

external tests. The results showed that all the performance of SVR is slightly better than that of MLR and PLS, with its determination coefficient (R^2) of 0.80 and standard error of estimate (SEE) of 0.31 for test sets. The prediction abilities of the MLR and PLS are relatively weak, exhibiting 0.60 and 0.64 for the training set with SEE of 0.40 and 0.31, respectively. Our results showed that MLR-, PLS-, and SVR-based *in silico* models have good potential in the prediction of OB and may facilitate the drug design. Generally, the compounds meeting the criteria of OB ≥ 30% are considered as potential active compounds with satisfactory pharmacological properties. The comparisons between the tools of the prediction of OB developed by the other groups and PreOB model are summarized in **Table 1**. More importantly, the PreOB model has been successfully applied for material-based analysis of many Chinese medicines (Li et al., 2012b; Liu et al., 2013a).

Systematic Identification of Multiple Toxin–Target Interaction (SysTox)

For the novel drug development, many efforts are being devoted to evaluate the toxicity properties of drugs. Due to the vastness of chemical space (toxins) and the diversity of biological systems (targets), the prediction of the toxin–target interface remains difficult. Recently, several novel approaches have been proposed to achieve this goal. For example, a chemical genomics approach that focuses on how similar ligands may interact with similar proteins has been applied to predict novel bioactive compounds of a target (Klabunde, 2010; Yamanishi et al., 2010). In addition, Yu et al. have used the network method to explore ligand–target interactions from high-dimensional biological data (Yu et al., 2012). However, the prediction of toxicity information of a variety of compounds by experimental methods remains difficult, and a systems-level analysis of multiple toxin–target associations is still lacking up to now. Therefore, in our previous study, we established a novel systems toxicology approach SysTox (Zhou et al., 2013) to predict the toxin targets and their related networks, which is based on a large-scale database of 33,800 poison–target interactions through the integration of chemical, genomic, and toxicological information and systems biology technologies. The procedures of SysTox are as follows: 1) a systematic model integrating the extracted chemical and genomic features has been developed to predict the multiple toxin–target interactions with its reliability and robustness estimated by support vector machine (SVM) and random forest (RF) methods. And according to the phenotypic diseases, the qualitative classification of targets has been applied to further explore the biological significance of targets, as well as to validate the robustness of the *in silico* models. 2) As an example, a genome-scale toxin–target–disease network of cardiovascular disease is constructed. 3) The topological analysis of the network is implemented to identify drug targets that are most susceptible to attracting the most critical toxins, as well as to uncover the toxin-specific mechanisms. The advantage of our SysTox approach is that it can be used to predict the toxin–target interactions even for targets with unknown 3D structure. It is worth to note that the toxin–target interaction network can help us to identify new toxins and new target proteins simultaneously and infer novel links from the information of known links. The limitation of the SysTox approach is that the drug targets involving DNA or RNA were not integrated into the model due to the insufficiency of toxin–target information. So the prediction of toxins that target RNA or DNA may be an extension in the following work. The approaches to evaluate the toxicity properties of drugs are listed in **Table 2**.

The Prediction of Half-Life (HL)

The biological half-life of a drug is defined as the time required for the human body to metabolize or eliminate 50% of an initial

TABLE 2 | The approaches for the prediction of the toxicity properties of drugs.

Number	Model name	Description of the model	Reference
1	A chemical genomics approach	Similar ligands that may interact with similar proteins were used to predict the novel compounds of a target	(Klabunde, 2010; Yamanishi et al., 2010)
2	Network method	Predict ligand–target interactions from high-dimensional biological data	(Yu et al., 2012)
3	SysTox approach	Based on a large-scale database of 33,800 poison–target interactions through the integration of chemical, genomic, toxicological information and systems biology technologies	(Zhou et al., 2013)

drug dosage. It is noteworthy that measuring and predicting the half-life of a given drug are important for the safe and accurate dosage of the drug (Berezhkovskiy, 2013). At present, several models were proposed to predict the half-lives of drugs. For example, Sharma et al. have proposed the prediction model for peptide half-life (HLP) in intestine-like environment based on 10mer (HL10) and 16mer (HL16) peptides dataset, which helps in estimating half-lives of peptides relatively rather than in absolute terms (Sharma et al., 2014). With the help of seven machine learning methods and molecular descriptors, Lu et al. have proposed an approach to predict elimination of half-life in humans (Lu et al., 2016). In addition, Turner et al. predicted human half-lives of 20 cephalosporins by integrating constitutional, topological, and quantum-chemical descriptors (Turner et al., 2010). Moreover, Arnot et al. developed two half-life prediction models in humans based on molecular fragments and an automated iterative fragment selection method (Arnot et al., 2014). In summary, most models of prediction of half-life were based on drug structures, while the PreHL model was constructed on only eight molecular descriptors of drugs by principal component analysis (PCA). However, it is difficult and time-consuming to predict the half-life of a specific drug.

In a previous study, we have proposed the PreHL model for TCM injection systems (Yang et al., 2014), which is a systematic decision-making model to predict long or short half-lives of drugs by the C-partial least square (C-PLS) algorithm (Boulesteix, 2004; Kidron et al., 2012). More specifically, the PreHL model was built in three steps: 1) *Dataset collection:* One hundred sixty-nine drugs (injection formulation) with their half-life values, DrugBank ID, chemical name, and Chemical Abstracts Service (CAS) number were collected from DrugBank database (Knox et al., 2011), and they were divided into two subsets: a training set (n = 126) used to build the model and an independent test set (n = 43) to validate the accuracy of the model. 2) *Descriptor calculation and selection:* Molecular descriptors were first calculated to construct the model, and then 43 objective features were selected based on forward stepwise algorithm. Finally, by PCA, only eight of them were applied for C-PLS modeling process. 3) *Model performance:* For internal validation, the model was evaluated by the leave-one-out (LOO) methodology. Bedsides, external validation was performed by all models. The performance of the model was evaluated by short half-life and long half-life accuracies. For internal validation and external validation, the overall accuracy, long half-life accuracy, and short half-life prediction accuracy are all approximately 85–87%. According to the PreHL model, a half-life higher than 4 h is considered as a satisfactory metabolism property of drugs. Furthermore, the PreHL model was successfully used to assess the half-lives of the potential bioactive components of reduning injection (Yang et al., 2014). The models or approaches of half-life are listed in **Table 3**. Compared with other models, PreHL is a more systematic decision-making model addressing the plasma protein binding, active transport across the membrane, absorption, BBB permeability, drug metabolism, and half-life in the body.

Identification of Drug Targets

The identification of drug targets of TCM is a basic problem in the processes of drug development, as well as an essential factor for the dissection of the holistic mechanisms of action of TCM (Cao et al., 2012). Currently, the LBVS, SBVS, and the text mining-based approach are widely used to predict the target–ligand interactions. In brief, LBVS aims to identify novel compounds by comparing candidate ligands with the known drugs of a target protein (Byvatov et al., 2003; Krejsa et al., 2003). Nevertheless, if the number of known active compounds for a target is small, the performance of LBVS is poor. In addition, it is difficult to identify drugs with novel structural scaffolds that differ from the known molecules. As for SBVS, it is constrained by the available crystallographic structure of target, thus hampering the prescreening process of drugs. And it is particularly limited for those membrane proteins, like the GPCRs (G-protein coupled receptors), whose 3D structure information is still unavailable up to now (Ballesteros and Palczewski, 2001).

Therefore, to predict the drug–target interactions, we have developed three models, including systematic drug–target identification technology (SysDT) (Yu et al., 2012), weighted ensemble similarity (WES) (Zheng et al., 2015) method, and Pred-binding method (Shar et al., 2016). All the methods of the prediction of drug targets are listed in **Table 4**. In the following part, we will review these methods.

The SysDT Model

The SysDT model was developed as a systematic approach for the prediction of the drug–target interactions that integrated artificial intelligence computing methods systems biology, chemical genomics, and structural genomics, which are based on two powerful methods, RF and SVM (Yu et al., 2012) The model was constructed by 6,707 drugs and 4,228 targets with known drug–target interactions in the DrugBank

TABLE 3 | The models or approaches for the prediction of half-life.

Number	Model name or approaches of half-life	Description of the models	Reference
1	Model of peptide half-life (HLP)	For HLP in intestine-like environment based on 10mer (HL10) and 16mer (HL16) peptides dataset	(Sharma et al., 2014)
2	An approach to predict elimination half-life in human	Seven machine learning methods and molecular descriptors	(Lu et al., 2016)
3	The prediction model of 20 cephalosporins	By the integration of constitutional, topological, and quantum-chemical descriptors	(Turner et al., 2010)
4	Two half-life prediction models in humans	Based on molecular fragments and an automated iterative fragment selection method	(Arnot et al., 2014)
5	PreHL model	The C-partial least square (C-PLS) algorithm	(Yang et al., 2014)

database, which constructed the positive samples. The negative samples were obtained by three steps: I) re-coupling all drugs and targets in the benchmark dataset into pairs, II) discarding those drug–protein pairs that appeared in the positive samples and keeping the remaining pairs to represent the non-interaction space, and III) randomly selecting the negative pairs from the non-interaction space to ensure the same number as the positive pairs. Then, by SVM, numerical vectors of the drug–target pairs (for both positive and negative samples) by concatenating chemical descriptors and protein descriptors were mapped into a higher dimensional feature space, which is a maximal margin hyper-plane that separates the positive from the negative samples by using a kernel function. Another method, RF, was also used to build a model, which is an ensemble of unpruned classification or regression tree. Finally, the performance of the models was evaluated by internal five-fold cross-validation and four external independent validations with the known drug–target interactions.

Our results showed that the optimal models by SVM showed impressive prediction performance, with a concordance of 82.83%, a sensitivity of 81.33%, and a specificity of 93.62%. Both SVM and RF demonstrate the reliability and robustness of the obtained models. Compared with the structure-based simulation methods, the SysDT approach is not restricted by the 3D structure of targets. More importantly, the advantage of the SysDT model is that it enables to identify the unrelated targets that may share structure similarity of a chemical with ligands. Moreover, it can promote the multi-target drug discovery by recognizing the proteins targeted by a particular ligand. Therefore, the SysDT approach may provide a reliable analysis tool for drug target identification of the herbal molecules on human proteins. Although the SysDT model is effective for the prediction of the drug-target interactions, it is limited by the information of the 3D structure features of the ligand-binding domains. Therefore, novel optimal approaches are still needed to be proposed in further research.

The WES Method

The available computational approaches mainly focus on the prediction of indirect targets of drugs or direct targets of drugs in a small scale. To further improve the drug target prediction systems, we have successfully developed two optical mathematical models: 1) a WES method and 2) a Pred-binding approach (**Figure 3**) to identify the direct targets of drugs based on large scale of drug–target interactions.

The WES approach was proposed on the theory that the systematic features of ligands could accurately reflect the ligand–receptor binding pattern. The WES method was constructed based on over 900,000 drug–target relations, including three steps: 1) identifying the key ligand structural features that strongly related to the pharmacological properties in a framework of ensemble; 2) confirming the targets of drugs by the evaluation of the overall similarity (ensemble) rather than a single ligand judgment; 3) obtaining the overall similarity with the ligand set by integrating the standardized ensemble similarities (*Z* score) by Bayesian network and multi-variate kernel approach; and 4) evaluating and validating the performance of the approach by leave-one-out cross-validation (LOOCV) and the ligand-binding assay test experiments. The WES method exhibits good reliability with a good specificity and sensitivity [Area Under The Curve (AUC) = 0.85] and external [both the binding (positive sample) and non-binding data (negative sample)] and experimental test (ligand-binding assay test) accuracies of 70% and 71%, respectively. Notably, it is able to distinguish the direct binding or indirect binding relationships between drugs and targets, which is of great benefit for drug repositioning and discovery (Zheng et al., 2015).

The advantages of WES includes the following: 1) the structural features based on statistical tests and optimization analysis were integrated into a framework of ensemble to reduce dimensionality of dataset and eliminate data noise. 2) The ensemble concept was proposed to ensure the model to predict the target of the drug based on the drug's similarity with the whole feature of an ensemble. The one nearest neighbor (1NN) model evaluates the probability of drug targets based only on the maximum similarity to the known ligands

TABLE 4 | The methods for the prediction of drug targets.

Number	Model or method name	Description of the model	Reference
1	The ligand-based virtual screening (LBVS)	By comparing candidate ligands with the known drugs of a target protein	(Byvatov et al., 2003; Krejsa et al., 2003)
2	Structured-based virtual screening (SBVS)	Based on the available crystallographic structure of target	(Ballesteros and Palczewski, 2001)
3	Ligand-based approach	Based on the families or subfamilies of targets	(Huang et al., 2013b)
4	Target-based approach	Divide the receptors and pooled together the known ligands into clusters	(Nagamine and Sakakibara, 2007)
5	*In silico* model for predicting the drug–target interactions	By the integration of the amino acid sequences, two-dimensional chemical structures, and mass spectrometry data, as well as the chemical functional groups and biological features	(He et al., 2010)
6	The SysDT model	By the integration of artificial intelligence computing methods systems biology, chemical genomics, and structural genomics, which are based on two powerful methods, random forest (RF) and support vector machine (SVM)	(Yu et al., 2012)
7	Weighted ensemble similarity (WES) method	Based on the theory that the systematic features of ligands that could accurately reflect the ligand–receptor binding pattern	(Zheng et al., 2015)
8	Pred-binding method	Based on 1,589 Dragon descriptors of ligands and 1,080 protein descriptors, by SVM and RF	(Shar et al., 2016)

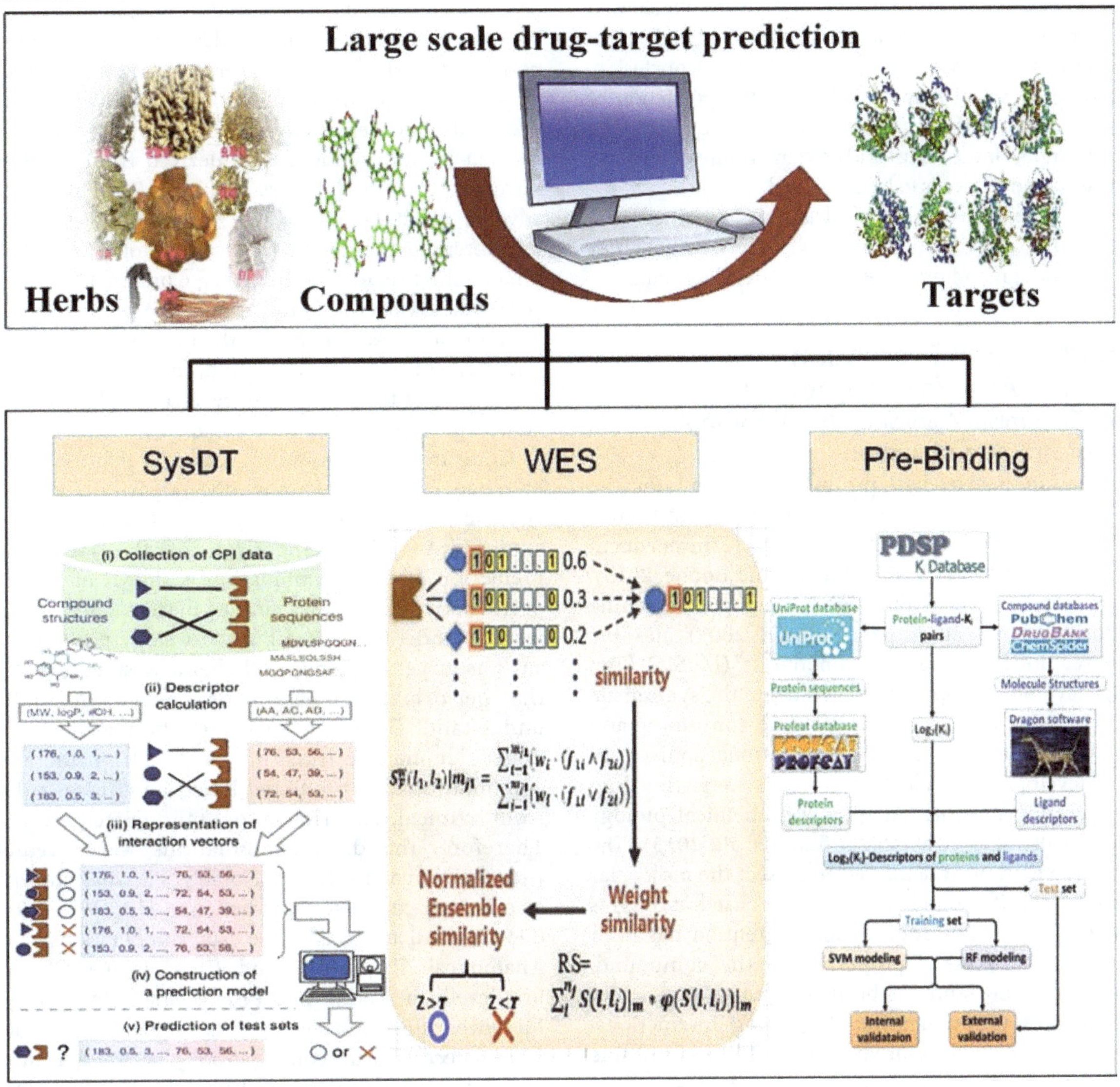

FIGURE 3 | Drug target identification approaches of systematic drug–target identification technology (SysDT), weighted ensemble similarity (WES), and Pred-binding models.

of the target. Compared with the 1NN model, WES is better in predicting drug targets for various structurally diverse compounds.

Pred-Binding Approach

Drug–target interactions are important for exploring biological activities of these proteins. In fact, some drugs may bind to multiple target proteins and sometimes improperly bind to unwanted off-targets (Wang et al., 2013), leading to severe harmful side effects. Therefore, identifying the satisfactory targets of drugs is an urgent task for drug development. In our previous study, we have developed the Pred-binding model to accurately predict the binding strength between drugs and targets (Shar et al., 2016). The Pred-binding model includes the following: 1) *Dataset construction:* The ligand and target dataset information with known binding affinity abstracted from Psychoactive Drug Screening Program (PDSP) Ki database was used to build the model (Roth et al., 2000). After the exclusion of ligand–target–Ki entries with the repeat number of Ki of more than 70, finally, a dataset consisting of 9,948 ligand–target–Ki pairs was constructed. And 1,589 Dragon descriptors of ligands and 1,080 protein descriptors were obtained for further analysis. 2) *Training set and test set construction:* The dataset was split into training (used to build the model) and test (used to validate the model's accuracy) sets, and they were randomly split into five subsets with equal number, and one subset was selected as the test set, and the others were considered as the training set. 3) *Model building:* Two *in silico* models based on SVM and RF were proposed to predict the binding affinity. 4) *Model validation:* As mentioned above, first, each subset was selected as the test set, and the other four subsets serve as the training set for validating model. The processes were repeated five times. Second, five external independent validations were performed for all models using different test sets. Third, the comparison of the performance of RF model and SVM model by *F* test was performed. The results showed that the cross-validation coefficient was 0.6079 for SVM and 0.6267 for RF, exhibiting a good potent Ki predictability. In conclusion, the Pred-binding approach may contribute to the prediction of novel potential targets, further guiding the drug development. The limitation of the model is the robust and efficient features; therefore, a better regression model needs to be developed.

In summary, the above three models have provided new approaches for the identification of drug targets, which may benefit the drug design and promote the drug development.

Drug Combination Prediction and Dynamic Analysis Approach

Probability Ensemble Approach (PEA) for the Prediction of Drug Combination

Drug combination has been a promising strategy for the treatment of complex diseases with higher efficacy and fewer side effects than has the single-drug treatment (Zimmermann et al., 2007; Al-Lazikani et al., 2012; Roemer and Boone, 2013). *In vitro* approaches, such as the high-throughput screening method (Borisy et al., 2003; Lehár et al., 2009) and the "multiplex screening for interacting compounds" (MuSIC) (Tan et al., 2012), have been proposed to investigate the synergistic drug pairs. However, these methods are time-consuming and cost intensive. Alternatively, several computational approaches have been developed to identify novel synergistic drug pairs by integrating network analysis and chemical biology data (Chou, 2010; Zhao et al., 2011; Tang et al., 2013). The majority of these methods are limited to dissect the molecular mechanisms or identify combinatorial drugs based on targets with multiple diseases. In addition, some attention has been focused on pharmacokinetic properties of the compound, pharmacodynamic constants, or both pharmacokinetics and pharmacodynamics to predict the drug–drug interactions. But the systematic analysis for predicting the efficacy and side effects of the known or novel drug pairs is still lacking.

To clarify the issue, we have proposed the probability ensemble approach (PEA model) (Li et al., 2015b), by the integration of the molecular chemical space, the pharmacological space, the gene annotations, and the biological networks, for the prediction of drug combinations (**Figure 4**). First, by the integration of drug molecular and pharmacological phenotypes, a Bayesian network model based on a similarity algorithm was developed for the prediction of both clinical efficacy and adverse effects. The performance of PEA showed that the combination efficacy of drugs with high specificity and sensitivity (AUC = 0.90), which was further verified by independent data derived from the literature or novel experimental assays. Second, PEA also assesses the adverse effects (AUC = 0.95) quantitatively and predicts the potential therapeutic indications of drug combinations. Finally, the PreDC (Predict Drug Combination) database was constructed with 1,571 known and 3,269 predicted optimal drug combinations associated with their therapeutic indications and potential side effects. In addition, the standalone software and web server of the PreDC are freely available at http://lsp.nwu.edu.cn/predc.php.

Compared with the simple feature-enrich method proposed by Zhao et al. (2011), the PEA algorithm exhibited good advantages with high training efficiency and extensive applicability (the comparison of the methods for the prediction of drug combination is shown in **Table 5**). More particularly, PEA shows similar performances as the whole-feature model by integrating the weakly predictive features, such as target sequence and chemical structure, to improve the performance, making it convenient and easy to understand. Generally, owing to the unknown underlying molecular mechanisms of combination therapies, drug combinations are predicted based on clinical rules derived from clinical experience or randomized clinical trials. Therefore, the drug combinations were predicted only with the similar functions. Notably, PEA has shown that 43% of our high-confidence predictions (with P1 ≥ 0.9 and P2 ≤ 0.1) are predicted as effective drug combinations with different Anatomical Therapeutic and Chemical (ATC) classes (the first level), indicating that PEA is not restrained by the rule. Moreover, PEA model was experimentally validated by 10 novel effective drug combinations that are a combination of antibacterial and anticancer drugs, showing that 80% pairs are synergistic to cancer models. Moreover, the PEA algorithm has incorporated the clinical efficacy and adverse effect evaluation to identify the potential drug combinations effectively. The limitation of the PEA is that the dosage was not integrated into the model; therefore, it should be taken into account to improve the prediction of drug combinations.

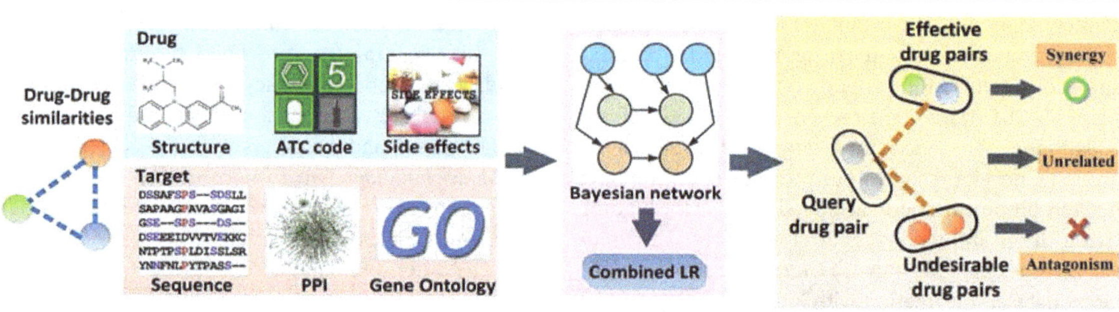

FIGURE 4 | Design processes of the drug combination prediction approach [probability ensemble approach (PEA) model] (Li et al., 2015b).

TABLE 5 | The approaches for the prediction of drug combination.

Number	Approach name	Description	Reference
1	High-throughput screening method	*In vitro* approaches	(Borisy et al., 2003; Lehár et al., 2009)
2	Multiplex screening for interacting compounds (MuSIC)	*In vitro* approaches	(Tan et al., 2012)
3	Several computational approaches	By integrating network analysis and chemical biology data	(Chou, 2010; Zhao et al., 2011; Tang et al., 2013)
4	Simple feature-enrich method	By simple feature-enrich method to predict drug combinations	(Zhao et al., 2011)
5	Probability ensemble approach (PEA model)	By the integration of the molecular chemical space, the pharmacological space, the gene annotations, and the biological networks	(Li et al., 2015b)

Network Elementary Subgraphs and Dynamic Modeling Analysis (NetSyner)

TCM is a complex system with multiple compounds and multiple targets; particularly, natural products derived from TCM with weak binding affinity have been proved to have satisfactory therapeutic efficacy through the regulation of the coordination equilibrium of the whole biological network (Zhu and Xu, 2003; Tan, 2007; Huang et al., 2013a). Recently, nearly ~110,000 small molecules with low binding affinity have been reported in the public database (Liu et al., 2007). However, a suitable strategy to discover the low-binding-affinity molecules is yet to be constructed.

In a previous study, we have developed a systematic approach NetSyner, which is based on the dynamics of target networks and the dynamics of formula structure to predict the response of perturbation of multiple nodes by cell signaling networks (**Figure 5**) (Wang et al., 2016b). The approach includes three steps: First, dynamic models for a series of three-component elementary subgraphs were built, and 33 elementary subgraphs were performed to determine the desired topology and dynamic parameters among targets. And elementary subgraphs were modeled by a set of ordinary differential equations (ODEs) including the rate laws of mass action and the complete Michaelis–Menten reaction kinetics. The combination index (CI) was used to evaluate whether the two targets in an elementary subgraph can have a synergistic effect. Specially, the mitogen-activated protein kinase (MAPK) pathway is an evolutionarily conserved and well-studied signaling pathway involved in regulating fundamental cellular processes in response to stress and inflammation (Johnson and Lapadat, 2002; Sabio and Davis, 2014). As an example, through the application of the elementary subgraphs to the MAPK pathway, several optimal target combinations were predicted. Then, all the targets of the formula were mapped into the elementary subgraphs; both the modes (synergistic, antagonistic, or unrelated) and extent (synergistic index) of interactions between the bioactive compounds were calculated by the dynamic analysis. Moreover, molecular dynamics simulation and molecular mechanics Poisson–Boltzmann surface area (MM-PBSA) methods were employed to evaluate the binding free energies between the compound and the targets. Furthermore, to experimentally validate the prediction of NetSyner, analyses of the inhibitory effects of the two natural products (luteolin and tanshinone IIA) and the four known selective inhibitors on IL-6 and TNF-α production were carried out. The results indicated that multi-weak perturbations of luteolin and tanshinone IIA against the MAPK signaling pathway can potentially decrease the inflammatory response. In conclusion, weak-binding drugs exhibit favorable efficiency and few adverse reactions, which may offer a promising future for novel drug discovery. Nevertheless, due to the parameter independent model of NetSyner, it is applicable to those pathways that must be satisfied by two conditions: 1) pathways must be evolutionarily conserved and 2) the parameters of the pathway must be intact.

APPLICATION OF SYSTEMS PHARMACOLOGY IN TCM

Construction of TCM Systems Pharmacology Software and Databases

At present, several databases have been established for the investigation of TCM from different aspects. (The database of TCMs were listed in **Table 6**.) For example, TCM Database@ Taiwan (Chen, 2011) and TCM-ID (Chen et al., 2010) have provided a large number of herbal ingredients with 3D structures and functional properties. TCMID (Xue et al., 2013) consists of TCM formulae, herbs, ingredients, and their related targets and diseases. Both ChemTCM (Ehrman et al., 2007) and HIT (Ye et al., 2011) focus on herbal ingredients and their corresponding targets. The CVDHD database (Gu et al., 2013) focuses on natural products associated with cardiovascular diseases and targets. But there is lack of systematic network pharmacology analysis among these databases.

Therefore, our team proposed a unique systems pharmacology platform of TCM-TCMSP (Ru et al., 2014; Liu et al., 2016) (http://lsp.nwu.edu.cn/tcmsp.php). The database consists of more than 36,000 chemical molecules and forms a complete library of Chinese medicine ingredients. In addition, the database integrated 12 ADME key properties like human oral bioavailability, half-life, drug-likeness, Caco-2 permeability, blood–brain barrier and Lipinski's rule of five, and the drug-likeness analysis of compounds, with more than 4,000 targets and 1,000 types of disease information. More importantly, "drug–target–disease" network pharmacology analysis tools were developed as a novel tool for the identification of the specific targets and the specific diseases of active molecules/groups in TCM. In summary, the particular strengths of TCMSP are the large number of herbal ingredients with ADME properties and their ability to analyze

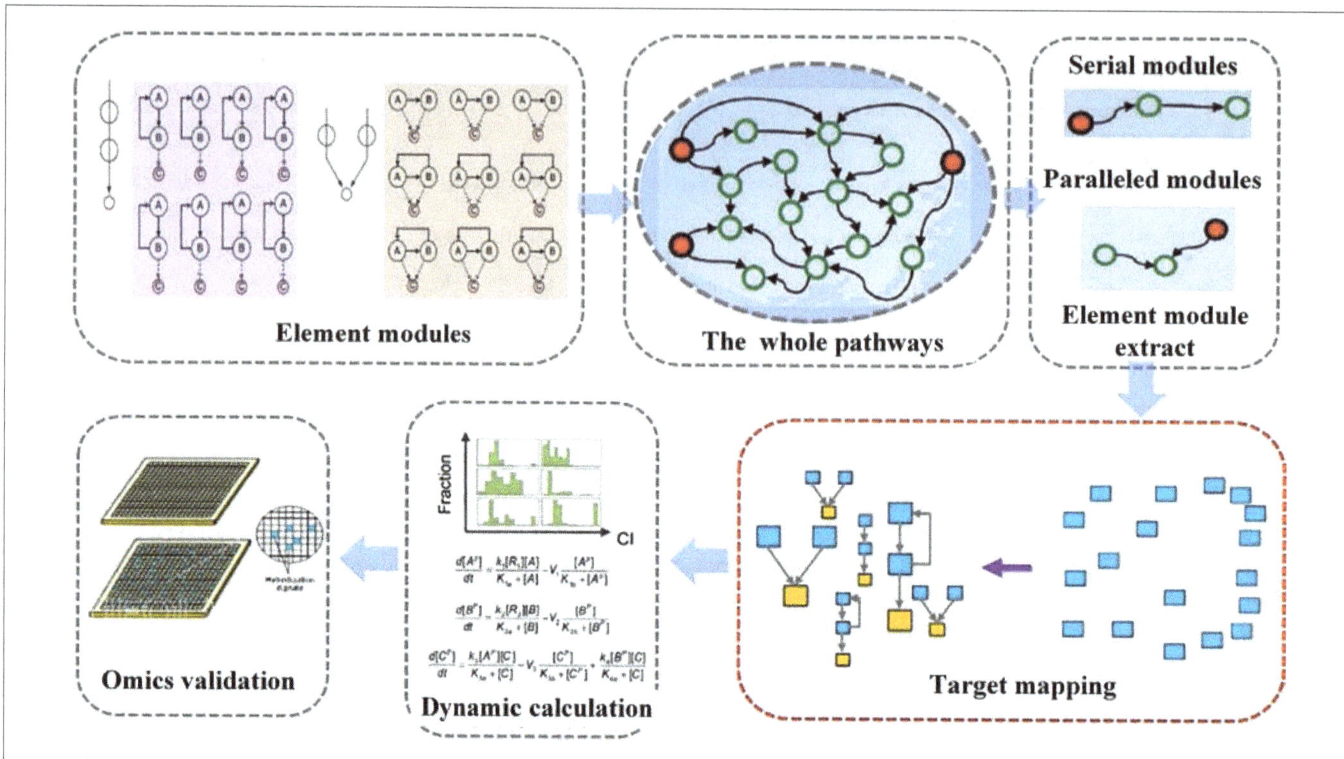

FIGURE 5 | Flowchart of network elementary subgraphs and dynamic modeling analysis (NetSyner) (Wang et al., 2016b).

TABLE 6 | The database of TCMs.

Number	Database name	Description	Reference
1	TCM Database@Taiwan	Provides a large number of herbal ingredients with 3D structures and functional properties	(Chen, 2011)
2	TCM-ID		(Chen et al., 2010)
3	TCMID database	Consists of TCM formulae, herbs, ingredients and their related targets and diseases, drug–target networks, and drug–disease networks	(Xue et al., 2013)
4	ChemTCM	Focuses on herbal ingredients and their corresponding targets	(Ehrman et al., 2007)
5	HIT		(Ye et al., 2011)
6	CVDHD database	Focuses on natural products associated with cardiovascular diseases and targets	(Gu et al., 2013)
7	TCMSP database	Consists of herbs, their chemical molecules, ADME properties, targets, and disease information	(Ru et al., 2014)
8	SymMap database	Focuses on TCM symptoms and their relationships to herbs and diseases	(Wu et al., 2019)
9	ECTM database	Includes the herbs' basic property and quality control standard, formula composition, ingredient drug-likeness, the gene targets of the ingredients, and related pathways or diseases.	(Xu et al., 2019)

drug–target networks and drug–disease networks, thus providing a platform to dissect the mechanisms of action of TCM, uncover nature of TCM theory, and develop novel herbal-oriented drugs. Moreover, the related software can be used to search the information in the database conveniently. Recently, two novel databases, SymMap (Wu et al., 2019) and ETCM databases (Encyclopedia of Traditional Chinese Medicine) (Xu et al., 2019), were built. SymMap is an integrative database of TCM enhanced by symptom mapping. SymMap is an integrative database, consisting of the information of TCM symptoms and related herbs, diseases and associated symptoms, herbal ingredients, and gene targets. Furthermore, SymMap could be applied to predict component pairwise relationships by statistical tests to filter promising results to guide drug discovery. Actually, SymMap was focused on TCM symptoms and their relationships to herbs and diseases, which provides both candidate leads and screening directions for phenotypic drug discovery. As for the ETCM database, it contains comprehensive and standardized information of 403 TCM herbal species, 3,962 TCM formulae, 7,274 herbal ingredients, 2,266 validated or predicted drug targets, and 3,027 related diseases. ETCM is convenient to obtain the information of the herbs' basic property and quality control standard, formula composition, ingredient drug-likeness, the gene targets of the ingredients, and related pathways or diseases.

Compared with SymMap, TCMSP is a more comprehensive database that integrated all the herbs and their related compounds, the compound ADME properties, potential targets, and diseases, which can automatically establish the compound–target and target–disease networks to analyze the drugs' mechanisms of action and promote the TCM drug development. The limitation of TCMSP is that it lacks some medicinal and pharmacological data, the dose–effect relationship of ingredients, and the drug action modes: stimulation or inhibition, drug combination for various diseases, and tissues and organs that the compounds target. To improve these limitations, the ETCM database provides the habitat and quality control information of herbs, which may become a major data warehouse for TCM to promote TCM drug development.

Although tremendous efforts have been made in the past to provide databases containing cancer-related information, to our knowledge, no such dedicated comprehensive repository of anticancer herbs and anticancer herb-originating natural products has been developed currently as yet. Some databases like CancerDR (Kumar et al., 2013) and CancerPPD (Tyagi et al., 2015) have been made in the past to provide comprehensive data involved in anticancer ingredients. However, the CancerDR mainly focuses on FDA-approved and experimental drugs, and CancerPPD is a database of anticancer peptides and proteins. Considering the bleak situation of cancer and absence of systematic database for anticancer herbal products, for the first time, we have developed a comprehensive repository named anticancer herbs database of systems pharmacology (CancerHSP). The CancerHSP database provides information of 2,439 anticancer herbs, 2,439 anticancer active compounds, the molecular structure of each compound, and antitumor activity data based on 492 different cell lines (Tao et al., 2015). Furthermore, the database also consists of natural products with anticancer effects, their related ADME properties, antitumor activity, and target information, which not only helps to dissect the underlying molecular mechanisms of anticancer drugs but also provides basic data support for the development of anticancer drugs.

Synergistic Effects of the Active Components in TCM

Multi-Target Synergistic Effects of TCM

Based on network pharmacological methods, scientists discovered that TCM exhibits multi-target synergistic effects. For example, Violeta et al. have built a computer multiphase pharmacology fingerprint (CPF) based on the Gauss integration screening method (GES) to encode the corresponding multiple target fingerprint atlas of drugs. Besides, the approach successfully found that drugs can interact with multiple targets, which provides a novel method for the discovery of new preclinical and clinical drug candidates (Violeta et al., 2014). In fact, if one drug could act on multiple targets, the drug molecules may exhibit better therapeutic effects through targeting on multiple targets under the synergistic effects (Hopkins, 2007; Hopkins, 2008). Recently, Huang et al. successfully dissected the molecular mechanisms of TCM with multiple targets for the treatment of depression; for example, several antidepressant drugs acted on more than 20 targets (Huang et al., 2013a). In addition, Liu et al. illustrated the mechanisms of action for the herb licorice, and the potential bioactive components were identified by the systems pharmacology. For instance, liquiritigenin, licochalcone B, naringenin, and kaempferol were considered as the bioactive compounds that acted on 22 targets related to cough, including ADRB1 (β-1 adrenergic receptor), ADRB2 (β-2 adrenergic receptor), CALM1 (calmodulin-1), PDE4B (cAMP-specific 3′,5′-cyclic phosphodiesterase 4B), PDE4D (cAMP-specific 3′,5′-cyclic phosphodiesterase 4D), HSP90AA1 (heat shock protein HSP 90-α), HSP90AB1 (heat shock protein HSP 90-β), PPARG (peroxisome proliferator-activated receptor γ), and THRB (thyroid hormone receptor β). The flavonoids, including isoliquiritigenin, liquiritigenin, and liquiritin, exerted synergistic therapeutic effects on thrombosis through the regulation of the proteins F2 (prothrombin), F10 (coagulation factor X), and PTGS2 (prostaglandin G/H synthase 2), which are closely involved in the processes of thrombosis. In addition, licochalcone A and licoisoflavanone acted on the proteins 5-hydroxytryptamine 1A receptor (HTR1A), ADRB1, cell division protein kinase 5 (CDK5), D opioid receptor (OPRD1), GSK3B, and HRH1; therefore, they may exert synergetic effects to achieve anti-ischemic effects to treat ischemic heart disease (Liu et al., 2013a).

Moreover, we identified some novel targets, 5-hydroxytryptamine 2A receptor (5-HT2A) and aldose reductase (AKR1B1), which are associated with diabetes. Also, several bioactive compounds in licorice could target proteins of the nervous system, such as monoamine oxidase type B (MAOB), D2 and D3 dopaminergic receptors, and mitogen-activated protein kinase 10 (MAPK10) (Liu et al., 2013a). Notably, we dissected the detoxification mechanism of licorice; for example, the compounds liquiritin and licochalcone G can target the metalloelastase to destroy bacteria and strengthen the tissue macrophages, thus defending against external invasions. In summary, with the aid of systems pharmacology, we generated a novel perspective for better understanding of single herbal medicine for treating various diseases from the molecular level to the systems level. More importantly, it also explained why licorice is a popular herb, as well as the mechanisms of detoxification of the licorice (Liu et al., 2013a).

Multi-Pathway Interactions of Herbs

To comprehensively investigate the interactions between herbal ingredients and their related biological processes, a drug–target–pathway network was generated (Chen et al., 2009). The most important pathways are the cellular signaling pathways, which can interact with each other. In addition, various stimuli appear to activate the same downstream targets, thus exhibiting the same cellular functions. For example, Gong et al. identified alternative pathways based on experimental data, which are involved in regulating cell functions (Gong and Zhang, 2005). In the target–pathway network, targets that appear in multiple pathways are often considered as potential key targets for the treatment of complex diseases.

In addition, by a systematic genetic analysis of 24 types of cancers, scientists found that 67–100% of tumor cells were involved in 12 cellular signaling pathways and related carcinogenesis processes (Jones et al., 2008). Li et al. found that multiple compounds were involved in multiple pathways in Compound Danshen Formula: 58 compounds were associated with the glucocorticoid and inflammatory signaling pathways; 56 compounds acted on the l-arginine/NO signaling pathways; 35 compounds disturbed the renin–angiotensin–aldosterone pathways; and 31 compounds regulated signaling pathways associated with platelet aggregation. Interestingly, all these signaling pathways are closely related to inflammation and coagulation, indicating that Compound Danshen Formula may synergistically regulate these signaling pathways to treat cardiovascular diseases effectively (Li et al., 2012b). Therefore, multi-target drugs of TCM are likely to be involved in alternative pathways or biological processes to treat complex disease effectively instead of single-target drugs.

Combinations of Herbal Compounds Acting on Multiple Organs

TCM is a part of holistic medicine, which concentrates on systematic health care for the whole human body rather than one part of the body (**Figure 6A**) (Ventegodt et al., 2014); however, to understand the mechanisms of action of TCM at a systems level is still difficult. Indeed, there are two key problems: 1) If the compound and the person are considered as whole entities, how do they interact with each other? 2) How do the molecules, tissues, and organs of the body respond to different molecules or molecule groups in a formula under holistic frameworks? To solve these problems, in the previous studies, we have examined the molecular basis of some diseases associated with different organs, such as cardio-cerebral diseases and cardiovascular diseases (CVDs) and gastrointestinal disorders (GIDs). The systems pharmacology model consists of four modules (**Figure 6B**): 1) an ADME evaluation model, including oral bioavailability prediction, drug-likeness evaluation, human intestinal absorption, half-life, and BBB permeability prediction; 2) network target fishing and pathway analysis; 3) compound–pathway analysis; and 4) drug–organ enrichment and interaction model (Wang et al., 2015).

Take Xinnaoxin Pill and Sanhe Decoction as examples; with the help of systems pharmacology, we dissected the scientific connotations of simultaneous treatment for cardio-cerebral diseases, and CVDs and GIDs. More specifically, we found that several components in Xinnaoxin Pill exhibited good BBB permeability, suggesting that it may be beneficial for the cardiovascular system. Besides, it could act on several organs involved in multiple biological processes and multiple pathways associated with multiple functions, such as inflammation, myocardial contraction, and angiogenesis, thus allowing the simultaneous treatment of cardio-cerebral diseases.

Moreover, by ADME system evaluation, we identified 59 potential active compounds in Sanhe Decoction (Zhang et al., 2016). Seventy target proteins of these compounds were predicted by target fishing. The compound–pathway network analysis revealed that multiple drugs were simultaneously involved in several pathways, such as calcium ion signaling pathway, cGMP-dependent protein kinase (PKG) signaling pathway, and vascular smooth muscle contractions (**Figure 7A**), suggesting that these drugs tend to exhibit multi-target synergetic or additive effects. The target tissue distribution network indicated that the compounds of Sanhe Decoction acted on multiple tissues or organs simultaneously, the majority of which were associated with heart and stomach, thereby achieving therapeutic effects on CVDs and GIDs (**Figure 7B**). Furthermore, Sanhe Decoction significantly alleviates the myocardial conditions compared with those of the control group in a rat model of myocardial ischemia, verifying the reliability of the theoretical model (Zhang et al., 2016).

In conclusion, the systems pharmacology approach provides a holistic strategy for rational drug design for complex associated diseases, promoting the drug development.

Bidirectional Regulation of TCM for the Treatment of Diseases

Reduning injection, derived from the experience of ancient Chinese medicine doctors, consists of three herbs: *Artemisia annua* L. (genus *Artemisia*, Asteraceae), *Gardenia jasminoides* J.Ellis (genus *Gardenia*, Rubiaceae), and *Lonicera japonica* Thunb. (genus *Lonicera*, Caprifoliaceae), which are mainly used for the treatment of influenza-like diseases, including viral infections, fever, respiratory diseases, and inflammation (Yang et al., 2014). The target network indicated that different diseases may have the same symptoms and can be cured by the same combination of herbs (Lin, 1998). The mechanisms of reduning injection were illustrated by systems pharmacology. The compound–target network of reduning injection is shown in **Figure 8**. We noticed that arachidonate 5-lipoxygenase (ALOX5) is one of the key enzymes in the formation of proinflammatory eicosanoids from arachidonic acid (Albert et al., 2002), which transforms essential fatty acids into leukotrienes (such as leukotriene B4, C4, D4, and E4). Actually, leukotriene B4 is an effective activator of the chemotactic reaction in white blood cells. In the network, ALOX5 is a common pharmaceutical target against various diseases that interacted with several compounds, such as quercetin and luteolin. Moreover, reduning injection might also control the virus infection by directly targeting viral proteins, such as DNA topoisomerase 2-alpha (TOP2A) to inhibit the virus replication (Wang et al., 2012). The cell experiments also showed that the herbal ingredients reduced the inflammatory response through the regulation of inflammatory cytokines and proinflammatory mediators, such as IL-6, IL-8, TNF-α, and COX2. More importantly, the bioactive compounds in reduning can directly kill the virus through the inhibition of virus expression. In summary, the systems pharmacology-based analysis revealed that the dual regulation of reduning injection not only inhibited virus replication but also exerted anti-inflammatory activities to promote body recovery.

Application of Systems Pharmacology in the Examination of "Jun-Chen-Zuo-Shi" in the Combination Principles of Formula

"Jun-Chen-Zuo-Shi" Combination Principle of Mahuang Decoction and Yujin Formula

"Jun-Chen-Zuo-Shi" is one of the basic principles of herbal formulae. It has been found that there was a clear difference in the structure and biological activity of each ingredient in different herbs and even ingredients in the same herb; however, only some bioactive compounds exhibit therapeutic activities (Zhao et al., 2010). Given the numerous components of a TCM, the interpretation of the rules of combination is difficult. In the previous study, taking Mahuang Decoction as an example, we explored the scientific connotation of the combination principle of TCM (Yao et al., 2013). Mahuang

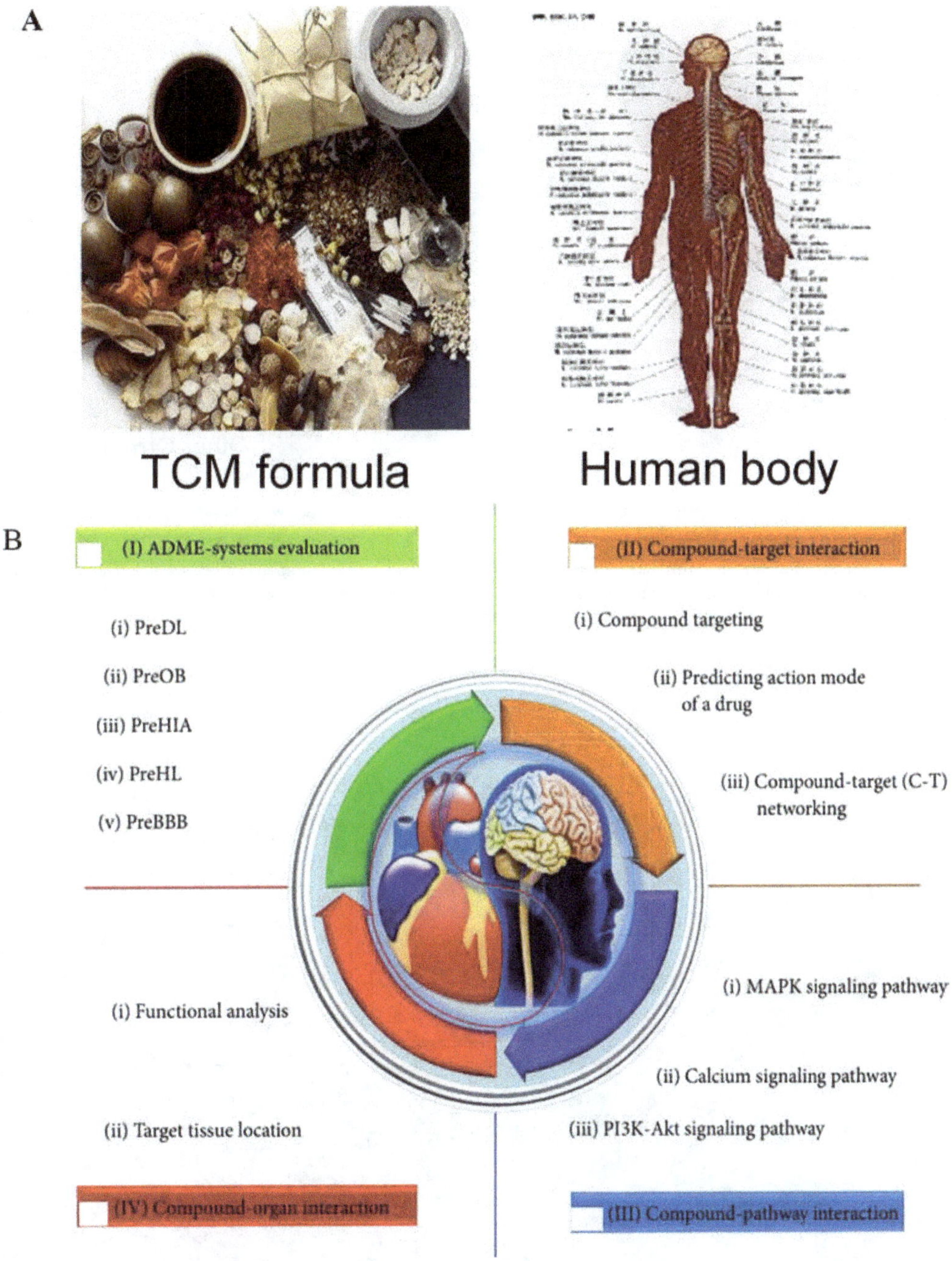

FIGURE 6 | Multi-organ interactions of the multiple compounds in TCMs. **(A)** The holistic herb–human interactions. **(B)** The strategy of systems pharmacology of TCMs for the treatment of complex diseases (Wang et al., 2015).

Decoction consists of four herbs: ephedra, cinnamon, almond, and licorice. By the developed systems pharmacology model, the different roles of the four herbs in the prescription were deciphered through the integration of pharmacokinetic interactions, the drug–target network, and the target–disease network from the molecular level to the systems level (**Figure 9**). The main findings were as follows: 1) 45 active compounds were screened by ADME system; among these, 14 potential bioactive compounds belonged to ephedra, including ephedrine, pseudoephedrine, N-methyl ephedrine, and quercetin; 10 compounds were from cinnamon, including cinnamic aldehyde, cinnamic acid, and coumarin; and 9 compounds were from almonds, such as bitter amygdalin and soybean sterol. Licorice has 12 active molecules, which include glycyrrhizic acid, 18-beta-glycyrrhizic acid, and glycyrrhizin; 2) the herb ephedrine plays a prominent role as the "Jun" herb, which mainly stimulates the body heat and asthma through targeting on epinephrine receptor; 3) the "Chen" herb cinnamon can act on the same targets as the "Jun" herb ephedrine, which enhances therapeutic effects. For example, the

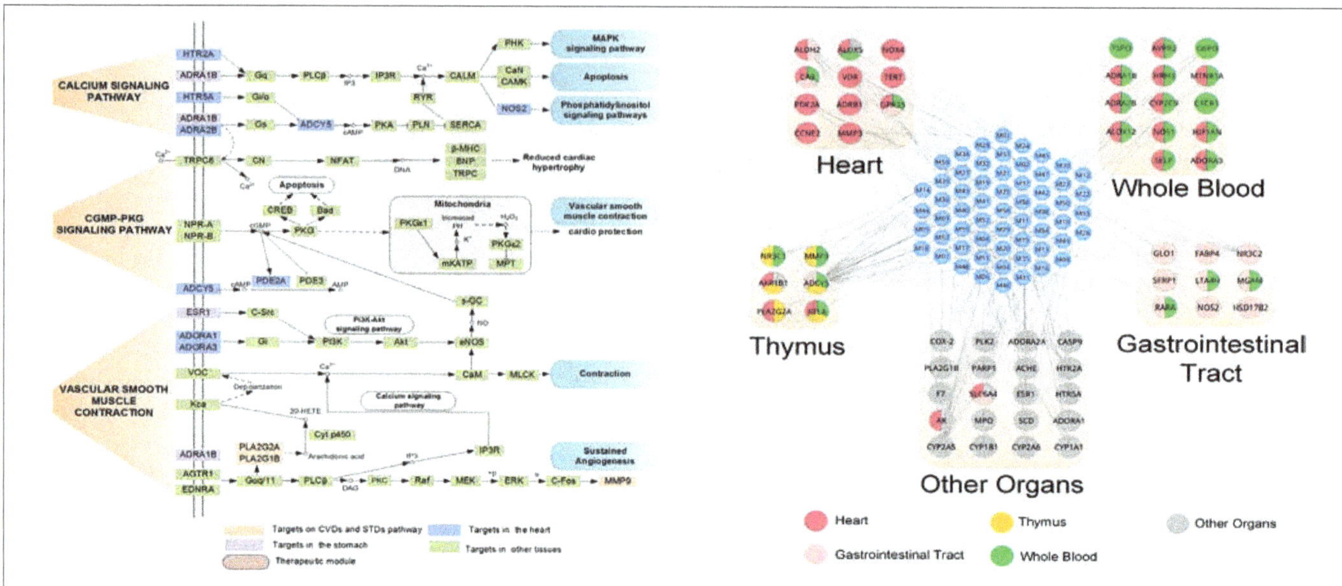

FIGURE 7 | Composition of TCMs has effects on a combination of multiple organs. **(A)** Pathways and therapeutic modules associated with cardiovascular–gastrointestinal diseases. **(B)** The target organ location map; the node represents the organ where the target is located (Zhang et al., 2016).

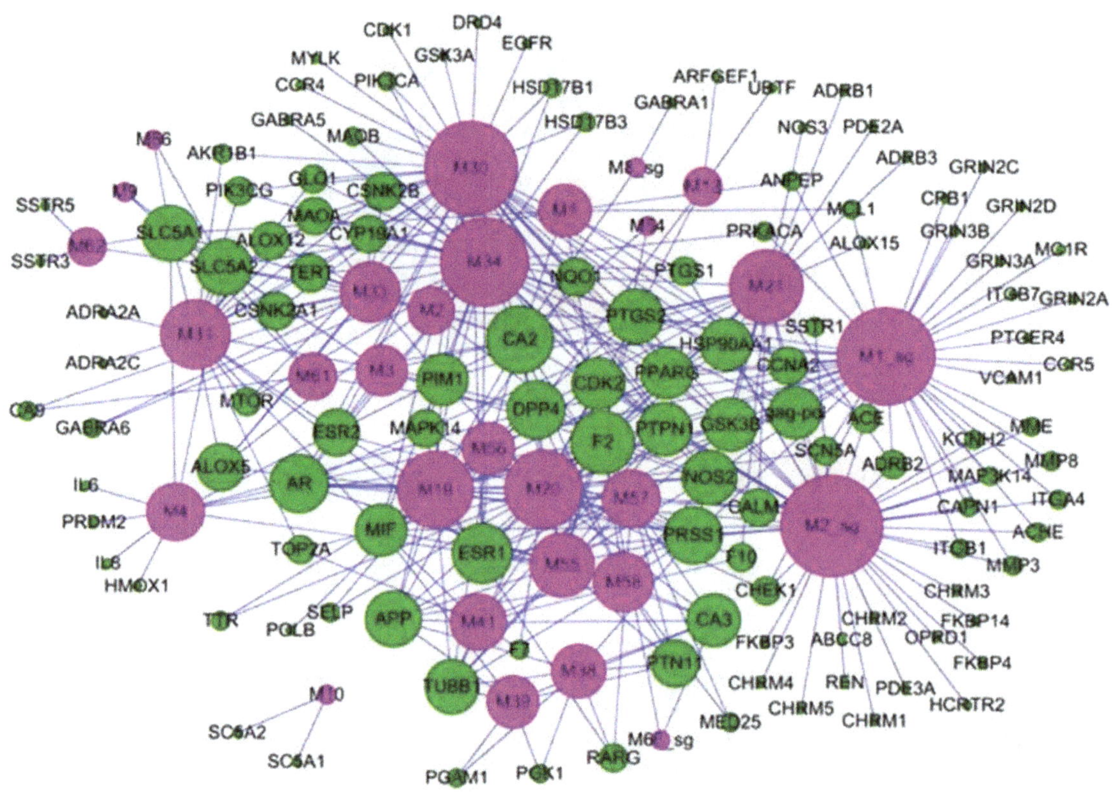

FIGURE 8 | Bidirectional regulation of TCM for the treatment of diseases; the target–disease network of the reduning injection. It is composed of 49 target nodes (round, purple) and 11 disease nodes (square, green), and the size of the circle is the degree of the node (Yang et al., 2014).

herb cinnamon also acted on both the beta 1-adrenergic receptor and the beta 2-adrenergic receptor, thus reducing the dose of the "Jun" herb ephedrine required. 4) The "Zuo" and "Shi" herbs almond and licorice helped to improve the bioavailability of the "Jun" and "Chen" herbs and to coordinate all the drug activities to promoting synergistic effects of four herbs.

Moreover, we have dissected the famous prescription Yujin Formula for treating cardiovascular diseases to clarify the "Jun-Chen-Zuo-Shi" combination principle in Chinese medicine (Li et al., 2012a). From the Yujin Formula, 58 potential bioactive compounds were identified by ADME screening. The compound–target network indicated that the "Jun" herb *Curcuma aromatic* possessed the most bioactive compounds, which acted on the targets associated with CVDs; the "Chen" herb *Fructus Gardeniae* has fewer bioactive compound and targets and shared 15 targets with the "Jun" herb *C. aromatic* to enhance the therapeutic effects; both the "Zuo" "Shi" herbs musk and borneol play assistant roles by decreasing the toxicity and targeting the ingredients to corresponding organs. In the Yujin Formula, target–disease network (**Figure 10B**) showed that most targets were associated with CVDs (44/147); moreover, they were distributed in tumors (40/147), neurological diseases (13/147), and nutritional metabolic diseases (9/147). These results indicated that Yujin Formula may be applied not only for the treatment of CVDs but also for tumors, nervous system diseases, nutritional or metabolic disease, and other diseases. In summary, the scientific connotations of the "Jun-Chen-Zuo-Shi" combination principle were illustrated, which are of great significance for understanding the mechanisms of TCM.

Pathogenesis of Vitiligo and Its Treatment by Qubaibabuqi Formula

Vitiligo is an acquired, pigmentary skin disease that is disfiguring and difficult to treat. Clinically, many TCM prescriptions possess significant effects on vitiligo. Previously, we examined the

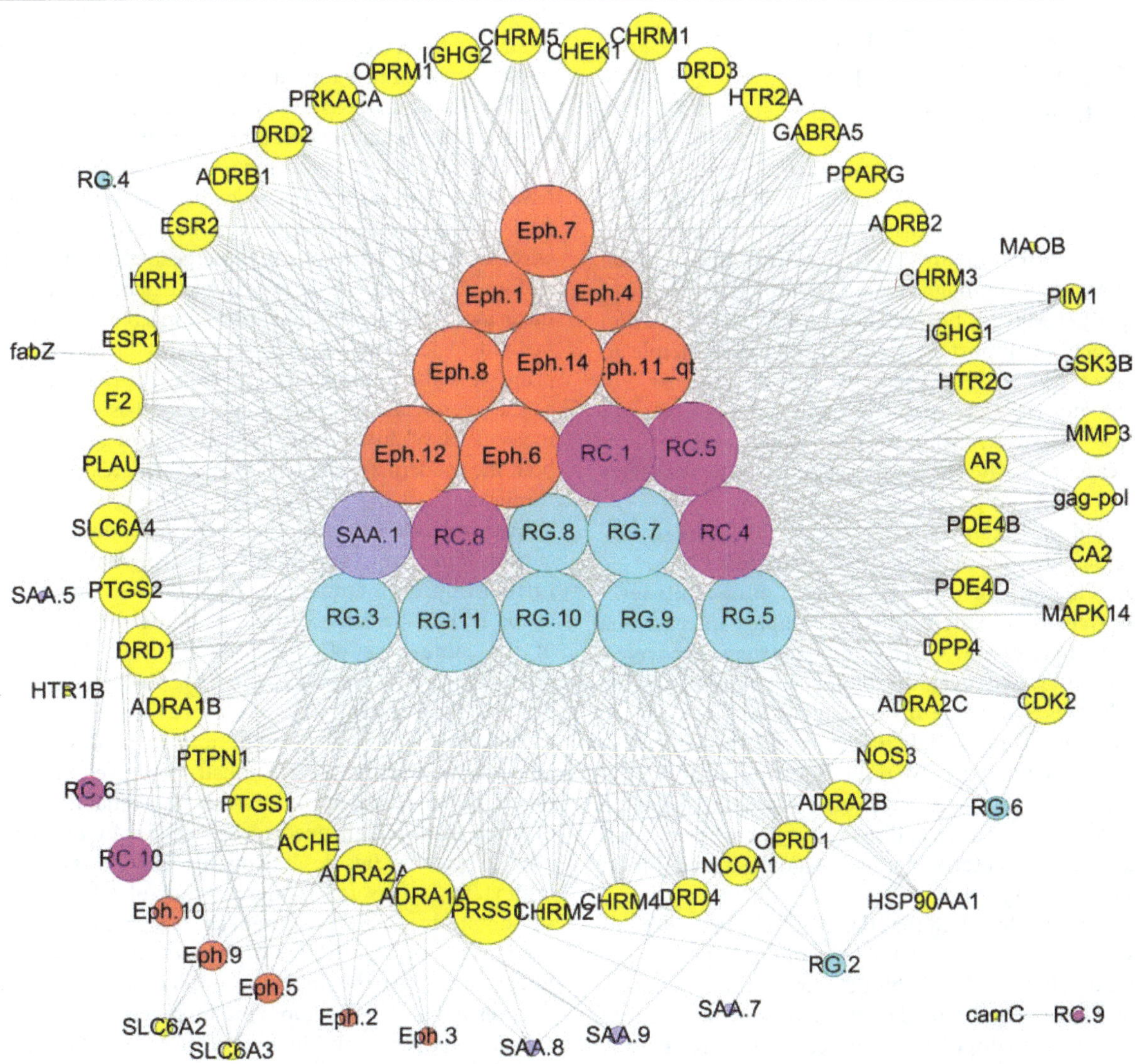

FIGURE 9 | Schematic diagram of the principle of "Jun-Chen-Zuo-Shi" combination principle of Mahuang Decoction. The Eph represents the "Jun" herb ephedra, the RC is the "Chen" (minister) herb cinnamon, the SAA is the "Zuo" (adjuvant) herb almond, and the RG represents the "Shi" (guide) herb licorice (Yao et al., 2013).

potential pathogenic mechanisms of vitiligo and its treatment by Qubaibabuqi formula by the systems pharmacology (Pei et al., 2016). Fifty-six active ingredients were identified as the active compounds, including buritin, bubonin, kaempferol, and cholesterol, which played important roles in the treatment of vitiligo. They acted on 83 target ADCY1 (adenylate cyclase type 1), SCD (stearoyl-coenzyme A desaturase), and BCHE (butyrylcholinesterase) to enhance immune response, increase melanin synthesis, and equilibrate the nervous system. In addition, the analysis of the target network and integration of vitiligo pathways showed that the Qubaibabuqi formula may be involved in modules such as immune-related modules, nervous system-related modules, and melanin synthesis-related modules, exhibiting synergistic effects on vitiligo. The study systematically analyzed the potential molecular mechanisms of Qubaibabuqi formula and pathogenesis of vitiligo from the molecular, network, and pathway levels, deepening our understanding of vitiligo and extending the application of TCM in modern medicine.

DISSECTION OF SYNDROME DIFFERENTIATION THEORY AND QI-BLOOD THEORY

TCM is derived from ancient medical practices that integrate the integrity of the body and the natural environment. The concept of entirety and the method of treatment with syndrome differentiation in TCM is distinctive, which provides a basis for the diagnosis and treatment of diseases (Jiang et al., 2012). More importantly, syndrome differentiation has always been an important pharmacological principle to guide the prescription. For example, Liuwei Dihuang Pill and Jinkui Shenqi Pill were developed under the guidance of the syndrome. However, owing to little evidence of the link between diseases and efficacy, the therapeutic strategies under syndrome are still lacking.

With the aid of systems pharmacology, the "drug–gene–targets–disease subtype" network associated with CVDs was established. Therein, the drugs, targets, and multi-level interactions were illuminated, and the complex interactions between disease genes and CVDs' subtypes were discovered (Li et al., 2014). To uncover the biological basis of CVDs' syndrome, "CVDs syndrome of qi stagnation, blood stasis, qi deficiency, and blood deficiency" were implemented. Combined with the related TCM and refined prescription, the "syndrome–gene–target–drug" network was established to clarify the molecular network and pathways in coronary heart disease with the characteristic of qi stagnation and blood stasis (Zhou and Wang, 2014).

Furthermore, we identified that the qi-tonifying medicines were involved in the enhancement of immunity, the promotion of energy metabolism, and blood circulation, whereas blood-tonic Chinese herbs tended to improve and promote the function of hematopoietic stem cells (**Figure 11**). A computational method was built to distinguish the molecular characteristics of qi-tonifying and blood-tonic molecules, with a prediction accuracy higher than 80%, providing a new tool for the material-based analysis of qi-blood theory and the discovery of new drugs (Liu et al., 2013b).

CONCLUSIONS AND PROSPECTS

TCM is a complex mixed system with multiple components and multiple targets; thus, the identification of the potential bioactive molecules and the dissection of the underlying mechanisms of action to establish the optical drug combinations are the essential tasks of TCM. Fortunately, the advent of systems pharmacology framework provides powerful tools for TCM studies: 1) new methods for identification of active components/groups of TCM from the whole perspective. More than 10 mathematical models, including PreOB and PreHF, have been developed, which overcome the limitation of TCM in pharmacokinetic and pharmacodynamic experiments, providing convenient approaches for the discovery of effective substances; 2) large-scale target prediction systems of TCM, with three approaches (SysDT, WES, and Pred-binding) as new tools for drug target discovery; 3) the probability ensemble approach (PEA) model as a novel tool for the dissection of mechanisms of action and the prediction of new indications of TCM; and 4) a novel network of elementary subgraphs and a dynamic model was proposed for the large-scale screening of weak-binding compound in TCM.

With the aid of the systems pharmacology method above, we have built a systems pharmacology database and analysis platform for TCM, which has been applied for the illustration of the synergetic effects of drug combinations, the synergetic effects of multiple targets, pathways and organs, and the bidirectional regulation of Chinese medicine. Moreover, the systems pharmacology of TCM provides methodological guidance for the dissection of the combination principle and syndrome differentiation of herbal formulae, as well as the interpretation of the qi and blood basis of TCM from the molecular level to the systems level. It is of great significance to both the modernization of TCM and the development of modern medicine.

Although the systems pharmacology approach has achieved certain applications and results, the theory and methods require further improvements in the future; for example, the dose of herbs should be added into the model because the efficacy of the same herb obviously differs with different dosages. Therefore, it is necessary to integrate the drug dosage into the systems pharmacology models to provide guidance for clinical applications and further validation. In addition, the systems pharmacology models were constructed predominantly based on computer predictions; however, the reliability and validity of these models still need to be verified by experiments and clinical practice. Besides, the quality of TCM is one of the most important factors for modernization of Chinese medicines, so the study on its genuineness is of great significance for the efficacy of TCM. How to assess the quality of TCM and integrate it into the in silico model should be considered. Furthermore, the development of precision medicine, TCM combination, or a combination of TCM and Western medicine (WM) has obvious advantages. Mass clinical data showed that the complementary advantages of combined TCM and WM can significantly improve the efficacy of treatment for

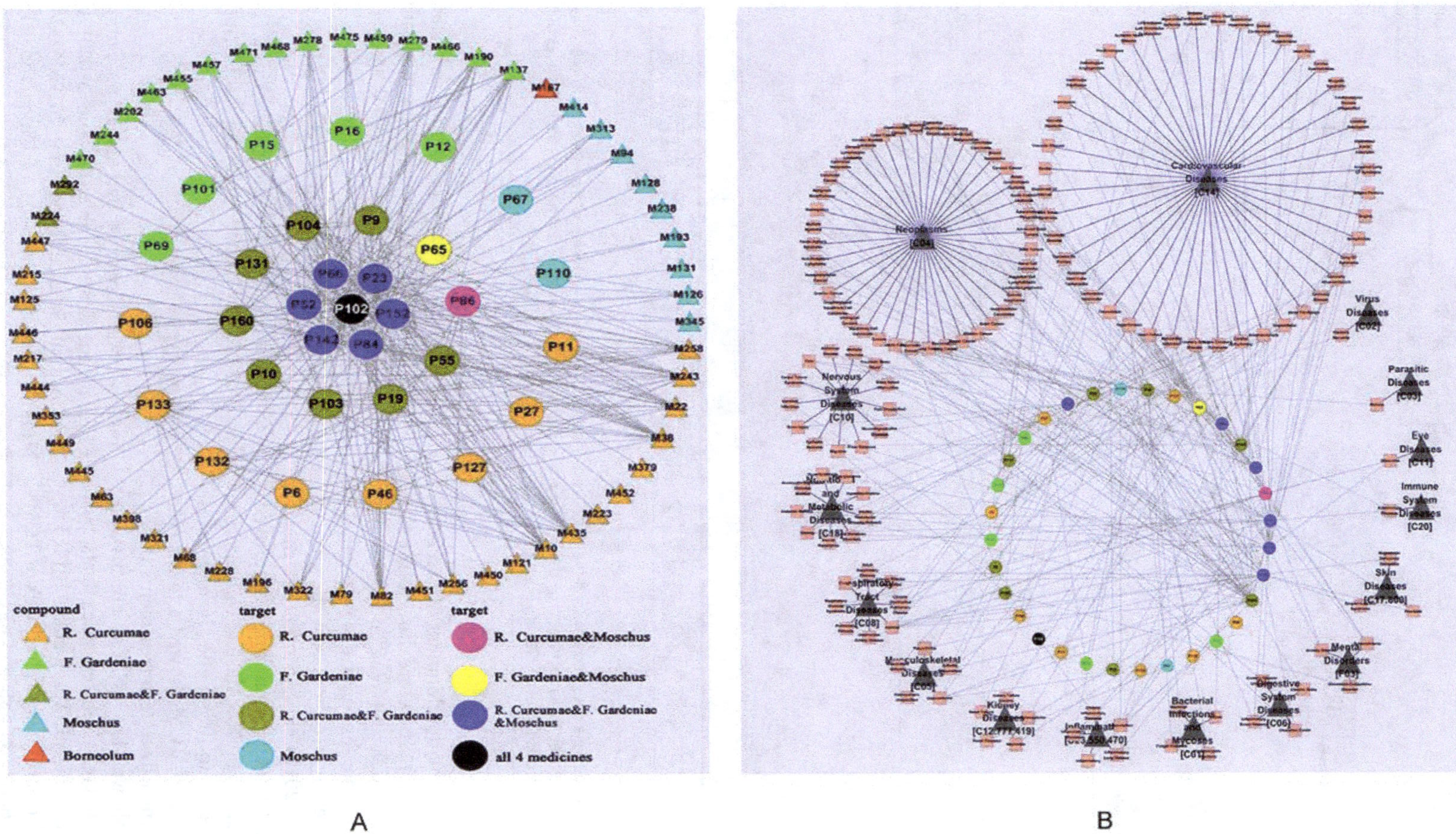

FIGURE 10 | Dissection of the "Jun-Chen-Zuo-Shi" combination principle of Yujin Formula. **(A)** The potential molecule–target networks constructed by 58 potential active components (triangles) and 32 potential targets associated with cardiovascular diseases (CVDs) (round). **(B)** Target–disease network, linked by 32 potential targets (the middle circles were marked with a variety of colors, as in **Figure 2**) and 147 kinds of diseases (red squares), which were divided into 16 types (black triangles) (Li et al., 2012a).

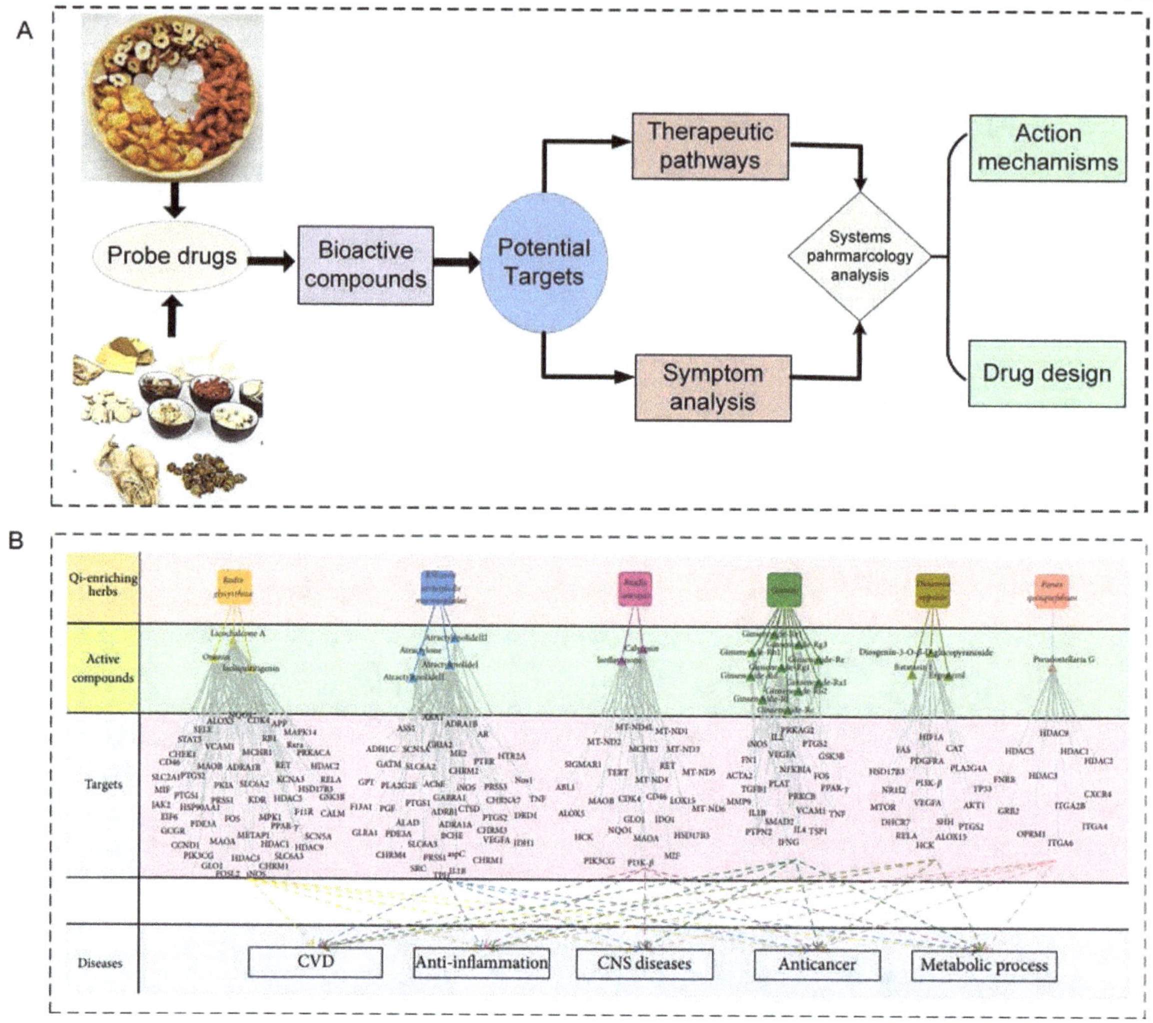

FIGURE 11 | Study of the mechanism of disease and syndrome and the theory of qi and blood. **(A)** The relationship at the molecular level between the different subtypes of cardiovascular disease and the distribution of targets on the pathway; blue indicates blood stasis syndrome, and red indicates qi deficiency syndrome. **(B)** Study of the material basis of qi and bloods (Liu et al., 2013b).

many diseases and contribute to the development of precision medicine (Wang and Zhang, 2017). Therefore, how to predict the drug combination of these TCM and WM and assess the efficacy and side effects is valuable for novel drug design. At present, RCTs have been generally used to assess the clinical efficacy of TCM (Hu et al., 2017). For example, a meta-analysis of RCTs has shown that TCM significantly improved analog scale, Western Ontario and McMaster Universities Osteoarthritis Index (WOMAC), and total effectiveness rates of knee osteoarthritis. In addition, TCM showed a lower risk of adverse events than did standard western treatments (Chen et al., 2016). Studies have shown that TCM is effective in treating atrial fibrillation and has relatively few side effects, but the mechanism of action is still unclear (Wang et al., 2011; Liu et al., 2014; Cai et al., 2017). However, respective RCTs of TCM are limited, because there has been no English meta-analysis of TCM treatment for some diseases.

In the future, we will further improve systems pharmacology and provide extended guidance for the modernization of Chinese medicine and the development of new drugs.

AUTHOR CONTRIBUTIONS

WZ wrote the first draft of the manuscript. YH drew the figures. ZM, AQ, and YW helped revise the manuscript.

FUNDING

This work was supported by Fund of the Fundamental Research Funds for the Central Universities (no. 3102017OQD050), China's Post-doctoral Science Fund (no. 2017M623249), the National Natural Science Foundation of China (no. 31570940), and the Key Research and Development Project of Shaanxi Province (no. 2018SF-363).

REFERENCES

Agoram, B., Woltosz, W. S., and Bolger, M. B. (2001). Predicting the impact of physiological and biochemical processes on oral drug bioavailability. *Adv. Drug Deliv. Rev.* 50 Suppl 1, S41–67. doi: 10.1016/S0169-409X(01)00179-X

Ai, C. Z., Li, Y., Wang, Y. H., Chen, Y., and Yang, L. (2009). Insight into the effects of chiral isomers quinidine and quinine on CYP2D6 inhibition. *Bioorg. Med. Chem. Lett.* 19, 803–806. doi: 10.1016/j.bmcl.2008.12.016

Ai, C. Z., Li, Y., Wang, Y. H., Li, W., Dong, P. P., Ge, G. B., et al. (2010). Investigation of binding features: effects on the interaction between cyp2a6 and inhibitors. *J. Comput. Chem.* 31, 1822–1831. doi: 10.1002/jcc.21455

Albert, D., Zündorf, I., Dingermann, T., Müller, Walter, E., Steinhilber, D., and Werz, O. (2002). Hyperforin is a dual inhibitor of cyclooxygenase-1 and 5-lipoxygenase. *Biochem. Pharmacol.* 64, 1767–1775. doi: 10.1016/S0006-2952(02)01387-4

Al-Lazikani, B., Banerji, U., and Workman, P. (2012). Combinatorial drug therapy for cancer in the post-genomic era. *Nat. Biotechnol.* 30, 679–692. doi: 10.1038/nbt.2284

Aller, S. G., Yu, J., Ward, A., Weng, Y., Chittaboina, S., Zhuo, R., et al. (2009). Structure of P-glycoprotein reveals a molecular basis for poly-specific drug binding. *Science* 323, 1718–1722. doi: 10.1126/science.1168750

Arnot, J. A., Brown, T. N., and Wania, F. (2014). Estimating screening-level organic chemical half-lives in humans. *Environ. Sci. Technol.* 48, 723–730. doi: 10.1021/es4029414

Balakin, K. V., Tkachenko, S. E., Lang, S. A., Okun, I., Ivashchenko, A. A., and Savchuk, N. P. (2003). Property-based design of GPCR-targeted library. *Cheminform* 34, 1332–1342. doi: 10.1002/chin.200304210

Ballesteros, J., and Palczewski, K. (2001). G protein-coupled receptor drug discovery: implications from the crystal structure of rhodopsin. *Curr. Opin. Drug Discov. Devel.* 4, 561–574.

Berezhkovskiy, L. M. (2013). Prediction of drug terminal half-life and terminal volume of distribution after intravenous dosing based on drug clearance, steady-state volume of distribution, and physiological parameters of the body. *J. Pharm. Sci.* 102, 761–771. doi: 10.1002/jps.23396

Borisy, A. A., Elliott, P. J., Hurst, N. W., Lee, M. S., Lehar, J., Price, E. R., et al. (2003). Systematic discovery of multicomponent therapeutics. *Proc. Natl. Acad. Sci.* 100, 7977–7982. doi: 10.1073/pnas.1337088100

Boulesteix, A. (2004). PLS dimension reduction for classification with microarray data. *Stat. Appl. Genet. Mol. Biol.* 3, 1–30. doi: 10.2202/1544-6115.1075

Byvatov, E., Fechner, U., Sadowski, J., and Schneider, G. (2003). Comparison of support vector machine and artificial neural network systems for drug/nondrug classification. *J. Chem. Inf. Comput. Sci.* 43, 1882–1889. doi: 10.1021/ci0341161

Cabrera-Pérez, M. Á., and Pham-The, H. (2018). Computational modeling of human oral bioavailability: what will be next? *Expert. Opin. Drug Discov.* 13, 509–521. doi: 10.1080/17460441.2018.1463988

Cai, X. L., Wang, Y. P., Li, Z. Q., Zhang, Y., Wang, D. W., and Yan, X. (2017). Chinese herbal medicine for patients with atrial fibrillation: protocol for a systematic review and meta-analysis. *Medicine* 96, e9228. doi: 10.1097/MD.0000000000009228

Cao, D. S., Liu, S., Xu, Q. S., Lu, H. M., Huang, J. H., Hu, Q. N., et al. (2012). Large-scale prediction of drug-target interactions using protein sequences and drug topological structures. *Anal. Chim. Acta* 752, 1–10. doi: 10.1016/j.aca.2012.09.021

Chen, B., Wild, D., and Guha, R. (2009). Pubchem as a source of polypharmacology. *J. Chem. Inf. Model.* 49, 2044–2055. doi: 10.1021/ci9001876

Chen, B., Zhan, H. S., Marszalek, J., Chung, M., Lin, X., Zhang, M., et al. (2016). Traditional Chinese medications for knee osteoarthritis pain: a meta-analysis of randomized controlled trials. *Am. J. Chin. Med.* 44, 677–703. doi: 10.1142/S0192415X16500373

Chen, X., Zhou, H., Liu, Y. B., Wang, J. F., Li, H., Ung, C. Y., et al. (2010). Database of traditional Chinese medicine and its application to studies of mechanism and to prescription validation. *Br. J. Pharmacol.* 149, 1092–1103. doi: 10.1038/sj.bjp.0706945

Chen, Y. C. (2011). TCM Database. Taiwan: the world's largest traditional Chinese medicine database for drug screening in silico. *PLoS One* 6, e15939. doi: 10.1371/journal.pone.0015939

Chou, T. C. (2010). Drug combination studies and their synergy quantification using the Chou-Talalay method. *Cancer Res.* 70, 440–446. doi: 10.1158/0008-5472.CAN-09-1947

Ehrman, T. M., Barlow, D. J., and Hylands, P. J. (2007). Phytochemical databases of Chinese herbal constituents and bioactive plant compounds with known target specificities. *J. Chem. Inf. Model.* 47, 254–263. doi: 10.1021/ci600288m

Fang, J., Cai, C., Wang, Q., Lin, P., Zhao, Z., and Cheng, F. (2017). Systems pharmacology-based discovery of natural products for precision oncology through targeting cancer mutated genes. CPT. *Pharmacometrics Syst. Pharmacol.* 6, 177–187. doi: 10.1002/psp4.12172

Frimurer, T. M., Ulven, T., Elling, C. E., Gerlach, L. O., Kostenis, E., and Högberg, T. (2005). A physicogenetic method to assign ligand-binding relationships between 7TM receptors. *Bioorg. Med. Chem. Lett.* 15, 3707–3712. doi: 10.1016/j.bmcl.2005.05.102

Gong, Y. C., and Zhang, Z. L. (2005). Alternative signaling pathways: when, where and why? *FEBS Lett.* 579, 0–5274. doi: 10.1016/j.febslet.2005.08.062

Gu, J. Y., Gui, Y. S., Chen, L. R., Yuan, G., and Xu, X. J. (2013). CVDHD: a cardiovascular disease herbal database for drug discovery and network pharmacology. *J. Cheminform.* 5, 51. doi: 10.1186/1758-2946-5-51

Hao, M., Li, Y., Wang, Y., and Zhang, S. (2011). A classification study of human β, 3-adrenergic receptor agonists using bcut descriptors. *Mol. Divers.* 15, 877–887. doi: 10.1007/s11030-011-9321-6

He, Z., Zhang, J., Shi, X. H., Hu, L. L., Kong, X., Cai, Y. D., et al. (2010). Predicting drug-target interaction networks based on functional groups and biological features. *PLoS One* 5 (3), e9603. doi: 10.1371/journal.pone.0009603

Hopkins, A. L. (2007). Network pharmacology. *Nat. Biotechnol.* 25, 1110–1111. doi: 10.1038/nbt1007-1110

Hopkins, A. L. (2008). Network pharmacology: the next paradigm in drug discovery. *Nat. Chem. Biol.*, 4, 682–690. doi: 10.1038/nchembio.118

Hou, T. J., and Xu, X. J. (2002). ADME evaluation in drug discovery: 1. applications of genetic algorithms to the prediction of blood–brain partitioning of a large set of drugs. *J. Mol. Model.* 8, 337–349. doi: 10.1007/s00894-002-0101-1

Hu, J., Liu, S., Liu, W. H., Zhang, H. N., Chen, J., and Shang, H. C. (2017). Establishing an evaluation mode with multiple primary outcomes based on combination of diseases and symptoms in TCM clinical trials. *Ann. Transl. Med.* 5, 420. doi: 10.21037/atm.2017.06.06

Huang, C., Zheng, C. L., Li, Y., Wang, Y. H., and Yang, L. (2013a). Systems pharmacology in drug discovery and therapeutic insight for herbal medicines. *Brief. Bioinformatics* 15, 710–733. doi: 10.1093/bib/bbt035

Huang, S. H., Xia, H. W., Chi, F., and Khalaf, N. K. (2013b). Chemoinfectomics in drug design and development. *Antiinfect. Agents* 11, 100–108. doi: 10.2174/2211352511311020003

Jain, A. N. (2003). Surflex: fully automatic flexible molecular docking using a molecular similarity-based search engine. *J. Med. Chem.* 46, 499–511. doi: 10.1021/jm020406h

Jiang, M., Lu, C., Zhang, C., Yang, J., Tan, Y., Lu, A. P., et al. (2012). Syndrome differentiation in modern research of traditional Chinese medicine. *J. Ethnopharmacol.* 140, 634–642. doi: 10.1016/j.jep.2012.01.033

Johnson, G. L., and Lapadat, R. (2002). Mitogen-activated protein kinase pathways mediated by ERK, JNK, and p38 protein kinases. *Science* 298,1911–1912. doi: 10.1126/science.1072682

Jones, S., Zhang, X., Parsons, D. W., Lin, J. C., Leary, R. J., and Angenendt, P. (2008). Core signaling pathways in human pancreatic cancers revealed by global genomic analyses. *Science* 26, 321:1801–1806. doi: 10.1126/science.1164368

Kassel, D. B. (2004). Applications of high-throughput ADME in drug discovery. *Curr. Opin. Chem. Biol.* 8, 339–345. doi: 10.1016/j.cbpa.2004.04.015

Kidron, H., Amo, E. M. D., Vellonen, K. S., and Urtti, A. (2012). Prediction of the vitreal half-life of small molecular drug-like compounds. *Pharm. Res.* 29, 3302–3311. doi: 10.1007/s11095-012-0822-5

Klabunde, T. (2010). Chemogenomic approaches to drug discovery: similar receptors bind similar ligands. *Br. J. Pharmacol.* 152, 5–7. doi: 10.1038/sj.bjp.0707308

Knox, C., Law, V., Jewison, T., Liu, P., Ly, S., Frolkis, A., et al. (2011). DrugBank 3.0: a comprehensive resource for 'omics' research on drugs. *Nucleic Acids Res.* 39, D1035–D1041. doi: 10.1093/nar/gkq1126

Krejsa, C. M., Horvath, D., Rogalski, S. L., Penzotti, J. E., Mao, B., Barbosa, F., et al. (2003). Predicting ADME properties and side effects: the BioPrint approach. *Curr. Opin. Drug Discov. Devel.* 6, 470–480. doi: 10.2174/0929867033457386

Kumar, R., Chaudhary, K., Gupta, S., Singh, H., Kumar, S., Gautam, A., et al. (2013). CancerDR: cancer drug resistance database. *Sci. Rep.* 3, 1445. doi: 10.1038/srep01445

Lehár, J., Krueger, A. S., Avery, W., Heilbut, A. M., Johansen, L. M., Price, E. R., et al. (2009). Synergistic drug combinations tend to improve therapeutically relevant selectivity. *Nat. Biotechnol.* 27, 659–666. doi: 10.1038/nbt.1549

Li, S. (2009). Network systems underlying traditional Chinese medicine syndrome and herb formula. *Curr. Bioinform.* 4, 188–196. doi: 10.2174/157489309789071129

Li, B. H., Xu, X., Wang, X., Yu, H., Li, X. X., Tao, W. Y., et al. (2012a). A systems biology approach to understanding the mechanisms of action of Chinese herbs for treatment of cardiovascular disease. *Int. J. Mol. Sci.* 13, 13501–13520. doi: 10.3390/ijms131013501

Li, J. S., Zhao, P., Li, Y., Tian, Y. G., and Wang, Y. H. (2015a). Systems pharmacology-based dissection of mechanisms of Chinese medicinal formula Bufei Yishen as an effective treatment for chronic obstructive pulmonary disease. *Sci. Rep.* 5, 15290. doi: 10.1038/srep15290

Li, P., Fu, Y., Ru, J. L., Huang, C., Du, J. F., Zheng, C. L., et al. (2014). Insights from systems pharmacology into cardiovascular drug discovery and therapy. *BMC Syst. Biol.* 8, 141. doi: 10.1186/s12918-014-0141-z

Li, P., Huang, C., Fu, Y. X., Wang, J. N., Wu, Z. Y., Ru, J. L., et al. (2015b). Large-scale exploration and analysis of drug combinations. *Bioinformatics* 31, 2007–2016. doi: 10.1093/bioinformatics/btv080

Li, P., Yang, L. P., and Gong, Y. W. (2009). Application of systems biology technology in research of traditional Chinese medicine. *J. Tradit. Chin. Med.* 29, 153–157. doi: 10.1016/S0254-6272(09)60054-6

Li, X. X., Xu, X., Wang, J. N., Yu, H., Wang, X., Yang, H. J., et al. (2012b). A system-level investigation into the mechanisms of Chinese traditional medicine: compound Danshen formula for cardiovascular disease treatment. *PLoS One* 7, e43918. doi: 10.1371/journal.pone.0043918

Lin, Q. C. (1998). The present state and prospect of the study of syndrome. *Chin. J. Integr. Med.* 4, 242–246. doi: 10.1007/BF02935463

Lipinski, C. A., Lombardo, F., Dominy, B. W., and Feeney, P. J. (2012). Experimental and computational approaches to estimate solubility and permeability in drug discovery and development settings. *Adv. Drug Deliv. Rev.* 64, 4–17. doi: 10.1016/j.addr.2012.09.019

Liu, H., Wang, J. N., Zhou, W., Wang, Y. H., and Yang, L. (2013a). Systems approaches and polypharmacology for drug discovery from herbal medicines: an example using licorice. *J. Ethnopharmacol.* 146, 773–793. doi: 10.1016/j.jep.2013.02.004

Liu, J. L., Pei, M. J., Zheng, C. L., Li, Y., Wang, Y. H., Lv, A. P., et al. (2013b). A systems-pharmacology analysis of herbal medicines used in health improvement treatment: predicting potential new drugs and targets. *Evid. Based Complement. Altern. Med.* 2013, 938764. doi: 10.1155/2013/938764

Liu, J. L., Pei, T. L., Mu, J. X., Zheng, C. L., Chen, X. T., Huang, C., et al. (2016). Systems pharmacology uncovers the multiple mechanisms of Xijiao Dihuang decoction for the treatment of viral hemorrhagic fever. *Evid. Based Complement. Altern. Med.* 2016, 1–17. doi: 10.1155/2016/9025036

Liu, T. Q., Lin, Y. M., Wen, X., Jorissen, R. N., and Gilson, M. K. (2007). Bindingdb: a web-accessible database of experimentally determined protein–ligand binding affinities. *Nucleic Acids Res.* 35, 198–201. doi: 10.1093/nar/gkl999

Liu, Y. F., Li, N., Jia, Z. H., Lu, F., and Pu, J. L. (2014). Chinese medicine shensongyangxin is effective for patients with bradycardia: results of a randomized, double-blind, placebo-controlled multicenter trial. *Evid. Based Complement. Altern. Med.* 2014, 605714, 1–6. doi: 10.1155/2014/605714

Lu, J., Lu, D., Zhang, X. C., Bi, Y., Cheng, K. G., Zheng, M. Y., et al. (2016). Estimation of elimination half-lives of organic chemicals in humans using gradient boosting machine. *Biochim. Biophys. Acta Gen. Subj.* 1860, 2664–2671. doi: 10.1016/j.bbagen.2016.05.019

Ma, Y., Zhou, K., Fan, J., and Sun, S. (2016). Traditional Chinese medicine: potential approaches from modern dynamical complexity theories. *Front. Med.* 10, 28–32. doi: 10.1007/s11684-016-0434-2

MacCoss, M., and Baillie, T. A. (2004). Organic chemistry in drug discovery. *Science* 303, 1810–1813. doi: 10.1126/science.1096800

Nagamine, N., and Sakakibara, Y. (2007). Statistical prediction of protein–chemical interactions based on chemical structure and mass spectrometry data. *Bioinformatics* 23, 2004–2012. doi: 10.1093/bioinformatics/btm266

Pei, T. L., Zheng, C. L., Huang, C., Chen, X. T., Guo, Z. H., Fu, Y. X., et al. (2016). Systematic understanding the mechanisms of vitiligo pathogenesis and its treatment by Qubaibabuqi formula. *J. Ethnopharmacol.* 190, 272–287. doi: 10.1016/j.jep.2016.06.001

Roemer, T., and Boone, C. (2013). Systems-level antimicrobial drug and drug synergy discovery. *Nat. Chem. Biol.* 9, 222–231. doi: 10.1038/nchembio.1205

Rognan, D. (2007). Chemogenomic approaches to rational drug design. *Br. J. Pharmacol.* 152, 38–52. doi: 10.1038/sj.bjp.0707307

Roth, B. L., Lopez, E., Patel, S., and Kroeze, W. K. (2000). The multiplicity of serotonin receptors: uselessly diverse molecules or an embarrassment of riches? *Neuroscientist* 6, 252–262. doi: 10.1177/107385840000600408

Ru, J. L., Li, P., Wang, J. N., Zhou, W., Li, B. H., Huang, C., et al. (2014). TCMSP: a database of systems pharmacology for drug discovery from herbal medicines. *J. Cheminform.* 6, 13. doi: 10.1186/1758-2946-6-13

Sabio, G., and Davis, R. J. (2014). TNF and MAP kinase signaling pathways. *Semin. Immunol.* 26, 237–245. doi: 10.1016/j.smim.2014.02.009

Shar, P. A., Tao, W. Y., Gao, S., Huang, C., Li, B. H., Zhang, W. J., et al. (2016). Pred-binding: large-scale protein–ligand binding affinity prediction. *J. Enzyme Inhib. Med. Chem.* 31, 1443–1450. doi: 10.3109/14756366.2016.1144594

Sharma, A., Singla, D., Rashid, M., and Raghava, G. P. S. (2014). Designing of peptides with desired half-life in intestine-like environment. *BMC Bioinformatics* 15, 282. doi: 10.1186/1471-2105-15-282

Su, X. Y., Kong, L., Lei, X. Y., Hu, L. H., Ye, M. L., and Zou, H. F. (2007). Biological fingerprinting analysis of traditional Chinese medicines with targeting ADME/Tox property for screening of bioactive compounds by chromatographic and MS methods. *Mini Rev. Med. Chem.* 7, 87–98. doi: 10.2174/138955707779317830

Talete, S. (2011) Dragon for windows (software for molecular descriptor calculations), version 5.4. Available online: http://www.talete.mi.it (accessed on 20 May 2011).

Tan, L. T. (2007). Bioactive natural products from marine cyanobacteria for drug discovery. *Phytochemistry* 68, 954–979. doi: 10.1016/j.phytochem.2007.01.012

Tan, X., Hu, L., Luquette, L. J., Gao, G., Liu, Y. F., Qu, H. J., et al. (2012). Systematic identification of synergistic drug pairs targeting HIV. *Nat. Biotechnol.* 30, 1125–1130. doi: 10.1038/nbt.2391

Tang, F., Zhang, Q. L., Nie, Z., Yao, S. Z., and Chen, B. (2009). Sample preparation for analyzing traditional Chinese medicines. *Trac-Trend Anal. Chem.* 28, 1253–1262. doi: 10.1016/j.trac.2009.09.004

Tang, J., Karhinen, L., Xu, T., Szwajda, A., Yadav, B., Wennerberg, K., et al. (2013). Target inhibition networks: predicting selective combinations of druggable targets to block cancer survival pathways. *PLoS Comput. Biol.* 9 (9), e1003226. doi: 10.1371/journal.pcbi.1003226

Tao, W. Y., Li, B. H., Gao, S., Bai, Y. F., Shar, P. A., Zhang, W. J., et al. (2015). CancerHSP: anticancer herbs database of systems pharmacology. *Sci. Rep.* 5, 11481. doi: 10.1038/srep11481

Turner, J. V., Maddalena, D.J., Cutler, D. J., and Agatonovic, K. S. (2010). Multiple pharmacokinetic parameter prediction for a series of cephalosporins. *J. Pharm. Sci.* 92, 552–559. doi: 10.1002/jps.10314

Tyagi, A., Tuknait, A., Anand, P., Gupta, S., Sharma, M., Mathur, D., et al. (2015). CancerPPD: a database of anticancer peptides and proteins. *Nucleic Acids Res.* 43, D837–D843. doi: 10.1093/nar/gku892

Ventegodt, S., Andersen, N. J., and Merrick, J. (2014). Holistic medicine: scientific challenges. *Sci. World J.* 3, 1108–1116. doi: 10.1100/tsw.2003.96

Vesanto, J. (2002). Clustering of the self-organizing map. *IEEE Trans. Neural Netw.* 11, 586–600. doi: 10.1109/72.846731

Violeta, I. P.-N., Karaboga, A. S., Souchet, M., and Ritchie, D. W. (2014). GES polypharmacology fingerprints: a novel approach for drug repositioning. *J. Chem. Inf. Model.* 54, 720–734. doi: 10.1021/ci4006723

Wang, J., and Zhang, T. (2017). Integration of traditional Chinese medicine and western Medicine in the era of precision medicine. *J. Integr. Med.* 15 (1), 1–760314–5. doi: 10.1016/S2095-4964(17)60314-5

Wang, Y. H., and Li, Y., (2016a). *Systems pharmacology of traditional Chinese medicine. The theory, approaches and application of systems pharmacology.* Dalian, Liaoning: Dalian University of Technology Press, 9–22.

Wang, Y. H., and Yang, L. (2013). Systems pharmacology-based research framework of traditional Chinese medicine. *J. World Chin. Med.* 8, 801–808. doi: 10.3969/j.issn.1673-7202.2013.07.032

Wang, A. H., Pu, J. L., Qi, X. Y., Miao, W. L., Hou, Z. S., Cong, H. L., et al. (2011). Evaluation of shensongyangxin capsules in the treatment of paroxysmal atrial fibrillation: a randomized, double blind and controlled multicenter trial. *Zhonghua Yi Xue Za Zhi* 91, 1677–1681. doi: 10.3760/cma.j.issn.0376-2491.2011.24.006

Wang, G. X., Li, Y., Liu, X. L., and Wang, Y. H. (2009). Understanding the aquatic toxicity of pesticide: structure–activity relationship and molecular descriptors to distinguish the ratings of toxicity. *Mol. Inform.* 28, 1418–1431. doi: 10.1002/qsar.200960050

Wang, J. H., Li, Y., Yang, Y. F., Du, J., Zhao, M. Q., Lin, F., et al. (2017). Systems pharmacology dissection of multi-scale mechanisms of action for herbal medicines in treating rheumatoid arthritis. *Mol. Pharm.* 14, 7b00505. doi: 10.1021/acs.molpharmaceut.7b00505

Wang, J. N., Guo, Z. H., Fu, Y. X., Wu, Z. Y., Huang, C., Zheng, C. L., et al. (2016b). Weak-binding molecules are not drugs?—Toward a systematic strategy for finding effective weak-binding drugs. *Brief. Bioinformatics* 1–12. doi: 10.1093/bib/bbw018

Wang, K. J., Sun, J. Z., Zhou, S. F., Wan, C. L., Qin, S. Y., Li, C., et al. (2013). Prediction of drug-target interactions for drug repositioning only based on genomic expression similarity. *PLoS Comput. Biol.* 9, e1003315. doi: 10.1371/journal.pcbi.1003315

Wang, X., Xu, X., Tao, W. Y., Li, Y., Wang, Y. H., and Yang, L. (2012). A systems biology approach to uncovering pharmacological synergy in herbal medicines with applications to cardiovascular disease. *Evid. Based Complement. Altern. Med.* 2012, 519031. doi: 10.1155/2012/519031

Wang, Y. H., Zheng, C. L., Huang, C., Chen, X. T., Wu, Z. Y., Wang, Z. Z., et al. (2015). Systems-pharmacology dissecting holistic medicine for treatment of complex diseases: an example using cardio-cerebrovascular diseases treated by TCM. *Evid. Based Complement. Altern. Med.* 2015, 1–19. doi: 10.1155/2015/980190

Wu, Y., Zhang, F. L., Yang, K., Fang, S. S., Bu, D. C., Li, H., et al. (2019). SymMap: an integrative database of traditional Chinese medicine enhanced by symptom mapping. *Nucleic Acids Res.* 47, D1110–D1117. doi: 10.1093/nar/gky1021

Xia, Z., Zhou, X. B., Sun, Y. X., and Wu, L. Y. (2009). Semi-supervised drug–protein interaction prediction from heterogeneous spaces. *In The Third International Symposium on Optimization and Systems Biology.* 11, 123–131.

Xu, H. Y., Zhang, Y. Q., Liu, Z. M., Chen, T., Lv, C. Y., and Tang, S. H. (2019). ETCM: an encyclopaedia of traditional Chinese medicine. *Nucleic Acids Res.* 47, D976–D982. doi: 10.1093/nar/gky987

Xu, X., Fu, J., Wang, H., Zhang, B., Wang, X., and Wang, Y. H. (2011a). Influence of p-glycoprotein on embryotoxicity of the antifouling biocides to sea urchin (Strongylocentrotus intermedius). *Ecotoxicology* 20, 419–428. doi: 10.1007/s10646-011-0593-5

Xu, X., Li, Y., Wang, Y., and Wang, Y. H. (2011b). Assessment of toxic interactions of heavy metals in multi-component mixtures using sea urchin embryo-larval bioassay. *Toxicol. In Vitro* 25, 294–300. doi: 10.1016/j.tiv.2010.09.007

Xu, X., Zhang, W. X., Huang, C., Li, Y., Yu, H., Wang, Y., et al. (2012). A novel chemometric method for the prediction of human oral bioavailability. *Int. J. Mol. Sci.* 13, 6964–6982. doi: 10.3390/ijms13066964

Xue, R. C., Fang, Z., Zhang, M. X., Yi, Z. H., Wen, C. P., and Shi, T. L. (2013). TCMID: traditional Chinese medicine integrative database for herb molecular mechanism analysis. *Nucleic Acids Res.* 41, D1089–D1095. doi: 10.1093/nar/gks1100

Yamanishi, Y., Kotera, M., Kanehisa, M., and Goto, S. (2010). Drug-target interaction prediction from chemical, genomic and pharmacological data in an integrated framework. *Bioinformatics* 26, i246–i254. doi: 10.1093/bioinformatics/btq176

Yamanishi, Y., Pauwels, E., Saigo, H., and Stoven, V. (2011). Extracting sets of chemical substructures and protein domains governing drug-target interactions. *J. Chem. Inf. Model.* 51 (5), 1183–1194. doi: 10.1021/ci100476q

Yang, H. X., Zhang, W. J., Huang, C., Zhou, W., Yao, Y., Wang, Z., et al. (2014). A novel systems pharmacology model for herbal medicine injection: a case using reduning injection. *BMC Complement. Altern. Med.* 14, 430. doi: 10.1186/1472-6882-14-430

Yang, Y. F., Li, Y., Wang, J. H., Sun, K., Tao, W. Y., Wang, Z. H., et al. (2017). Systematic investigation of Ginkgo biloba leaves for treating cardio-cerebrovascular diseases in an animal model. *ACS Chem. Bio.* 12, 1363–1372. doi: 10.1021/acschembio.6b00762

Yao, Y., Zhang, X. D., Wang, Z. Z., Zheng, C. L., Li, P., Huang, C., et al. (2013). Deciphering the combination principles of traditional Chinese medicine from a systems pharmacology perspective based on Ma-huang Decoction. *J. Ethnopharmacol.* 150, 619–638. doi: 10.1016/j.jep.2013.09.018

Ye, H., Ye, L., Kang, H., Zhang, D. F., Tao, L., Tang, K. L., et al. (2011). HIT: linking herbal active ingredients to targets. *Nucleic Acids Res.* 39, D1055–D1059. doi: 10.1093/nar/gkq1165

Yoshida, F., and Topliss, J. G. (2000). QSAR model for drug human oral bioavailability. *J. Med. Chem.* 43,2575–2585. doi: 10.1021/jm0000564

Yu, L. X. (1999). An integrated model for determining causes of poor oral drug absorption. *Pharm. Res.* 16, 1883–1887. doi: 10.1023/A:1018911728161

Yu, H., Chen, J. X., Xu, X., Li, Y., Zhao, H. H., Fang, Y. P., et al. (2012). A systematic prediction of multiple drug-target interactions from chemical, genomic, and pharmacological data. *PLoS One* 7, e37608. doi: 10.1371/journal.pone.0037608

Zhang, Q. W., Lin, L. G., and Ye, W. C. (2018). Techniques for extraction and isolation of natural products: a comprehensive review. *Chin. Med.* 13, 20. doi: 10.1186/s13020-018-0177-x

Zhang, W. J., and Wang, Y. H. (2015). The principle, methods and the application of systems pharmacology in the traditional Chinese medicine. *J. World Chin. Med.* 2, 280–286. doi: 10.3969/j.issn.1673-7202.2015.02.033

Zhang, W. J., Tao, Q., Guo, Z. H., Fu, Y. X., Chen, X. T., Shar, P. A., et al. (2016). Systems pharmacology dissection of the integrated treatment for cardiovascular and gastrointestinal disorders by traditional Chinese medicine. *Sci. Rep.* 6, 32400. doi: 10.1038/srep32400

Zhao, J., Jiang, P., and Zhang, W. D. (2010). Molecular networks for the study of TCM pharmacology. *Brief Bioinformatics* 11, 417–430. doi: 10.1093/bib/bbp063

Zhao, X. M., Iskar, M., Zeller, G., Kuhn, M., Van Noort, V., and Bork, P. (2011). Prediction of drug combinations by integrating molecular and pharmacological data. *PLoS Comput. Biol.* 7, e1002323. doi: 10.1371/journal.pcbi.1002323

Zheng, C. L., Guo, Z. H., Huang, C., Wu, Z. Y., Li, Y., Chen, X. T., et al. (2015). Large-scale direct targeting for drug repositioning and discovery. *Sci. Rep.* 5, 11970. doi: 10.1038/srep11970

Zhou, W., and Wang, Y. H. (2014). A network-based analysis of the types of coronary artery disease from traditional Chinese medicine perspective: potential for therapeutics and drug discovery. *J. Ethnopharmacol.* 151, 66–77. doi: 10.1016/j.jep.2013.11.007

Zhou, W., Huang, C., Li, Y., Duan, J. Y., Wang, Y. H., and Yang, L. (2013). A systematic identification of multiple toxin–target interactions based on chemical, genomic and toxicological data. *Toxicology* 304, 173–184. doi: 10.1016/j.tox.2012.12.012

Zhu, L. L., and Xu, X. J. (2003). Selective separation of active inhibitors of epidermal growth factor receptor from Caragana jubata by molecularly imprinted solid-phase extraction. *J. Chromatogr. A* 991, 151–158. doi: 10.1016/S0021-9673(03)00207-3

Zhu, D. N., Chen, C., Wang, S. M., and Wang, Y. F. (2018). Advances in the application of network pharmacology in traditional Chinese medicine. *Guangdong Chem. Eng.* 22, 67–70. doi: CNKI:SUN:GDHG.0.2018-07-067

Zimmermann, G. R., Lehar, J., and Keith, C. T. (2007). Multi-target therapeutics: when the whole is greater than the sum of the parts. *Drug Discov. Today* 12, 34–42. doi: 10.1016/j.drudis.2006.11.008

9

WTD Attenuating Rheumatiod Arthiritis *via* Suppressing Angiogenesis and Modulating the PI3K/AKT/mTOR/HIF-1α Pathway

*Xin Ba[1], Ying Huang[1,2], Pan Shen[1], Yao Huang[1], Hui Wang[3], Liang Han[1], Wei Ji Lin[1], Hui Jia Yan[1], Li Jun Xu[1], Kai Qin[2], Zhe Chen[1,2] and Sheng Hao Tu[1,2]**

[1]Institute of Integrated Traditional Chinese and Western Medicine, Tongji Hospital, Tongji Medical College, Huazhong University of Science and Technology, Wuhan, China, [2]Department of Integrated Traditional Chinese and Western Medicine, Tongji Hospital, Tongji Medical College, Huazhong University of Science and Technology, Wuhan, China, [3]Rehabilitation and Sports Medicine Research Institute of Zhejiang Province, Zhejiang Provincial People's Hospital, People's Hospital of Hangzhou Medical College, Hangzhou, China

***Correspondence:**
Sheng Hao Tu
shtu@tjh.tjmu.edu.cn

Background: Wutou Decoction (WTD), as a classic prescription, has been generally used to treat rheumatoid arthritis (RA) for two thousand years in China. However, the potential protective effects of WTD on rheumatoid arthritis and its possible mechanism have rarely been reported.

Purpose: The aim of this study was to explore the possible mechanism of WTD against RA and a promising alternative candidate for RA therapy.

Methods: A model of collagen-induced arthritis (CIA) was constructed in rats to assess the therapeutic effects of WTD. Histopathological staining, immunofluorescence, and western blotting of synovial sections were conducted to detect the antiangiogenic effects of WTD. Then, cell viability assays, flow cytometry, scratch healing assays, and invasion assays were conducted to explore the effects of WTD on MH7A human fibroblast-like synoviocyte (FLS) cell proliferation, apoptosis, migration, and invasion *in vitro*. The ability of WTD to induce blood vessel formation after MH7A cell and human umbilical vein endothelial cell line (HUVEC) coculture with WTD intervention was detected by a tube formation assay. The mechanisms of WTD were screened by network pharmacology and confirmed by *in vivo* and *in vitro* experiments.

Results: WTD ameliorated the symptoms and synovial pannus hyperplasia of CIA rats. Treatment with WTD inhibited MH7A cell proliferation, migration, and invasion and promoted MH7A apoptosis. WTD could inhibit MH7A cell expression of proangiogenic factors, including VEGF and ANGI, to induce HUVEC tube formation. Furthermore, the PI3K-AKT-mTOR-HIF-1α pathway was enriched as a potential target of WTD for the treatment of RA through network pharmacology enrichment analysis. Finally, it was confirmed *in vitro* and *in vivo* that WTD inhibits angiogenesis in RA by interrupting the PI3K-AKT-mTOR-HIF-1α pathway.

Conclusion: WTD can inhibit synovial hyperplasia and angiogenesis, presumably by inhibiting the migration and invasion of MH7A cells and blocking the production of proangiogenic effectors in MH7A cells. The possible underlying mechanism by which WTD ameliorates angiogenesis in RA is the PI3K-AKT-mTOR-HIF-1α pathway.

Keywords: rheumatoid arthritis, fibroblast-like synoviocytes, wutou decoction, angiogenesis, collagen-induced arthritis, network pharmacology

INTRODUCTION

Rheumatoid arthritis (RA) is a chronic autoimmune disease with the characteristic pathological changes of persistent synovitis, hyperplastic synovial pannus tissue formation, the destruction of cartilage and bone, and the presence of autoantibodies (especially rheumatoid factor and citrullinated peptide) (Mcinnes and Schett, 2011). Multiple genetic factors (e.g., HLA-DRB1 and PTPN22) and environmental risks (e.g., smoking) are closely related to the development of RA (Smolen et al., 2016). RA affects approximately 1% of the global population, especially elderly individuals and women, with 5–50 per 100,000 individuals newly diagnosed with RA annually (Myasoedova et al., 2010; Tobon et al., 2010). In recent decades, disease-modifying antirheumatic drugs (DMARDs) have been the predominant therapeutic agents for RA. The leading DMARD is methotrexate, which is widely accepted as a first-line regimen due to its superior efficacy and economic advantages. Biological agents and small molecule targeted drugs are used when RA cannot be controlled or toxic side effects arise with DMARD treatment (Smolen et al., 2017; Sparks et al., 2021). However, biological targeted DMARDs are expensive and may increase the risk of infection (Burmester and Pope, 2017). More than 30% of patients still cannot satisfactorily control this disease after using the drugs mentioned above (Singh et al., 2015; Favalli et al., 2017; Aletaha and Smolen, 2018). Therefore, it is necessary to find new drugs or therapeutic strategies for RA patients.

Angiogenesis in synovial tissue is considered an important early event in the development of RA (Elshabrawy et al., 2015). Angiogenesis is mediated by proangiogenic factors and the corresponding receptors on the surface of endothelial cells, including growth factors, proinflammatory cytokines, chemokines, and others (Latacz et al., 2020). In particular, hypoxia-inducible factor-1 (HIF-1) and vascular endothelial growth factor (VEGF) are considered major mediators of angiogenesis. In an inflammatory or hypoxic environment, the expression of HIF-1 increases to mediate angiogenesis. HIF-1 is a transcription factor composed of constitutive expression of the β subunit and oxygen-regulated α subunit, which mainly determines HIF-1 activation. HIF-1α is quickly degraded under normal oxygen conditions but stabilized under hypoxic conditions when it quickly translocates to the nucleus, where it induces the expression of VEGF. VEGF then promotes the activation of endothelial cells to induce inflammation and thereby establish crosstalk between vascular production and articular inflammation in RA (Ferrara, 2004). An increase in the number of blood vessels can provide more oxygen and nutrients to synovial tissue, but abnormal vessels facilitate inflammatory cell migration and pannus formation, thus destroying neighboring cartilage and bones, as observed in RA (Paleolog and Miotla, 1998). Fibroblast-like synoviocytes (FLSs) are a key component of the proliferative synovial membrane and play a crucial role in the pathogenesis of RA (Nygaard and Firestein, 2020). Notably, proangiogenic factors are mainly produced by RA synovial tissue macrophages and fibroblasts. The RA synovial tissue lining layer plays an indispensable role in maintaining synovitis through neovascularization. A recent study indicated that RA-FLSs are closely involved in synovial angiogenesis (Wei et al., 2020). Therefore, modulation of the angiogenesis induced by FLSs is a promising strategy for the treatment of RA (Bottini and Firestein, 2013).

Wutou decoction (WTD), a traditional Chinese medicine (TCM), has been used to treat RA for two thousand years in China, and it has been gradually accepted by clinicians due to its excellent efficacy and few side effects (Moudgil and Berman, 2014). WTD contains five traditional drugs, including *Glycyrrhizae Radix Preparata*, *Ephedrae Herba*, *Paeoniae Radix Alba*, *Aconiti Radix Cocta*, and *Astragali Radix*. Modern pharmacological studies have shown that WTD has anti-inflammatory effects, regulates immunity, relieves pain, and has antiangiogenic effects (Lu et al., 2015; Guo et al., 2020). However, the underlying mechanism by which WTD alleviates RA is still unknown, which impedes its further clinical application.

In the past, due to the multiple components, targets, and channels that are characteristic of TCM compounds, their mechanisms of action have been difficult to clarify (Yuan et al., 2020). Network pharmacology is considered a promising method for complicated mechanistic studies and new drug discovery from TCMs (Tao et al., 2013). TCM network pharmacology methods establish a drug-gene-disease network in combination with existing clinical drug targets to predict the target spectrum and pharmacological effects of herbal compounds and to explain the combination rules and network regulation of herbal formulas (Guo et al., 2017). Therefore, we carried out this study based on network pharmacology to investigate the mechanism by which WTD ameliorates angiogenesis in RA.

MATERIALS AND METHODS

Preparation of Wutou decoction

WTD contains five traditional drugs, including 6 g of *Aconiti Radix* (*Aconitum carmichaeli* Debeaux.), 9 g of *Ephedrae Herba* (*Ephedra sinica* Stapf), 9 g of *Paeoniae Radix Alba* (*Paeonia lactiflora* Pall.), 9 g of *Astragali Radix* (*Astragalus mongholicus* Bunge), and 9 g of *Glycyrrhiza Radix Preparata* (*Glycyrrhiza uralensis* Fisch. ex DC.). The composition of WTD is shown in **Table 1**. The herbs were purchased from Tongji Hospital Pharmacy Department (Wuhan, China). WTD was prepared as previously described (Zhang et al., 2015). All herbs were soaked in 2 L of pure water for 2 h in advance. First, *Aconiti Radix Cocta* was boiled for 0.5 h. Then, the remaining drugs were added and boiled for 0.5 h. The decoction was filtered through a strainer, and the filtrate was collected. The herbs were boiled for 0.5 h with 2 L of water, and the filtrates were extracted following the above method. The filtrates were combined and concentrated to a concentration of 0.75 g/ml. For *in vitro* experiments, the pH of the decoction was adjusted to neutral, the penetrating pressure of the decoction was adjusted to 310 mmol/L, and then the freeze-dried powder was condensed. Subsequently, the filtrate was filtered through 0.22 μm sterile filters, and this filtrate was collected and stored at 4°C for no more than 1 week. Finally, the decoction was diluted to the appropriate concentration with saline for the *in vivo* experiments and with PBS for the *in vitro* experiments before use.

High-Performance Liquid Chromatography (HPLC) Fingerprinting of Wutou decoction

HPLC fingerprint analysis was used to identify the main chemical components of the WTD extract. The extract was dissolved in water at a concentration of 1.92 g/ml (w/v) and further diluted to 0.96 g/ml (w/v) with methanol-water (50:50). Samples were passed through an Acclaim™ 120 C18 column (4.6 mm × 250 mm, 5 μm) at a flow rate of 1.0 ml/min with the mobile phases of methanol (A) and 0.1% phosphoric acid (B). HPLC signals were measured at a detection wavelength of 240 nm with gradient elution as detailed in **Table 1**. Ephedrine hydrochloride, pseudoephedrine hydrochloride, paeoniflorin, verbasil-7-O-glucoside, glycyrrhizin, benzoylaconitine, benzoylneoaconitine, benzoylhypoaconitine, and glycyrrhizinate were purchased from Chengdu MUST Biotechnology Co., Ltd. (Chengdu, China). The TCM compound solution was evenly mixed by vortexing, 200 μL of the solution was accurately measured, and 1 ml of methanol: water (8:2, V/V) was added, and the mixture was vortexed. After centrifugation for 10 min at 4°C and 20,000×g, the supernatant was filtered through a 0.22 μm filter membrane and the filtrate was collected for analysis.

Construction of a Collagen-Induced Arthritis Rat Model and Wutou decoction Treatment

Fifty male Wistar rats (6 weeks of age, 160–200 g) were provided by the Hubei Provincial Centers for disease Control and Prevention (Animal Certificate of Conformity: SCXK (Hubei) 2015–0,018). Rats were kept under normal illumination conditions, and the room temperature was maintained at 22 ± 4°C. Bovine type II collagen (Chondrex Inc. Redmond, WA, United States of America) was mixed with complete Freund's adjuvant (Sigma, United States of America) at a proportion of 1:1. Each rat was injected with 0.3 ml of the emulsion at the end of the tail and on the back, and a second injection was administered on the seventh day. The study program was approved by the Ethical Committee of Tongji Hospital, Tongji Medical College, Huazhong University of Science and Technology (TJ-A20170502).

The level of arthritis in the rats was graded with the following evaluation system, and the highest grade was 16 points. The arthritis severity was expressed with a visual semiquantitative score system for each paw from 0 to 4 according to the following criteria: 0, normal joints; 1, slight swelling or a digital red spot; 2, red skin and slight swelling in the ankles and feet; 3, moderate swelling and erythema; and 4, severe swelling and erythema involving the entire posterior claw or precipitation (Kollias et al., 2011). On day 14, successfully modelled rats with arthritis scores over 6 were randomly allocated to 4 groups: the Control, the CIA, WTD at low-dose (WTD-L), and WTD at high-dose (WTD-H) groups according to a random number table. Treatment was given daily for 28 days from day 14 to day 42. According to the human adult (body weight of 70 kg) dosage of 42 g/d (the conversion factor used for conversion of human to rat is 6), the dosage of WTD (3.75 and 7.5 g/kg/day) was selected for the rats. This low dosage of WTD is nearly equivalent to the daily RA patient dosage. The WTD groups were given intragastric with corresponding doses of WTD (3.75 and 7.5 g/kg/day). The control group and the model group were given intragastric saline. The animals were sacrificed with 2% pentobarbital on day 42. Blood, knee synovial tissues, and hind paw ankles were excised from the rat.

Cell Viability Assay

The human FLS cell line MH7A (RIKEN Cell Bank, Japan) was incubated in sterile DMEM supplemented with 10% FBS, 100 U/mL penicillin, and 80 U/mL streptomycin. MH7A cells (1×10^4 cells/mL) were seeded in 96-well plates and incubated in sterile DMEM with different concentrations of WTD (1 or 10 mg/ml) for 24, 36, or 48 h. Cell viability was determined by the 3-(4,5-dimethyl-2-thiazolyl)-2,5-diphenyl-2 H-tetrazolium bromide (MTT) method. The OD value was measured at a wavelength of 570 nm with a microplate reader (United States of America, Bio-Tek), and the inhibition rate was calculated. Three independent experiments were performed.

Cell Apoptosis Analysis by Flow Cytometry

MH7A cells were seeded in 6-well plates and incubated with different concentrations of WTD (1 or 10 mg/ml) for 24 h. Adherent MH7A cells were digested with trypsin without EDTA. The cells were resuspended in 200 μL of 1× binding buffer in a centrifuge tube, and the concentration of cells was adjusted to 1×10^6 cells/ml. Then, apoptosis was detected with an Annexin V-PE/7-AAD staining kit (BD Biosciences) and assayed by flow cytometry (BD FACS caliber; BD Biosciences). Data analysis was conducted using FlowJo software.

Scratch Healing Assay

MH7A cells were seeded in a 12-well plate (5×10^5 cells in 200 μL of DMEM per well). Wounds were made using a pipette tip at time 0 h. After washing with PBS, DMEM containing 5% FBS with or without TNFα (40 ng/ml) and different concentrations of

TABLE 1 | The composition of Wutou decoction (WTD)

Herbal medicine	Chinese name	Plant part	Occupied percent	Week usage (g)
Aconiti Radix	Chuanwu	Root	14.28%	24
Ephedra Herba	Mahuang	stems	21.43%	36
Paeoniae Radix Alba	Baishao	Root	21.43%	36
Hedysarum Multijugum Maxim	Huangqi	Root	21.43%	36
Glycyrrhiza Radix Preparata	Gancao	Root	21.43%	36

WTD (1 or 10 mg/ml) were added to the wells. The cells were placed in a 37°C, 5% CO_2 incubator for culture. Then, photographs of the wells were taken immediately at 0 h and at 24 and 48 h, and the distance and area of each scratch was measured. Three independent experiments were performed.

Invasion Assay

The upper surfaces of Transwell inserts were prepared with Matrigel (1.25 mg/ml, 20 μL/well) for 45 min at 37°C. All groups except the blank group were treated with or without TNFα (40 ng/ml) and different concentrations of WTD (1 or 10 g/ml) for 24 h at 37°C and 5% CO2. After 24 h of incubation, the noninvasive cells on the upper membrane surface were removed by wiping with a cotton swab. The cells were stained with crystal violet staining solution and photographed under a phase-contrast microscope at 200 × magnification. Five random fields were imaged, and the experiment was repeated three times.

Tube Formation Assay

To examine the inhibitory effects of WTD on MH7A-induced HUVEC tube formation, a tube formation assay was performed as described previously. Matrigel (10 mg/ml, 35 μL/well) was spread on the bottom of a 96-well plate and placed in a 37°C incubator for 45 min. After it solidification, Matrigel was added (10 mg/ml, 15 μL/well) to cover the bottom of the 96-well plate to ensure that the liquid was level, and the plate was placed in a 37°C incubator overnight. Human umbilical vein endothelial cells (HUVECs) were inoculated on the bottom of a 24-well plate, and 600 μL of DMEM containing 10% serum was added. After digestion of the MH7A cells with or without TNFα (40 ng/ml) and different concentrations of WTD (1 or 10 g/ml) for 24 h in advance, the HUVECs were seeded on the upper chamber surface of a 24-well Transwell chamber, and 200 μL of DMEM containing 10% serum was added. HUVECs and FLSs were cocultured for 24 h at 37°C with 5% CO_2. Then, HUVECs were seeded on 96-well plates with Matrigel at a density of 2×10^4 cells per well. After incubation for 6 h, the capillary tube formation of each well was imaged with a phase-contrast microscope. Quantitation of the antiangiogenic activity of WTD on tube formation was performed by counting the number of branch points. Three independent assays were performed.

Immunohistochemical and Immunofluorescence Staining

Synovial tissue was fixed in 4% paraformaldehyde and embedded in paraffin. It was then heated in an oven at 60°C for 1 h, dewaxed in dimethyl benzene, polarized with descending concentrations of alcohol (100, 95, and 75%), and washed with water. Endogenous peroxidase activity was prevented by incubation at room temperature with a 3% H2O2 solution. The antigenic epitope was blocked by incubation with 20% normal goat serum for 1 h followed by incubation with primary antibodies at 4°C for 12 h. After washing with water three times, the slides were incubated with a HRP-conjugated secondary antibody for 1 h at room temperature. Then, the slides were visualized with DAB, and counterstaining was performed with hematoxylin. Images were taken with an Olympus fluorescence microscope system, with at least 5 random overlaps of each portion.

For immunofluorescence staining, preparation of the slides followed the same method as that for IHC. However, in contrast, an Alexa powder 488- or 594-conjugated secondary antibody (1: 1,000) was used instead of the HRP-conjugated secondary antibody, and nuclei were dyed using a DAPI solution. There was no need for visualization with DAB, and counterstaining was performed with hematoxylin.

Western Blot

MH7A cells were pretreated with WTD for 24 h and subsequently treated with or without TNFα (40 ng/ml) and different concentrations of WTD (1 or 10 g/ml). Total protein was extracted from the synovial tissue, and the protein concentration was quantified with a bicinchoninic acid protein assay kit. Each protein sample (30 μg/lane) was separated by 8–15% SDS-PAGE (80 V, for 1 h) and then transferred to a 0.22 μm nitrocellulose filter membrane (280 mA, 1 kD/min). The membrane was blocked with 5% skim milk for 1 h at room temperature and incubated overnight at 4°C with primary antibodies against β-actin, PI3K, AKT, p-AKT, mTOR, p-mTOR, VEGF, ANG1, VEGFR2, TEK (1:1,000, ABclonal, China), and HIF-1α (1: 1,000, CST, United States of America). Subsequently, the membranes were incubated with secondary antibiotics at room temperature for 1 h. Finally, the membranes were visualized with an Odyssey Infrared Imaging system (LI-COR Biosciences, United States of America). The images was quantified using ImageJ software and standardized against β-actin. Three independent assays were performed.

Network Pharmacology-Based Analysis of Wutou decoction

All chemical compounds from the five herbs in WTD were obtained from the TCMSP database (https://tcmspw.com/tcmsp.php) (Ru

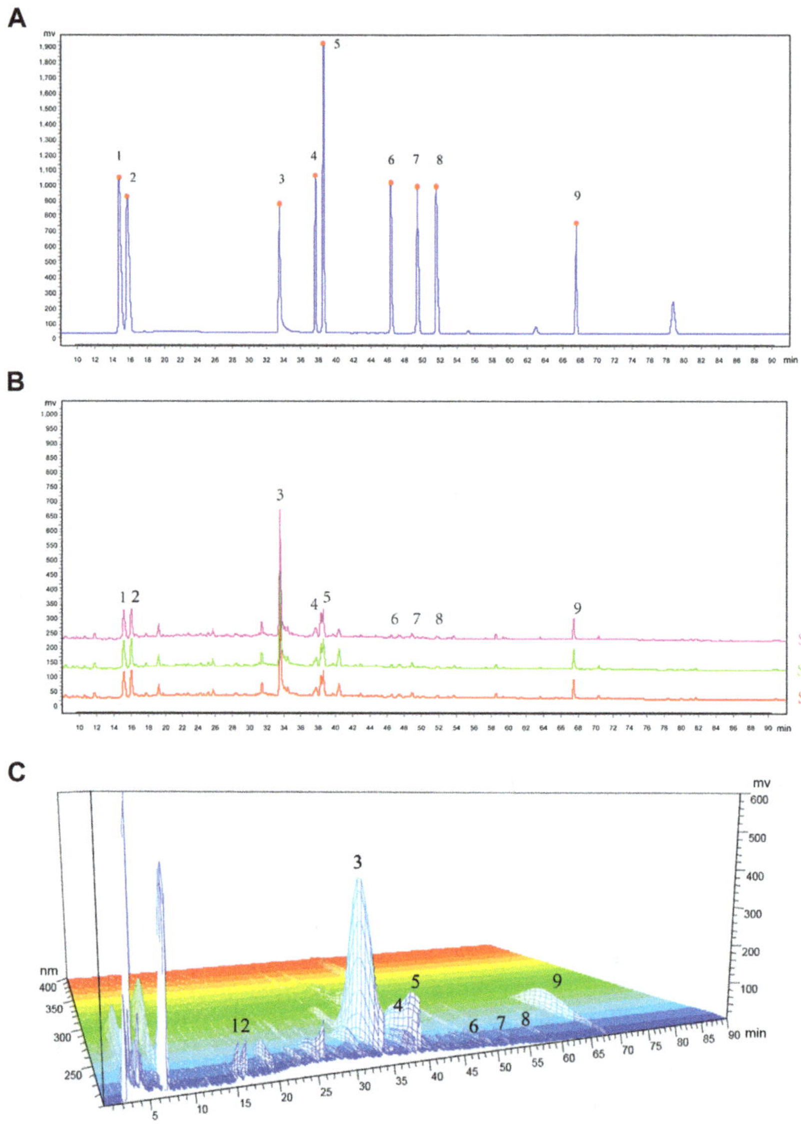

FIGURE 1 | HPLC fingerprinting of WTD. **(A)** HPLC fingerprinting chromatograms of the reference standards. **(B)** HPLC fingerprinting chromatograms of the WTD extracts. In the chromatograms the peaks are labeled as follows: 1) ephedrine hydrochloride; 2) pseudoephedrine hydrochloride; 3) paeoniflorin; 4) verbasil-7-O-glucoside; 5) glycyrrhizin; 6) benzoylaconitine; 7) benzoylneoaconitine; 8) benzoylhypoaconitine; and 9) glycyrrhizinate. **(C)** HPLC 3D fingerprinting chromatograms of the WTD extracts.

et al., 2014) and the Bioinformatics Analysis Tool for Molecular Mechanism of Traditional Chinese Medicine (BATMAN-TCM, http://bionet.ncpsb.org/batman-tcm/) (Liu et al., 2016). Before target prediction, the candidate components should meet the following parameters: oral bioavailability (OB) < 30% and drug-likeness (DL) < 0.18 to obtain compounds with higher oral absorption, utilization, and biological characteristics. Then, the compounds from multiple databases were combined, and duplicated items were removed. The target proteins were converted into genes *via* UniProt (http://www.UniProt.org/).

For disease target identification, RA-related target proteins were screened from the DrugBank (Wishart et al., 2018), OMIM (Amberger et al., 2015), pharmGK (Barbarino et al., 2018), Therapeutic Target database (Wang et al., 2020), DisGeNET (Pinero et al., 2017) and GeneCards (Stelzer et al., 2016) databases by using the keyword "RHEUMATOID ARTHRITIS". The overlapping WTD targets and RA targets were considered WTD-regulated RA targets (**Supplementary Table S1**). The "compound-target" network was established with Cytoscape 3.8 software. The 348 overlapping target genes were considered potential targets of WTD for the treatment of RA and were used to construct a PPI network. Gene ontology (GO) and Kyoto Encyclopedia of Genes and Genomes (KEGG) pathway enrichment analysis of the WTD-regulated RA target network was conducted by the Metascape database (http://metascape.org/gp/index.html) (Zhou et al., 2019). Finally, the KEGG pathway map was drawn by using KEGG mapper (https://www.genome.jp/kegg/) (Kanehisa et al., 2017).

TABLE 2 | HPLC fingerprinting of WTD

Herb name	Main chemical composition	RT (min)	Sample RT (min)			Constent estimation (μg/ml)		
			S1	S2	S3	S1	S2	S3
Aconiti Radix Cocta	Benzoylaconitine	49.621	48.941	48.958	48.917	88.2295	95.72827	95.94493
	Benzoylneoaconitine	46.532	46.554	46.567	46.531	37.71674	41.45507	41.23415
	Benzoylhypoaconitine	51.761	51.845	51.864	51.817	46.46893	51.20894	51.51884
Ephedrae Herba	Ephedrine Hydrochloride	15.190	15.188	15.181	15.18	429.4898	467.1652	483.6357
	Pseudoephedrine hydrochloride	16.071	16.06	16.053	16.05	351.8483	394.7957	402.0504
Paeoniae Radix Alba	Paeoniflorin	33.535	33.557	33.558	33.531	3341.241	3688.472	3739.668
Astragali Radix	Verbasil-7-0-glucoside	37.697	37.798	37.823	37.785	226.2418	236.1833	237.9742
Glycyrrhiza Radix Preparata	Glycyrrhizinate	67.544	67.542	67.566	67.546	522.187	579.8064	587.9906
	Glycyrrhizin	38.623	38.631	38.652	38.616	92.3727	100.6486	101.4226

Statistical Analysis

Statistical analyses were performed using GraphPad Prism 8.0. Data from multiple repeat experiments are presented as the means ± standard deviation (SD). Significant differences among the groups were evaluated by one-way analysis of variance (ANOVA) and Dunnett's *t*-test, and $p < 0.05$ was considered statistically significant. The number of replicates and/or the total number of animals are shown in the figure legends or within the figures.

RESULTS

High-Performance Liquid Chromatography Fingerprinting of Wutou decoction

A total of nine chemical components in WTD were determined, including benzoylaconitine (CW), benzoylneoaconitine (CW), benzoylhypoaconitine (CW), ephedrine hydrochloride (MH), pseudoephedrine hydrochloride (MH), paeoniflorin (BS), verbasil-7-O-glucoside (HQ), glycyrrhizinate (GC), and glycyrrhizin (GC). The HPLC fingerprint results of the standard are shown in **Figure 1A** and the sample is shown in **Figure 1B**. Three different batches of medicinal materials were repeated to confirm that these nine substances could be stably detected. The relative content of each substance in WTD was calculated and the detection of nine compounds in different wavelength ranges were better shown by 3D HPLC fingerprint (**Figure 1C**). The retention times and contents of the main chemical components of WTD are shown in **Table 2**.

Wutou decoction Treatment Ameliorates Arthritis in Collagen-Induced Arthritis Rats

To verify the efficacy of WTD against RA, a CIA rat model, which is widely used to clarify the mechanisms of RA and to explore potential therapeutic targets, was established and the rats were treated with two dosing regimens of WTD (**Figure 2A**). The body weights, arthritis scores, and synovial H&E analysis results were used to evaluate the treatment effects of WTD in CIA rats. Compared with the control group, the limbs of rats in the treated and model groups were obviously swollen on day 14 (**Figures 2B,C**). After 28 days of WTD treatment, the joint swelling in the treatment group was significantly improved (**Figure 2B**), and the arthritis score decreased (**Figure 2C**). The body weights of the rats decreased and could not be changed by WTD treatment (**Figure 2D**). From the results of H&E staining, the model group lining layer slide was significantly thickened (shown as blue arrowheads), and the number of small blood vessels (shown as red arrowheads) increased compared to the control group. Synovial hyperplasia and angiogenesis in the WTD treatment group were significantly improved.

Wutou decoction Inhibited Angiogenesis in the Synovial Tissue of Collagen-Induced Arthritis Rats

Angiogenesis is a very important in the pathogenesis of RA. To study angiogenesis in CIA rats, immunohistochemical staining of synovial tissue was performed after 28 days of WTD treatment. Compared with the control group, the expression levels of CD31 and vWF were upregulated in the model group. However, WTD treatment at either the low or high dose significantly reduced the expression of both CD31 and vWF (**Figures 3A–C**), which have been identified as vascular markers (Latacz et al., 2020). In addition to detecting vascular hyperplasia, we also determined the expression of vascular generation factors and their corresponding receptors in the synovial membrane by immunofluorescence and western blot analyses. Compared to the model group, the expression of VEGF and ANG1 (**Figures 3F–H**), as well as their related receptors (VEGFR2 and TEK) (**Figure 3M–O**), was downregulated in the treatment group by western blot. The effects of WTD high-dose treatment on the inhibition of angiogenesis was better than that of the low-dose group. The immunofluorescence results further verified the above conclusions. These results suggested that WTD might ameliorate angiogenesis in CIA rats by reducing vascular generation factors in synovial tissue.

The Effects of Wutou decoction on the Proliferation, Apoptosis, Migration, and Invasion of MH7A Cells

To explore the mechanism of WTD against RA, a series of experiments were conducted in MH7A cells that interfered with WTD treatment. Abnormal hyperplasia and apoptosis resistance in fibroblasts are the main causes of synovial hyperplasia. In this study, we explored the role of WTD in MH7A cell proliferation and apoptosis. The cell proliferation experiment found that when the concentration of WTD

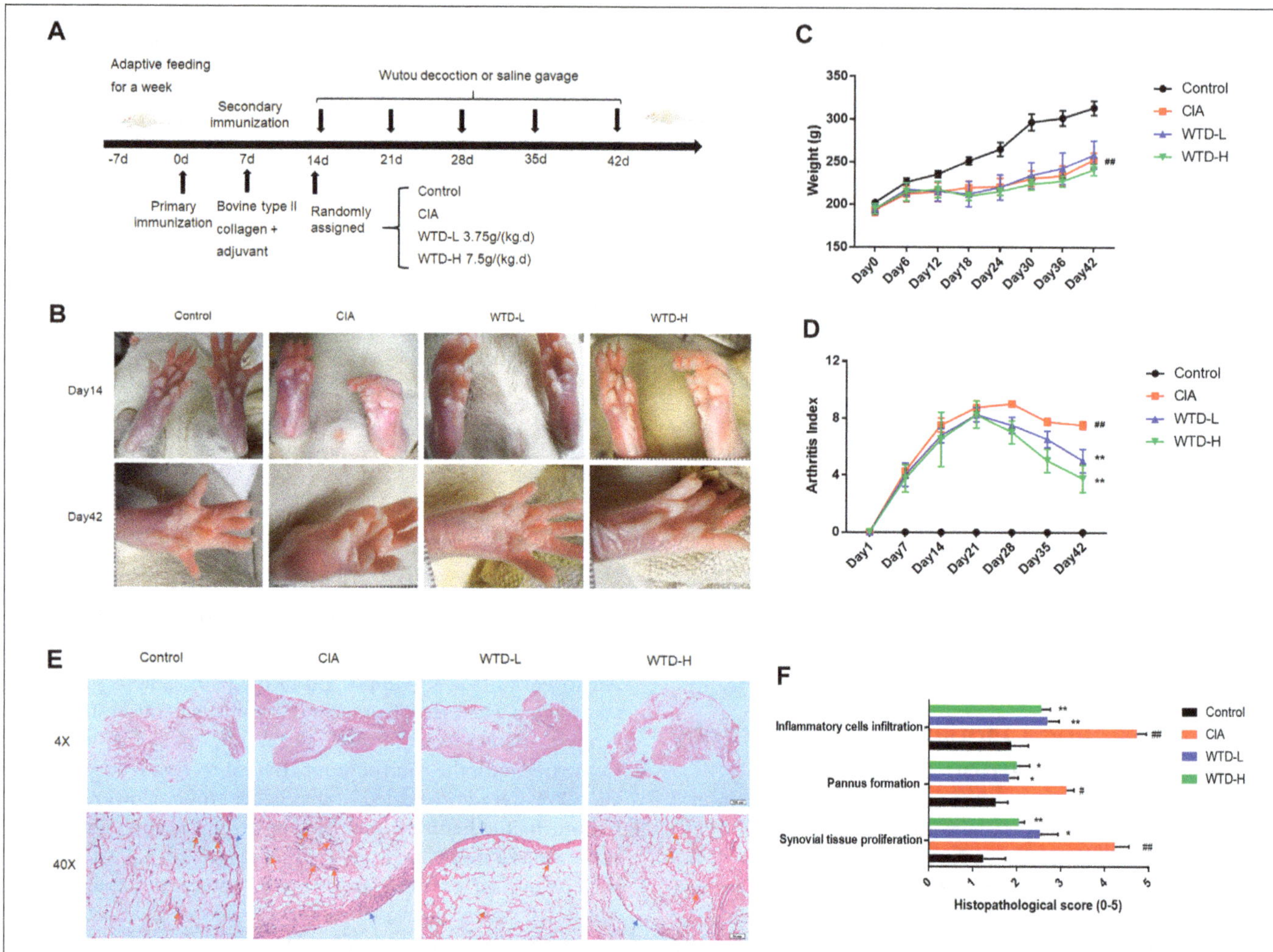

FIGURE 2 | WTD treatment ameliorated CIA rats. **(A)** Schematic of CIA rat model induction and WTD intervention. **(B)** Representative images of the hind paws from the different groups. **(C)** The weights and **(D)** arthritis indexes of CIA rats treated with PBS, WTD-L (3.75 g/kg) or WTD-H (7.5 g/kg) were monitored every 6 days. **(E)** The synovium of the knee joint was sectioned for hematoxylin-eosin staining. Representative joint tissue sections are shown (original magnification, ×40 and ×200). **(F)** The histology scores of synovial tissue proliferation, pannus formation, and inflammatory cell infiltration. The results were expressed as mean ± SE. $N = 6$. #$p < 0.05$, ##$p < 0.01$ versus the control group; *$p < 0.05$, **$p < 0.01$ versus the CIA group. CIA, The Collagen-induced arthritis group; WTD-L, the low dose Wutou decoction group (3.75 g/kg/day); WTD-H, the high dose Wutou decoction group (7.5 g/kg/day).

was greater than 1 mg/ml, inhibition of MH7A cells began to be seen, exhibiting dose- and time-dependence (**Figure 4A**). According to the cell proliferation results, 1 mg/ml and 10 mg/ml WTD were selected for subsequent experiments. Flow cytometry detection found that WTD could promote apoptosis in MH7A cells (**Figures 4B,C**). Due to their migratory and invasive characteristics, FLSs can migrate to the sublining layer of the synovial membrane, where they promote angiogenesis. TNFα promoted MH7A cell migration, but WTD intervention inhibited MH7A cell migration, as shown by the cell scratch experiments (**Figures 4D–F**). Furthermore, WTD intervention inhibited MH7A cell invasion induced by TNFα (**Figures 4G,H**).

The Effects of Wutou decoction on the Ability of MH7A Cells to Induce Human Umbilical Vein Endothelial Cell Angiogenesis

Blood vessels are mainly composed of vascular endothelial cells and pericyte cells. However, vascular hyperplasia is affected by inflammatory factors and proangiogenic factors, which are secreted by the surrounding cells. To further confirm the mechanism by which WTD affects synovial angiogenesis, MH7A cells and HUVECs were cocultured in Transwell chambers, and HUVEC tube formation was detected after WTD was used to treat MH7A cells. The tube formation experiment showed that the ability of MH7A cells to induce HUVEC

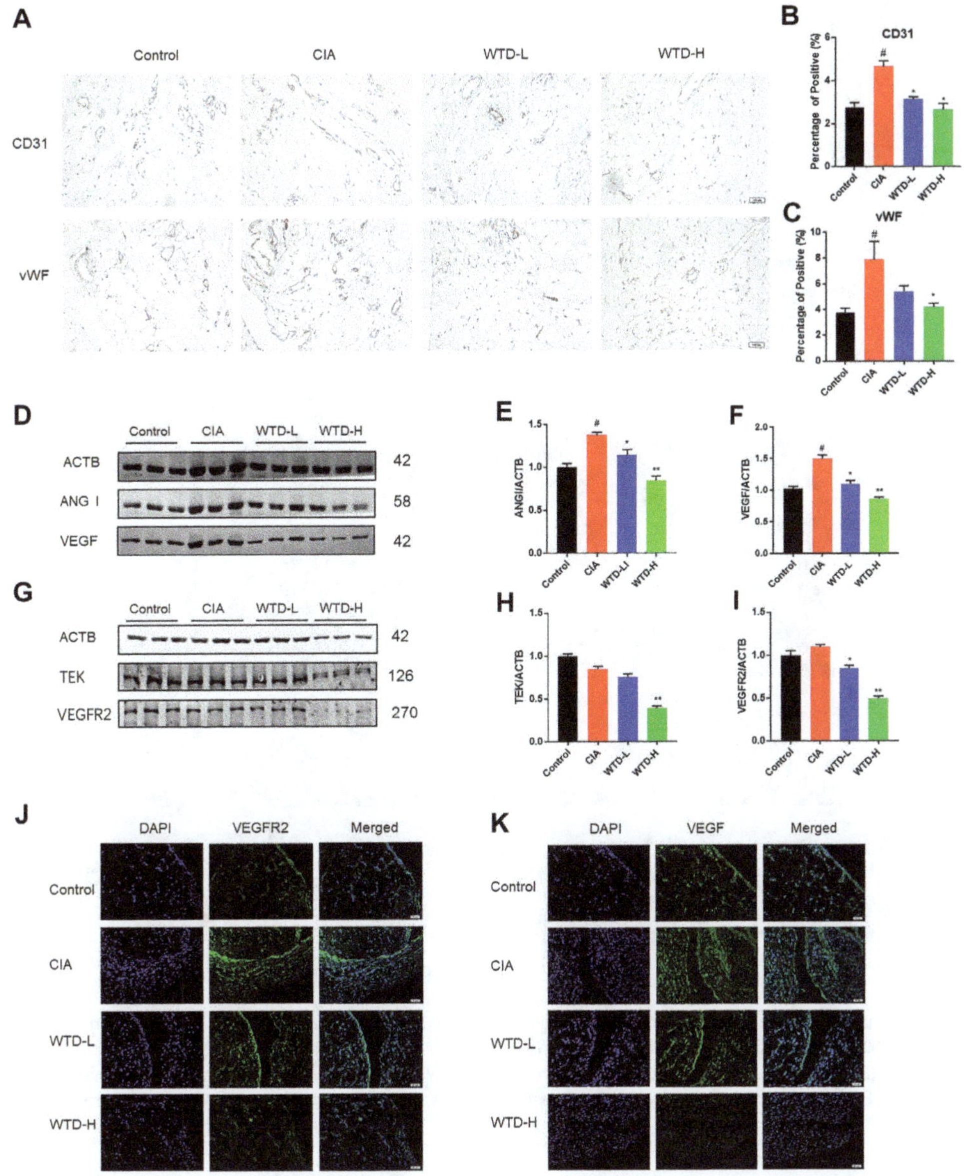

FIGURE 3 | WTD inhibited angiogenesis in the synovial tissues of CIA rats. **(A)** Representative immunohistochemical staining for CD31 and vWF in synovial sections. Scale bar: 100 μm. **(B–C)** Quantitative analysis of immunohistochemical staining for CD31 and vWF in synovial tissue. **(D)** Representative western blots showing VEGF and ANGI after WTD treatment. **(E–F)** Quantitative analysis of VEGF and ANGI. **(G)** Representative western blots showing VEGFR2 and TEK after WTD treatment. **(H–M)** Quantitative analysis of the VEGFR2 and TEK western blots after WTD treatment. **(N–O)** Representative immunofluorescence staining of VEGF and VEGFR2 in synovial sections. Scale bar: 50 μm. The results were expressed as mean ± SE. *N* = 6. #*p* < 0.05, ##*p* < 0.01 versus the control group; **p* < 0.05, ***p* < 0.01 versus the CIA group. CIA, The Collagen-induced arthritis group; WTD-L, the low dose Wutou decoction group (3.75 g/kg/day); WTD-H, the high dose Wutou decoction group (7.5 g/kg/day).

tube formation significantly increased after TNFα stimulation, and WTD reduced the ability of MH7A cells to induce HUVEC tube formation (**Figures 5A,B**). Furthermore, WTD inhibited the expression of the proangiogenic factors VEGF and Ang1 (**Figures 5C,D**) produced by MH7A cells. The expression of the corresponding homologous receptors VEGFR2 and TEK in HUVECs also decreased (**Figures 5E,F**). From these results, we concluded that WTD could suppress the expression of proangiogenic factors in FLSs and inhibit angiogenesis in synovial tissue.

Network Pharmacology Analysis Shows That Wutou decoction Exerts Its Antiangiogenic Effects Through the PI3K-AKT-mTOR Pathway

To clarify the molecular mechanism underlying the effects of WTD against RA, we established a WTD-target-RA network. A total of 863 potential targets of WTD were discovered, and 2,147 genes related to RA were obtained after deleting

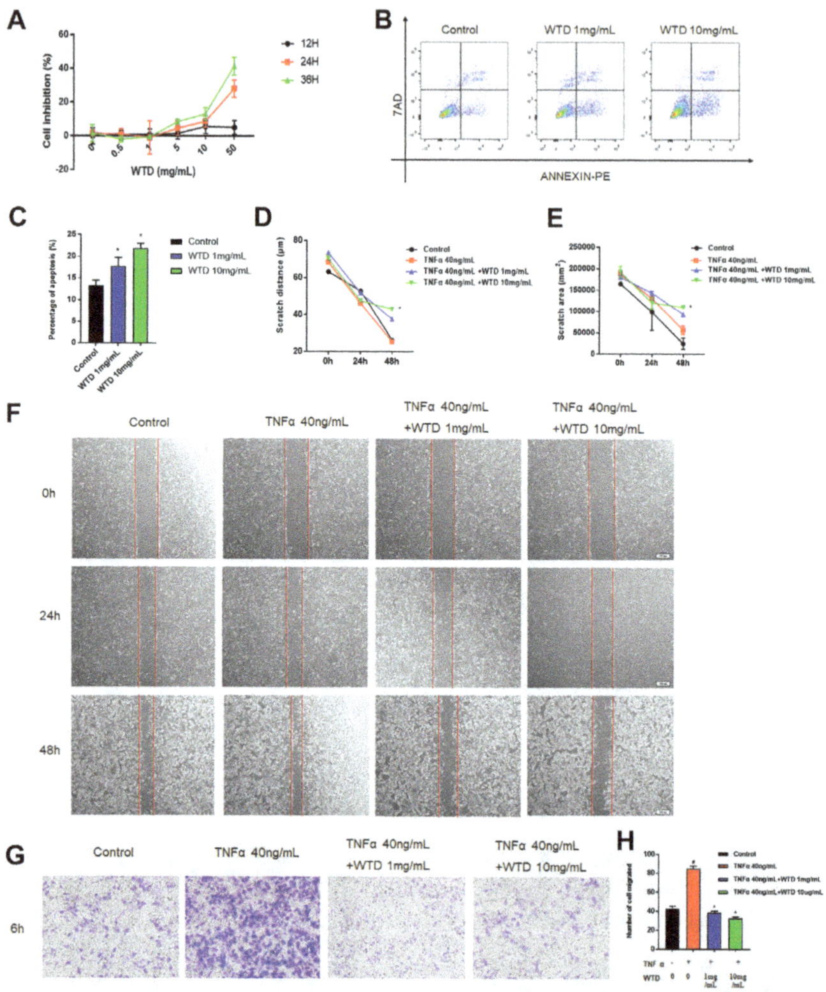

FIGURE 4 | The effects of WTD on the proliferation, apoptosis, migration and invasion of MH7A cells. **(A)** Effects of WTD intervention on MH7A cell proliferation at 12, 24, and 36 h **(B–C)** Effects of MH7A cell apoptosis after WTD intervention. **(D)** Effects of MH7A cell migration at 0, 24, and 48 h after WTD intervention. Statistical diagram of € scratch distance and **(F)** scratch area. **(G)** Effects of MH7A cell invasion after WTD intervention. **(H)** Statistical results of the number of migrated cells. The results were expressed as mean ± SE. All experimental results were repeated three times. #$p < 0.05$, ##$p < 0.01$ versus the control group; *$p < 0.05$, **$p < 0.01$ versus the TNFα 40 ng/ml group.

redundant data (**Figure 6A** and **Supplementary Table S1**). A total of 863 potential targets of WTD were compared to 2147 RA-related candidate targets, and 348 overlapping targets were found (**Figures 6B,C**), such as PI3K, AKT, mTOR, VEGF, and HIF-1α (**Supplementary Table S2**). These targets show the possible mechanism of WTD against RA angiogenesis. To identify relevant pathways and functions, KEGG pathway enrichment and GO functional analyses were performed for these 348 targets using Metascape (**Figures 6D,E**). The enriched target proteins are mainly related to tumors, metabolic disease, immunomodulation, and angiogenesis. Moreover, the PI3K-AKT and HIF-1α signaling pathways associated with angiogenesis were enriched. These 384 targets were ranked by their degree value, and the top 10 targets, including PIK3CA and AKT1, are shown in **Figure 6F**. The PI3K-AKT pathway plays an important role in the regulation of cellular functions, including cell growth, proliferation, differentiation, apoptosis, and angiogenesis. This result is consistent with the PI3K-AKT pathway target map of WTD (**Figure 6G**) and was verified by experiments *in vitro in vivo.* Therefore, these data indicate that the therapeutic mechanism of WTD on RA may be through these signaling pathways.

The Effects of Wutou decoction on PI3K-AKT-mTOR-HIF1α *in vivo*

After combining the of GO and KEGG analysis results, WTD was found to probably ameliorate RA through the PI3K-AKT and HIF-1α signaling pathways. Western blot analysis was used to measure the protein expression of the PI3K-AKT and HIF-1α pathways, including PI3K, AKT, p-AKT, mTOR, p-mTOR, and HIF-1α. PI3K-AKT-mTOR signaling in CIA rats was strengthened compared with the control group, and the WTD group showed inhibited PI3K-AKT-mTOR signaling compared with the CIA group. The

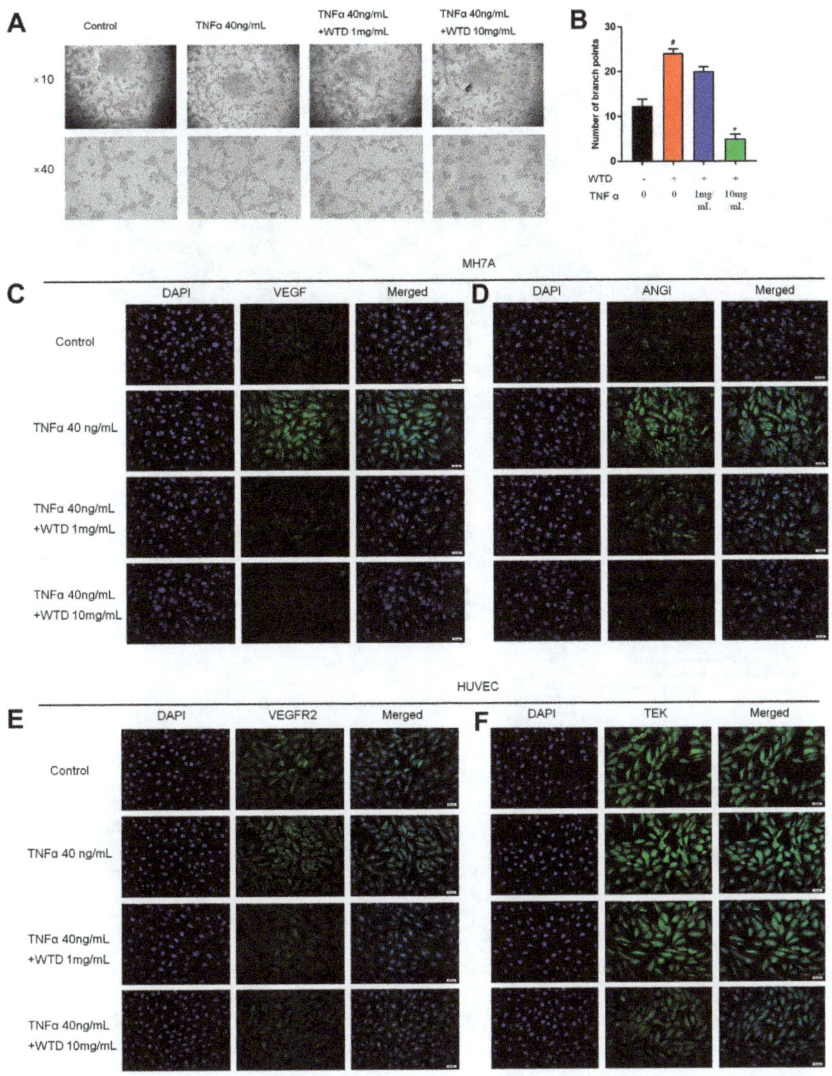

FIGURE 5 | The effects of WTD on the ability of MH7A cells to induce HUVEC angiogenesis. **(A)** Representative HUVEC tube formation sections after 6 h of cocultivation with MH7A cells (original magnification,×100 and ×400). **(B)** Quantification of the number of branch points for **(A)**. **(C–D)** Representative immunofluorescence staining for VEGF and ANGI in MH7A cell sections. Scale bar: 50 μm. **(E–F)** Representative immunofluorescence staining for VEGFR2 and TEK in HUVEC sections. Scale bar: 50 μm. The results are expressed as mean ± SE. All experimental results were repeated three times. #$p < 0.05$, ##$p < 0.01$versus the Control group; *$p < 0.05$, **$p < 0.01$ versus the TNFα 40 ng/ml group.

downregulation of PI3K-AKT-mTOR signaling further led to a reduction in the HIF-1α protein expression (**Figures 7A–G**). Immunofluorescence verified that WTD could downregulate the expression of HIF-1α in the synovium of CIA rats (**Figure 7H**). Moreover, HIF-1α is an important transcription factor for the expression of pro-angiogenesis genes. Therefore, PI3K-AKT-mTOR-HIF1α could be a possible underlying mechanism by which WTD inhibits angiogenesis in the synovium of CIA rats.

The Effects of Wutou decoction on PI3K-AKT-mTOR-HIF1α *in vitro*

To further confirm the involvement of WTD in the PI3K-AKT-mTOR-HIF1α pathway, we investigated the protein expression of the abovementioned molecules in TNFα-induced MH7A cells. Notably, WTD effectively inhibited the upregulation of phosphorylated Akt and mTOR induced by TNFα *in vitro* (**Figures 8A–G**). Moreover, the expression of HIF-1α was inhibited in MH7A cells treated with WTD (**Figure 8H**). These data indicated that WTD suppressed TNFα-induced angiogenesis by downregulating PI3K-AKT-mTOR-HIF1α signaling in MH7A cells.

DISCUSSION

RA is a chronic systematic disease in which angiogenesis can promote inflammatory cell infiltration into the joints, leading to

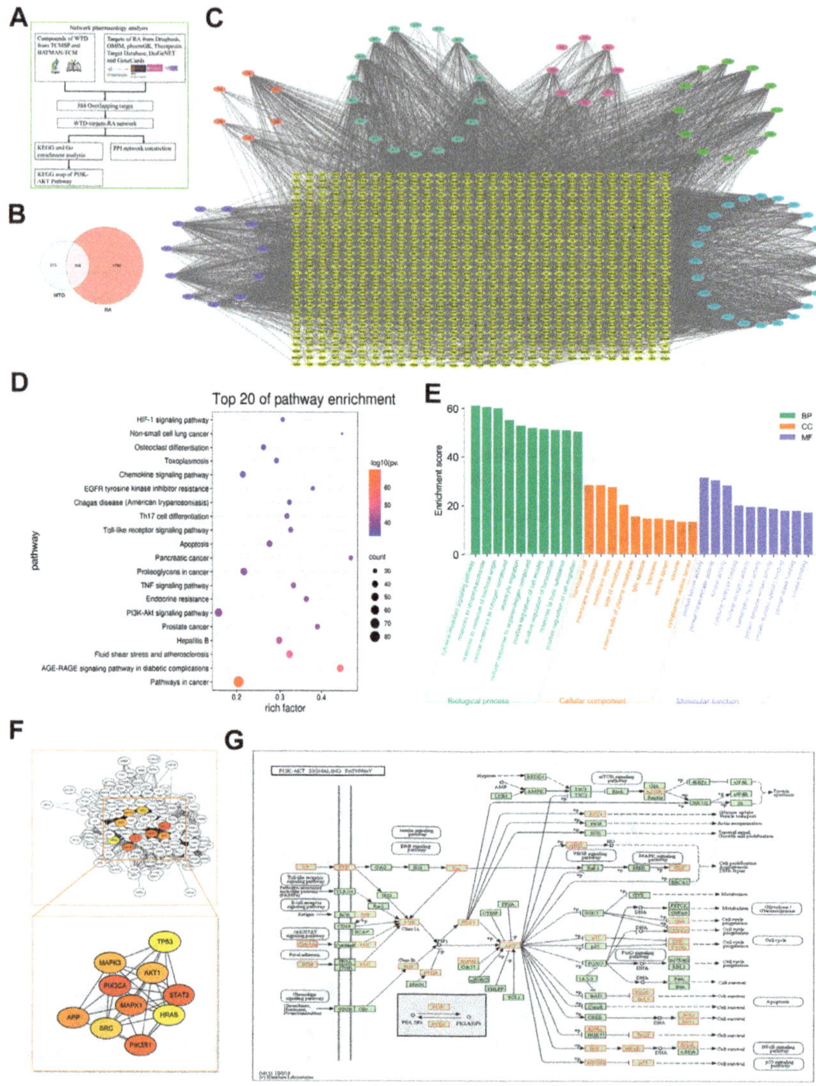

FIGURE 6 | Network pharmacology analysis indicated that WTD could exert antiangiogenic effects through the PI3K-AKT-mTOR pathway. **(A)** Network Pharmacology analysis flowchart of WTD-regulated RA. **(B)** Venn diagram showing that 348 targets overlapped between WTD and RA, which were selected as the WTD-regulated RA targets. **(C)** The compound-target network was established by Cytoscape 3.8 software; the blue ellipse represents *Glycyrrhiza Radix Preparata,* the light *blue* ellipse represents *Ephedrae Herba,* the pink ellipse represents *Paeoniae Radix Alba,* the red ellipse represents *Aconiti Radix Cocta*, the green ellipse represents *Astragali Radix*, the purple ellipse represents the ingredients shared with two or more herbs, and the yellow diamonds represent WTD-regulated RA targets. **(D)** KEGG enrichment analysis and **(E)** GO enrichment analysis for the 348 WTD-regulated RA targets performed by the Metascape database. **(F)** Hub targets were identified from the PPI network using the Cytoscape plug-in MCODE. **(G)** The KEGG map of WTD-regulated targets in the PI3K-AKT-mTOR pathway. RA, Rheumatoid Arthritis; WTD, Wutou decoction; CW, Chuanwu; MH, Mahuang; BS, Baishao; HQ, Huangqi; GC, Gancao; BP, Biological process; CC, Cellular component; MF, Molecular function.

synovial inflammation, hyperplasia, and progressive bone destruction (Mcinnes and Schett, 2011). Currently, the main treatment for RA is nonsteroidal anti-inflammatory drugs, DMARDs and glucocorticoids (Smolen and Aletaha, 2015; Chatzidionysiou et al., 2017; Palmowski et al., 2017). However, from a long-term perspective, only DMARDs, including conventional synthetic DMARDs, biological DMARDs, and targeted synthetic DMARDs, are considered to be able to target synovial inflammation and mitigate the progression of joint damage (Buttgereit et al., 2015). In recent years, there has been great progress in the development of new antirheumatic drugs for rheumatoid arthritis, such as TNFα inhibitors, IL-6 receptor antagonists, and inhibitors targeting the JAK pathway. These new drugs have considerably delayed RA progression and improved the quality of life of RA patients (Ramiro et al., 2017). However, conventional synthetic DMARDs have liver and kidney toxicity, and biological DMARDs and targeted synthetic DMARDs have more adverse events, including the occurrence of serious infections and cancer (Ranganath et al., 2015; Silva-Fernandez et al., 2016; Pawar et al., 2019; Van Mulligen et al., 2019).

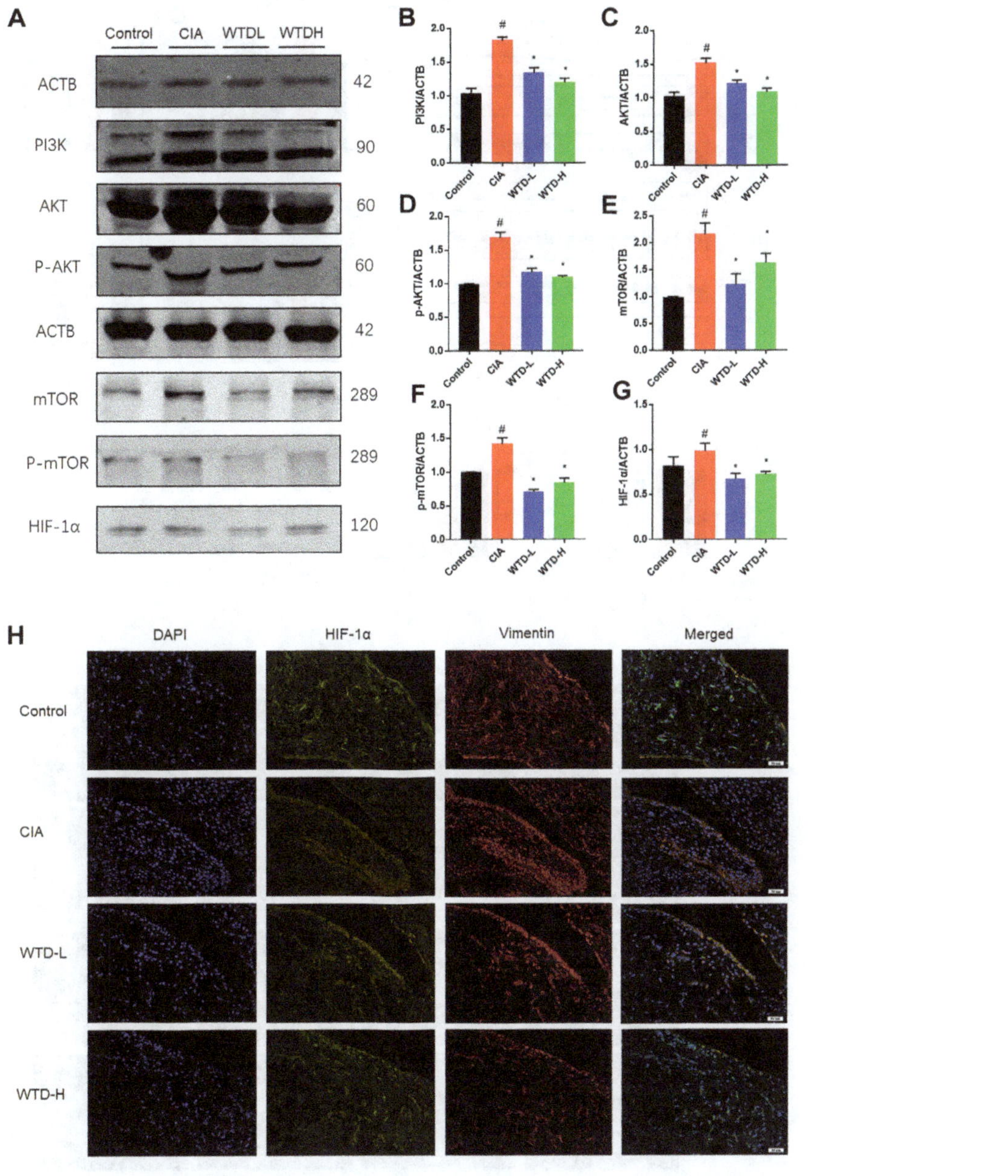

FIGURE 7 | The effects of WTD on the PI3K-AKT-mTOR-HIF-1α pathway *in vivo*. **(A)** Representative western blots showing the components of the PI3K-AKT-mTOR-HIF-1α pathway after WTD treatment in CIA rats. **(B–G)** Quantitative analysis of the western blots after WTD treatment in CIA rats. **(H)** Representative immunofluorescence staining for HIF1α in the synovium of CIA rats. The results are expressed as mean ± SE. $N = 6$. #$p < 0.05$, ##$p < 0.01$ versus the control group; *$p < 0.05$, **$p < 0.01$ versus the CIA group. CIA, The Collagen-induced arthritis group; WTD-L, the low dose Wutou decoction group (3.75 g/kg/day); WTD-H, the high dose Wutou decoction group (7.5 g/kg/day). ACTB, β-actin; PI3K, Phosphatidylinositide 3-kinases; AKT, protein kinase B; p-AKT, Phosphorylated protein kinase B; mTOR, Mammalian target of rapamycin; p-mTOR, Phosphorylated Mammalian target of rapamycin; HIF-1α, Hypoxia-induced factor 1α.

As a classic prescription, WTD has been generally used to treat Bi Zheng for two thousand years in China, and its clinical efficacy has been confirmed (Qi et al., 2014). Modern pharmacological studies have shown that WTD has anti-inflammatory effects, regulates immunity, and relieves pain. Additionally, WTD has been reported to have higher safety and no side effects compared with DMARDs, including liver and kidney toxicity, infection, and tumors. Furthermore, a variety of pharmacological studies have confirmed that ingredients in WTD were effective in the treatment of RA (Zhang et al., 2015; Guo et al., 2017). Benzoylacetone, extracted from *Aconiti Radix Cocta*, can reduce the expression of TNFα, IL-1β, and NF-κB-p65 in activated macrophages to inhibit NF-κB signaling pathways (Gai et al., 2020). Glycyrrhizin was extracted from *Glycyrrhiza Radix Preparata*, which has been proven to regulate high mobility group 1 protein, Beclin-1, and nuclear factor—inflammatory improvement factor 2, thus improving articular inflammation (Shafik et al., 2019). Glycyrrhizic acid is also the main bioactive

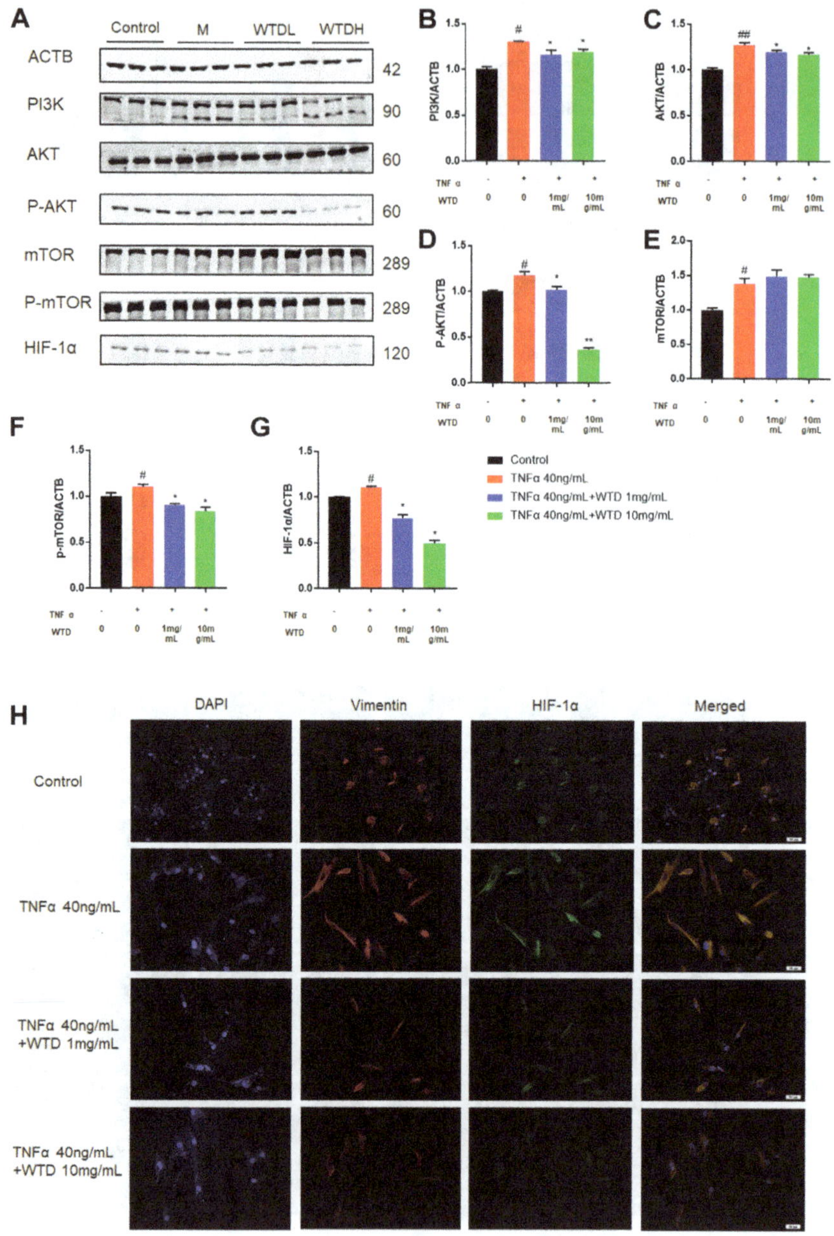

FIGURE 8 | The effects of WTD on the PI3K-AKT-mTOR-HIF-1α pathway *in vitro*. **(A)** Representative western blots showing the components of the PI3K-AKT-mTOR-HIF1α pathway after WTD treatment in MH7A cells. M: TNFα 40 ng/ml; WTD-L: TNFα 40 ng/ml + WTD 1 mg/ml; WTD-H: TNFα 40 ng/ml + WTD 1 mg/ml **(B–G)** Quantitative analysis of the western blots after WTD treatment in MH7A cells. **(H)** Representative immunofluorescence staining for HIF1α in MH7A cell sections. The results are expressed as mean ± SE. #$p < 0.05$, ##$p < 0.01$versus the Control group; *$p < 0.05$, **$p < 0.01$ versus the TNFα 40 ng/ml group. ACTB, β-actin; PI3K, Phosphatidylinositide 3-kinases; AKT, protein kinase B; p-AKT, Phosphorylated protein kinase B; mTOR, Mammalian target of rapamycin; p-mTOR, Phosphorylated Mammalian target of rapamycin; HIF-1α, Hypoxia-induced factor 1α.

component of *Glycyrrhiza Radix Preparata*, which has been reported to inhibit articular inflammation (Qu et al., 2019). Total glucosides of peony and total glycosides extracted from the dry roots of *Paeoniae Radix Alba* are widely used to treat RA due to their anti-inflammatory, immunomodulatory and analgesic effects (Xu et al., 2018; Zhai et al., 2018; Zhang and Wei, 2020). In addition, paeoniflorin and Talatizinine, the main ingredients of *Paeoniae Radix Alba*, could be combined with PPAR-γ, C-JUN, MMP13, and TGF-β1, which are candidate targets of the mechanism of WTD against RA (Mao et al., 2020). Collectively, these studies show that WTD or its ingredients have obvious anti-inflammatory, immunomodulatory, and analgesic effects, which may be an important in the mechanism of RA treatment by WTD. However, little is known about the role of WTD in the regulation of synovial angiogenesis.

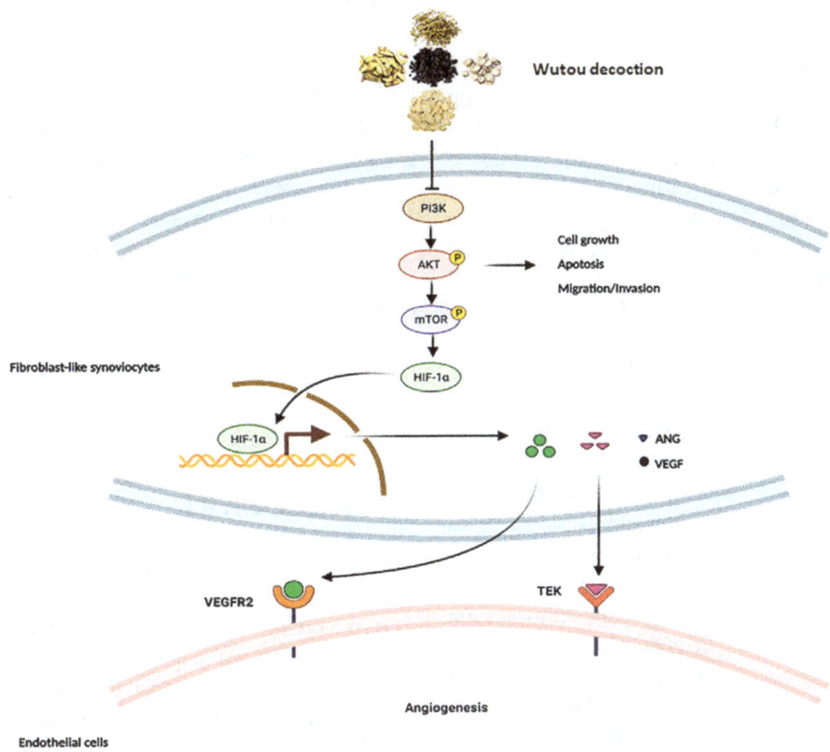

FIGURE 9 | The mechanism of WTD against angiogenesis in RA. Overview of the underlying mechanisms of WTD treatment by the PI3K/AKT/mTOR signaling pathway. Activation of PI3K by receptor tyrosine kinases promotes cell growth, proliferation, migration and invasion as well as angiogenesis. PI3K signaling can activate and phosphorylate AKT, and p-AKT can inhibit the expression of apoptosis-related genes to allow the cells to survive while promoting the expression of genes related to cell proliferation, migration, and invasion. More importantly, p-AKT can activate mTOR to upregulate the expression of HIF1α. HIF-1α is stabilized under hypoxic conditions and quickly translocated to the nucleus, where it facilitates the expression of the associated genes VEGF and ANGI). However, VEGF and ANGI can bind corresponding homologous receptors coupled to endothelial cells to promote synovial angiogenesis. PI3K, Phosphatidylinositide 3-kinases; AKT, protein kinase B; mTOR, Mammalian target of rapamycin; HIF-1α, Hypoxia-induced factor 1α; VEGF, Vascular endothelial growth factor; VEGFR2, Vascular endothelial growth factor receptor 2; ANG1, Angiopoietin 1; TEK, Angiopoietin-1 receptor.

Angiogenesis is crucial for the pathogenesis of arthritis in RA. The angiogenesis process includes endothelial cell migration, sprouting, and tube formation, followed by the wrapping of pericyte cells around the tube to promote blood vessel stability. In this process, various cytokines participate, such as proangiogenic factors, proinflammatory cytokines, matrix metalloproteases, and adhesion molecules (Elshabrawy et al., 2015). The process of angiogenesis begins with growth factors, such as VEGF, and its combination with its homologous receptor VEGFR2 on endothelial cells to stimulate the proliferation, migration, and sprouting of endothelial cells. Then, the blood vessels are stabilized by the factors generated, such as ANG1, and pericyte cells are incorporated into the newly formed substrate film to promote the blood flow process (Ferrara, 2004; Heinolainen et al., 2017). Single-cell spatial transcription group sequencing has indicated that FLSs are distributed with a spatial gradient distribution within the blood vessels in the synovial membrane (Wei et al., 2020). A variety of cellular activation processes, including cell migration and invasion, are involved in tube formation (Zhu et al., 2020). RA-FLSs exhibit aggressive features, including excessive proliferation, apoptotic resistance, and high invasion, and have long been considered to be an attractive treatment target. Activated RA-FLSs can not only migrate and invade adjacent unaffected joints, causing degradation of the articles, but also migrate to the lower layer of the synovial lining to promote angiogenesis and exacerbate synovial hyperplasia and bone destruction (Ma et al., 2019; Zhang et al., 2019). Our study shows that 10 mg/ml WTD can inhibit RA-FLS proliferation, migration, and invasion and promote apoptosis. Moreover, WTD improved CIA rat joint synovial hyperplasia and relieved joint swelling. This is consistent with the results of a previous study (He et al., 2018). Additionally, we focused on the role of WTD in the regulation of synovial angiogenesis. MH7A cells were cocultured with HUVECs, and MH7A cells secreted the hypoxia-induced factor HIF-1α after TNFα stimulation, which generated VEGF and Ang1. Additionally, the expression levels of the corresponding homologous receptors VEGFR2 and TEK in HUVECs were upregulated. FLSs can facilitate synovial angiogenesis through VEGF-VEGFR2 and then further promote blood vessel stability by Ang1-TEK. Tube formation assays in HUVECs further proved that WTD can inhibit MH7A cell-induced angiogenesis. In addition, *in vivo* experiments confirmed that FLS-induced synovial vascular hyperplasia can be blocked by WTD, but the specific mechanism is not clear. Determination of the potential mechanism of Chinese herbal medicines can not only discover the potential goals of disease treatment but also clarify the effective ingredients in the Chinese herbal medicines to provide a scientific basis for their clinical use.

With the development of bioinformatics, modern network pharmacology is considered to be a very important tool to explore the complex mechanism of TCM compounds (Ru et al., 2014). This study identified the main components of WTD by querying the traditional Chinese medicine database TCM-SP and collecting the main targets. Combined with modern pharmacological study of RA disease treatment targets and the targets of WTD, the main KEGG pathways of WTD in the treatment of RA include the AGE-RAGE signaling pathway, PI3K-AKT signaling pathway, TNF signaling pathway, Toll-like receptor signaling pathway, and HIF-1α signaling pathway.

The PI3K-AKT pathway plays important roles in cell proliferation, apoptosis, and differentiation (Karar and Maity, 2011). In this study, we found that WTD can inhibit MH7A cell proliferation and promote MH7A cell apoptosis. WTD can also inhibit the invasion and migration of activated MH7A cells induced by TNFα. However, further experiments are needed to verify whether WTD affects the PI3K-AKT pathway to inhibit MH7A cell proliferation and reduce apoptosis resistance. Additionally, we focused on the role of WTD in angiogenesis in the synovial tissues during RA. Many inhibitors targeting the PI3K-AKT pathway have shown the effects of downregulating the expression of VEGF and suppressing angiogenesis. The PI3K-AKT pathway plays an important role in regulating angiogenesis in RA. The connection between the PI3K-AKT pathway and angiogenesis has been confirmed in many studies. Ginsenoside RG1 facilitates cerebrovascular generation and increases ischemic stroke by increasing the expression of VEGF through the PI3K-AKT-mTOR signaling pathway (Chen et al., 2019). Shikonin (SKN), the main chemical component separated from zicao (*Lithospermum erythrorhizon Sie*b), has an antiangiogenic effect by impeding the PI3K-AKT signaling pathways in RA. Artesunate can suppress inflammation and prevent cartilage and bone destruction in collagen-induced arthritis models in rats (Ma et al., 2019). Many ingredients in WTD have also been confirmed to have pharmacological effects within the PI3K-AKT pathway (Liu et al., 2020). Studies have shown that glycyrrhizenic acid is produced by adjusting autophagy and inhibiting the PI3K/AKT/mTOR pathway after induction by inflammatory factors in ALI, which can provide new therapies for Ali GA (Qu et al., 2019). Studies have shown that astragalus IV (AS-IV) treatment promotes cell proliferation and tube formation and induces activation of the PTEN/PI3K/AKT signaling pathway (Cheng et al., 2019). Paeoniflorin can inhibit mesangial cell proliferation and the inflammatory response through the PI3K/Akt/GSK-3β pathway. Inflammation or hypoxic stimulation results in the expression and stabilization of HIF-1α, increasing vascular endothelial growth factor expression (VEGF) (Park et al., 2007). Is there a similar mechanism by which WTD ameliorates angiogenesis in RA? The PI3K/AKT pathway can increase VEGF secretion through both hypoxia-induced factor 1 (HIF-1)-dependent and HIF-1-independent mechanisms (Karar and Maity, 2011; Li et al., 2018; Chen et al., 2019; Zhu et al., 2020). In this study, WTD interrupted the PI3K-AKT pathway and suppressed HIF-1α expression. Therefore, the PI3K-AKT-mTOR-HIF-1α pathway could be the underlying mechanism by which WTD ameliorates angiogenesis in RA (**Figure 9**).

There are some limitations in of this study. The concentration of the WTD extract used in this experiment was 1–10 mg/ml, which seems to have no pharmacological significance. However, the compound ingredients of traditional Chinese medicine are complicated. This is a total concentration of a mixed drug not a concentration of a chemical component. According to the quantification of fingerprint, the content of the main components of WTD we calculate (supplement 4) is pharmacological significance.

CONCLUSION

In conclusion, we demonstrated that WTD could treat RA by inhibiting MH7A cell proliferation, migration, invasion, and promotion of angiogenesis. The underlying mechanism by which WTD ameliorated angiogenesis in RA was associated with the inhibition of the PI3K-AKT-mTOR-HIF1α signaling pathway. This experiment can provide a scientific explanation for the clinical applications of WTD and facilitate the discovery of natural drugs for treating RA. Furthermore, it may complement existing RA drug treatments from the viewpoint of angiogenesis rather than suppressing inflammation and regulating immunity. This experiment suggests WTD could be considered as a promising alternative candidate for RA characterized by joint swelling and synovial vascular hyperplasia.

AUTHOR CONTRIBUTIONS

ST designed the study. XB performed the experiments and wrote the manuscript. YH, PS, and YH contributed to the analysis of the data. Lijun Xu made lyophilized powder of WTD. LH, WL, JY, and ZC reviewed and edited the manuscript. All authors read and approved the manuscript.

FUNDING

This work was supported by the National Natural Science Foundation of China (No. 81573802 and No.81874383).

REFERENCES

Aletaha, D., and Smolen, J. S. (2018). Diagnosis and Management of Rheumatoid Arthritis: A Review. *JAMA* 320, 1360–1372. doi:10.1001/jama.2018.13103

Amberger, J. S., Bocchini, C. A., Schiettecatte, F., Scott, A. F., and Hamosh, A. (2015). OMIM.org: Online Mendelian Inheritance in Man (OMIM®), an Online Catalog of Human Genes and Genetic Disorders. *Nucleic Acids Res.* 43, D789–D798. doi:10.1093/nar/gku1205

Barbarino, J. M., Whirl-Carrillo, M., Altman, R. B., and Klein, T. E. (2018). PharmGKB: A Worldwide Resource for Pharmacogenomic Information. *Wiley Interdiscip. Rev. Syst. Biol. Med.* 10, e1417. doi:10.1002/wsbm.1417

Bottini, N., and Firestein, G. S. (2013). Duality of Fibroblast-like Synoviocytes in RA: Passive Responders and Imprinted Aggressors. *Nat. Rev. Rheumatol.* 9, 24–33. doi:10.1038/nrrheum.2012.190

Burmester, G. R., and Pope, J. E. (2017). Novel Treatment Strategies in Rheumatoid Arthritis. *Lancet* 389, 2338–2348. doi:10.1016/S0140-6736(17)31491-5

Buttgereit, F., Smolen, J. S., Coogan, A. N., and Cajochen, C. (2015). Clocking in: Chronobiology in Rheumatoid Arthritis. *Nat. Rev. Rheumatol.* 11, 349–356. doi:10.1038/nrrheum.2015.31

Chatzidionysiou, K., Emamikia, S., Nam, J., Ramiro, S., Smolen, J., Van Der Heijde, D., et al. (2017). Efficacy of Glucocorticoids, Conventional and Targeted Synthetic Disease-Modifying Antirheumatic Drugs: a Systematic Literature Review Informing the 2016 Update of the EULAR Recommendations for the Management of Rheumatoid Arthritis. *Ann. Rheum. Dis.* 76, 1102–1107. doi:10.1136/annrheumdis-2016-210711

Chen, J., Zhang, X., Liu, X., Zhang, C., Shang, W., Xue, J., et al. (2019a). Ginsenoside Rg1 Promotes Cerebral Angiogenesis via the PI3K/Akt/mTOR Signaling Pathway in Ischemic Mice. *Eur. J. Pharmacol.* 856, 172418. doi:10.1016/j.ejphar.2019.172418

Chen, Y., Zhao, B., Zhu, Y., Zhao, H., and Ma, C. (2019b). HIF-1-VEGF-Notch Mediates Angiogenesis in Temporomandibular Joint Osteoarthritis. *Am. J. Transl Res.* 11, 2969–2982.

Cheng, S., Zhang, X., Feng, Q., Chen, J., Shen, L., Yu, P., et al. (2019). Astragaloside IV Exerts Angiogenesis and Cardioprotection after Myocardial Infarction via Regulating PTEN/PI3K/Akt Signaling Pathway. *Life Sci.* 227, 82–93. doi:10.1016/j.lfs.2019.04.040

Elshabrawy, H. A., Chen, Z., Volin, M. V., Ravella, S., Virupannavar, S., and Shahrara, S. (2015). The Pathogenic Role of Angiogenesis in Rheumatoid Arthritis. *Angiogenesis* 18, 433–448. doi:10.1007/s10456-015-9477-2

Favalli, E. G., Raimondo, M. G., Becciolini, A., Crotti, C., Biggioggero, M., and Caporali, R. (2017). The Management of First-Line Biologic Therapy Failures in Rheumatoid Arthritis: Current Practice and Future Perspectives. *Autoimmun. Rev.* 16, 1185–1195. doi:10.1016/j.autrev.2017.10.002

Ferrara, N. (2004). Vascular Endothelial Growth Factor: Basic Science and Clinical Progress. *Endocr. Rev.* 25, 581–611. doi:10.1210/er.2003-0027

Gai, W., Hao, X., Zhao, J., Wang, L., Liu, J., Jiang, H., et al. (2020). Delivery of Benzoylaconitine Using Biodegradable Nanoparticles to Suppress Inflammation via Regulating NF-Kb Signaling. *Colloids Surf. B Biointerfaces* 191, 110980. doi:10.1016/j.colsurfb.2020.110980

Guo, Q., Mizuno, K., Okuyama, K., Lin, N., Zhang, Y., Hayashi, H., et al. (2020). Antineuropathic Pain Actions of Wu-tou Decoction Resulted from the Increase of Neurotrophic Factor and Decrease of CCR5 Expression in Primary Rat Glial Cells. *Biomed. Pharmacother.* 123, 109812. doi:10.1016/j.biopha.2020.109812

Guo, Q., Zheng, K., Fan, D., Zhao, Y., Li, L., Bian, Y., et al. (2017). Wu-tou Decoction in Rheumatoid Arthritis: Integrating Network Pharmacology and *In Vivo* Pharmacological Evaluation. *Front. Pharmacol.* 8, 230. doi:10.3389/fphar.2017.00230

He, L., Liu, C., Sun, C., Wang, J., Zhi, K., Sun, D., et al. (2018). Wu-tou Decoction Inhibits Angiogenesis in Experimental Arthritis by Targeting VEGFR2 Signaling Pathway. *Rejuvenation Res.* 21, 442–455. doi:10.1089/rej.2017.2011

Kanehisa, M., Furumichi, M., Tanabe, M., Sato, Y., and Morishima, K. (2017). KEGG: New Perspectives on Genomes, Pathways, Diseases and Drugs. *Nucleic Acids Res.* 45, D353–D361. doi:10.1093/nar/gkw1092

Karar, J., and Maity, A. (2011). PI3K/AKT/mTOR Pathway in Angiogenesis. *Front. Mol. Neurosci.* 4, 51. doi:10.3389/fnmol.2011.00051

Kollias, G., Papadaki, P., Apparailly, F., Vervoordeldonk, M. J., Holmdahl, R., Baumans, V., et al. (2011). Animal Models for Arthritis: Innovative Tools for Prevention and Treatment. *Ann. Rheum. Dis.* 70, 1357–1362. doi:10.1136/ard.2010.148551

Latacz, E., Caspani, E., Barnhill, R., Lugassy, C., Verhoef, C., Grünhagen, D., et al. (2020). Pathological Features of Vessel Co-option versus Sprouting Angiogenesis. *Angiogenesis* 23, 43–54. doi:10.1007/s10456-019-09690-0

Li, Y., Liu, Y., Wang, C., Xia, W. R., Zheng, J. Y., Yang, J., et al. (2018). Succinate Induces Synovial Angiogenesis in Rheumatoid Arthritis through Metabolic Remodeling and HIF-1α/VEGF axis. *Free Radic. Biol. Med.* 126, 1–14. doi:10.1016/j.freeradbiomed.2018.07.009

Liu, C., He, L., Wang, J., Wang, Q., Sun, C., Li, Y., et al. (2020). Anti-angiogenic Effect of Shikonin in Rheumatoid Arthritis by Downregulating PI3K/AKT and MAPKs Signaling Pathways. *J. Ethnopharmacol* 260, 113039. doi:10.1016/j.jep.2020.113039

Liu, Z., Guo, F., Wang, Y., Li, C., Zhang, X., Li, H., et al. (2016). BATMAN-TCM: a Bioinformatics Analysis Tool for Molecular mechANism of Traditional Chinese Medicine. *Sci. Rep.* 6, 21146. doi:10.1038/srep21146

Lü, S., Wang, Q., Li, G., Sun, S., Guo, Y., and Kuang, H. (2015). The Treatment of Rheumatoid Arthritis Using Chinese Medicinal Plants: From Pharmacology to Potential Molecular Mechanisms. *J. Ethnopharmacol* 176, 177–206. doi:10.1016/j.jep.2015.10.010

Ma, J. D., Jing, J., Wang, J. W., Yan, T., Li, Q. H., Mo, Y. Q., et al. (2019). A Novel Function of Artesunate on Inhibiting Migration and Invasion of Fibroblast-like Synoviocytes from Rheumatoid Arthritis Patients. *Arthritis Res. Ther.* 21, 153. doi:10.1186/s13075-019-1935-6

Mao, X., Li, W., Chen, W., Li, Y., Wang, Q., Wang, X., et al. (2020). Exploring and Characterizing a Novel Combination of Paeoniflorin and Talatizidine for the Treatment of Rheumatoid Arthritis. *Pharmacol. Res.* 153, 104658. doi:10.1016/j.phrs.2020.104658

Mcinnes, I. B., and Schett, G. (2011). The Pathogenesis of Rheumatoid Arthritis. *N. Engl. J. Med.* 365, 2205–2219. doi:10.1056/NEJMra1004965

Moudgil, K. D., and Berman, B. M. (2014). Traditional Chinese Medicine: Potential for Clinical Treatment of Rheumatoid Arthritis. *Expert Rev. Clin. Immunol.* 10, 819–822. doi:10.1586/1744666X.2014.917963

Myasoedova, E., Crowson, C. S., Kremers, H. M., Therneau, T. M., and Gabriel, S. E. (2010). Is the Incidence of Rheumatoid Arthritis Rising?: Results from Olmsted County, Minnesota, 1955-2007. *Arthritis Rheum.* 62, 1576–1582. doi:10.1002/art.27425

Paleolog, E. M., and Miotla, J. M. (1998). Angiogenesis in Arthritis: Role in Disease Pathogenesis and as a Potential Therapeutic Target. *Angiogenesis* 2, 295–307. doi:10.1023/a:1009229508096

Palmowski, Y., Buttgereit, T., Dejaco, C., Bijlsma, J. W., Matteson, E. L., Voshaar, M., et al. (2017). "Official View" on Glucocorticoids in Rheumatoid Arthritis: A Systematic Review of International Guidelines and Consensus Statements. *Arthritis Care Res. (Hoboken)* 69, 1134–1141. doi:10.1002/acr.23185

Park, S. Y., Jeong, K. J., Lee, J., Yoon, D. S., Choi, W. S., Kim, Y. K., et al. (2007). Hypoxia Enhances LPA-Induced HIF-1alpha and VEGF Expression: Their Inhibition by Resveratrol. *Cancer Lett.* 258, 63–69. doi:10.1016/j.canlet.2007.08.011

Pawar, A., Desai, R. J., Solomon, D. H., Santiago Ortiz, A. J., Gale, S., Bao, M., et al. (2019). Risk of Serious Infections in Tocilizumab versus Other Biologic Drugs in Patients with Rheumatoid Arthritis: a Multidatabase Cohort Study. *Ann. Rheum. Dis.* 78, 456–464. doi:10.1136/annrheumdis-2018-214367

Piñero, J., Bravo, À., Queralt-Rosinach, N., Gutiérrez-Sacristán, A., Deu-Pons, J., Centeno, E., et al. (2017). DisGeNET: a Comprehensive Platform Integrating Information on Human Disease-Associated Genes and Variants. *Nucleic Acids Res.* 45, D833–D839. doi:10.1093/nar/gkw943

Qi, Y., Li, S., Pi, Z., Song, F., Lin, N., Liu, S., et al. (2014). Chemical Profiling of Wu-tou Decoction by UPLC-Q-TOF-MS. *Talanta* 118, 21–29. doi:10.1016/j.talanta.2013.09.054

Qu, L., Chen, C., He, W., Chen, Y., Li, Y., Wen, Y., et al. (2019). Glycyrrhizic Acid Ameliorates LPS-Induced Acute Lung Injury by Regulating Autophagy through the PI3K/AKT/mTOR Pathway. *Am. J. Transl Res.* 11, 2042–2055.

Ramiro, S., Sepriano, A., Chatzidionysiou, K., Nam, J. L., Smolen, J. S., Van Der Heijde, D., et al. (2017). Safety of Synthetic and Biological DMARDs: a Systematic Literature Review Informing the 2016 Update of the EULAR Recommendations for Management of Rheumatoid Arthritis. *Ann. Rheum. Dis.* 76, 1101–1136. doi:10.1136/annrheumdis-2016-210708

Ranganath, V. K., Motamedi, K., Haavardsholm, E. A., Maranian, P., Elashoff, D., Mcqueen, F., et al. (2015). Comprehensive Appraisal of Magnetic Resonance Imaging Findings in Sustained Rheumatoid Arthritis Remission: a Substudy. *Arthritis Care Res. (Hoboken)* 67, 929–939. doi:10.1002/acr.22541

Ru, J., Li, P., Wang, J., Zhou, W., Li, B., Huang, C., et al. (2014). TCMSP: a Database of Systems Pharmacology for Drug Discovery from Herbal Medicines. *J. Cheminform* 6, 13. doi:10.1186/1758-2946-6-13

Shafik, N. M., El-Esawy, R. O., Mohamed, D. A., Deghidy, E. A., and El-Deeb, O. S. (2019). Regenerative Effects of Glycyrrhizin And/or Platelet Rich Plasma on Type-II Collagen Induced Arthritis: Targeting Autophay Machinery Markers, Inflammation and Oxidative Stress. *Arch. Biochem. Biophys.* 675, 108095. doi:10.1016/j.abb.2019.108095

Silva-Fernández, L., Lunt, M., Kearsley-Fleet, L., Watson, K. D., Dixon, W. G., Symmons, D. P., et al. (2016). The Incidence of Cancer in Patients with Rheumatoid Arthritis and a Prior Malignancy Who Receive TNF Inhibitors or Rituximab: Results from the British Society for Rheumatology Biologics Register-Rheumatoid Arthritis. *Rheumatology (Oxford)* 55, 2033–2039. doi:10.1093/rheumatology/kew314

Singh, J. A., Cameron, C., Noorbaloochi, S., Cullis, T., Tucker, M., Christensen, R., et al. (2015). Risk of Serious Infection in Biological Treatment of Patients with Rheumatoid Arthritis: a Systematic Review and Meta-Analysis. *Lancet* 386, 258–265. doi:10.1016/S0140-6736(14)61704-9

Smolen, J. S., Aletaha, D., and Mcinnes, I. B. (2016). Rheumatoid Arthritis. *Lancet* 388, 2023–2038. doi:10.1016/S0140-6736(16)30173-8

Smolen, J. S., and Aletaha, D. (2015). Rheumatoid Arthritis Therapy Reappraisal: Strategies, Opportunities and Challenges. *Nat. Rev. Rheumatol.* 11, 276–289. doi:10.1038/nrrheum.2015.8

Smolen, J. S., Landewé, R., Bijlsma, J., Burmester, G., Chatzidionysiou, K., Dougados, M., et al. (2017). EULAR Recommendations for the Management of Rheumatoid Arthritis with Synthetic and Biological Disease-Modifying Antirheumatic Drugs: 2016 Update. *Ann. Rheum. Dis.* 76, 960–977. doi:10.1136/annrheumdis-2016-210715

Sparks, J. A., Jin, Y., Cho, S. K., Vine, S., Desai, R., Doyle, T. J., et al. (2021). Prevalence, Incidence and Cause-specific Mortality of Rheumatoid Arthritis-Associated Interstitial Lung Disease Among Older Rheumatoid Arthritis Patients. *Rheumatology* 60, 3689–3698. doi:10.1093/rheumatology/keaa836

Stelzer, G., Rosen, N., Plaschkes, I., Zimmerman, S., Twik, M., Fishilevich, S., et al. (2016). The GeneCards Suite: From Gene Data Mining to Disease Genome Sequence Analyses. *Curr. Protoc. Bioinformatics* 54, 13031–13033. doi:10.1002/cpbi.5

Tao, W., Xu, X., Wang, X., Li, B., Wang, Y., Li, Y., et al. (2013). Network Pharmacology-Based Prediction of the Active Ingredients and Potential Targets of Chinese Herbal Radix Curcumae Formula for Application to Cardiovascular Disease. *J. Ethnopharmacol* 145, 1–10. doi:10.1016/j.jep.2012.09.051

Tobón, G. J., Youinou, P., and Saraux, A. (2010). The Environment, Geo-Epidemiology, and Autoimmune Disease: Rheumatoid Arthritis. *J. Autoimmun.* 35, 10–14. doi:10.1016/j.jaut.2009.12.009

Van Mulligen, E., De Jong, P. H. P., Kuijper, T. M., Van Der Ven, M., Appels, C., Bijkerk, C., et al. (2019). Gradual Tapering TNF Inhibitors versus Conventional Synthetic DMARDs after Achieving Controlled Disease in Patients with Rheumatoid Arthritis: First-Year Results of the Randomised Controlled TARA Study. *Ann. Rheum. Dis.* 78, 746–753. doi:10.1136/annrheumdis-2018-214970

Wang, Y., Zhang, S., Li, F., Zhou, Y., Zhang, Y., Wang, Z., et al. (2020). Therapeutic Target Database 2020: Enriched Resource for Facilitating Research and Early Development of Targeted Therapeutics. *Nucleic Acids Res.* 48, D1031–D1041. doi:10.1093/nar/gkz981

Wei, K., Korsunsky, I., Marshall, J. L., Gao, A., Watts, G. F. M., Major, T., et al. (2020). Notch Signalling Drives Synovial Fibroblast Identity and Arthritis Pathology. *Nature* 582, 259–264. doi:10.1038/s41586-020-2222-z

Wishart, D. S., Feunang, Y. D., Guo, A. C., Lo, E. J., Marcu, A., Grant, J. R., et al. (2018). DrugBank 5.0: a Major Update to the DrugBank Database for 2018. *Nucleic Acids Res.* 46, D1074–D1082. doi:10.1093/nar/gkx1037

Xu, H., Cai, L., Zhang, L., Wang, G., Xie, R., Jiang, Y., et al. (2018). Paeoniflorin Ameliorates Collagen-Induced Arthritis via Suppressing Nuclear Factor-kappaB Signalling Pathway in Osteoclast Differentiation. *Immunology* 154, 593–603. doi:10.1111/imm.12907

Yuan, N., Gong, L., Tang, K., He, L., Hao, W., Li, X., et al. (2020). An Integrated Pharmacology-Based Analysis for Antidepressant Mechanism of Chinese Herbal Formula Xiao-Yao-San. *Front. Pharmacol.* 11, 284. doi:10.3389/fphar.2020.00284

Zhai, W., Ma, Z., Wang, W., Song, L., and Yi, J. (2018). Paeoniflorin Inhibits Rho Kinase Activation in Joint Synovial Tissues of Rats with Collagen-Induced Rheumatoid Arthritis. *Biomed. Pharmacother.* 106, 255–259. doi:10.1016/j.biopha.2018.06.130

Zhang, L., and Wei, W. (2020). Anti-inflammatory and Immunoregulatory Effects of Paeoniflorin and Total Glucosides of Paeony. *Pharmacol. Ther.* 207, 107452. doi:10.1016/j.pharmthera.2019.107452

Zhang, Q., Liu, J., Zhang, M., Wei, S., Li, R., Gao, Y., et al. (2019). Apoptosis Induction of Fibroblast-like Synoviocytes Is an Important Molecular-Mechanism for Herbal Medicine along with its Active Components in Treating Rheumatoid Arthritis. *Biomolecules* 9. doi:10.3390/biom9120795

Zhang, Y., Bai, M., Zhang, B., Liu, C., Guo, Q., Sun, Y., et al. (2015). Uncovering Pharmacological Mechanisms of Wu-tou Decoction Acting on Rheumatoid Arthritis through Systems Approaches: Drug-Target Prediction, Network Analysis and Experimental Validation. *Sci. Rep.* 5, 9463. doi:10.1038/srep09463

Zhou, Y., Zhou, B., Pache, L., Chang, M., Khodabakhshi, A. H., Tanaseichuk, O., et al. (2019). Metascape Provides a Biologist-Oriented Resource for the Analysis of Systems-Level Datasets. *Nat. Commun.* 10, 1523. doi:10.1038/s41467-019-09234-6

Zhu, Y., Liu, X., Zhao, P., Zhao, H., Gao, W., and Wang, L. (2020). Celastrol Suppresses Glioma Vasculogenic Mimicry Formation and Angiogenesis by Blocking the PI3K/Akt/mTOR Signaling Pathway. *Front. Pharmacol.* 11, 25. doi:10.3389/fphar.2020.00025

10

Anti-Endometriosis Mechanism of *Jiawei Foshou San* Based on Network Pharmacology

Yi Chen[1,2,3†], Jiahui Wei[1,2,3†], Ying Zhang[1,2,3], Wenwei Sun[1,2,3], Zhuoheng Li[1,2,3], Qin Wang[4], Xiaoyu Xu[1,2,3], Cong Li[5*] and Panhong Li[1,2,3*]*

[1] College of Pharmaceutical Sciences and Chinese Medicine, Southwest University, Chongqing, China, [2] Chongqing Key Laboratory of New Drug Screening from Traditional Chinese Medicine, Chongqing, China, [3] Pharmacology of Chinese Materia Medica – the Key Discipline Constructed by the State Administration of Traditional Chinese Medicine, Chongqing, China, [4] Department of Traditional Chinese Medicine and Pharmacy, Chongqing Hospital of Traditional Chinese Medicine, Chongqing, China, [5] Department of Obstetrics and Gynecology, First Affiliated Hospital of Chongqing Medical University, Chongqing, China

***Correspondence:**
Yi Chen
rachelcy@swu.edu.cn
Cong Li
b05104@126.com
Panhong Li
1311636767@qq.com*

† These authors have contributed equally to this work.

Jiawei Foshou San (JFS) is the new formula originated from classic *Foshou San* formula, composed with ligustrazine, ferulic acid, and tetrahydropalmatine. Previously JFS inhibited the growth of endometriosis (EMS) with unclear mechanism, especially in metastasis, invasion, and epithelial–mesenchymal transition. In this study, network pharmacology was performed to explore potential mechanism of JFS on EMS. Through compound–compound target and compound target–EMS target networks, key targets were analyzed for pathway enrichment. MMP–TIMP were uncovered as one cluster of the core targets. Furthermore, autologous transplantation of EMS rat's model were used to evaluate *in vivo* effect of JFS on invasion, metastasis and epithelial–mesenchymal transition. JFS significantly suppressed the growth, and reduced the volume of ectopic endometrium, with modification of pathologic structure. In-depth study, invasion and metastasis were restrained after treating with JFS through decreasing MMP-2 and MMP-9, increasing TIMP-1. Meanwhile, JFS promoted E-cadherin, and attenuated N-cadherin, Vimentin, Snail, Slug, ZEB1, ZEB2, Twist. In brief, anti-EMS effect of JFS might be related to the regulation of epithelial–mesenchymal transformation, thereby inhibition of invasion and metastasis. These findings reveal the potential mechanism of JFS on EMS and the benefit for further evaluation.

Keywords: *Jiawei Foshou San*, endometriosis, network pharmacology, invasion and metastasis, epithelial–mesenchymal transition

INTRODUCTION

Endometriosis is known as the growth of the active endometrial tissue outside the uterus. Even though EMS is considered as a benign gynecological disease, there are malignant performance of invasiveness, angiogenesis, recurrence, and malignant transformation (Ma et al., 2016; Mihailovici et al., 2017). However, the mechanism of EMS is unclear, the reflux theory of menstruation is most

Abbreviations: CPPI, core protein–protein interaction; CT–DT, compound target–disease target; EMS, endometriosis; JFS, *Jiawei Foshou San*; TCM, traditional Chinese medicine.

widely accepted. It is suggested that invasion and metastasis is a very important step in flowing endometrial tissue (Borrelli et al., 2015; Chui et al., 2017).

In TCM, blood stasis and obstruction of uterus are considered as the main cause of EMS (Shan et al., 2017; Wen et al., 2017). So the treatment of EMS is based on activating blood circulation to dissipate blood stasis (Zhao, 2018). *Foshou San* formula is one of the famous *Huoxue Huayu* recipes, originally reported in *Puji Benshi Fang*. JFS is the new formula originated from classic *Foshou San* formula, composed with ligustrazine, ferulic acid, and tetrahydropalmatine. In previous experiment, good efficiency of JFS has been recovered, including diminishing the growth of EMS, suppression of E_2, anti-inflammation and anti-angiogenesis (Tang et al., 2014). However, the effect of JFS on invasion, metastasis, and epithelial–mesenchymal transformation has not been reported in EMS.

Traditional Chinese medicine formula has the complicate characteristic of poly-component with poly-target through poly-pathway (Wang et al., 2017). Network pharmacology is a new discipline combined systems biology with drug efficacy, generally describing the connection of multi-component with multi-target and multi-pathway (Ning et al., 2017). So application of network pharmacology on TCM will contribute to illustrate the utility of TCM.

In this study, compound–compound target and compound target–EMS target networks were established through network pharmacology data bases. Key targets and pathway enrichment were analyzed. Then autologous transplantation of EMS rat's model were used to evaluate *in vivo* effect of JFS on EMS. Furthermore, the influence of JFS on invasion, metastasis, and epithelial–mesenchymal transition were investigated (**Figure 1**).

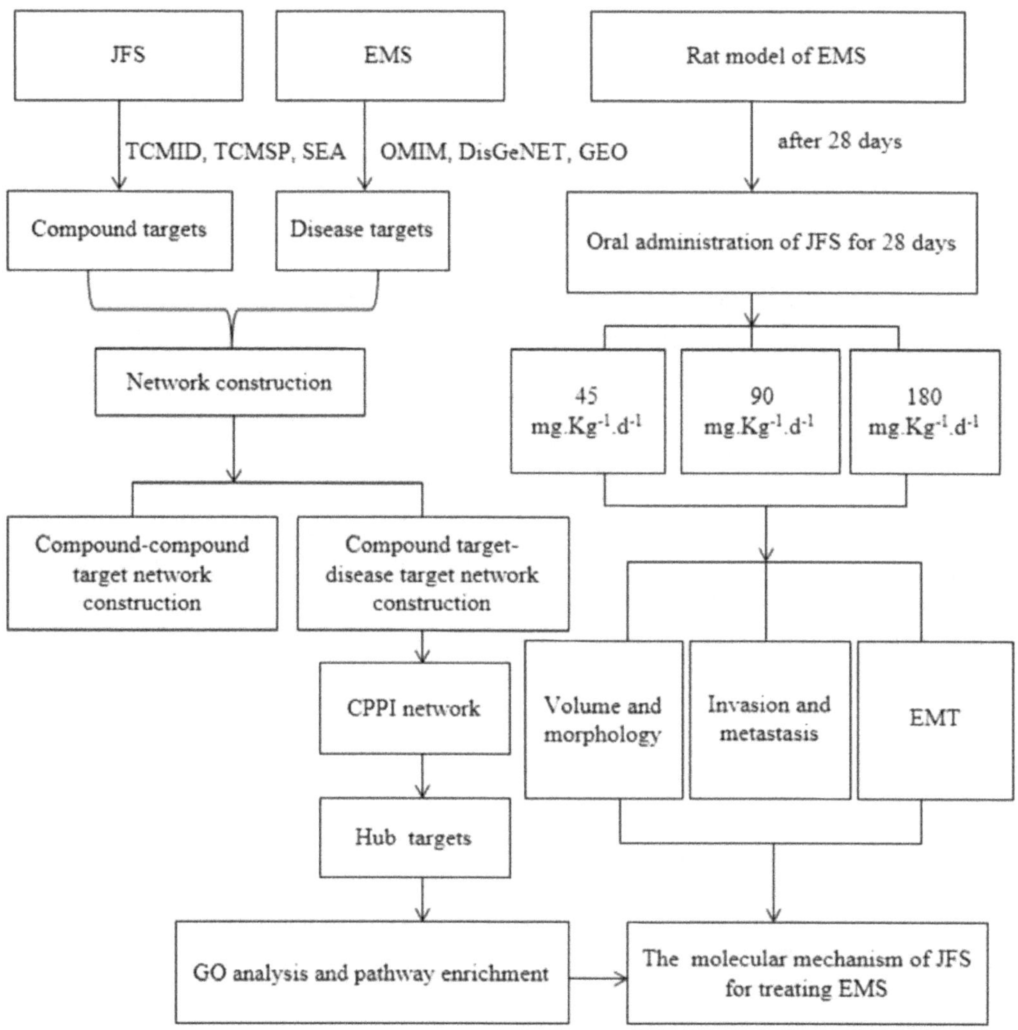

FIGURE 1 | The flowchart of this study based on an integration strategy of network pharmacology and experimental verification. EMS, endometriosis; JFS, *Jiawei Foshou San*; TCMID, Traditional Chinese Medicines Integrated Database; TCMSP, Traditional Chinese Medicine Systems Pharmacology Database and Analysis Platform; SEA, Similarity ensemble approach database; OMIM, Online Mendelian Inheritance in Man; DisGeNET, a database of gene–disease associations; GEO, Gene Expression Omnibus; CPPI, core protein–protein interaction.

MATERIALS AND METHODS

Collection of Potential Targets for Jiawei Foshou San

In order to collect potential targets of three compounds in JFS as many as possible, the following three databases were used: Traditional Chinese Medicines Integrated Database (TCMID)[1], Traditional Chinese Medicine Systems Pharmacology Database and Analysis Platform (TCMSP)[2], and the Similarity ensemble approach (SEA) database[3].

Collection of Potential Targets in EMS

The potential targets for EMS were obtained from the three resources using "Endometriosis" as the keyword: Online Mendelian Inheritance in Man (OMIM)[4], a database of gene–disease associations (DisGeNET)[5], and Gene Expression Omnibus (GEO)[6].

ID Conversion for Searched Targets

All JFS-related and EMS-related targets obtained from databases were aggregated together, and the duplicate ones were removed. Simultaneously, the UniProtKB search function in the protein database UniProt[7] was used to modify the searched targets to their official names. By entering the target name and limiting the species to "*Homo sapiens*," multifarious ID types of the targets were converted into UniProt IDs.

Protein–Protein Interaction Data

The STRING database furnishes both predicted protein-protein interaction information and the data which have been experimentally proven (Szklarczyk et al., 2011). The version 10.5 of STRING[8] was employed to search for the protein–protein interaction data, with the species limited to "*Homo sapiens*" and a confidence score >0.4 (Tang et al., 2016).

Network Construction and Analysis

The compound–compound target and compound target–EMS target networks were constructed based on their interaction data and visualized by Cytoscape 3.5.0 software. In the generated networks, nodes represented targets and compounds, edges represented the relationship between them. The targets without interaction were excluded from the network. Afterward, the Network Analyzer, a plugin of Cytoscape, was applied to analyze the topological parameters of each node in the network. Among the topological parameters, degree and betweenness centrality were used as crucial factors to describe the most influential nodes in networks (Li et al., 2015; Tang et al., 2015). Thus, the nodes with higher or equal degrees and betweenness than the average were chosen as the hubs.

[1]http://www.megabionet.Org/tcmid/search/
[2]http://lsp.nwu.edu.cn/tcmsp.php, updated on May 31, 2014
[3]http://sea.bkslab.org/
[4]https://omim.org/, updated on Oct 31, 2017
[5]http://www.disgenet.org/, last updated May 28, 2017
[6]https://www.ncbi.nlm.nih.gov/geo/
[7]http://www.uniprot.org/, last modified June 22, 2017
[8]https://string-db.org/

GO Enrichment and Pathway Analysis

The Database for Annotation, Visualization and Integrated Discovery (DAVID)[9] and the Protein Analysis Through Evolutionary Relationships database (PANTHER)[10] were applied for Gene Ontology (GO) enrichment and pathway analysis. The specific operation steps were as following, inputting the protein ID and restricting the species to "*Homo sapiens*," then utilizing the functional annotation tool to make GO enrichment and pathway analysis.

Animals and Chemicals

Female Sprague-Dawley rats aged 6–7 weeks were purchased from Experimental Animals Institute of Chongqing Academy of Chinese Materia (Certification No: SCXK [yu] 2012-0006). The rats were housed at a *Ta* of 20 ± 2°C and 12 h light/dark cycle, free access to food and water in the Experimental Center, College of Pharmaceutical Sciences, Southwest University. This study was carried out in strict accordance with the recommendations in the Guide for the Care and Use of Laboratory Animals of Southwest University (Approval No. 0002183).

Ferulic acid, ligustrazine, and tetrahydropalmatine with the purity of 99.8, 99.3, and 98.1% separately, were provided by

[9]https://david.ncifcrf.gov/, version 6.8
[10]http://pantherdb.org, version 13.1

TABLE 1 | qPCR primer sequence.

Genes		5′–3′
MMP-2	Forward	GGCCCTGTCACTCCTGAGAT
	Reverse	GGCATCCAGGTTATCGGGGA
MMP-9	Forward	TGGACGATGCCTGCAACGTG
	Reverse	GTCGTGCGTGTCCAAAGGCA
TIMP-1	Forward	CAATTCCGACCTCGTCATCAG
	Reverse	CTTGGAACCCTTTATACATCTTGG
E-cadherin	Forward	CTGGACCGAGAGAGTTACCC
	Reverse	GGCACCGACCTCATTCTCAA
N-cadherin	Forward	GCTTCTGGCGGCCTTGCTTCA
	Reverse	GCGTACACTGTGCCGTCCTCATCC
Vimentin	Forward	CCTTGACATTGAGATTGCCA
	Reverse	GTATCAACCAGAGGGAGTGA
Snail	Forward	TTACCTTCCAGCAGCCCTAC
	Reverse	GCTTCGGATGTGCATCTTG
Slug	Forward	ATCTGACCCGTCGACG
	Reverse	CGTCACGACGGGTCAGAT
ZEB1	Forward	GATGGGGCTGCGGATGAG
	Reverse	GCAGGGTGCTCTGGGTCATA
ZEB2	Forward	TCTGCGACATAAATACGA
	Reverse	GAGTGAAGCCTTGAGTGC
Twist	Forward	ACCCTCACACCTCTGCATTC
	Reverse	CAGTTTGATCCCAGCGTTTT
GAPDH	Forward	AGACAGCCGCATCTTCTTGT
	Reverse	CTTGCCGTGGGTAGAGTCAT

Nanjing Zelang Medical Technology Co., Ltd. (Nanjing, China). They were mixed by a ratio of 10:5:3, then suspended in CMC-Na to constitute JFS. Gestrinone was purchased from Zizhu Pharmaceutical Co., Ltd. (Beijing, China).

Rat Endometriosis Model

Sixty rats with estrus were surgically induced EMS by auto-transplantation of uterine tissue. All operational procedures were conducted as described by Tang et al. (2014) with slight modification. Briefly under sterile condition, uterine horns of anesthetized rats were separated and cut into 5 mm × 5 mm fragments. The uterine segments were suspended in sterile PBS, then sutured onto the inner peritoneum near blood vessels. The incisions were closed and disinfected.

After 28 days of transplantation, the growth of the ectopic endometrium were observed on gross and microscopic examination. The volume of ectopic endometrium were detected by Vernier caliper with volume formula (0.52 × length × width × height) (Pinar et al., 2017). The rats were included with following criteria, viable and well vascularized endometrial explants, and graft volume $\geq$20 mm^3 in the second laparotomy.

Experimental Design

After 28 days of auto-transplantation, EMS model were successfully established in 50 from 60 rats. The success rate of the model was 83%. Those rats were randomly divided into EMS group, low, medium, and high JFS groups and gestrinone group. There were no significant difference in endometriotic volume of each group before treatment (**Table 3**). Another 10 normal female rats were treated as control group without transplantation. 0.5% CMC-Na were administered in control and EMS group. Low, medium, and high JFS groups were given with 45, 90, and 180 $mg.kg^{-1}.d^{-1}$ JFS, respectively. A 50 $mg.kg^{-1}.d^{-1}$ gestrinone was given in gestrinone group. All the above groups were administered consecutive 28 days by gavage.

Hematoxylin and Eosin Staining

Eutopic endometrium in control group and ectopic endometrium in other groups were collected and fixed in paraformaldehyde in the end of administration. Then sections from different groups were stained with hematoxylin and eosin (H&E). Endometrial glands and stroma were identified as the essential criteria for diagnosis. The morphological structure were examined and photographed under a microscope (DFC310 FX, Leica, Germany).

RNA Isolation and Real-Time PCR

The process for RNA isolation and real-time PCR were performed as described previously (Chen et al., 2012). Briefly, TRIzol reagent (Invitrogen, CA, United States) were used for mRNA extraction from the tissues with acid phenol extraction. RT-PCR was carried out using a PrimeScript™ RT reagent Kit

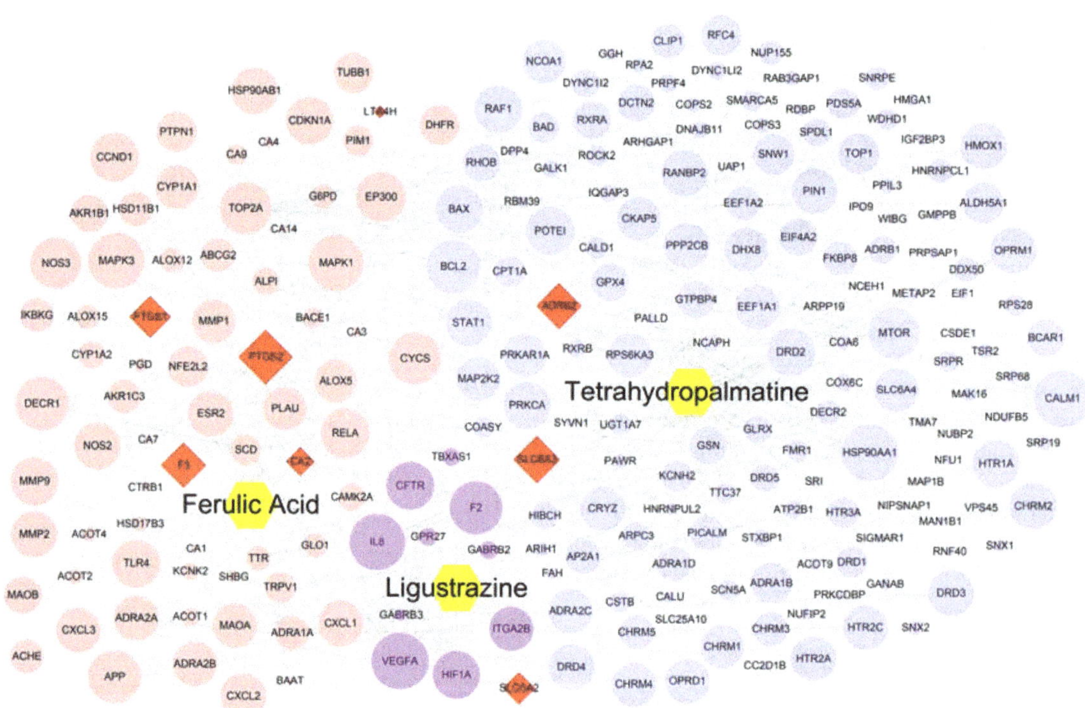

FIGURE 2 | The compound–compound target network. Purple circles, pink circles, blue circles, and red diamonds represented the targets of ligustrazine, ferulic acid, tetrahydropalmatine, and the common targets for all three components, respectively. Yellow hexagons represented the three compounds of *Jiawei Foshou San*. The size of circles and diamonds represented nodes degree value.

(Takara, China) according to the manufacturer's protocols. Real-time PCR was performed with CFX96 Real-Time System (Bio-Rad, United States) with SYBR^{TM} Green Master Mix (Thermo Fisher Scientific, United States). Rat specific primers were synthesized by Dingguo Changsheng Biotechnology (Beijing, China) (**Table 1**). Each PCR was carried out with the following conditions: 95°C for 2 min, 40 cycles of 95°C for 15 s and 60°C for 1 min. Melt curves were analyzed at the end of each assay to confirm the specificity. Fold change was determined using the $2^{-\Delta\Delta CT}$ method normalized with endogenous control GAPDH.

Western Blot Analysis

The protein were separated and extracted from eutopic endometrium in control group and ectopic endometrium in other groups. The tissue lysates were prepared as described previously (Chen et al., 2015, 2017). Briefly quantified protein lysates were separated by SDS-PAGE, transferred to polyvinylidene difluoride membrane (Millipore, United States) and probed with primary rabbit anti-MMP-2, rabbit anti-MMP-9 (1:100 dilution; Boster Biological Technology, Wuhan, China), rabbit anti-TIMP-1 (1:300 dilution; Proteintech Biotechnology, Wuhan, China), rabbit anti-E-cadherin, rabbit anti-Vimentin, rabbit anti-Snail, rabbit anti-Slug (1:1000 dilution; Cell Signaling Technology, Beverly, MA, United States), rabbit anti-β-actin (1:5000 dilution; Proteintech Biotechnology, Wuhan, China) overnight at 4°C. Then the membranes were blotted with an appropriate horseradish peroxidase-linked goat secondary antibody (1:2000 dilution; Zhongshan Golden Bridge

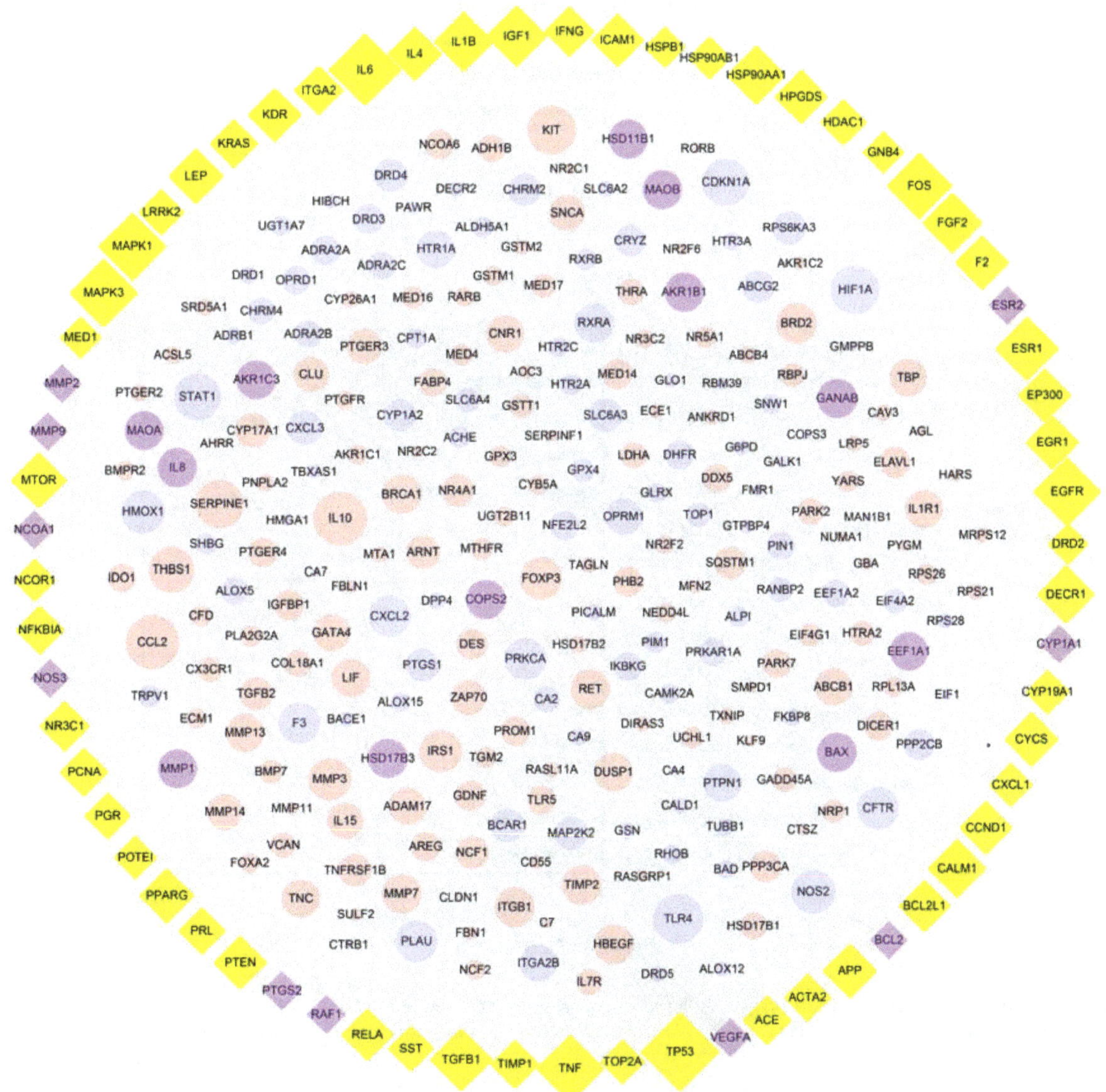

FIGURE 3 | The core protein–protein interaction network. Pink circles, blue circles, Purple circles and yellow diamonds showed for the targets of disease, targets of compounds, 22 common targets, and 66 candidate targets, respectively. Purple diamonds represented the intersection between 66 candidate targets and 22 common targets. The size of circles and diamonds indicated nodes degree value.

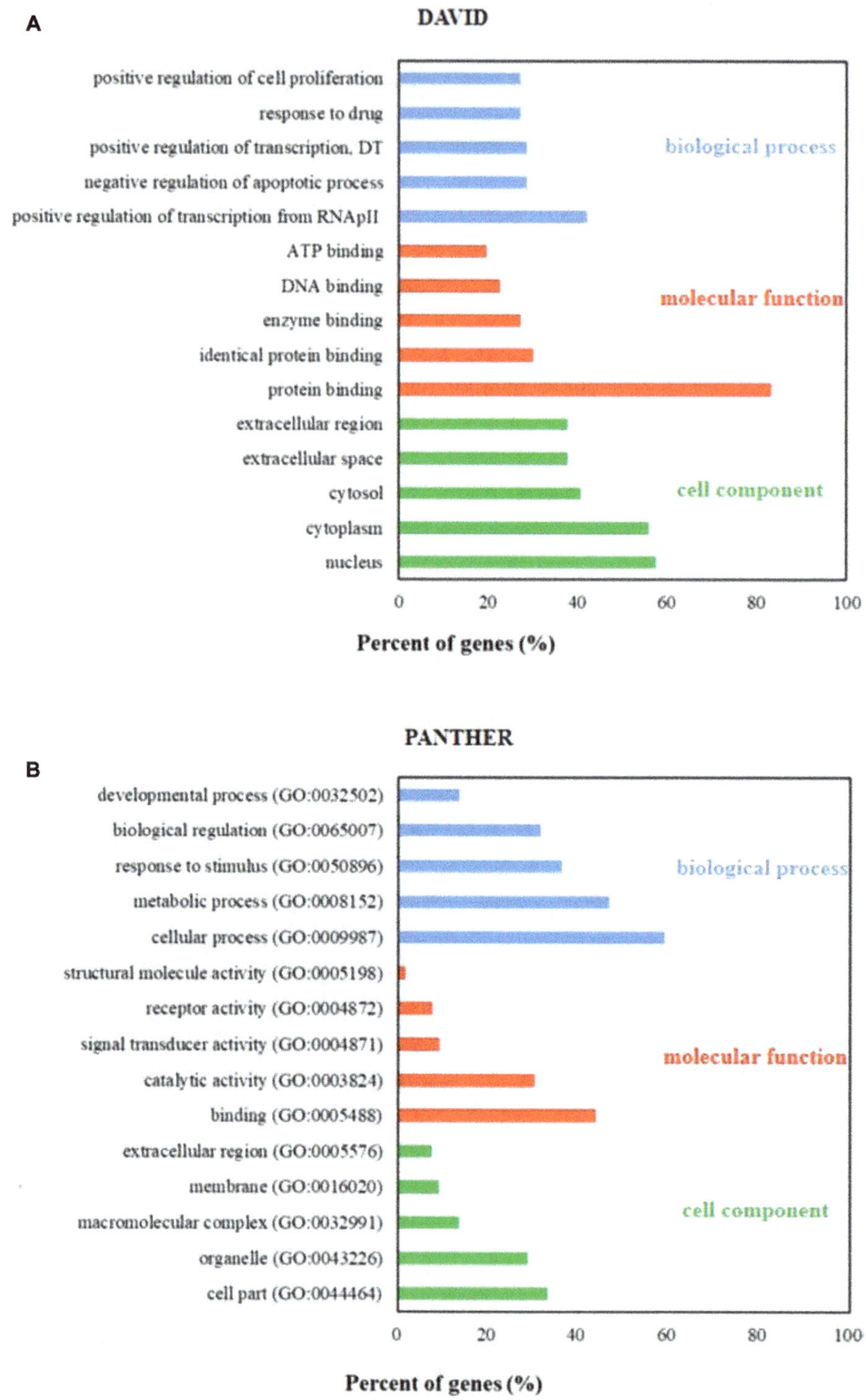

FIGURE 4 | Gene ontology (GO) analysis of candidate targets. GO enrichment analysis in DAVID **(A)** and PANTHER **(B)** database showed the five remarkably enriched items in the biological processes, cell component, and molecular function. RNApII, RNA polymerase II promoter; DT, DNA-templated.

Biotechnology, Beijing, China). Electrochemiluminescence was performed according to the manufacturer's instructions with Tanon 5200 imaging system (Tanon, China). β-Actin was used as endogenous control.

Statistical Analysis

Data were represented as the arithmetic mean ± SD and compared by one-way ANOVA test using SPSS software (Version 21). $P < 0.05$ was considered statistically significant.

TABLE 2 | Pathway including MMP-2, MMP-9, and TIMP-1

Pathway name	Gene name
Pathways in cancer	MMP-2, MMP-9
Proteoglycans in cancer	MMP-2, MMP-9
Estrogen signaling pathway	MMP-2, MMP-9
GnRH signaling pathway	MMP-2
Bladder cancer	MMP-2, MMP-9
Hepatitis B	MMP-9
TNF signaling pathway	MMP-9
Transcriptional misregulation in cancer	MMP-9
MicroRNAs in cancer	MMP-9
HIF-1 signaling pathway	TIMP-1
CCKR signaling map	MMP-9
Plasminogen activating cascade	MMP-9

RESULTS

Compound–Compound Target Network Construction and Analysis

A total of 275 potential targets were obtained for three JFS compounds, 10 for ligustrazine, 86 for ferulic acid, and 179 for tetrahydropalmatine. Detailed information is described in **Supplementary Table S1**. The compound–compound target network consisted of 235 nodes and 1508 edges. In this network, most targets belonged to a single compound, while the targets, such as ADRB2, CA2, F3, LTA4H, PTGS1, PTGS2, SLC6A2, and SLC6A3, belonged to more than one compound (**Figure 2**). It was suggested that these uniform targets might be the foundation of synergistic therapeutic effect of TCM.

Compound Target–Disease Target Network Construction and Analysis

By integrating data from disease databases, 401 EMS-related targets were acquired (**Supplementary Table S2**). The CT–DT network consisted of 592 nodes and 6166 edges. Targets of compounds were mapped to the EMS targets to obtain 22 common targets (**Supplementary Table S3**). Then a CPPI network including 22 targets and their first neighbors was extracted from the CT–DT network. The CPPI network comprised 315 nodes and 4703 edges (**Figure 3**). Subsequently, the average values of "Degree" and "Betweenness" for nodes were 29.8603 and 0.0039 in the CPPI network. The 66 nodes with "Degree" ≥ 29.8603 and "Betweenness" ≥ 0.0039 were chosen as the key targets (**Supplementary Table S4**). Interestingly, the 22 common targets were not completely contained in 66 key targets.

Pathway Enrichment Analysis for Key Targets

In order to further study the molecular mechanism of JFS on EMS, GO analysis and pathway enrichment of the 66 candidate targets were performed with KEGG and PANTHER database. The results of GO analysis were described by biological process (BP), cell component (CC), and molecular function (MF) terms. In KEGG database, 340 of 417 BPs, 34 of 42 CCs, and 60 of 76 MFs enriched for these targets were recognized as $P < 0.05$. Twelve BPs, six CCs, and five MFs were enriched from PANTHER database. An overview of the GO analysis was explored with top 5 remarkably enriched terms in the BP, CC, and MF categories (**Figure 4**). According to the results of pathway enrichment, 115 and 76 target-related pathways have been found in KEGG (**Supplementary Table S5**) and PANTHER database (**Supplementary Table S6**). Subsequently, remarkable 12 pathways were presented including MMP/TIMP (**Table 2**).

Jiawei Foshou San Inhibited the Volume of Ectopic Endometrium

After continuous gavage for 28 days, the volume of ectopic endometrium were evaluated and compared with pretreatment. There were no significantly varieties observed in EMS and JFS 45 mg.kg^{-1}.d^{-1} groups. Using 90 or 180 mg.kg^{-1}.d^{-1} JFS, the transplants became smaller, less adhesion and blood vessels outside, lower height of effusion. The volume of ectopic endometrium were 36.32 ± 11.78 and 17.90 ± 5.17 mm^3, significantly reduced by 48.68 ± 12.19 and 65.29 ± 9.15 mm^3, respectively ($P < 0.01$). Gestrinone diminished the volume of ectopic endometrium tissue from 81.92 ± 19.20 to 16.01 ± 5.53 mm^3 ($P < 0.01$) (**Table 3** and **Figures 5A–E**). This suggests that JFS restrained the growth of ectopic endometrium in a dose-dependent manner.

Improvement of Ectopic Endometrium Morphology by *Jiawei Foshou San*

In H&E staining, the ectopic endometrium in EMS group had a similar structure with eutopic endometrium in control group.

TABLE 3 | Effect of JFS on ectopic endometrium volume (n = 6).

Groups	Doses	Volume(mm^3)		Volume changes (mm^3)
		Pretreatment	Post-treatment	
EMS	–	80.94 ± 18.97	66.55 ± 16.01	14.39 ± 6.31
JFS	45 mg.kg^{-1}.d^{-1}	84.44 ± 17.03	74.54 ± 17.88	9.90 ± 2.48
	90 mg.kg^{-1}.d^{-1}	85.00 ± 18.42	36.32 ± 11.78**	48.68 ± 12.19
	180 mg.kg^{-1}.d^{-1}	83.19 ± 12.27	17.90 ± 5.17**	65.29 ± 9.15
GTN	50 mg.kg^{-1}.d^{-1}	81.92 ± 19.20	16.01 ± 5.53**	65.91 ± 14.34

*JFS, Jiawei Foshou San; GTN, gestrinone. Values were mean ± SD. * P < 0.05, **P < 0.01 vs. pretreatment.*

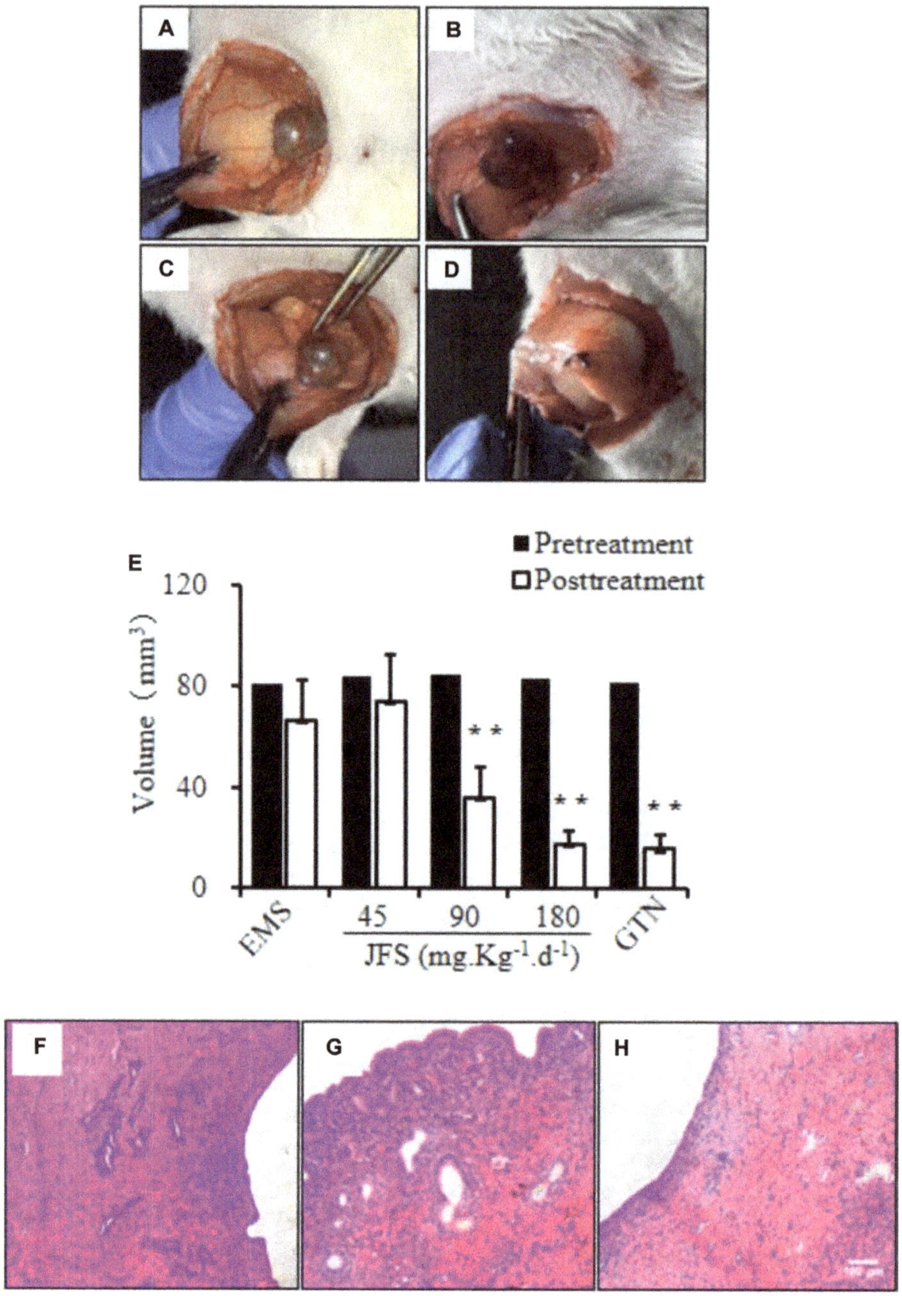

FIGURE 5 | Regulation of JFS on volume and morphology of ectopic endometrium. The ectopic endometrium were observed before and after administration for 28 days in EMS group **(A,B)** and 180 mg.kg^{-1}.d^{-1} JFS **(C,D)**. **(E)** The volume of ectopic endometrium were detected by Vernier caliper in rat endometriosis model. The morphological change of structure were found in eutopic endometrium in control **(F)**, ectopic endometrium in EMS **(G)**, and 180 mg.kg^{-1}.d^{-1} JFS **(H)** in H&E staining. $^{**}P < 0.01$ to pretreatment. Columns, mean ($n = 6$). Bars, SD. Magnification, ×100. EMS, endometriosis; JFS, *Jiawei Foshou San*; GTN, gestrinone.

The ectopic endometrium were constituted with endometrial glandular epithelial cell, endometrial stromal cell, and fibrous connective tissue. After gavage of 90 and 180 mg.kg^{-1}.d^{-1} JFS, the amelioration of ectopic endometrium structure were found, such as thinner ectopic endometrium, looser cell arrangement, less pseudoglandular, decreased blood vessels and inflammatory cells (**Figures 5F–H**).

Jiawei Foshou San Suppressed Invasion and Metastasis

MMP-2, MMP-9, and TIMP-1 are considered as the important roles in invasion and metastasis (Li et al., 2017). The gene and protein expression of MMP-2, MMP-9, and TIMP-1 were tested in our study. The mRNA levels of MMP-2 and MMP-9 significantly rose in EMS group ($P < 0.05$), while the mRNA level

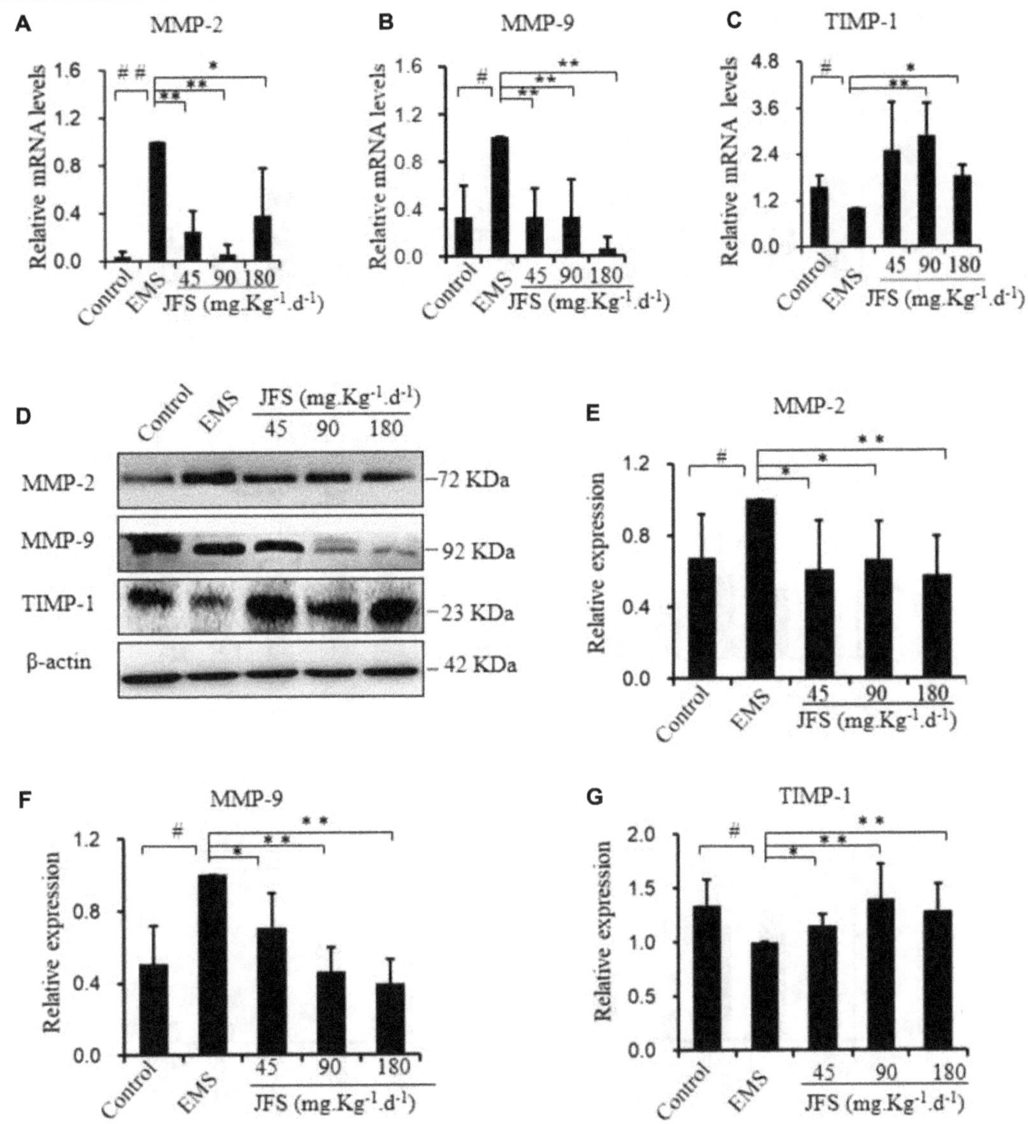

FIGURE 6 | Effect of JFS on invasion and metastasis. **(A–C)** The mRNA levels of MMP-2, MMP-9, and TIMP-1 were detected by qPCR in different groups. **(D–G)** The protein levels of MMP-2, MMP-9, and TIMP-1 were detected by western blotting, and the ratio of MMP-2, MMP-9, and TIMP-1 with β-actin were shown. $^{\#}P < 0.05$ to control, $^{\#\#}P < 0.01$ to control, $^{*}P < 0.05$ to EMS, $^{**}P < 0.01$ to EMS. Columns, mean ($n = 3$). Bars, SD. EMS, endometriosis; JFS, *Jiawei Foshou San*.

of TIMP-1 declined ($P < 0.05$). On the contrary, JFS obviously inhibited the gene expression of MMP-2 ($P < 0.05$) and MMP-9 ($P < 0.01$) compared with EMS group. Meanwhile the mRNA level of TIMP-1 was significantly upregulated in 90 and 180, not 45 $mg.kg^{-1}.d^{-1}$ JFS group, compared with EMS group ($P < 0.05$) (**Figures 6A–C**). Remarkably higher protein levels of MMP-2 and MMP-9 were founded in EMS group, with lower protein level of TIMP-1 than those in control group ($P < 0.05$). While treated with JFS, MMP-2, MMP-9 protein were decreased significantly in a dose-dependent manner ($P < 0.05$). The protein level of TIMP-1 was increased in three JFS groups vs. EMS group ($P < 0.05$) (**Figures 6D–G**). This suggests that the abatement of invasion and metastasis by JFS were connected with increasing MMP-2, MMP-9, and decreasing TIMP-1.

Reverse of Epithelial–Mesenchymal Transition by *Jiawei Foshou San*

Epithelial-mesenchymal transition is related with invasion and metastasis (Zheng et al., 2015). E-cadherin gene expressed significantly lower in EMS group vs. control group ($P < 0.01$). In contrast, N-cadherin, Vimentin, Snail, Slug, ZEB1, ZEB2, and Twist mRNA were significantly higher in EMS group than those in control group ($P < 0.05$). Since administration of JFS, the transition from epithelial phenotype to mesenchymal phenotype were reversed, for instance, upregulated mRNA level of E-cadherin, downregulated mRNA levels of N-cadherin, Vimentin, Snail, Slug, ZEB1, ZEB2, Twist compared with EMS group ($P < 0.05$) (**Figure 7**). Remarkably higher protein levels of Vimentin, Snail, and Slug were founded in EMS group,

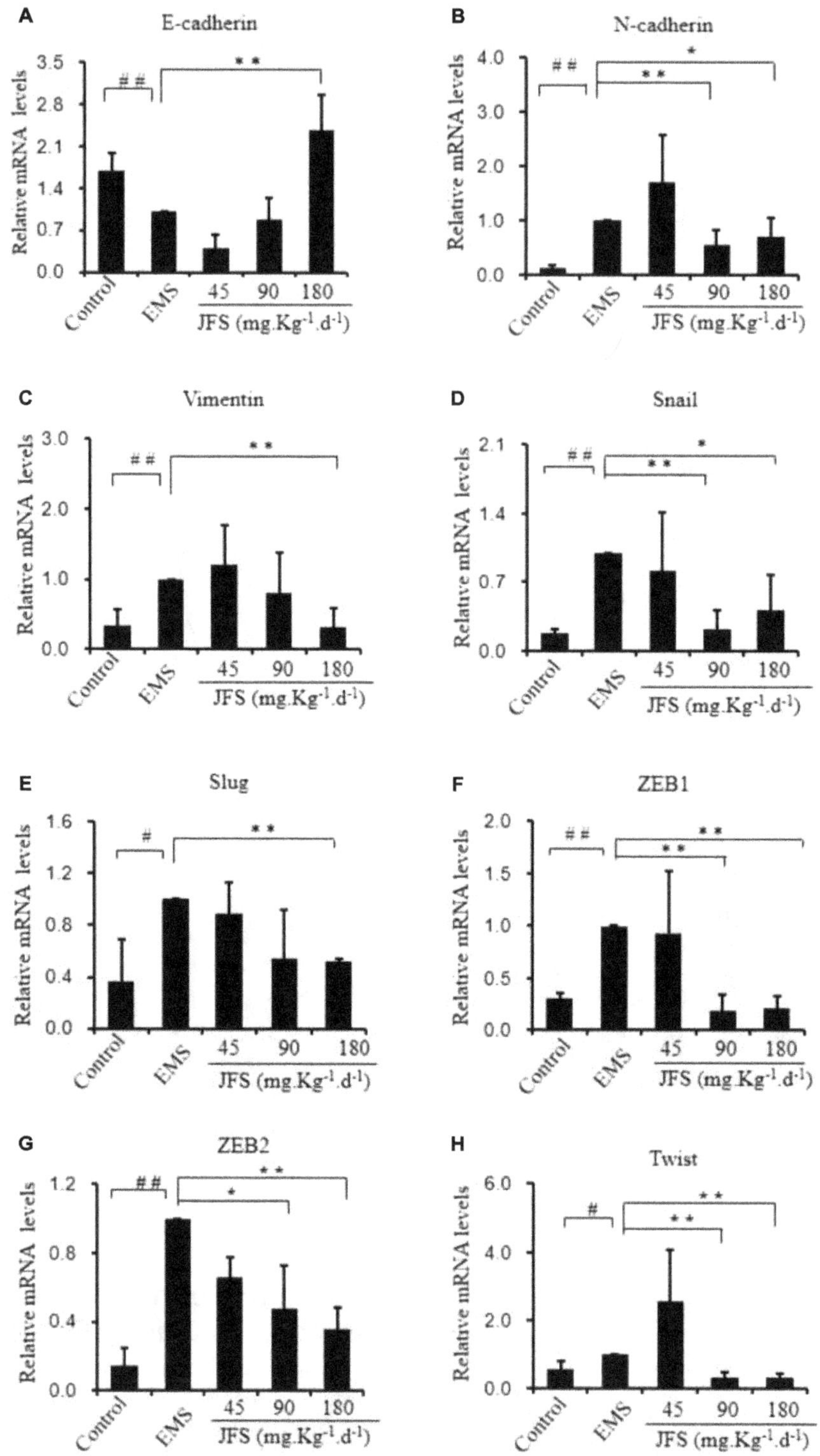

FIGURE 7 | Gene expression of epithelial–mesenchymal transition adjusted by JFS. **(A)** The epithelial marker E-cadherin mRNA level was measured by qPCR. **(B–H)** Mesenchymal genes expression of N-cadherin, Vimentin, Snail, Slug, ZEB1, ZEB2, and Twist using qPCR. $^{\#}P < 0.05$ to control, $^{\#\#}P < 0.01$ to control, $^{*}P < 0.05$ to EMS, $^{**}P < 0.01$ to EMS. Columns, mean ($n = 3$). Bars, SD. EMS, endometriosis; JFS, *Jiawei Foshou San*.

with lower protein level of E-cadherin than those in control group ($P < 0.05$). While using JFS, Vimentin, Snail, and Slug protein were decreased significantly in a dose-dependent manner ($P < 0.05$). The protein level of E-cadherin was increased in three JFS groups vs. EMS group ($P < 0.05$) (**Figure 8**).

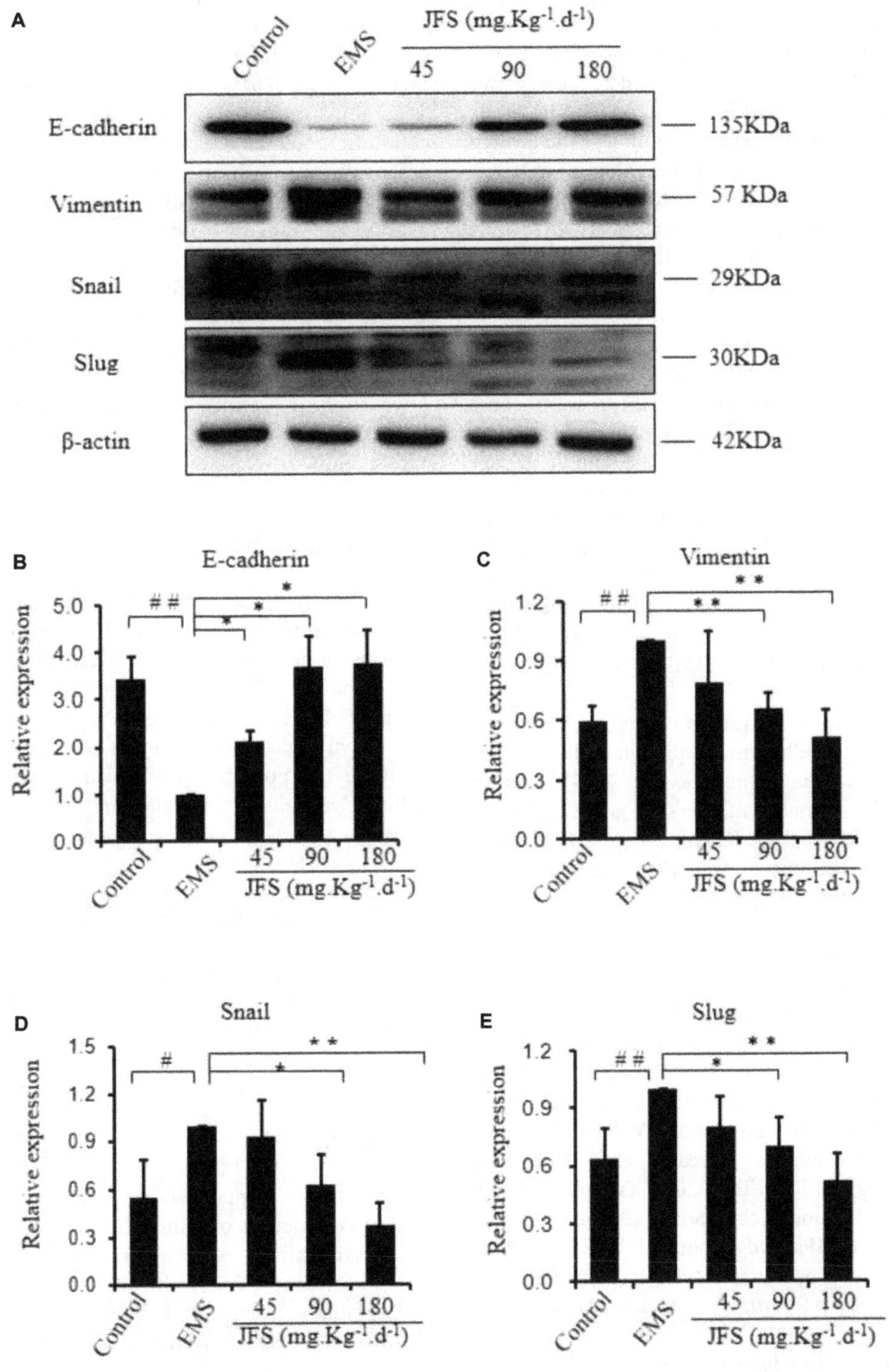

FIGURE 8 | Modification of epithelial–mesenchymal transition protein treating with JFS. **(A–E)** The protein levels of E-cadherin, Vimentin, Snail, and Slug were detected by western blotting, and the ratio of E-cadherin, Vimentin, Snail, and Slug with β-actin were shown. $^{\#}P < 0.05$ to control, $^{\#\#}P < 0.01$ to control, $^{*}P < 0.05$ to EMS, $^{**}P < 0.01$ to EMS. Columns, mean (n = 3). Bars, SD. EMS, endometriosis; JFS, *Jiawei Foshou San*.

DISCUSSION

According to the reflux theory of menstruation, invasion and metastasis of ectopic endometrium is the vital step in EMS, especially following with degradation of extracellular matrix. MMP-2, MMP-9, and TIMP-1 are the important factors in invasion and metastasis, and balance between them regulate degradation of extracellular matrix. In previous study, MMP-2 and MMP-9 increased, meanwhile TIMP-1 decreased in EMS (Huang et al., 2015; Yi et al., 2015; Jana et al., 2016; Szymanowski et al., 2016). The therapy, through suppressing MMP-2 and MMP-9, promoting TIMP-1, have been reported as the effective methods on EMS (Huang et al., 2015; Li et al., 2016; Kim et al., 2017). Consistently, in our experiment, JFS inhibited the growth of ectopic endometrium and recurred the pathological changes. It might be related with the regulation of MMP-2, MMP-9, and TIMP-1 to suppress invasion and metastasis. It is worthwhile to explore role of other MMP or TIMP, for example, MMP-1, MMP-7, TIMP-2 in EMS, and the effect of JFS on them in future.

Using network pharmacological analysis, the kernel targets were collected from the CPPI network for pathway enrichment. Interestingly, we found that there were some pathways related to MMP or TIMP, including estrogen, GnRH and TNF pathways. Estrogen, GnRH, and TNF are the pivotal mediators of endometrial homeostasis (Granese et al., 2015; Leavy, 2015; Simmen and Kelley, 2016; Tosti et al., 2017). Furthermore, MMP and TIMP are regulated by these three pathways (Raga et al., 1999; Voloshenyuk and Gardner, 2010; Yang et al., 2012). In our previous study, JFS suppressed GnRH, estrogen, and TNF (Tang et al., 2014). These might be the reasons of regulating MMP/TIMP balance by JFS.

Epithelial–mesenchymal transition presents the features, loss of polarity, and cellular adhesion in epithelial cells, convert into mesenchymal phenotype (Thiery et al., 2009). During this process, epithelial surface markers (e.g., E-cadherin, keratin) lose, mesenchymal markers (e.g., Vimentin, N-cadherin) express, and more migration and invasion subsequently emerge. Snail, Slug, ZEB1, ZEB2, and Twist, as the transcription factors, induce epithelial–mesenchymal transition through depressing E-cadherin (Cano et al., 2000; Zhang et al., 2006; Chen et al., 2010). Recently, lower E-cadherin, and higher Vimentin, N-cadherin, Snail, Slug, ZEB1, ZEB2, and Twist have been demonstrated in EMS (Furuya et al., 2017; Chatterjee et al., 2018; Wang et al., 2018). Interestingly, epithelial–mesenchymal transition has been inhibited with decline of MMP expression (Wu et al., 2018). We also found that E-cadherin increased, and Vimentin, N-cadherin, Snail, Slug, ZEB1, ZEB2, and Twist decreased. JFS restrained epithelial–mesenchymal transition, at the same time suppressed MMPs and promoted TIMP-1. These consistent data indicated a potential mechanism of increasing invasion and metastasis by JFS through epithelial–mesenchymal transition.

Foshou San formula is composed of *Ligusticum chuanxiong* Hort and *Angelica sinensis.* Ligustrazine from *L. chuanxiong* Hort, ferulic acid from *A. sinensis*, and tetrahydropalmatine are mixed to JFS with the certain proportion. Firstly, in previous study, ligustrazine has the anti-metastatic effects through decreasing MMP-2, MMP-9, MMP-3, MMP-13, increasing TIMP-1, TIMP-2 (Liang et al., 2014; Jiang et al., 2017; Fang et al., 2018). But up-regulating expression of MMP-2 and MMP-9 is found in bone marrow mesenchymal stem cells by ligustrazine (Wang et al., 2016). These results suggest that ligustrazine might have the different influence on metastasis in different diseases. Tetramethylpyrazine also inhibits epithelial–mesenchymal transition progression (Luan et al., 2016). Secondly, treated with ferulic acid alone or combination with other drugs, its role in suppression of metastatic potential are regulated by the reversal of epithelial–mesenchymal transition (Wei et al., 2015; Zhang et al., 2016). Thirdly, tetrahydropalmatine had a negative effect against invasion in cancer (Yodkeeree et al., 2013). While levo-tetrahydropalmatine attenuates blood–brain barrier injury and brain edema, but inhibits MMP-2/9 (Mao et al., 2015). In our study, JFS restrained metastasis through accumulating TIMP-1 and attenuating MMP-2, MMP-9. In addition, epithelial–mesenchymal transition were recovered. With all above confused results, the mechanism of JFS on metastasis and epithelial–mesenchymal transition need for further investigation.

CONCLUSION

In conclusion, these results showed that CPPI network was established through analysis of JFS targets with EMS targets. Then 66 kernel targets were selected for pathway enrichment. In EMS model, JFS was able to inhibit growth and pathological change. Furthermore, the modification of MMP/TIMP balance and down-regulation of epithelial–mesenchymal transition might be the potential mechanisms for JFS on EMS. These findings provide logical support for further evaluation of JFS.

AUTHOR CONTRIBUTIONS

YC and JW performed the major research in equal contribution. YZ, WS, ZL, QW, and XX provided the technical support. CL contributed to final approval of the version to be published. PL designed the study and revised the manuscript.

FUNDING

This work was supported by grants from National Natural Science Foundation of China (Nos. 81773984 and 81402441), traditional Chinese medicine research project of Chongqing Health Bureau (No. zy201602125), Southwest University Undergraduate Science and Technology Innovation Fund (No. 20162902003), SWU National Experimental Demonstration Center of Pharmacy (Nos. XY2017-CXZD-04 and YX2017-CXYB-01), and Chongqing Science and Technology Commission of China (No. CSTC2014JCYJA1038).

SUPPLEMENTARY MATERIAL

TABLE S1 | Detail and interaction information of targets for JFS compounds.

TABLE S2 | EMS-related targets and interaction information with JFS-related targets.

TABLE S3 | 22 common targets obtained from JFS-related targets and EMS-related targets.

TABLE S4 | 66 key targets extracted from a core protein–protein interaction network.

TABLE S5 | GO analysis and KEGG pathway enrichment of 66 key targets from DAVID database.

TABLE S6 | GO analysis and pathway analysis of 66 key targets from PANTHER database.

REFERENCES

Borrelli, G. M., Abrao, M. S., Taube, E. T., Darb-Esfahani, S., Kohler, C., Kaufmann, A. M., et al. (2015). Immunohistochemical investigation of metastasis-related chemokines in deep-infiltrating endometriosis and compromised pelvic sentinel lymph nodes. *Reprod. Sci.* 22, 1632–1642. doi: 10.1177/1933719115592711

Cano, A., Perez-Moreno, M. A., Rodrigo, I., Locascio, A., Blanco, M. J., del Barrio, M. G., et al. (2000). The transcription factor snail controls epithelial-mesenchymal transitions by repressing e-cadherin expression. *Nat. Cell Biol.* 2, 76–83. doi: 10.1038/35000025

Chatterjee, K., Jana, S., DasMahapatra, P., and Swarnakar, S. (2018). EGFR-mediated matrix metalloproteinase-7 up-regulation promotes epithelial-mesenchymal transition via ERK1-AP1 axis during ovarian endometriosis progression. *FASEB J.* doi: 10.1096/fj.201701382RR [Epub ahead of print].

Chen, Y. J., Li, H. Y., Huang, C. H., Twu, N. F., Yen, M. S., Wang, P. H., et al. (2010). Oestrogen-induced epithelial-mesenchymal transition of endometrial epithelial cells contributes to the development of adenomyosis. *J. Pathol.* 222, 261–270. doi: 10.1002/path.2761

Chen, Y., Sun, W. W., He, R., Zhang, F. Y., Wang, H. Y., Li, P. H., et al. (2017). Lidamycin decreases CD133 expression in hepatocellular carcinoma via the Notch signaling pathway. *Oncol. Lett.* 14, 7889–7895. doi: 10.3892/ol.2017.7248

Chen, Y., Yu, D. K., Zhang, C. X., Shang, B. Y., He, H. W., Chen, J. J., et al. (2015). Lidamycin inhibits tumor initiating cells of hepatocellular carcinoma Huh7 through GSK3 beta/beta-catenin pathway. *Mol. Carcinogen.* 54, 1–8. doi: 10.1002/mc.22069

Chen, Y., Yu, D. K., Zhang, H., He, H. W., Zhang, C. X., Zhao, W. L., et al. (2012). CD133(+)EpCAM(+) phenotype possesses more characteristics of tumor initiating cells in hepatocellular carcinoma Huh7 cells. *Int. J. Biol. Sci.* 8, 992–1004. doi: 10.7150/ijbs.4454

Chui, M. H., Wang, T. L., and Shih, I. M. (2017). Endometriosis: benign, malignant, or something in between? *Oncotarget* 8, 78263–78264. doi: 10.18632/oncotarget.21051

Fang, M., Mei, X., Yao, H., Zhang, T., Zhang, T., Lu, N., et al. (2018). beta-elemene enhances anticancer and anti-metastatic effects of osteosarcoma of ligustrazine in vitro and in vivo. *Oncol. Lett.* 15, 3957–3964. doi: 10.3892/ol.2018.7788

Furuya, M., Masuda, H., Hara, K., Uchida, H., Sato, K., Sato, S., et al. (2017). ZEB1 expression is a potential indicator of invasive endometriosis. *Acta Obstet. Gynecol. Scand.* 96, 1128–1135. doi: 10.1111/aogs.13179

Granese, R., Perino, A., Calagna, G., Saitta, S., De Franciscis, P., Colacurci, N., et al. (2015). Gonadotrophin-releasing hormone analogue or dienogest plus estradiol valerate to prevent pain recurrence after laparoscopic surgery for endometriosis: a multi-center randomized trial. *Acta Obstet. Gynecol. Scand.* 94, 637–645. doi: 10.1111/aogs.12633

Huang, Y., Shen, L., Cai, A., and Xiao, J. (2015). Effect of warming Yang and removing blood stasis method on matrix metalloproteinases/tissue inhibitor metalloproteinases levels secreted by cultured endometrial cells from patients with endometriosis. *J. Tradit. Chin. Med.* 35, 571–576. doi: 10.1016/S0254-6272(15)30141-2

Jana, S., Chatterjee, K., Ray, A. K., DasMahapatra, P., and Swarnakar, S. (2016). Regulation of matrix metalloproteinase-2 activity by COX-2-PGE2-pAKT axis promotes angiogenesis in endometriosis. *PLoS One* 11:e0163540. doi: 10.1371/journal.pone.0163540

Jiang, L., Pan, C. L., Wang, C. Y., Liu, B. Q., Han, Y., Hu, L., et al. (2017). Selective suppression of the JNK-MMP2/9 signal pathway by tetramethylpyrazine attenuates neuropathic pain in rats. *J. Neuroinflamm.* 14:174. doi: 10.1186/s12974-017-0947-x

Kim, J. H., Woo, J. H., Kim, H. M., Oh, M. S., Jang, D. S., and Choi, J. H. (2017). Anti-endometriotic effects of pueraria flower extract in human endometriotic cells and mice. *Nutrients* 9:212. doi: 10.3390/nu9030212

Leavy, O. (2015). Reproductive immunology evading immunosurveillance in endometriosis. *Nat. Rev. Immunol.* 15, 729–729. doi: 10.1038/nri3942

Li, F., Lv, Y. N., Tan, Y. S., Shen, K., Zhai, K. F., Chen, H. L., et al. (2015). An integrated pathway interaction network for the combination of four effective compounds from ShengMai preparations in the treatment of cardio-cerebral ischemic diseases. *Acta Pharmacol. Sin.* 36, 1337–1348. doi: 10.1038/aps.2015.70

Li, Z., Liu, H., He, Z., Zhang, G., and Lang, J. (2016). Effects of cisplatin and letrozole on surgically induced endometriosis and comparison of the two medications in a rat model. *Eur. J. Pharm. Sci.* 93, 132–140. doi: 10.1016/j.ejps.2016.07.018

Li, Z., Takino, T., Endo, Y., and Sato, H. (2017). Activation of MMP-9 by membrane type-1 MMP/MMP-2 axis stimulates tumor metastasis. *Cancer Sci.* 108, 347–353. doi: 10.1111/cas.13134

Liang, Q. Q., Ding, D. F., Xi, Z. J., Chen, Y., Li, C. G., Liu, S. F., et al. (2014). Protective effect of ligustrazine on lumbar intervertebral disc degeneration of rats induced by prolonged upright posture. *Evid. Based Complement. Alternat. Med.* 2014:508461. doi: 10.1155/2014/508461

Luan, Y., Liu, J. L., Liu, X. L., Xue, X., Kong, F., Sun, C., et al. (2016). Tetramethypyrazine inhibits renal cell carcinoma cells through inhibition of NKG2D signaling pathways. *Int. J. Oncol.* 49, 1704–1712. doi: 10.3892/ijo.2016.3670

Ma, X., Hui, Y., Lin, L., Wu, Y., Zhang, X., and Qin, X. (2016). Possible relevance of tumor-related genes mutation to malignant transformation of endometriosis. *Eur. J. Gynaecol. Oncol.* 37, 89–94.

Mao, X. W., Pan, C. S., Huang, P., Liu, Y. Y., Wang, C. S., Yan, L., et al. (2015). Levo-tetrahydropalmatine attenuates mouse blood-brain barrier injury induced by focal cerebral ischemia and reperfusion: involvement of Src kinase. *Sci. Rep.* 5:11155. doi: 10.1038/srep11155

Mihailovici, A., Rottenstreich, M., Kovel, S., Wassermann, I., Smorgick, N., and Vaknin, Z. (2017). Endometriosis-associated malignant transformation in abdominal surgical scar: a PRISMA-compliant systematic review. *Medicine (Baltimore)* 96:e9136. doi: 10.1097/MD.0000000000009136

Ning, K., Zhao, X., Poetsch, A., Chen, W. H., and Yang, J. (2017). Computational molecular networks and network pharmacology. *Biomed. Res. Int.* 2017:7573904. doi: 10.1155/2017/7573904

Pinar, N., Karapinar, O. S., Ozcan, O., Ozgur, T., and Bayraktar, S. (2017). Effect of alpha-lipoic acid on endometrial implants in an experimental rat model. *Fundam. Clin. Pharmacol.* 31, 506–512. doi: 10.1111/fcp.12293

Raga, F., Casan, E. M., Wen, Y., Huang, H. Y., Bonilla-Musoles, F., and Polan, M. L. (1999). Independent regulation of matrix metalloproteinase-9, tissue inhibitor of metalloproteinase-1 (TIMP-1), and TIMP-3 in human endometrial stromal cells by gonadotropin-releasing hormone: implications in early human implantation. *J. Clin. Endocrinol. Metab.* 84, 636–642. doi: 10.1210/jcem.84.2.5464

Shan, J., Cheng, W., Zhai, D. X., Zhang, D. Y., Yao, R. P., Bai, L. L., et al. (2017). Meta-analysis of chinese traditional medicine bushen huoxue prescription for endometriosis treatment. *Evid. Based Complement Alternat. Med.* 2017:5416423. doi: 10.1155/2017/5416423

Simmen, R. C., and Kelley, A. S. (2016). Reversal of fortune: estrogen receptor-beta in endometriosis. *J. Mol. Endocrinol.* 57, F23–F27. doi: 10.1530/JME-16-0080

Szklarczyk, D., Franceschini, A., Kuhn, M., Simonovic, M., Roth, A., Minguez, P., et al. (2011). The STRING database in 2011: functional interaction networks of proteins, globally integrated and scored. *Nucleic Acids Res.* 39(Database issue), D561–D568. doi: 10.1093/nar/gkq973

Szymanowski, K., Mikolajczyk, M., Wirstlein, P., and Dera-Szymanowska, A. (2016). Matrix metalloproteinase-2 (MMP-2), MMP-9, tissue inhibitor of matrix metalloproteinases (TIMP-1) and transforming growth factor-beta2 (TGF-beta2) expression in eutopic endometrium of women with peritoneal endometriosis. *Ann. Agric. Environ. Med.* 23, 649–653. doi: 10.5604/12321966.1226861

Tang, F., Tang, Q., Tian, Y., Fan, Q., Huang, Y., and Tan, X. (2015). Network pharmacology-based prediction of the active ingredients and potential targets of Mahuang Fuzi Xixin decoction for application to allergic rhinitis. *J. Ethnopharmacol.* 176, 402–412. doi: 10.1016/j.jep.2015.10.040

Tang, H., He, S., Zhang, X., Luo, S., Zhang, B., Duan, X., et al. (2016). A network pharmacology approach to uncover the pharmacological mechanism of xuanhusuo powder on osteoarthritis. *Evid. Based Complement Alternat. Med.* 2016:3246946. doi: 10.1155/2016/3246946

Tang, Q., Shang, F. H., Wang, X. C., Yang, Y., Chen, G., Chen, Y., et al. (2014). Combination use of ferulic acid, ligustrazine and tetrahydropalmatine inhibits the growth of ectopic endometrial tissue: a multi-target therapy for endometriosis rats. *J. Ethnopharmacol.* 151, 1218–1225. doi: 10.1016/j.jep.2013.12.047

Thiery, J. P., Acloque, H., Huang, R. Y., and Nieto, M. A. (2009). Epithelial-mesenchymal transitions in development and disease. *Cell* 139, 871–890. doi: 10.1016/j.cell.2009.11.007

Tosti, C., Biscione, A., Morgante, G., Bifulco, G., Luisi, S., and Petraglia, F. (2017). Hormonal therapy for endometriosis: from molecular research to bedside. *Eur. J. Obstet. Gynecol. Reprod. Biol.* 209, 61–66. doi: 10.1016/j.ejogrb.2016.05.032

Voloshenyuk, T. G., and Gardner, J. D. (2010). Estrogen improves TIMP-MMP balance and collagen distribution in volume-overloaded hearts of ovariectomized females. *Am. J. Physiol. Regul. Integr. Compar. Physiol.* 299, R683–R693. doi: 10.1152/ajpregu.00162.2010

Wang, C., Zhang, J., Fok, K. L., Tsang, L. L., Ye, M., Liu, J., et al. (2018). CD147 induces epithelial-to-mesenchymal transition by disassembling CAS/E-cadherin/beta-catenin complex in human endometriosis. *Am. J. Pathol.* 188, 1597–1607. doi: 10.1016/j.ajpath.2018.03.004 doi: 10.1016/j.ajpath.2018.03.004

Wang, J., Qu, T. B., Chu, L. S., Li, L., Ren, C. C., Sun, S. Q., et al. (2016). Ligustrazine promoted the migration of bone marrow mesenchymal stem cells by up-regulating MMP-2 and MMP-9 expressions. *Zhongguo Zhong Xi Yi Jie He Za Zhi* 36, 718–723.

Wang, Y., Lin, W., Li, C., Singhal, S., Jain, G., Zhu, L., et al. (2017). Multipronged therapeutic effects of chinese herbal medicine qishenyiqi in the treatment of acute myocardial infarction. *Front. Pharmacol.* 8:98. doi: 10.3389/fphar.2017.00098

Wei, M. G., Sun, W., He, W. M., Ni, L., and Yang, Y. Y. (2015). Ferulic acid attenuates TGF-beta1-induced renal cellular fibrosis in NRK-52E cells by inhibiting smad/ILK/snail pathway. *Evid. Based Complement Alternat. Med.* 2015:619720. doi: 10.1155/2015/619720

Wen, Y., Wang, Y., Feng, T.T., and Wei, S. B. (2017). Differential proteomics analysis of endometriosis in blood stasis syndrome. *Chin J Integr Med.* doi: 10.1007/s11655-017-2401-4 [Epub ahead of print].

Wu, R. F., Huang, Z. X., Ran, J., Dai, S. J., Lin, D. C., Ng, T. W., et al. (2018). Lipoxin A4 suppresses estrogen-induced epithelial-mesenchymal transition via ALXR-dependent manner in endometriosis. *Reprod. Sci.* 25, 566–578. doi: 10.1177/1933719117718271

Yang, Y. N., Wang, F., Zhou, W., Wu, Z. Q., and Xing, Y. Q. (2012). TNF-alpha stimulates MMP-2 and MMP-9 activities in human corneal epithelial cells via the activation of FAK/ERK signaling. *Ophthalmic Res.* 48, 165–170. doi: 10.1159/000338819

Yi, K. W., Kim, S. H., Ihm, H. J., Oh, Y. S., Chae, H. D., Kim, C. H., et al. (2015). Increased expression of p21-activated kinase 4 in adenomyosis and its regulation of matrix metalloproteinase-2 and-9 in endometrial cells. *Fertil. Steril.* 103, U1089–U1303. doi: 10.1016/j.fertnstert.2014.12.124

Yodkeeree, S., Wongsirisin, P., Pompimon, W., and Limtrakul, P. (2013). Anti-invasion effect of crebanine and O-methylbulbocapnine from *Stephania venosa* via down-regulated matrix metalloproteinases and urokinase plasminogen activator. *Chem. Pharm. Bull. (Tokyo)* 61, 1156–1165. doi: 10.1248/cpb.c13-00584

Zhang, H., Niu, Y. D., Feng, J., Guo, H. F., Ye, X., and Cui, H. (2006). Use of proteomic analysis of endometriosis to identify different protein expression in patients with endometriosis versus normal controls. *Fertil. Steril.* 86, 274–282. doi: 10.1016/j.fertnstert.2006.01.028

Zhang, X., Lin, D., Jiang, R., Li, H., Wan, J., and Li, H. (2016). Ferulic acid exerts antitumor activity and inhibits metastasis in breast cancer cells by regulating epithelial to mesenchymal transition. *Oncol. Rep.* 36, 271–278. doi: 10.3892/or.2016.4804

Zhao, R.H. (2018). Strategies for activating blood circulation-regulating gan (Liver)-tonifying shen (Kidney) sequential therapy of endometriosis-associated infertility. *Chin. J Integr Med.* doi: 10.1007/s11655-018-2931-9 [Epub ahead of print].

Zheng, X. F., Carstens, J. L., Kim, J., Scheible, M., Kaye, J., Sugimoto, H., et al. (2015). Epithelial-to-mesenchymal transition is dispensable for metastasis but induces chemoresistance in pancreatic cancer. *Nature* 52, 525–530. doi: 10.1038/nature16064

11

Analysis of Antidepressant Activity of Huang-Lian Jie-Du Decoction Through Network Pharmacology and Metabolomics

Shu-Yue Qu[1†], *Xiao-Yue Li*[2†], *Xia Heng*[1], *Yi-Yu Qi*[1], *Ping-Yuan Ge*[1], *Sai-jia Ni*[2], *Zeng-Ying Yao*[2], *Rui Guo*[3], *Nian-Yun Yang*[1], *Yi Cao*[4], *Qi-Chun Zhang*[1,2]* *and Hua-Xu Zhu*[1]*

[1]*Jiangsu Key Laboratory for High Technology Research of TCM Formulae, Nanjing University of Chinese Medicine, Nanjing, China,* [2]*Jiangsu Key Laboratory for Pharmacology and Safety Evaluation of Chinese Materia Medica, School of Pharmacy, Nanjing University of Chinese Medicine, Nanjing, China,* [3]*School of Medicine and Holistic Integrative Medicine, Nanjing University of Chinese Medicine, Nanjing, China,* [4]*Institute of Literature in Chinese Medicine, Nanjing University of Chinese Medicine, Nanjing, China*

***Correspondence:**
Qi-Chun Zhang
zhangqichun@njucm.edu.cn
Hua-Xu Zhu
zhuhx@njucm.edu.cn

[†]*These authors have contributed equally to this work*

Depressive disorder is a common mental disorder characterized by depressed mood and loss of interest or pleasure. As the Herbal medicines are mainly used as complementary and alternative therapy for depression. This study aimed at exploring antidepressant activity of Huang-lian Jie-du Decoction (HLJDD), and evaluating active components and potential depression-associated targets. HLJDD was administered on chronic unpredictable mild stress-induced (CUMS) depressive mice. Behavior evaluation was performed through force swimming test (FST), novelty-suppressed feeding test (NSF), and open field test (OFT). Active components of HLJDD, potential targets, and metabolic pathways involved in depression were explored through systemic biology-based network pharmacology assay, molecular docking and metabonomics. FST assay showed that CUMS mice administered with HLJDD had significantly shorter immobility time compared with control mice. Further, HLJDD alleviated feeding latency of CUMS mice in NSFand increased moving distance and duration in OFT. In the following network pharmacology assay, thirty-eight active compounds in HLJDD were identified based on drug-like characteristics, and pharmacokinetics and pharmacodynamics profiles. Moreover, forty-eight molecular targets and ten biochemical pathways were uncovered through molecular docking and metabonomics. GRIN2B, DRD, PRKCA, HTR, MAOA, SLC6A4, GRIN2A, and CACNA1A are implicated in inhibition of depressive symptoms through modulating tryptophan metabolism, serotonergic and dopaminergic synaptic activities, cAMP signaling pathway, and calcium signaling pathway. Further network pharmacology-based analysis showed a correlation between HLJDD and tryptophan metabolism. A total of thirty-seven active compounds, seventy-six targets, and sixteen biochemical pathways were involved in tryptophan metabolism. These findings show that HLJDD acts on potential targets such as SLC6A4, HTR, INS, MAO, CAT, and FoxO, PI3K/Akt, calcium, HIF-1, and mTOR signaling pathways, and modulates serotoninergic and dopaminergic synaptic functions. In addition, metabonomics showed that tryptophan metabolism is the primary target for HLJDD in CUMS mice. The findings of the study show that HLJDD exhibited antidepressant effects. SLC6A4 and MAOA in tryptophan metabolism were modulated by berberine, baicalein, tetrahydroberberine, candicine and may be the main antidepressant targets for HLJDD.

Keywords: network pharmacology, huang-lian jie-du decoction, depression, tryptophan metabolism, metabolomics

HIGHLIGHTS

1. HLJDD ameliorates the depression-like behaviors in CUMS-induced depressive mice.
2. Tryptophan metabolic plays a key role in underpinning the antidepressant effect of HLJDD.
3. SLC6A4 and MAOA are the most potential targets for HLJDD on depression.

INTRODUCTION

Major depressive disorder (MDD) is a common and severe mental disorder. MDD patients present with depressed mood, pessimistic thinking, loss of enjoyment in usual activities and lack of energy. Worldwide, more than 350 million people are suffering from depression (Ge et al., 2020; Wigner et al., 2018). World Health Organization reports that depression is a major cause of disabilities in the world. Depression reduces quality of life, increases risk of death at any age, and is a health burden on families and society (Guo et al., 2017).

Hypertension patients treated with reserpine often present with depression (Freis, 1954), therefore, Joseph Schildkraut proposed the monoamine hypothesis of depression in 1965. Compounds targeting 5-HT metabolism have antidepressant activity. Newly synthesized 5-HT from tryptophan is transported into synaptic vesicles within presynaptic neurons. Upon stimulation, 5-HT is released from vesicles into the synaptic space where it interacts with several postsynaptic and presynaptic serotonin receptors. Transportation of 5-HT back into presynaptic neurons by SLC6A4 or breakdown of 5-HT into 5-hydroxyindoleacetic acid by MAOA terminates activity of 5-HT.

Although more than a dozen antidepressants are available, most individuals with depression do not respond to these treatments. Most antidepressants are associated with unfavorable long-term outcomes and paradoxical effects, such as induction of depression, worsening of symptoms and withdrawal symptoms (Chouinard and Chouinard, 2015; Fava, 2003). Multi-target chemicals such as paroxetine and vortioxetine

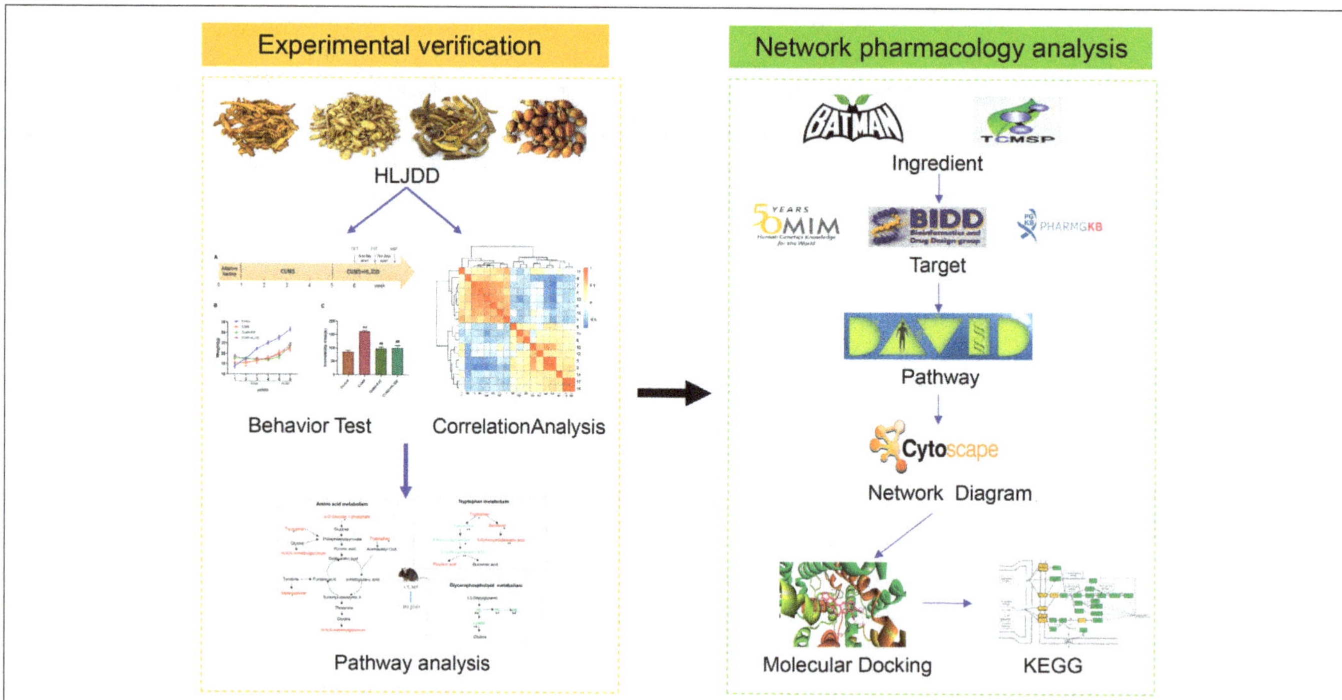

GRAPHICAL ABSTRACT | Antidepressant mechanism of HLJDD.

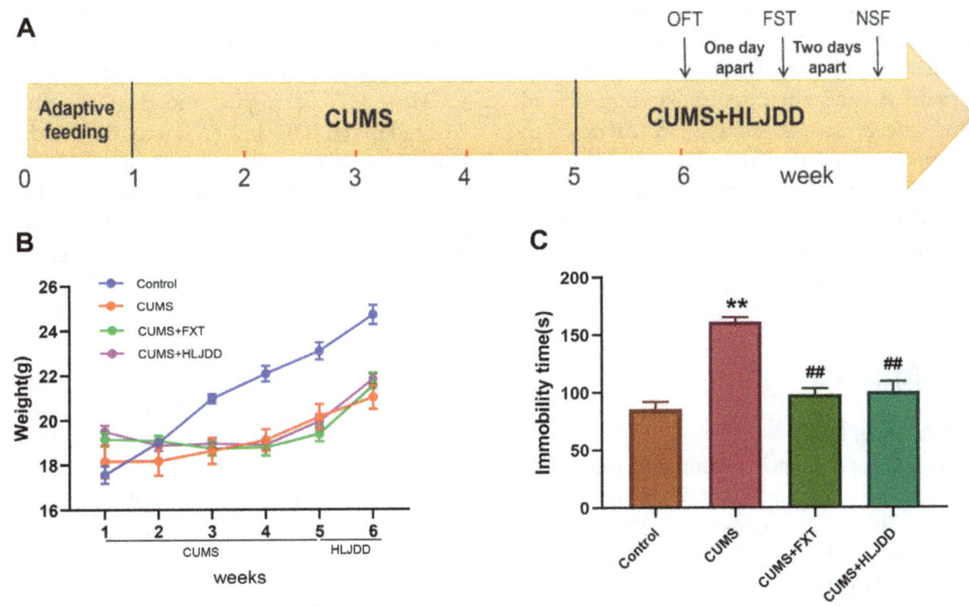

FIGURE 1 | FST results showing effect of HLJDD on behavior of CUMS mice. **(A)** Schematic diagram of the experimental process; **(B)** Body weight of mice in the control group and mice in HLJDD or FXT treatment groups after six weeks (n = 10, Mean ± SEM); **(C)** Immobility time of mice in the control group and HLJDD or FXT treated groups after carrying out FST 1 h after treatment (n = 10, Mean ± SEM). $^{*}p < 0.05$, $^{**}p < 0.01$, compared with Control; $^{\#\#}p < 0.01$, compared with CUMS via ANOVA.

have been developed to reduce side effects, intolerance and improve efficacy of antidepressant drugs (Bang-Andersen et al., 2011; Cipriani et al., 2018). Use of natural products that contain diverse chemical components and acceptable tolerance following long-term administration can be used as alternative therapy against depression.

In addition to use of complementary and alternative medicine as prophylactic interventions or treatments as, there is increased interest in use of Chinese herbal medicine for depression treatment. Huang-lian Jie-du decoction (HLJDD), is a well-known Chinese herbal initially recorded in Prescriptions for Emergent Reference over 1500 years ago (Zhouhou Beiji Fang, A.D. 341). HLJDD has heat dissipation and detoxification activities (Dai et al., 2018). It is a mixture of Coptis chinensis Franch, Scutellaria baicalensis Georgi, Phellodendron amurense Ruer and Gardenia jasminoides J. Ellis herbs with a weight ratio of 3:2:2:3. HLJDD is used for treatment of symptoms caused by heat toxins (Yue et al., 2014). Several studies report that HLJDD ameliorates multiple central nervous system diseases such as cerebral ischemia, Alzheimer's disease (AD) and mental disorder (Liu et al., 2019; Okamoto et al., 2013; Wang et al., 2013). The formula modulates monoamine metabolism and kynureninet metabolism which are both implicated in pathogenesis of depressive syndromes (Sasaki et al., 2000; Yu et al., 2015). Active components of the formulation such as berberine and baicalin exhibit antidepressant activities (Lee et al., 2012; Zhang et al., 2016). HLJDD is believed to improve depression through synergistic activities of the active components. However, specific relationships between depression and HLJDD, and potential mechanisms of action of specific components have not been fully elucidated.

Network pharmacology is an emerging approach for evaluating systematic mechanism of action for multi-target drugs based on biological network associating with a disease. The approach is used to explore biological basis of herbal formulae and bioactive ingredients present. Several herbal formulae for treatment of neurological or mental disorders have been developed through network pharmacology (Zhang et al., 2019). HLJDD modulates ischemic stroke through "shotgun-like" pharmacological mechanism (Wang et al., 2019). Tian-Ma-Gou-Teng-Yin ameliorates Alzheimer's disease through neuroprotective and anti-neuroinflammatory activities (Wang et al., 2018). Key active compounds and antidepressant mechanism Xiao-Yao-San in treatment of depression were explored through network pharmacology (Liu et al., 2020).

In this study, experience-based approach and evidence-based assay were used to explore antidepressant activities of HLJDD, a traditional Chinese medicine formula. We explored the symptoms for depression in CUMS-induced depressive animal model after treatment with HLJDD. Further, network pharmacology assay using bioinformatics tools, systems biology, and polypharmacology was performed to determine genes, proteins, and signaling pathways implicated in activity of HLJDD against depression (Zhang et al., 2019). Currently, application of network pharmacology successfully integrates systematic information on herbal medicines or formulas of TCM for various diseases (Zhang et al., 2019; Ge et al., 2020). Findings of this study indicate that HLJDD ameliorates depressive-like behaviors in CUMS mice. In addition, the formulation modulates serotonergic synapse function and tryptophan metabolism. Further, we determined interactions between candidate chemicals and their molecular targets and analyzed their binding energy scores. Finally, we carried out metabonomics analysis to verify underlying mechanisms of action for HLJDD against depression in mice. Findings of the study show that tryptophan metabolism is the main target for HLJDD. This information provides a basis to design and develop novel plant-based therapies against depression.

ANIMAL EXPERIMENTS

Chemicals and Materials

Rhizome Coptis (Coptis chinensis Franch., Ranunculaceae; batch number, 1711028050), RadixScutellariae (Scutellaria baicalensis Georgi, Lemnaceae; batch number, 1709019024), CortexPhellodendri amurensis (Phellodendron amurense Ruer., Rutaceae; batch number, 1709016005) and Fructus Gardeniae (Gardenia jasminoides Ellis., Rutaceae; batch number, 1711018022) were purchased from Fu Chun Tong Chinese Herbal Pieces Co., Ltd. (Anhui, China). Herbal materials were authenticated by Dr Qinan Wu (Professor of Pharmacognosy, College of Pharmacy, Nanjing University of Chinese Medicine, Nanjing, China). A voucher number was assigned to each specimen and voucher specimens were deposited in Nanjing University of Chinese Medicine. Fluoxetine HCL (FXT) was purchased from Beijing Yinuokai Technology Co., Ltd. (Beijing, China).

Preparation of Huang-Lian Jie-Du Decoction Extract

HLJDD extract was prepared according to a protocol described in our previous study (Zeng et al., 2010). Coptis chinensis Franch (270 g), Scutellaria baicalensis Georgi (180 g), Phellodendron amurense Ruer (180 g) and Phellodendron amurense Ruer (270 g) mixture was soaked in 9 L of distilled water for 1 h and then refluxed for 1.5 h. Dregs of the herbs were refluxed again in 7.2 L of water for 1 h. The two supernatants were mixed and filtered using gauze. The supernatant was concentrated to 1 L using a rotary evaporator. Further, the supernatant was frozen at −80°C for 12 h. The frozen was lyophilized using a freeze dryer resulting to 222 g of lyophilized powder. Analysis of the constituents of HLJDD was carried out using HPLC with berberine, baicalin and geniposide as standards (Agilent 1260, United States). Peak areas of the samples were substituted into a standard curve, and the abundances of berberine, baicalin, and geniposide in HLJDD were 7.67%, 11.46%, 2.42% respectively. HLJDD powder used for administration to mice was suspended in 0.50% carboxymethyl cellulose sodium salt (CMC-Na) aqueous solution.

Animals

SPF male C57BL/6 mice, weighing 18–22 g (Animal Multiplication Center of Qigong Mountain, Nanjing, China), were housed in a animal laboratory with regulated temperature and humidity of 25 ± 1°C and 60 ± 5%, respectively. Animal were acclimatized for a week and randomly divided into 4 groups: control group, model group (CUMS), fluoxetine hydrochloride group (CUMS + FXT, 20 mg/kg) and HLJDD group (CUMS + HLJDD, 590 mg/kg). HLJDD and FXT were dissolved in 0.5% CMC-Na. A total of 20 ml/kg body weight for both HLJDD and FXT was administered orally every week. Mice in the control and model group were given 0.5% CMC-Na. HLJDD dosage was calculated using dosage conversion relationship between mice and human and clinical dosage of HLJDD extract. Behavioral experiment was performed 1 h after the last administration and data were analyzed using Video Analysis System for Animal Behavior (JL, Shanghai, PRC). The study was carried out following recommendations provided by Guide for the Care and Use of Laboratory Animals of the National Institutes of Health (NIH Publication No. 80–23; revised 1978). The Animal Care and Use Committee of Nanjing University of Chinese Medicine approved the protocol and total number of mice used in this study.

Chronic Unpredictable Mild Stress Model of Depression

Chronic unpredictable mild stress (CUMS) mice model is developed by exposing animals to a set of unpredictable mild stressors for several weeks to induce depression-like phenotypes (Wu et al., 2012). In this study, mice were subjected to CUMS for 4 weeks using food deprivation (24 h), water deprivation (24 h), cage tilting at 45° without bedding (24 h), dampening sawdust with 125 ml of clean water (24 h), removing sawdust from the cage (24 h), subjecting animals to cold swim (4°C, 5 min), hot environment (45°C, 5 min), tail clip (2 min, 1 cm from the distal portion of the tail), physical restraint (2 h) and shaking the cage (40 min) as stressors. Each animal was exposed to two of the ten mentioned stressors each day. Induction of depression using different stressors was randomized. After subjection to stressors for each day, mice were placed in clean cages and returned to the housing facility.

Forced Swim Test

Mice exhibits behavioral despair under unavoidable stressors, which is similar to MDD phenotypes in human (Steru et al., 1985). Forced swim test (FST) is used for determination of efficacy of antidepressant treatments (Rubio et al., 2006). CUMS mice models were housed in the experimental room 2 h before the test for acclimatization. Oral administrations of the treatment and control were carried out 60 min before starting FST. FST was carried out by placing each animal at a depth of 10 cm in an open cylindrical container (12 cm diameter ×25 cm height) containing water (25 ± 1°C). Mice were not allowed to touch the bottom of the cylinder. Each animal was allowed a 6-min swim test session. Swimming behavior of each animal was recorded, and the last 4 min of the session analyzed.

Novelty-Suppressed Feeding Test

Novelty-suppressed feeding test (NSF) is an effective behavioral paradigm commonly used to evaluate depression-like behaviors in experimental animals after fasting. The test uses the conflict between feeding and fear of a novel environment (Dulawa and Hen, 2005). After subjecting mice to fasting for 24 h, they were acclimatized in the testing room f overnight. A platform with food pellets was placed at the center of a square open box (40 × 40 × 35 cm, length × width × height). Each animal was placed in the test apparatus and the same position and direction to the platform was maintained. Time taken for each animal to eat the food pellet (bite the food pellet with use of forepaws while sitting on its haunches) was recorded during the 5 min run time.

Open Field Test

Open field test (OFT) is used to measure of exploratory behavior, locomotor activity and general depressive-like activity (Bai et al., 2012). Mice were transported to the experimental room 2 h prior to the test to adapt to the environment. OFT apparatus was constructed using four cubic boxes (40 × 40 × 40 cm, length × width × height) made of blue plastic material leaving the top open. The bottom of each arena was divided into 16 square lattices. Mice were placed at the center of the arena 1 h after administration with HLJDD, FXT or vehicle. Mice were allowed to explore the arena for 5 min. Time taken for central movement, distance moved at the center, total duration and total distance of movement of CUMS mice were recorded and analyzed using automated video tracking to evaluate exploratory behavior and response to novelty.

Neurotransmitters Assay

Neurotransmitters including γ-aminobutyric acid (GABA), glutamic acid (Glu), 5-hydroxytryptamine (5-HT), dopamine (DA) and acetylcholine (Ach) in the hippocampus, cortex, striatum and amygdala were determined using LC-MS/MS. Accurately weighed cerebral tissues were added to 10-fold volume of 0.1% formic acid and completely homogenized for 3 min. 100 μL of the homogenate were added to 200 μL 0.2% formic acid acetonitrile, vortexed for 3 min and centrifuged at 12,000 rpm at 4°C for 10 min. Supernatants were concentrated and reconstituted with 0.1% formic acid.

A 2.1 mm × 100 mm, 2.7 μm chromatographic column (Infinity Lab Poroshell 120 EC-C18 , Agilent, United States) was used. Other chromatographic conditions were; mobile phase consisting of A, 0.1% formic acid in water, and B, acetonitrile; column temperature, 30°C; flow rate: 300 μL/min; injection volume, 2 μL; gradient elution conditions, 0–2 min, 98–95% A; 2–3.5 min, 95–40% A; 3.5–4 min, 40–98% A; 4–6.1 min, 98% **A**. Ionization source conditions were capillary voltage, 3.0 kV; sampling cone voltage, 30.0 V; source temperature, 150°C and desolvation temperature, 500°C.

Statistical Analyses

Data were presented as mean ± SD. Analysis of variance (ANOVA with a Fisher's LSD test) was carried out to determine differences between groups. $p < 0.05$ was considered statistically significant. Data analysis was carried out using SPSS 17.0 software.

NETWORK PHARMACOLOGY ANALYSIS

Databases and Software

TCMSP database (http://lsp.nwu.edu.cn/tcmsp.php), BATMAN-TCM database (http://bionet.ncpsb.org/batman-tcm/), PharmMapper database (http://lilab-ecust.cn/pharmmapper/index.html), OMIM database (http://www.omim.org), PharmGkb database (https://www.pharmgkb.org/), TTD (http://bidd.nus.edu.sg/BIDD- Databases/TTD/TTD.asp), System Dock database Site database (http://systemsdock.unit.oist.jp), String Version 10.5 server (https://string-db.org/), RCSB PDB database (http://www.rcsb.org/pdb/home/home. do), DAVID database (https://david.ncifcrf.gov/) and Pubchem database (https://pubchem.ncbi.nlm.nih. gov) were used for network pharmacology analysis. Cytoscape 3.8.0 software was used to construct an interaction network. AutoDock Vina software was used to predict the binding mode and binding energy scores between active compounds and molecular targets.

Screening of Chemical Ingredients

Active compounds were screened using TCMSP and BATMAN-TCM databases. TCMSP was used to predict ADME/T and other biological, chemical and physical parameters of active compounds using mathematical and computational models. SysDT model is used to find relevant targets, map diseases, tissues and organs, and to predict drug efficacy and toxicity mechanism (Ru et al., 2014). BATMAN-TCM database is an online tool for study of molecular mechanisms of traditional Chinese medicine. BATMAN-TCM compares submitted herbs to a list of reference ingredients saved in the database, to predict targets for the new ingredients (Liu et al., 2016). In this study, components of HLJDD Huangshan (Coptis chinensis Franch), Huangqin (Scutellaria baicalensis Georgi Scutellaria baicalensis Georgi), Huanghai (Phellodendron amurense Ruer), Zhizi (Gardenia jasminoides J. Ellis) were submitted to BATMAN-TCM and TCMSP database. Active compounds with a Score ≥20 and p-value ≤ 0.05 in BATMAN-TCM were selected. Oral bioavailability (OB) ≥ 30% and drug-likeness (DL) ≥ 0.18 parameters in TCMSP were used to screen BATMAN-TCM results. The final cluster of chemical ingredients of HLJDD was a combination of BATMAN-TCM and TCMSP results.

Screening Ingredient-Related Targets

Targets of the active compounds were predicted using BATMAN-TCM, TCMSP and PharmMapper databases. PharmMapper Server is an open-source web-server for identification of potential target for small molecules (drugs, natural products, or newly discovered compounds with unknown binding targets) using pharmacophore mapping approach (Liu et al., 2010). 3D structural SDF format (.sdf) of these candidate active ingredients of HLJDD were downloaded from PubChem database and submitted to PharmMapper for identification of potential targets.

Screening Disease-Associated Targets

OMIM database, TTD database, and PharmGkb database were used for identification of potential targets implicated in depression and tryptophan metabolism. Depressive, antidepressant, depressed, depression for depressive symptoms analysis, and tryptophan, and tryptophan metabolism for tryptophan metabolism assay were used as keywords in the three databases and *Homo sapiens* targets were selected for study.

Gene Ontology and Kyoto Encyclopedia Genes Genomes Enrichment Analysis

Gene Ontology (GO) and Kyoto Encyclopedia of Genes and Genomes (KEGG) were used to analyze signaling pathways and bioprocesses associated with depression that are modulated by HLJDD. Moreover, targets implicated in HLJDD activity and tryptophan metabolism were selected for enrichment assay. Enrichment assay was used to predict possible association between HLJDD and tryptophan metabolism. Further, predicted targets were submitted to DAVID database. OFFICIAL_GENE_SYMBOL item gene list were selected for analysis. GO enrichment analysis was performed together with KEGG pathways analysis.

Network Diagram Construction

Data files and attribute files of compound-target interaction, target-pathway of depressive disorders and tryptophan metabolism were saved in Microsoft Excel. Data files were subsequently imported to Cytoscape 3.2.1 software and ingredient-target interaction networks for depression and tryptophan metabolism constructed.

Protein-Protein Interaction and Molecular Docking

Interaction network for screened target proteins implicated in depression and tryptophan metabolism was constructed using String database. Top five important targets in the interaction network were selected for molecular docking. Molecular docking was used to predict interactions between protein receptors and HLJDD active compounds. Five important targets and related active compounds were selected using Dock website database for molecular docking. Molecular docking was performed by uploading the PDB ID of each target and 3D structure of active ingredients in SDF (.sdf) format. A cutoff value of 4.25 was set for the binding energy score to ensure good binding affinity of active compounds against selected targets. Binding energy scores greater than 5.0 implied stronger binding affinity. Moreover, molecular docking was carried out using AutoDock Vina (Trott and Olson, 2010). AutoDock Vina allows the ligand to be flexible whereas the target is rigid during molecular docking. Box center coordinates and size of the box were determined prior to docking experiments using. Binding energy for each active compound was determined using AutoDock Vina tool.

METABONOMICS ANALYSIS

Collection and Processing of Biological Samples

Mice were sacrificed with carbon dioxide immediately after behavioral assay. *Hippocampus* of each animal was isolated and frozen separately in liquid nitrogen. *Hippocampus* sample to be analyzed using LC-Q/TOF-MS was accurately weighed. ddH_2O was added to the weighed hippocampus sample and homogenized for 3 min. 100 μL homogenate was added to ice-cold 80% methanol solution (containing 4 μg/mL L-2-chlorophenylalanine as internal standard) and vortexed for 3 min. The mixture wascentrifuged at 13,000 rpm for 15 min at 4°C. The supernatants were transferred to a centrifuge concentrator for concentration and drying. The concentrated supernatant was reconstituted with 0.1% formic acid.

Chromatographic Conditions

A 2.1 mm × 100 mm, 2.7 μm chromatographic column was used (InfinityLab Poroshell 120 EC-C18 , Agilent, United States). The mobile phase consisted of A and B, A, 0.1% formic acid in water, B, 0.1% formic acid in acetonitrile. The column temperature was set at 30°C; flow rate at 400 μL/min; injection volume at 5 μL and gradient elution conditions at 0–0.5 min, 1% B; 0.5–4 min, 1–20% B; 4–8 min, 20–100% B; 8–9 min, 100% B; 9–9.5 min, 100–1% B; 9.5–12 min, 1% **B**.

Mass Spectrometry Conditions

Electrospray ionization source in positive mode and negative mode was used for the mass spectrometer (AB SCIEX Triple TOF™ 5600). Ionization source conditions were capillary voltage set at 3.0 kV; source temperature set at 120°C; desolvation temperature set at 350°C set at sampling cone voltage set at 30 V; ion energy at 1.0 V; cone gas flow set at 50 L/h; desolvent gas flow set at 600 L/h and mass scanning range was 100 ~ 1000 m/z.

Data Processing and Analysis

Data were normalized using MarkerView software, and then imported into SIMCA 14.1 software. Principal component analysis (PCA) and orthogonal partial least-squares discrimination analysis (OPLS-DA) were performed after standardization. Potential different metabolites were screened using VIP >1.0, correlation coefficient | *p*(corr)| > 0.58, and those with no significant difference ($p > 0.05$) were excluded. Spectrum structure of each metabolite was obtained using HMDB database. Potential endogenous metabolites were determined using PeakView software. MetaboAnalyst 4.0 was used to predict metabolic pathways implicated in depression.

RESULTS

Effect of Huang-Lian Jie-Du Decoction on Behavior of Chronic Unpredictable Mild Stress Mice as Shown by Force Swimming Test

Details on CUMS operation and behavior analysis are shown in **Figure 1A**. CUMS stressed mice showed significantly lower

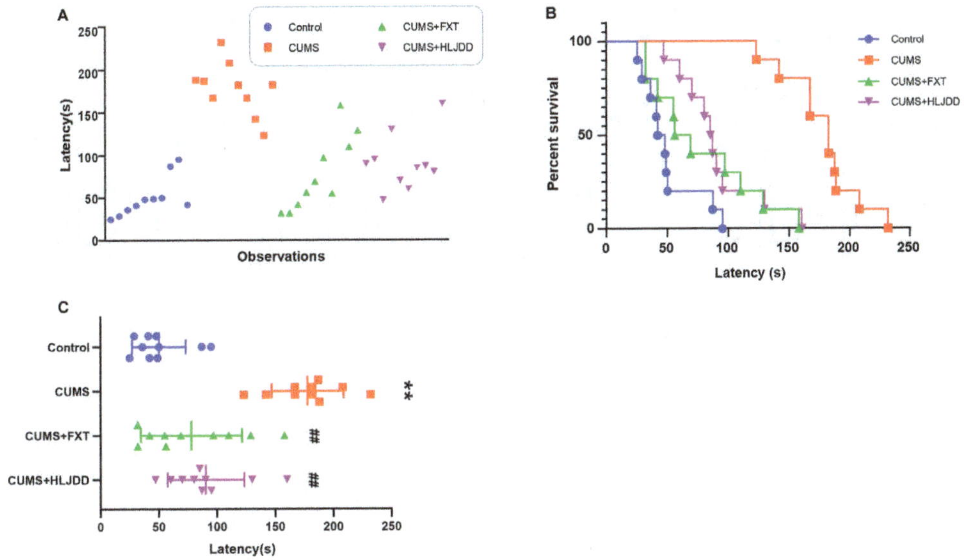

FIGURE 2 | NSF results showing effect of HLJDD on behavior of CUMS mice. **(A)** Individual response times for consuming food of mice in the three groups (*n* = 10); **(B)** Kaplan–Meier curves of latency in mice in the three groups (*n* = 10); **(C)** Latency of approaching and consuming food of mice in the three groups 1 h after administration (*n* = 10, Mean ± SEM). $^{**}p < 0.01$, compared with Control; $^{\#\#}p < 0.01$, compared with CUMS via ANOVA.

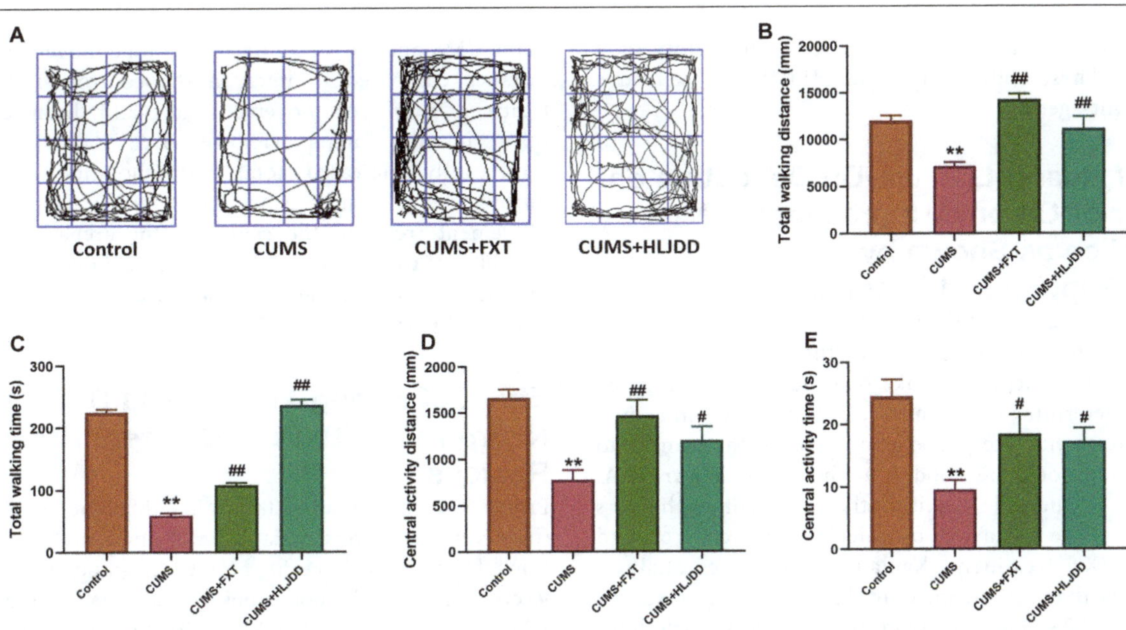

FIGURE 3 | OFT results showing effect of HLJDD on behavior of CUMS mice. **(A)** Trajectory of an individual mouse over a 5-min testing session in the OFT; **(B)** Total distance covered by mice in the three groups 1 h after treatment; **(C)** Total time of movement for mice in the three groups taken 1 h before the testing; **(D)** Distance covered by mice at the center of open field in all groups 1 h after oral gavage; **(E)** Time spent by mice to move at the center of arena with or without CUMS stress and CUMS mice with the treatment of HLJDD or FXT 1 h after oral gavage. Data are expressed as Mean ± SEM, *n* = 10 mice per group. $^{**}p < 0.01$, compared with Control; $^{\#}p < 0.05$, $^{\#\#}p < 0.01$, compared with CUMS via ANOVA.

body weight compared weight of mice in the control group ($p < 0.01$). One-week administration of HLJDD significantly increased weight in CUMS mice ($p < 0.01$) (**Figure 1B**). Mice in CUMS + HLJDD group exhibited shorter immobility time after one-week treatment with HLJDD as shown by FST results ($p < 0.01$). Mice in HLJDD and FXT

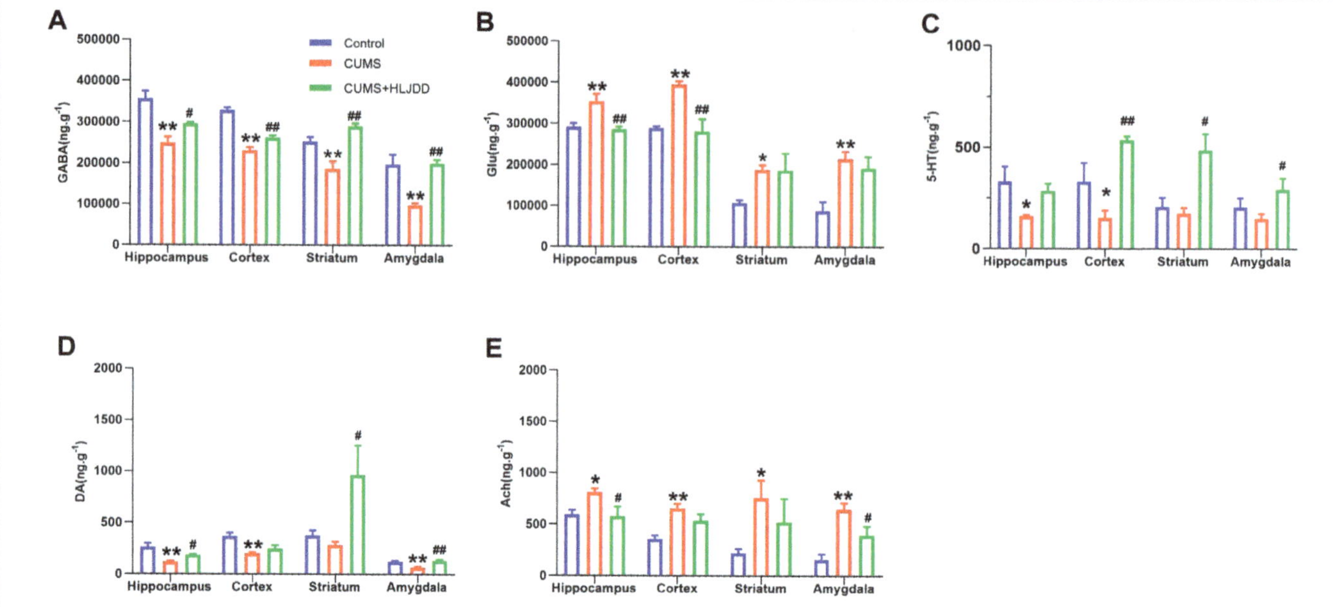

FIGURE 4 | Effect of HLJDD on neurotransmitters in different brain regions. Levels of GABA **(A)**, Glu **(B)**, 5-HT **(C)**, DA **(D)**, Ach **(E)** in the hippocampus, cortex, striatum and amygdala as detected using LC-MS/MS. Data are expressed as Mean ± SEM, $n = 10$ mice per group. *$p < 0.05$, **$p < 0.01$, compared with Control; #$p < 0.05$, ##$p < 0.01$, compared with CUMS via ANOVA.

groups showed no significant difference in immobility time (**Figure 1C**). These finding imply that HLJDD is an effective antidepressant agent.

Effect of Huang-Lian Jie-Du Decoction on Behavior of Chronic Unpredictable Mild Stress Mice as Shown by Novelty-Suppressed Feeding

The positive effect of HLJDD on behavior of CUMS mice shown by FST results prompted to further investigate effects of the formula on depressive-like behaviors. We conducted NSF test to determine aversion to eating by CUMS mice in a novel environment. Response times for each animal to approach and consume food are shown in **Figure 2A**. CUMS mice showed significantly different behaviors compared to the behavior of mice in the control and HLJDD or FXT treatment. Kaplan–Meier curves analyses demonstrated that 80% of mice in HLJDD group consumed food within 100 s. On the other hand, 80% CUMS mice without treatment consumed food in approximately 190 s (**Figure 2B**). Mice in HLJDD group showed significantly less time to consume food compared to mice in the control group ($p < 0.01$) (**Figure 2C**).

Effect of Huang-Lian Jie-Du Decoction on Behavior of Chronic Unpredictable Mild Stress Mice as Shown by Open Field Test

Mice with CUMS showed significantly shorter time and distance traveled in the center of open field. Further, OFT results showed that CUMS mice significantly shorter total movement time and distance compared to mice in the control group. HLJDD treatment improved movement time and distance taken by mice in the arena (**Figure 3A**). HLJDD treatment significantly increased total traveling time and distance during the 5-min session ($p < 0.01$) (**Figures 3B,C**). Movement trend in the center of the arena was observed. Notably, chronic HLJDD treatment significantly increased distance traveled at the center and travel duration of CUMS mice ($p < 0.05$) (**Figures 3D,E**).

Effect of Huang-Lian Jie-Du Decoction on Neurotransmitters in Different Brain Regions

Profile of neurotransmitters in different brain regions (hippocampus, cortex, striatum and amygdala) were analyzed using LC-MS/MS. Mice in the CUMS group showed reduced levels of GABA in hippocampus, cortex, striatum and amygdala. HLJDD restored GABA levels in the four brain regions (**Figure 4A**). On the contrary, CUMS mice showed higher Glu levels in hippocampus, cortex striatum and amygdala and HLJDD treatment significantly decreased Glu levels in hippocampus and cortex (**Figure 4B**). CUMS mice showed significantly lower 5-HT levels in hippocampus and cortex compared with the levels in mice in the control group. HLJDD administration improved 5-HT levels with a significant increase observed in cortex compared with the hippocampus. Although no significant difference in 5-HT was observed in striatum and amygdala of CUMS mice prior to treatment, HLJDD administration increased 5-HT levels in these two regions (**Figure 4C**). HLJDD administration restored

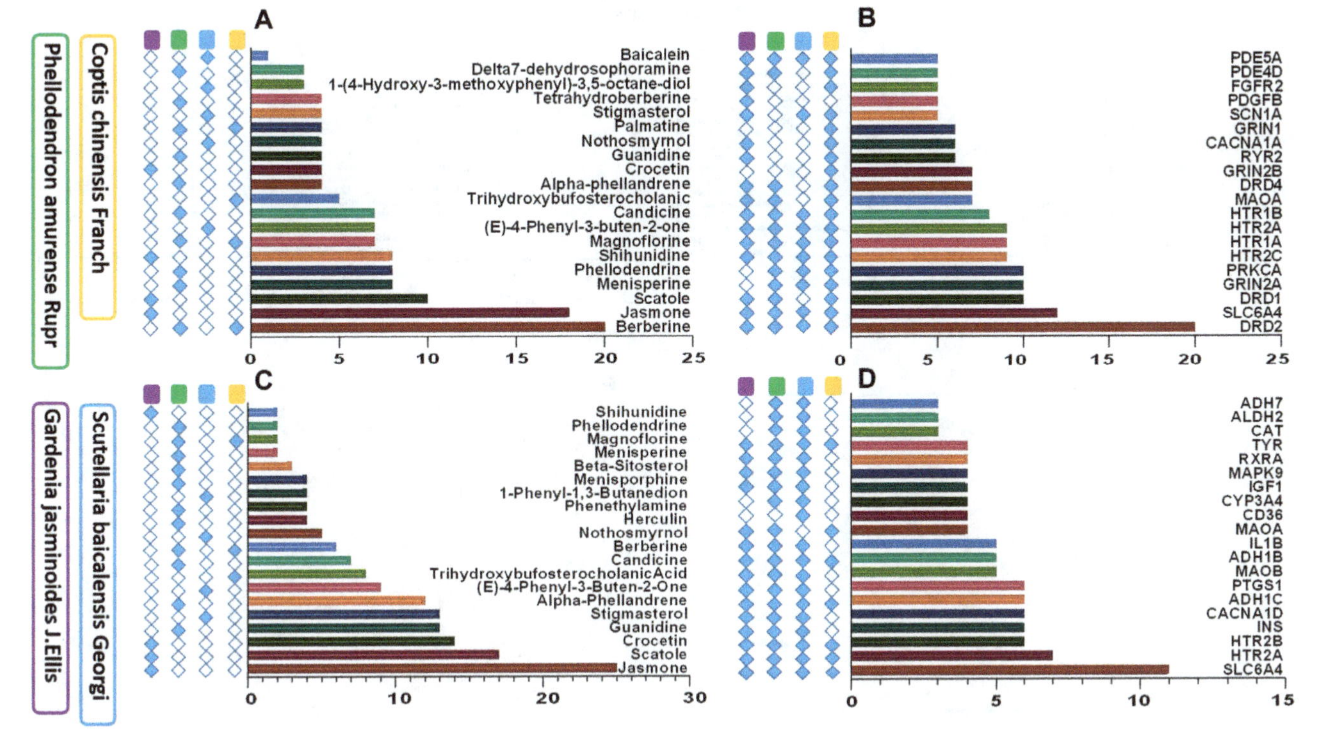

FIGURE 5 | Active compounds and targets of HLJDD against depression and tryptophan metabolism. **(A)** Active ingredients of HLJDD associated with depression; **(B)** HLJDD target proteins against depression; **(C)** Active compounds of HLJDD against tryptophan metabolism; **(D)** Target proteins of HLJDD associated with tryptophan metabolism.

DA levels in hippocampus, cortex, striatum and amygdala of CUMS mice. HJDD treatment significantly increased DA levels in the striatum (**Figure 4D**). Alternatively, HLJDD administration significantly lowered Ach levels in hippocampus and amygdala (**Figure 4E**).

Network Pharmacology Assay

Active Compounds and Targets of HLJDD on Depression and Tryptophan Metabolism

Area total of 1059 promising targets of HLJDD were identified after deleting duplicate targets within TCMSP, BATMAN-TCM and PharmMapper databases (161 with Coptis chinensis Franch; 684 with Scutellaria baicalensis Georgi; 612 with Phellodendron amurense Ruer, and 804 with Gardenia jasminoides J. Ellis). To explore the relationship between HLJDD and depression, 267 targets related to depressive disorders were retrieved from OMIM, TTD, and PharmGkb databases. area total of 48 common targets for HLJDD and depression were identified. Most common target proteins were D2 dopamine receptor (DRD2), Sodium-dependent serotonin transporter (SLC6A4), D1A dopamine receptor (DRD1), and Glutamate receptor ionotropic NMDA 2A (GRIN2A). A total of 67 active ingredients of HLJDD were correlated with the 48 proteins. A total of 38 active ingredients was shown to directly target the selected proteins. Common active compounds targeting the 48 proteins were Berberine, Jasmone, Skatole, Menisperine, Phellodendron, and Shihunidine. Top twenty depression-associated compounds and targets are listed in **Figures 5A,B**. A total of 1311 targets related to tryptophan metabolism were retrieved from OMIM, TTD, and PharmGkb databases. Out of these targets, 76 targets were common for HLJDD activity and tryptophan metabolism. Most frequently occurring target proteins were sodium-dependent serotonin transporter (SLC6A4), 5-hydroxytryptamine receptor 2A (HTR2A), 5-hydroxytryptamine receptor 2B (HTR2B) and voltage-dependent L-type calcium channel subunit alpha-1D (CACNA1D). A total of 67 active ingredients of HLJDD were implicated in binding of the selected 76 targets. Notably, a total of 37 active ingredients directly targeted the 76 target proteins. Common active ingredients against the 76 targets were Jasmone, Skatole, Crocetin, Guanidine, and Stigmasterol. These findings implied that tryptophan metabolism plays a key role in prognosis and treatment of depressive disorder. Top twenty tryptophan metabolism-associated active compounds and targets are shown in **Figures 5C,D**.

Gene Ontology Enrichment and Kyoto Encyclopedia Genes Genomes Pathways and Network Analysis of Targets Associated With Huang-Lian Jie-Du Decoction Activity on Depression

The 48 targets associated with HLJDD and depressive disorders were used for GO enrichment and KEGG pathway analysis using DAVID. Targets were analyzed under three levels, namely biological processes (BP), molecular function (MF) and cellular components (CC). Pathways that showed $p < 0.05$ were selected as potential pathways implicated in the activity of HLJDD against depression. Pathways identified under BP

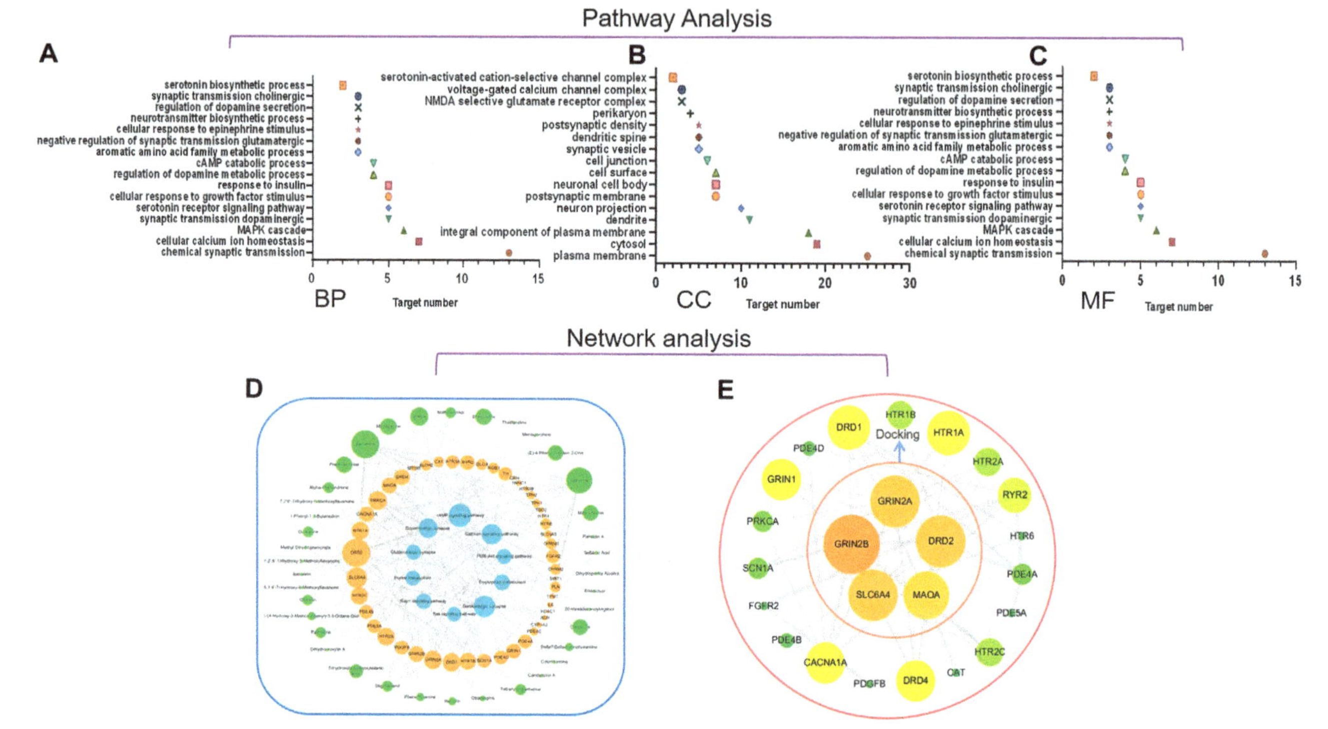

FIGURE 6 | (A–C) GO enrichment analysis of potential targets for primary active ingredients from HLJDD against depression. BP, biological process; CC, cellular components; MF, molecular function.; **(D)** HLJDD active compound-target-pathway network of depression; **(E)** Interaction network of HLJDD target proteins involved in depression.

category included serotonin receptor signaling pathway, serotonin biosynthetic process, neurotransmitter biosynthetic process and aromatic amino acid family metabolic process (**Figures 6A–C**). Two metabolic-related pathways, five signaling-related pathways and three synaptic-related pathways were identified suing In the KEGG pathway assay. These pathways are implicated in serotonergic synaptic and tryptophan metabolism pathway.

A compound-target-pathway network for active compounds in HLJDD implicated in treatment of depression was constructed using Cytoscape software (**Figure 6D**). The network showed 96 nodes with 48 of these nodes presented in orange. A larger the circle implied more active compounds and key pathways associated with depression. A total of 38 active ingredients were indicated in green, and 10 disease pathways were indicated in blue. Active compounds and pathways formed a complete network through 490 edge connections. Potential relationships between active compounds and targets or targets and pathways were expressed by edges. The degree represented the size of nodes, with a greater degree implying that the node plays a role in modulation of depression by HLJDD. Several active compounds were implicated in DRD1, DRD2, SLC6A4, and GRIN2A. Key pathways where these targets are involved in are cAMP signaling pathway, calcium signaling pathway, serotonergic synaptic pathway and dopaminergic synaptic pathway. Berberine had the most interactions as it interacted with twenty proteins and ten pathways.

In this study, interactions between anti-depressant targets and HLJDD active compounds were analyzed using String database. Interaction network of anti-depressant targets and HLJDD active compounds was constructed based on the degree value greater than medium of ranking. The network consisted of 24 nodes and 134 edges. Results were saved in TSV format and imported into Cytoscape for identification of key targets (**Figure 6E**). Higher degrees on nodes such as GRIN2B, GRIN2A, DRD2, SLC6A4, and MAOA implied that they play an important role in antidepressant activity.

Pathways and Network Analysis Huang-Lian Jie-Du Decoction Targets Associated With Tryptophan Metabolism

We further explored interaction network between HLJDD and tryptophan metabolism as tryptophan metabolism plays a key role in pathological process of depression. GO enrichment analysis and KEGG pathway analysis of the 76 targets involved in tryptophan metabolism was carried using DAVUD database. Pathways in which targets were implicated in were classified into three levels: BP, MF, and CC and those pathways with $p < 0.05$ were selected. Under the BP category pathways involved in drug response, regulation of insulin secretion and inflammatory response were identified. A total of 16 tryptophan metabolism-related pathways ($p < 0.05$) were screened in five categories using KEGG pathway analysis. Three pathways were metabolic-related pathways, nine were signaling-

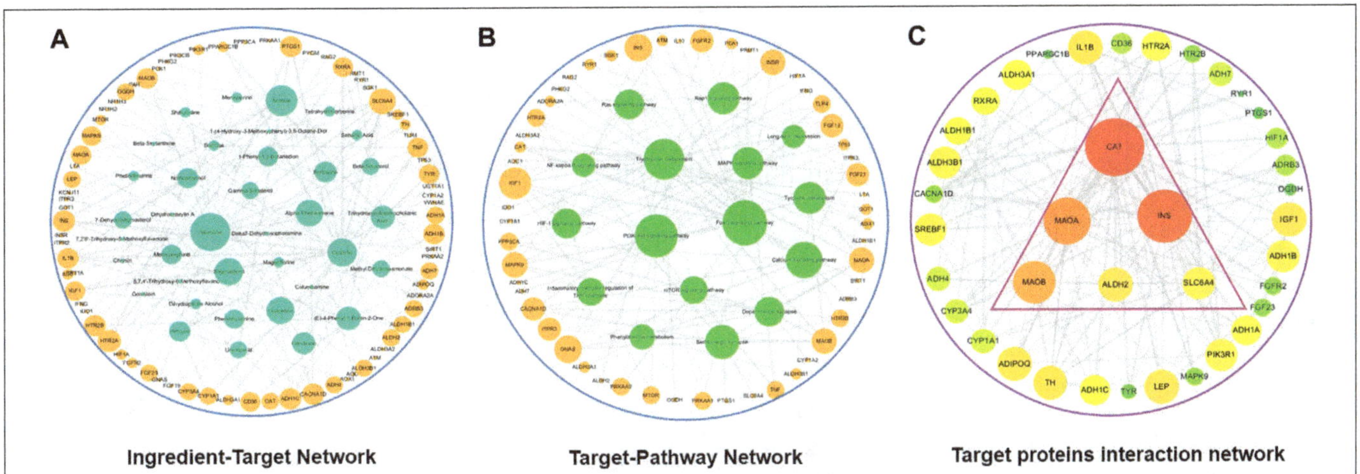

FIGURE 7 | Tryptophan metabolism network diagrams after HLJDD treatment. **(A)** HLJDD active ingredient-target network associated with tryptophan metabolism; **(B)** HLJDD target-pathway network associated with tryptophan metabolism; **(C)** Core HLJDD target proteins interaction network associated with tryptophan metabolism.

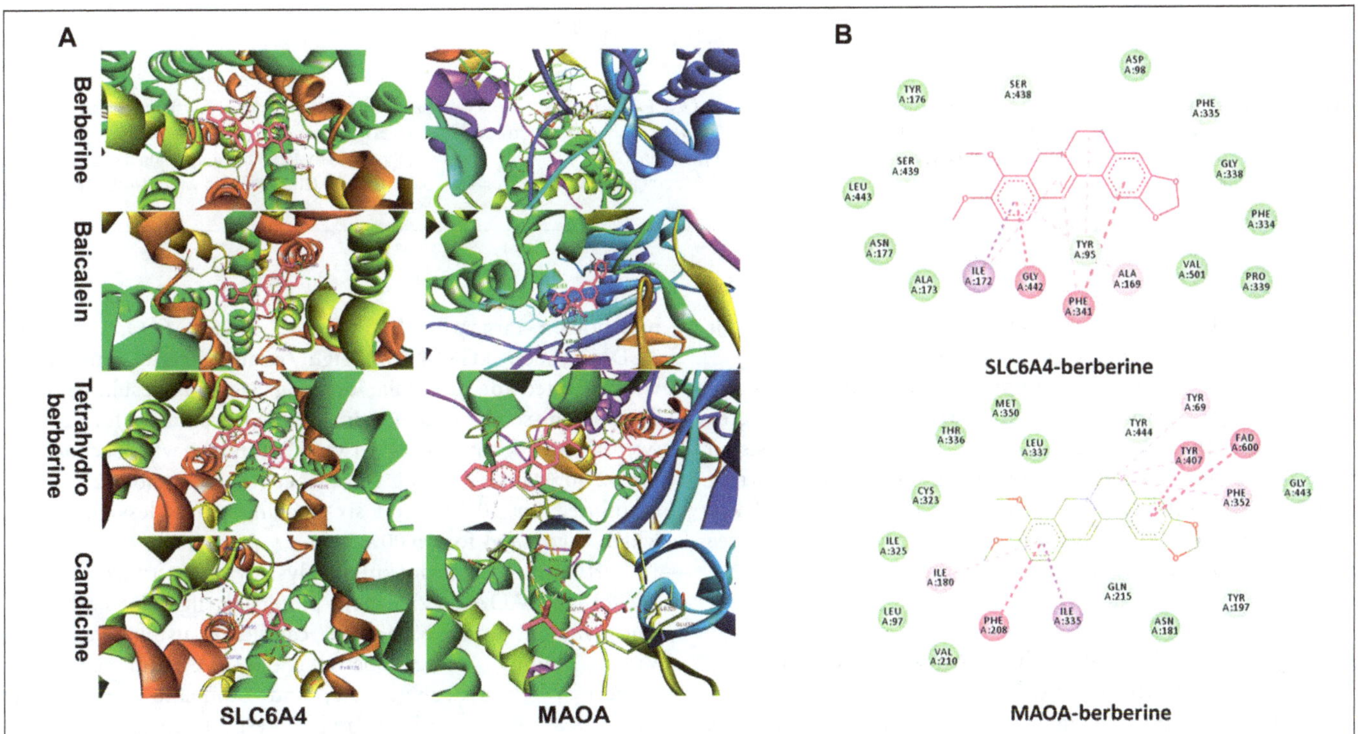

FIGURE 8 | (A) Stereoview of substrate/inhibitor binding of SLC6A4 and MAOA with berberine, baicalein, tetrahydroberberine, and candicine; **(B)** Biding poses of berberine at SLC6A4 and MAOA binding sites.

related pathways, two were synaptic-related pathways, one was a disease-related pathway and one inflammation pathway.

Compound-target network for tryptophan metabolism was constructed using Cytoscape based on active compounds and predicted target. The network had a total of 113 nodes. Out of these nodes, 37 were active compounds expressed in blue and 76 were targets expressed in orange. Active compounds and targets were connected by 372 edges. Main targets identified were SLC6A4, HTR2A, HTR2B, and INS which were mainly targeted by Jasmone, Skatole, berberine. SLC6A4 had the highest degree value among the selected targets (**Figure 7A**). In addition, a target-pathway network map of 92 nodes was constructed using Cytoscape. This network showed a total of 76 targets expressed in orange and 16 pathways expressed in green. 256 connecting edges formed the network. SLC6A4, HTR2A, HTR2B, and INS targets are involved in serotonergic synaptic

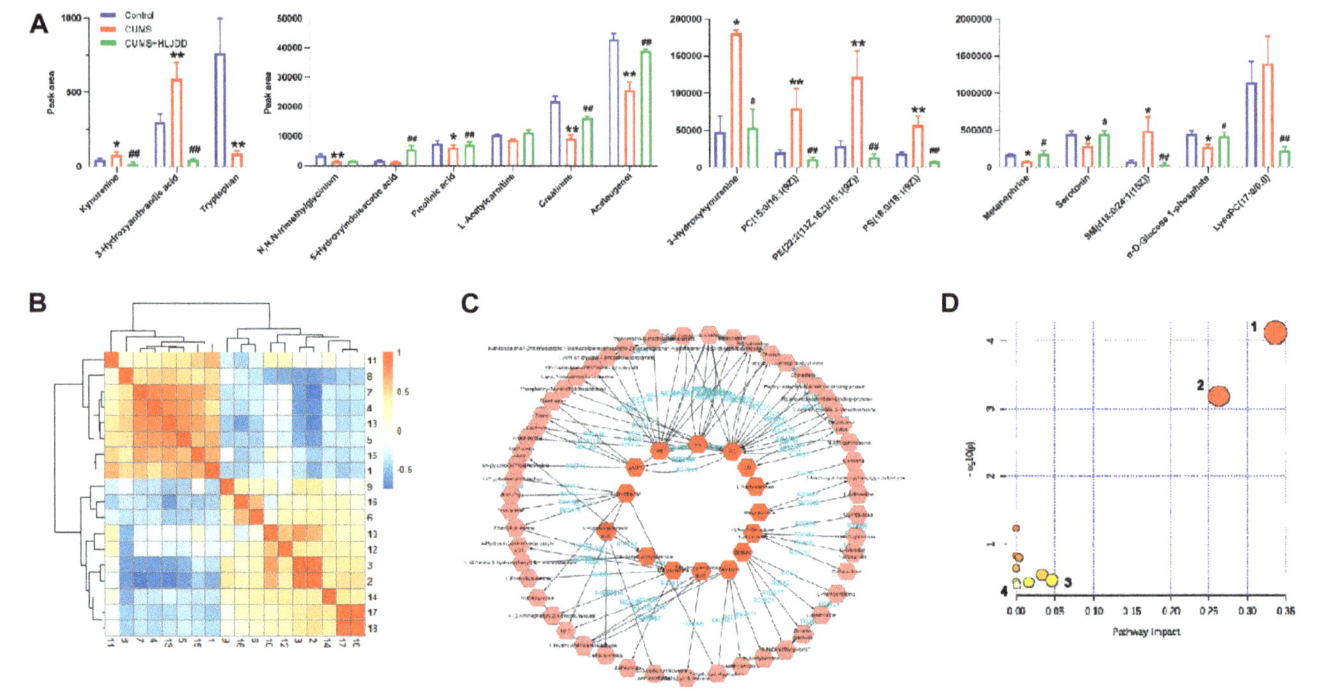

FIGURE 9 | Metabonomics analysis of hippocampus from CUMS mice using LC-Q/TOF-MS. **(A)** Metabolites associated with CUMS conditions with or without HLJDD; **(B)** Correlation heatmap of the 18 different metabolites; **(C)** Metabolic network of the metabolites constructed using MetScape; **(D)** Metabolic pathways as visualized using MetaboAnalyst. 1, tryptophan metabolism; 2, glycerol phospholipid metabolism; 3, glycine, serine and threonine metabolism; 4, tyrosine metabolism. Data are expressed as Mean ± SEM, n = 10 mice per group. $^{*}p < 0.05$, $^{**}p < 0.01$, compared with Control; $\#p < 0.05$, $\#\#p < 0.01$, compared with CUMS via ANOVA.

pathway, FoxO signaling pathway and inflammatory mediator regulation of TRP channels pathway (**Figure 7B**).

Interaction network of tryptophan metabolism targets and HLJDD active compounds was constructed using a degree value greater than the medium target. The network consisted of 38 nodes and 326 edges. Results were saved in TSV format and imported into Cytoscape software for selection of key targets (**Figure 7C**). Nodes with the highest degree represented targets that played an important role in the network.

Huang-Lian Jie-Du Decoction Active Compounds Target Proteins Implicated in Depression

Five important depression targets identified using the network map (GRIN2B, GRIN2A, DRD2, SLC6A4, and MAOA) and twenty-one related active compounds were selected for molecular docking. The PDB-ID for each target was retrieved from RCSB PDB database. The largest search term match score was selected as the optimal PDB-ID value. 3D structural formula of the active compounds were retrieved from Pubchem database. Four pair ingredient-target docking scores were greater than 7.0 and accounted for 3.81%. Seventy-one docking scores were between 7.0 and 5.0 and accounted for 67.62%. Further, sixteen docking scores were between 5.0 and 4.25 and accounted for 15.24% whereas fourteen docking scores were less than 4.25 and accounted for 13.33%. Five tryptophan metabolism targets including CAT, INS, MAOA, MAOB, ALDH2, and SLC6A4 and eight related active compounds were selected for molecular docking. Docking results showed five docking scores greater than 7.0 which accounted for 12.50%; twenty-five docking scores between 7.0 and 5.0 which accounted for 62.50%; four docking scores between 5.0 and 4.25 which accounted for 10.00% and six docking scores less than 4.25 which accounted for 15.00%.

Further molecular docking analysis was performed between SLC6A4, MAOA and their predicted ligands berberine, baicalein, tetrahydroberberine, candicine using AutoDock Vina. Binding energy between SLC6A and baicalein, berberine, tetrahydroberberine, and candicine were −10.1, −10, −8.8, and −6.5 kcal mol^{-1}, respectively for Binding energy scores of berberine, baicalein, tetrahydroberberine, and candicine against MAOA were −8.4, −8.4, −7.6, −6.2 kcal mol^{-1} (**Figure 7**). Berberine binds at the catalytic cavity of SLC6A4 and interacts with 17 amino acid residues. The interaction between berberine and Try-95 was a hydrogen bond. Moreover, berberine interacts with Try-176 through van der Waals force and Gly 342 and Phe-341 through a π–π interaction. Berberine interacts with 19 amino acid residues at the active site of MAOA. with the interaction between berberine and Tyr-197 was a hydrogen bond whereas interactions with Tyr-407, Fad-600 and Phe-208 were π–π interactions (**Figure 8**). A 2D representation the binding

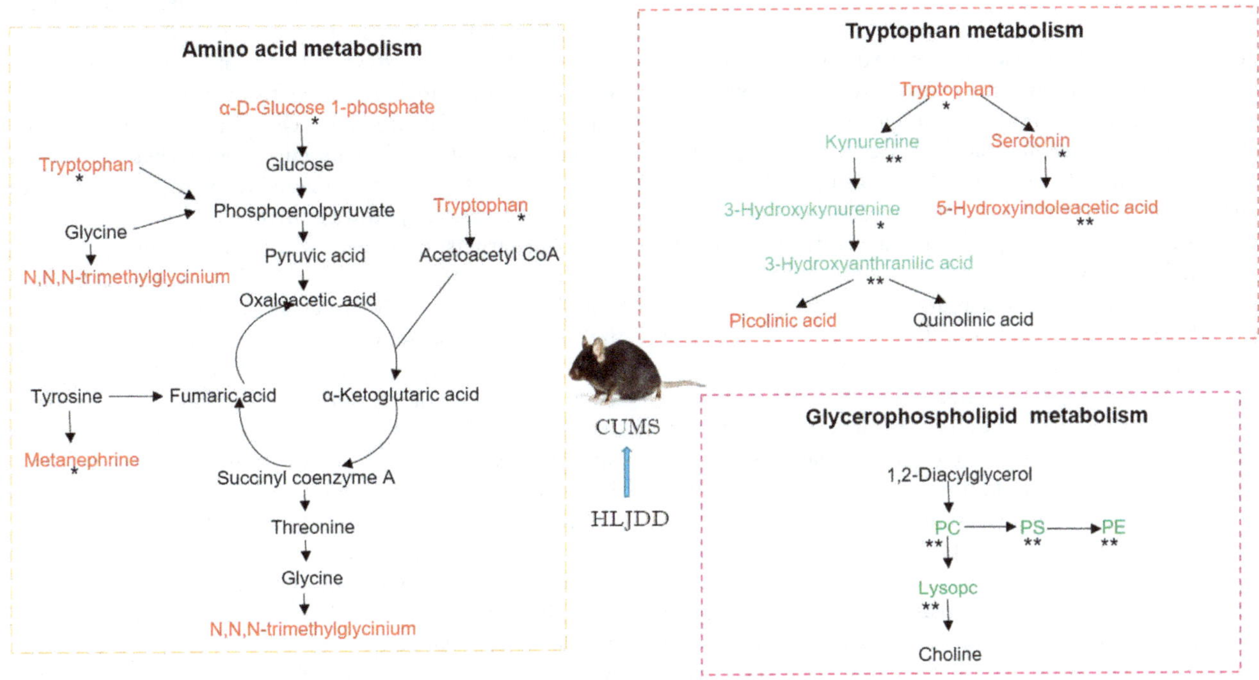

FIGURE 10 | Representative metabolic pathways demonstrated in metabonomics analysis, green represents pathways downregulated by HLJDD whereas red represents pathways upregulated by HLJDD.

poses and interactions between SLC6A4 and MAOA, and baicalein, tetrahydroberberine and candicine.

Hippocampal Metabolomics Analysis

LC-Q/TOF-MS metabolic profile data were analyzed using PCA in unsupervized mode. Data for the groups were completely separated within the two modes, ESI^+ and ESI^-. This implied that metabolic profile of hippocampal tissue for CUMS mice treated with HLJDD was significantly from the profile for untreated mice. To further identify the different metabolites, we used supervised mode OPLS-DA to reduce effect of intra-group differences on classification thus maximizing separation between groups. 200 permutation validations were performed to verify reliability of the model and prevent overfitting. All Q2 values on the left were lower than values on the right. The intersection value between the regression line of Q2 and the longitudinal axis was less than zero. In summary, the model was accurate in prediction of metabolites.

VIP≥1 in OPLS-DA mode, $|p(\text{corr})| > 0.58$ in S-Plot mode was used as the screening criteria for exploring different metabolites involved in depression using ANOVA ($p < 0.05$). A total of 18 different metabolites were identified based on secondary spectrum information and HMDB database in which 8 metabolites were up-regulated and 10 metabolites were down-regulated. Variation of the 18 metabolites was reversed by administration of HLJDD (**Figure 9A**). Kynurenic metabolism process involved in tryptophan metabolism was inhibited by HLJDD compounds by inhibition of kynurenine, 3-hydroxykynurenine and 3-hydroxyanthranilic acid. On the contrary, serotonin metabolism was promoted by HLJDD by increasing serotonin and 5-hydroxyindoleacetic acid.

Correlation analysis of 18 different metabolites were carried out and results presented as a heatmap using R software V3.6.3. Metabolites involved in serotonin metabolism (tryptophan, 5-hydroxyindoleacetic acid, tryptophan) showed a positive correlation with metabolites involved in kynurenine metabolism (kynurenine, 3-hydroxykynurenine, 3-hydroxyanthranilic acid). Serotonin metabolism showed a negative correlation with kynurenine metabolism was observed (**Figure 9B**). This implies that HLJDD promotes kynurenine metabolism and inhibits serotonin metabolism. MetScape, a Cytoscape plug-in was used to construct a composite network related to drug efficacy to further explore the mechanism of action of HLJDD active compounds. In the network, selected biomarkers were represented by a red hexagon, whereas metabolic reactions were represented by lines between the metabolites. The metabolic network consisted of 68 nodes and 110 edges (**Figure 9C**). The network shows internal connection between endogenous substances and presents antidepressant effect of HLJDD. Identified biomarkers were used to explore depression related metabolic pathways, including tryptophan metabolism, glycerol phospholipid metabolism, glycine, serine and threonine metabolism and tyrosine metabolism, using MetaboAnalyst database. (**Figure 9D**). Main metabolic pathways are shown in **Figure 10**.

DISCUSSION

Mood disorders, including major depressive disorder (MDD) and bipolar disorder (BD), are the most prevalent psychiatric conditions worldwide. World Health Organization predicted that MDD will be the leading cause of disease burden by 2030 (Reddy, 2012). Although neurological systems play a key role in development of MDD, the mechanism of action of specific neurological systems at onset, relapse and treatment of MDD are not fully known. Further, available antidepressant medications acting on monoaminergic systems are not effective. Therefore, poor understanding of pathophysiological process of MDD and lack of effective therapies limit attempts to eliminate MDD. The findings of this study imply that. There is need to come up with alternatives for treatment of MDD future. In addition, novel strategies should be designed to develop alternative MDD therapies. Further, studies should explore whether there are key pathways and targets implicated in pathogenesis and treatment of MDD in addition to tryptophan metabolism.

Herbal medicines have seen increased interest as promising complementary and alternative therapies for depressive disorders. Medicinal plants have been in use for several years as they have multiple active ingredients. Herbal medicines are widely adopted as therapy approaches against minor and mild depressive symptoms worldwide. *Hypericum* (St. John's wort, United Kingdom; Johanniskraut, Germany) showed significantly higher activity compared with placebo in the treatment of depression using Hamilton Depression Rating Scale. *Hypericum* mediates antidepressant effect by inhibiting reuptake of 5-HT, NA, and DA into the presynaptic neurons (Calapai et al., 2001). Other as antidepressant preparations inhibit transient receptor potential cation channel 2 channels and voltage-gated calcium channel-dependent Ca^{2+} mobilization, inhibit oxidative stress, and have anti-inflammatory activities against MDD related symptoms (Naziroglu et al., 2014). Herbal preparations have a myriad of pharmacological actions due to diversity of bioactive compounds (Jakovljevic et al., 2000). In China, herbal medicine has been in use for more than 8,000 years is increasingly been introduced for depressive treatment (Liu et al., 2015). Araliaceae elevates levels of 5-HT, NE, and DA in the brain, and upregulates CREB protein level (Jin et al., 2013). Antidepressant effects of Panax ginseng are mediated through modulation of monoamine neurotransmitters and neurotrophic factors, regulating the function of HPA axis, and anti-inflammatory activity (Jin et al., 2019). Herbal formula with several herbal medicines modulates more targets compared with single compound herbal preparation. Previous studies report activities of TCM formula such as Danzhi Xiaoyao powder, Gengnianchun, and Yixin Ningshen tablet against depression (Wu et al., 2020; Zhang et al., 2020; Zhu et al., 2020). The findings of our study show that HLJDD improves depressive disorders primarily through modulation of tryptophan metabolism, dopaminergic synaptic function, and cAMP, FoxO and calcium signaling pathways. Beside those pleiotropic pharmacological actions, herbal preparations and TCM formula have less side effects and are relatively affordable. Studies have shown that dysregulation or dysfunction of depression-associated metabolic or biochemical pathways play a key role in pathogenesis of depression. These findings form a basis for development of novel therapeutic approaches such as cocktail medicines, refined herbal medicines with multiple targets to inhibit the various pathways involved.

Multi-targets therapeutics are promising approaches for management of depressive disorders. Current drug design approaches are mainly target-based focusing on single target implicated in disease. Unfortunately, new candidates targeting first-in-class drug targets are less effective than first generation drugs and have more side effects. Moreover, discovery and development of novel molecular targets is a challenging and a slow process. Development of multi-target therapeutics will help overcome limitations of monotherapies through modulation of multiple cellular pathways (Borisy et al., 2003; Keith et al., 2005). Duloxetine (Cymbalta®) treats depression through inhibition of serotonin and norepinephrine reuptake. Brexpiprazole, a second-generation antidepressant, was approved by FDA in 2015 for treatment of MDD. As a novel antidepressant medicine, Brexpiprazole achieves its activity by modulating serotonin-dopamine activity. It partially activates dopamine D2 and serotonin 5HT1A receptors. Additionally, it has potent antagonistic activity against serotonin 5HT2A, noradrenergicα1B and α2C receptors (Beyer and Weisler, 2016). Multi-target therapies can be achieved through 3 approaches; 1) medicine cocktails acting on different targets that are involved in separate pathophysiological process or various nodes of the same signaling pathway; 2) one medicine with multicomponents delivered through a single system acting on the same target such as Synercid® (Manfredi and Sabbatani, 2010); 3) a single compound acting on multi-target. Exploration of the relationship between multiple ligands and multi-target through network pharmacology analysis is important in development of new drug candidates. The strategy is widely applicable for development of herbal medicines. In our study, HLJDD formula showed multi-target effects as an antidepressant (**Figure 8**). Dopamine D2 and D4 receptors of dopaminergic synapse and serotonin 5HT1A, 5HT2A, and 5HT4 receptors of serotonergic synapse are HLJDD targets for treatment of depressive disorder. Moreover, MAOA enzyme and SLC6A4 transporter associated with tryptophan metabolism play key role in mediating activity of HLJDD against depression. HLJDD consists of berberine, baicalein, tetrahydroberberine, and candicine compounds that target SLC6A4 and MAOA with good binding energy scores. Pharmacological activity of HLJDD against depression is due to multiple compound properties and multi-target action.

Currently, monoamine hypothesis of depression is the leading theory guiding drug discovery and clinical practice. The theory suggests assay of serotonin level in plasma and cerebrospinal fluid for diagnosis of depression (Perez-Caballero et al., 2019). First generation of antidepressant medicines modulate serotonin levels in synaptic space by inhibiting monoamine oxidase activity or neurotransmitter transporters. Follow-up antidepressants restore serotonin levels in synaptic cleft by selectively inhibiting serotonin reuptake and selective inhibition of noradrenaline reuptake (Jans et al., 2007). Current antidepressants target 5-hydroxytryptamine (5-HT) receptors. These drugs are either agonists or antagonists which are more effective than previous drugs and have rapid onset activity. Different 5-HT receptor subtypes play different roles in modulating mood, memory, sleep, appetite and circadian rhythms. 5-HT1A receptor antagonist and 5-HT4 receptor agonist increase cAMP levels and produce behavioral and neurochemical antidepressant-like effects. Canonical antidepressants have slow and moderate effects which can be overcome by modulators of glutamate receptor and 5-HT4R which have rapid and long-lasting antidepressant effects (Rosel et al., 2004; Valentine et al., 2011). Traditional antidepressants are characterized by withdraw and/or persistent side effects following long-term administration therefore, there is need to develop alternative pharmacological and non-pharmacological interventions. The findings of this study show that HLJDD modulates tryptophan metabolism and translocation. In addition, active compounds in HLJDD modulates activities of the serotonin receptors 5HT1A, 5HT2A, and 5HT4. Therefore, HLJDD mediates antidepressant activities through modulation of tryptophan metabolism and serotonergic synapse function.

An interaction network for depression-associated targets and corresponding compounds in HLJDD showed that several pathways are implicated in activity of HLJDD against MDD. In addition to tryptophan metabolism process and receptor modulation, dopamine receptors DRD2 and DRD4 are involved in therapeutic effects of HLJDD. Insulin signaling associated with glucose metabolism in neurons was identified, which is consistent with findings that intravenous insulin improves mood and cognition, and depression subjects have glucose disruption (Kozumplik and Uzun, 2011; Strachan, 2005). Although multi-targets actions mediate polypharmacology of HLJDD on depression disorder, action intensity and dynamics process on these targets should be explored through *in vitro* and *in vivo* experiments. Regulation of tryptophan metabolism by HLJDD is mediated through serotonin metabolism and kynurenine metabolism. Although, active phytochemicals were selected based on drug-like rules, novel available delivery system should be explored to improve bioavailability of compounds to specific brain regions. More studies on development of a multi-component therapy from HLJDD and explore different key targets for treatment of depression.

CONCLUSION

HLJDD, a TCM formula showed significant therapeutic effects on depressive disorder. HLJDD ameliorated depression-like behavior of CUMS mice using FST, NSF and OFT assays. Multiple pharmacological actions of HLJDD on depression are mainly achieved by modulation of tryptophan metabolism, monoamine nervous system function and energy metabolism. HLJDD provides scaffolds for development of a novel alternative antidepressant therapies.

AUTHOR CONTRIBUTIONS

Q-CZ acquired funding for the research; Q-CZ and H-XZ designed the work; S-YQ, XH, Y-YQ, and X-YL performed the experiment; S-YQ, P-YG, S-jN, Z-YY, and YC analyzed the network pharmacology data; S-YQ wrote the manuscript; Q-CZ, RG, and N-YY reviewed the manuscript. All of the authors reviewed and approved the submitted version of the paper.

FUNDING

This research was financially supported by the National Natural Science Foundation of China (Project Nos. 81873027; 81573635), the Qing-Lan Project of Jiangsu Province, the Open Project Program of Jiangsu Key Laboratory for Pharmacology and Safety Evaluation of Chinese Materia Medica (No. JKLPSE201820), the Project Funded by the Priority Academic Program Development of Jiangsu Higher Education Institutions (PAPD), the Project of the Innovation Research Team of Nanjing University of Chinese Medicine, and the Project Funded by the Six Talent Project in Jiangsu Province.

REFERENCES

Bai, M., Zhu, X., Zhang, Y., Zhang, S., Zhang, L., Xue, L., et al. (2012). Abnormal hippocampal BDNF and miR-16 expression is associated with depression-like behaviors induced by stress during early life. *PLoS One* 7, e46921. doi:10.1371/journal.pone.0046921

Bang-Andersen, B., Ruhland, T., Jorgensen, M., Smith, G., Frederiksen, K., Jensen, K. G., et al. (2011). Discovery of 1-[2-(2,4-dimethylphenylsulfanyl)phenyl]piperazine (Lu AA21004): a novel multimodal compound for the treatment of major depressive disorder. *J. Med. Chem* 54, 3206–3221. doi:10.1021/jm101459g

Beyer, J. L., and Weisler, R. H. (2016). Adjunctive brexpiprazole for the treatment of major depressive disorder. *Expet Opin. Pharmacother.* 17, 2331–2339. doi:10.1080/14656566.2016.1254188

Borisy, A. A., Elliott, P. J., Hurst, N. W., Lee, M. S., Lehar, J., Price, E. R., et al. (2003). Systematic discovery of multicomponent therapeutics. *Proc. Natl. Acad. Sci. U.S.A* 100, 7977–7982. doi:10.1073/pnas.1337088100

Calapai, G., Crupi, A., Firenzuoli, F., Inferrera, G., Squadrito, F., Parisi, A., et al. (2001). Serotonin, norepinephrine and dopamine involvement in the antidepressant action of hypericum perforatum. *Pharmacopsychiatry* 34, 45–49. doi:10.1055/s-2001-15180

Chouinard, G., and Chouinard, V. A. (2015). New classification of selective serotonin reuptake inhibitor withdrawal. *Psychother. Psychosom.* 84, 63–71. doi:10.1159/000371865

Cipriani, A., Furukawa, T. A., Salanti, G., Chaimani, A., Atkinson, L. Z., Ogawa, Y., et al. (2018). Comparative efficacy and acceptability of 21 antidepressant drugs for the acute treatment of adults with major depressive disorder: a systematic review and network meta-analysis. *Focus* 16, 420–429. doi:10.1176/appi.focus.16407

Dai, Y., Sun, L., and Qiang, W. (2018). A new strategy to uncover the anticancer mechanism of Chinese compound formula by integrating systems pharmacology and bioinformatics. *Evid Based Complement Alternat Med* 2018, 6707850. doi:10.1155/2018/6707850

Dulawa, S. C., and Hen, R. (2005). Recent advances in animal models of chronic antidepressant effects: the novelty-induced hypophagia test. *Neurosci. Biobehav. Rev.* 29, 771–783. doi:10.1016/j.neubiorev.2005.03.017

Fava, G. A. (2003). Can long-term treatment with antidepressant drugs worsen the course of depression?. *J. Clin. Psychiatr.* 64, 123–133. doi:10.4088/jcp.v64n0204

Freis, E. D. (1954). Mental depression in hypertensive patients treated for long periods with large doses of reserpine. *N. Engl. J. Med.* 251, 1006–1008. doi:10.1056/NEJM195412162512504

Ge, Q., Chen, L., Yuan, Y., Liu, L., Feng, F., Lv, P., et al. (2020). Network pharmacology-based dissection of the anti-diabetic mechanism of Lobelia chinensis. *Front. Pharmacol.* 11, 347. doi:10.3389/fphar.2020.00347

Guo, X., Qiu, W., Liu, Y., Zhang, Y., Zhao, H., and Chen, J. (2017). Effects of refined xiaoyaosan on depressive-like behaviors in rats with chronic unpredictable mild stress through neurosteroids, their synthesis and metabolic enzymes. *Molecules* 22, 1386. doi:10.3390/molecules22081386

Jakovljevic, V., Popovic, M., Mimica-Dukic, N., Sabo, A., and Gvozdenovic, L. (2000). Pharmacodynamic study of *Hypericum perforatum* L. *Phytomedicine* 7, 449–453. doi:10.1016/S0944-7113(00)80027-6

Jans, L. A., Riedel, W. J., Markus, C. R., and Blokland, A. (2007). Serotonergic vulnerability and depression: assumptions, experimental evidence and implications. *Mol. Psychiatr.* 12, 522–543. doi:10.1038/sj.mp.4001920

Jin, L., Wu, F., Li, X., Li, H., Du, C., Jiang, Q., et al. (2013). Anti-depressant effects of aqueous extract from Acanthopanax senticosus in mice. *Phytother Res.* 27, 1829–1833. doi:10.1002/ptr.4938

Jin, Y., Cui, R., Zhao, L., Fan, J., and Li, B. (2019). Mechanisms of Panax ginseng action as an antidepressant. *Cell Prolif* 52, e12696. doi:10.1111/cpr.12696

Keith, C. T., Borisy, A. A., and Stockwell, B. R. (2005). Multicomponent therapeutics for networked systems. *Nat. Rev. Drug Discov.* 4, 71–78. doi:10.1038/nrd1609

Kozumplik, O., and Uzun, S. (2011). Metabolic syndrome in patients with depressive disorder–features of comorbidity. *Psychiatr. Danub.* 23, 84–88. doi:10.1055/s-0030-1248553

Lee, B., Sur, B., Yeom, M., Shim, I., Lee, H., and Hahm, D. H. (2012). Effect of berberine on depression- and anxiety-like behaviors and activation of the noradrenergic system induced by development of morphine dependence in rats. *Korean J. Physiol. Pharmacl.* 16, 379–386. doi:10.4196/kjpp.2012.16.6.379

Liu, L. Y., Feng, B., Chen, J., Tan, Q. R., Chen, Z. X., Chen, W. S., et al. (2015). Herbal medicine for hospitalized patients with severe depressive episode: a retrospective controlled study. *J. Affect. Disord.* 170, 71–77. doi:10.1016/j.jad.2014.08.027

Liu, X., Ouyang, S., Yu, B., Liu, Y., Huang, K., Gong, J., et al. (2010). PharmMapper server: a web server for potential drug target identification using pharmacophore mapping approach. *Nucleic Acids Res.* 38, W609–W614. doi:10.1093/nar/gkq300

Liu, X., Wei, F., Liu, H., Zhao, S., Du, G., and Qin, X. (2020). Integrating hippocampal metabonomics and network pharmacology deciphers the antidepressant mechanisms of Xiaoyaosan. *J. Ethnopharmacol*, 268, 113549. doi:10.1016/j.jep.2020.113549

Liu, Y., Du, T., Zhang, W., Lu, W., Peng, Z., Huang, S., et al. (2019). Modified huang-lian-jie-du decoction ameliorates A. *Oxid. Med. Cell Longev.* 2019, 8340192. doi:10.1155/2019/8340192

Liu, Z., Guo, F., Wang, Y., Li, C., Zhang, X., Li, H., et al. (2016). BATMAN-TCM: a bioinformatics analysis tool for molecular mechANism of traditional Chinese medicine. *Sci. Rep.* 6, 21146. doi:10.1038/srep21146

Manfredi, R., and Sabbatani, S. (2010). Novel pharmaceutical molecules against emerging resistant gram-positive cocci. *Braz. J. Infect. Dis.* 14, 96–108. doi:10.1590/s1413-86702010000100020

Naziroglu, M., Cig, B., and Ozgul, C. (2014). Modulation of oxidative stress and Ca(2+) mobilization through TRPM2 channels in rat dorsal root ganglion neuron by *Hypericum perforatum*. *Neuroscience* 263, 27–35. doi:10.1016/j.neuroscience.2014.01.006

Okamoto, H., Chino, A., Hirasaki, Y., Ueda, K., Iyo, M., and Namiki, T. (2013). Orengedoku-to augmentation in cases showing partial response to yokukan-san treatment: a case report and literature review of the evidence for use of these Kamp herbal formulae. *Neuropsychiatric Dis. Treat.* 9, 151–155. doi:10.2147/NDT.S38318

Perez-Caballero, L., Torres-Sanchez, S., Romero-Lopez-Alberca, C., Gonzalez-Saiz, F., Mico, J. A., and Berrocoso, E. (2019). Monoaminergic system and depression. *Cell Tissue Res.* 377, 107–113. doi:10.1007/s00441-018-2978-8

Reddy, M. S. (2012). Depression - the global crisis. *Indian J. Psychol. Med.* 34, 201–203. doi:10.4103/0253-7176.106011

Rosel, P., Arranz, B., Urretavizcaya, M., Oros, M., San, L., and Navarro, M. A. (2004). Altered 5-HT2A and 5-HT4 postsynaptic receptors and their intracellular signalling systems IP3 and cAMP in brains from depressed violent suicide victims. *Neuropsychobiology* 49, 189–195. doi:10.1159/000077365

Ru, J., Li, P., Wang, J., Zhou, W., Li, B., Huang, C., et al. (2014). TCMSP: a database of systems pharmacology for drug discovery from herbal medicines. *J. Cheminf.* 6, 13. doi:10.1186/1758-2946-6-13

Rubio, J., Caldas, M., Davila, S., Gasco, M., and Gonzales, G. F. (2006). Effect of three different cultivars of Lepidium meyenii (Maca) on learning and depression in ovariectomized mice. *BMC Compl. Alternative Med.* 6, 23. doi:10.1186/1472-6882-6-23

Sasaki, K., Sudo, T., Kurusu, T., Kiuchi, T., and Yoshizaki, F. (2000). [The mechanism of alteration of monoamine metabolism in brain regions in marble burying behavior-isolated housing mice and effect of oren-gedoku-to on this alteration]. *Yakugaku Zasshi* 120, 559–567. doi:10.1248/yakushi1947.120.6_559

Steru, L., Chermat, R., Thierry, B., and Simon, P. (1985). The tail suspension test: a new method for screening antidepressants in mice. *Psychopharmacology (Berlin)* 85, 367–370. doi:10.1007/BF00428203

Strachan, M. W. (2005). Insulin and cognitive function in humans: experimental data and therapeutic considerations. *Biochem. Soc. Trans.* 33, 1037–1040. doi:10.1042/BST20051037

Trott, O., and Olson, A. J. (2010). Autodockvina: Improving the speed and accuracy of docking with a new scoring function, efficient optimization, and multithreading. *J. Comput. Chem.*, 31, 455–461. doi:10.1002/jcc.21334

Valentine, G. W., Mason, G. F., Gomez, R., Fasula, M., Watzl, J., Pittman, B., et al. (2011). The antidepressant effect of ketamine is not associated with changes in occipital amino acid neurotransmitter content as measured by [(1)H]-MRS. *Psychiatr. Res.* 191, 122–127. doi:10.1016/j.pscychresns.2010.10.009

Wang, P., Dai, L., Zhou, W., Meng, J., Zhang, M., Wu, Y., et al. (2019). Intermodule coupling analysis of huang-lian-jie-du decoction on stroke. *Front. Pharmacol.* 10, 1288. doi:10.3389/fphar.2019.01288

Wang, P. R., Wang, J. S., Zhang, C., Song, X. F., Tian, N., and Kong, L. Y. (2013). Huang-Lian-Jie-Du-Decotion induced protective autophagy against the injury of cerebral ischemia/reperfusion via MAPK-mTOR signaling pathway. *J. Ethnopharmacol.* 149, 270–280. doi:10.1016/j.jep.2013.06.035

Wang, T., Wu, Z., Sun, L., Li, W., Liu, G., and Tang, Y. (2018). A computational systems pharmacology approach to investigate molecular mechanisms of herbal formula tian-ma-gou-teng-yin for treatment of Alzheimer's disease. *Front. Pharmacol.* 9, 668. doi:10.3389/fphar.2018.00668

Wigner, P., Czarny, P., Galecki, P., SuK, P., and Sliwinski, T. (2018). Themolecular aspects of oxidative & nitrosative stress and the tryptophan catabolites pathway (TRYCATs) as potential causes of depression. *Psychiatry Res.*, 262, 566–574. doi:10.1016/j.psychres.2017.09.045

Wu, L. M., Hu, M. H., Tong, X. H., Han, H., Shen, N., Jin, R. T., et al. (2012). Chronic unpredictable stress decreases expression of brain-derived neurotrophic factor (BDNF) in mouse ovaries: relationship to oocytes developmental potential. *PLoS One* 7, e52331. doi:10.1371/journal.pone.0052331

Wu, R., Wang, H., Lv, X., Shen, X., and Ye, G. (2020). Rapid action of mechanism investigation of Yixin Ningshen tablet in treating depression by combinatorial use of systems biology and bioinformatics tools. *J. Ethnopharmacol.* 257, 112827. doi:10.1016/j.jep.2020.112827

Yu, D., Tao, B. B., Yang, Y. Y., Du, L. S., Yang, S. S., He, X. J., et al. (2015). The Ido inhibitor coptisine ameliorates cognitive impairment in a mouse model of Alzheimer's disease. *J Alzheimers Dis.* 43, 291–302. doi:10.3233/JAD-140414

Yue, G. H., Zhuo, S. Y., Xia, M., Zhang, Z., Gao, Y. W., and Luo, Y. (2014). Effect of huanglian jiedu decoction on thoracic aorta gene expression in spontaneous hypertensive rats. *Evid Based Complement Alternat Med.* 2014, 565784. doi:10.1155/2014/565784

Zeng, M. F., Pan, L. M., Zhu, H. X., Zhang, Q. C., and Guo, L. W. (2010). Comparative pharmacokinetics of baicalin in plasma after oral administration of Huang-Lian-Jie-Du-Tang or pure baicalin in MCAO and sham-operated rats. *Fitoterapia* 81, 490–496. doi:10.1016/j.fitote.2010.01.004

Zhang, K., Pan, X., Wang, F., Ma, J., Su, G., Dong, Y., et al. (2016). Baicalin promotes hippocampal neurogenesis via SGK1- and FKBP5-mediated glucocorticoid receptor phosphorylation in a neuroendocrine mouse model of anxiety/depression. *Sci. Rep.* 6, 30951. doi:10.1038/srep30951

Zhang, R., Zhu, X., Bai, H., and Ning, K. (2019). Network pharmacology databases for traditional Chinese medicine: review and assessment. *Front. Pharmacol.* 10, 123. doi:10.3389/fphar.2019.00123

Zhang, Y., Cao, Y., and Wang, L. (2020). The effects of a new, improved Chinese medicine, Gengnianchun formula granules, on hot flushes, depression, anxiety, and sleep in Chinese peri- and postmenopausal women: a randomized placebo-controlled trial. *Menopause.* 27, 899–905. doi:10.1097/GME.0000000000001558

Zhu, Y. L., Li, S. L., Zhu, C. Y., Wang, W., Zuo, W. F., and Qiu, X. J. (2020). Antidepressant metabonomics study of Danzhi Xiaoyao powder on rat model of chronic unpredictable mild stress(CUMS). *J. Ethnopharmacol.* 112832. doi:10.1016/j.jep.2020.112832

12

Cyclocarya paliurus Leaves Tea Improves Dyslipidemia in Diabetic Mice: A Lipidomics-Based Network Pharmacology Study

Lixiang Zhai[1], Zi-wan Ning[1], Tao Huang[1], Bo Wen[1,3], Cheng-hui Liao[3], Cheng-yuan Lin[1], Ling Zhao[1], Hai-tao Xiao[2] and Zhao-xiang Bian[1,3]**

[1] School of Chinese Medicine, Hong Kong Baptist University, Kowloon, Hong Kong, [2] School of Pharmaceutical Sciences, Health Science Center, Shenzhen University, Shenzhen, China, [3] Shenzhen Research Institute and Continuing Education, Hong Kong Baptist University, Shenzhen, China

***Correspondence:**
Hai-tao Xiao
xhaitao@szu.edu.cn
Zhao-xiang Bian
bzxiang@hkbu.edu.hk

Hyperlipidemia and hepatic steatosis afflict over 75% of patients with type 2 diabetes, causing diabetic dyslipidemia. *Cyclocarya paliurus* (CP) leaf is a herbal tea which has long been consumed by the Chinese population, particularly people suffering from obesity and diabetes. CP appears to exhibit a hypolipidemic effect in lipid loaded mice (Kurihara et al., 2003), although the detailed mechanisms and active ingredients for this hypolipidemic effect have not yet been answered. In this study, we investigated the beneficial effects of CP and predicted the mechanisms by utilizing lipidomics, serum-pharmacochemistry and network pharmacology approaches. Our results revealed that serum and hepatic levels of total triglyceride (TG), total cholesterol (T-CHO), low-density lipoproteins (LDL) and high-density lipoproteins (HDL), as well as 30 lipids including cholesterol ester (CE), diglyceride (DG), phosphatidylethanolamine (PE), phosphatidylcholine (PC), and sphingomyelin (SM) in CP-treated mice were improved in comparison with untreated diabetic mice. In parallel, 14 phytochemical compounds of CP were determined in mice serum after CP administration. Mechanistically, the network pharmacology analysis revealed the predicted targets of CP's active ingredients ALOX12, APP, BCL2, CYP2C9, PTPN1 and linked lipidome targets PLD2, PLA2G(s), and PI3K(s) families could be responsible for the CP effects on diabetic dyslipidemia. In conclusion, this study revealed the beneficial effects of CP on diabetic dyslipidemia are achieved by reducing accumulation of hepatic lipid droplets and regulating circulatory lipids in diabetic mice, possibly through PI3K signaling and MAPK signaling pathways.

Keywords: *Cyclocarya paliurus*, Diabetic dyslipidemia, hyperlipidemia, lipidomic, network pharmacology

---

Abbreviations: ALP, alkaline phosphatase; ALT, alanine aminotransferase; AST, aspartate aminotransferase; BUN, urea nitrogen; CE, cholesterol ester; CP, *Cyclocarya paliurus*; CREA, creatinine; DG, diglyceride; HDL, high-density lipoproteins; LDL, low-density lipoproteins; PC, phosphatidylcholine; PE, phosphatidylethanolamine; PPI, protein–protein interaction; SM, sphingomyelin; STZ, streptozotocin; T-CHO, total cholesterol; TG, total triglyceride.

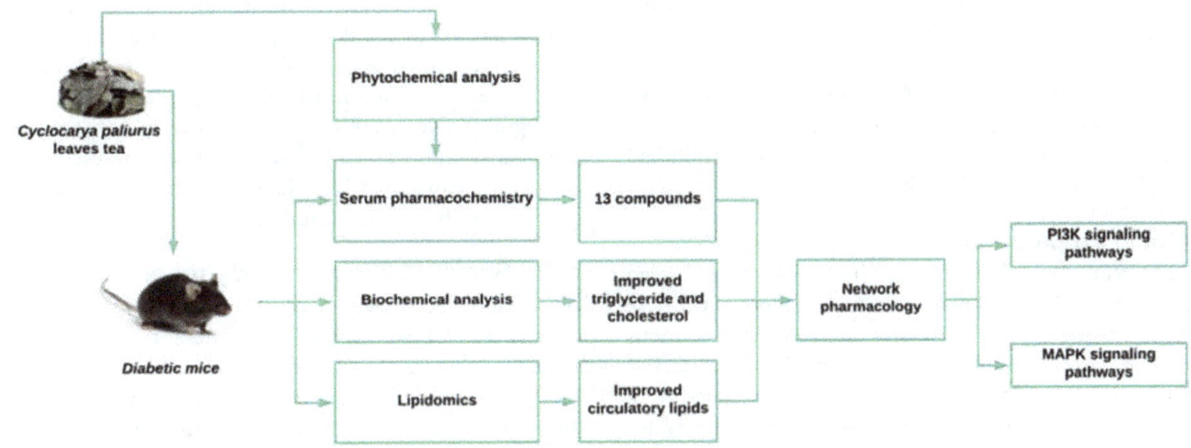

GRAPHICAL ABSTRACT | Work flow of the evaluation of the effects and mechanisms of *Cyclocarya paliurus* leaves tea on dyslipidemia in diabetic mice.

INTRODUCTION

Hyperlipidemia and hepatic steatosis are frequently found in the metabolic syndrome and type 2 diabetes (Jung and Choi, 2014; Perry et al., 2014). Hyperlipidemia is characterized as high T-CHO, TG, LDL, and low HDL levels (Richhariya et al., 2015), whilst hepatic steatosis is represented by high TG, T-CHO, AST, and ALT levels (Stern and Castera, 2017). Emerging evidence suggest that dyslipidemia is a significant risk factor for the development of type 2 diabetes (Andriankaja and Joshipura, 2014; Association, 2015), and pharmacological lipid-lowering therapy is effective to alleviate the complications of type 2 diabetes including hyperlipidemia, hepatic steatosis, coronary heart disease, etc. (Zafrir and Jain, 2014; Sattar et al., 2016; Spence et al., 2016). *Cyclocarya paliurus* (Batal.) Iljinskaja (Juglandaceae) is a native medicinal plant grown in the southwest of China. The leaves of *C. paliurus* (CP) have been used as a herbal tea in China for its special flavor and the benefits to the obese and diabetic Chinese populations. The bioactive components isolated from CP are flavonoids, triterpenoids, organic acids, and polysaccharides, these components contribute to its versatile biological properties including antihyperglycemia, antihyperlipidemia, and antihypertension (Jiang et al., 2015; Yoshitomi et al., 2017). Previous studies have investigated the anti-diabetic function and mechanism of CP leaves on STZ and high-fat diet-induced type 2 diabetic mice, and its potent hypoglycemic effect has been verified on diabetic mice (Wang Q. et al., 2013; Ma et al., 2015). Moreover, CP has also been reported with hypolipidemic effects *in vivo* (Yao et al., 2015; Lin et al., 2016; Yang et al., 2016). However, the mechanism of bioactive constituents of CP on diabetic dyslipidemia remain unknown. Therefore, our objective is to study the effects of CP on lipid disorders in diabetes and elucidate its mechanism-of-actions.

It is acknowledged that the majority of herbal medicines, including TCMs are orally delivered drugs of polypharmacy. Their active components are firstly absorbed into the bloodstream and then selectively and simultaneously interact with multiple targets at the root causes of the disease (Zhao et al., 2015). Serum pharmacochemistry is a rapid and reliable method using the UPLC-MS technique to track the components absorbed into the bloodstream and has been widely used to reveal the efficacy of TCMs (Yan et al., 2017). Moerover, metabolomics is an approach to analyze the metabolites, the intermediate products of metabolic reactions of living systems. This technology contains many subclasses based on the chemical characteristics of metabolites, namely lipidomics, amino metabolomics, and sugar metabolomics, etc. It has been widely used in the evaluation of the therapeutic effects and elucidation of the therapeutic mechanisms of herbal products (Wang X. et al., 2017). Metabolomics profiling can reveal whole metabolic profile changes of living systems in response to endogenous or exogenous stimuli such as drug treatment (Beger et al., 2016). Because any effects of herbal products are mediated by their constituents in a complex biological system, metabolomics can help us to analyze their action network comprehensively. Network pharmacology is a bioinformatics strategy to understand drug action and mechanisms by mapping drug-target-disease networks from the biological level (Li et al., 2014). To date, accumulating evidence suggest that network pharmacology approach is a powerful tool to study the molecular mechanisms of the complex components found in medicinal herbs.

Considering CP as a herbal tea with multiple components and diabetic dyslipidemia as a cluster of lipid abnormalities, we focused on the investigation of the beneficial effect of CP and its mechanisms against diabetic dyslipidemia using lipidomics, serum pharmacochemistry, and network pharmacology approaches.

MATERIALS AND METHODS

Chemicals and Materials

Regents and Standards

UPLC grade organic solvent was purchased from Merck (Darmstadt, Germany). Deionized water was obtained from a milli-Q system (Millipore, Billerica, MA, United States). Formic acid, ammonium formate, and phosphoric acid were obtained from Sigma (St. Louis, MO, United States). Lipids standards including a lipids mixture of TG, CE, DG, PE, PC, and SM, etc, were purchased from Avanti Polar Lipid (Alabaster, AL, United States). Strptomycin and glibenclamide was purchased from Sigma (St. Louis, MO, United States).

Plant Material Preparation

The leaves of *Cyclocarya paliurus* (Batal.) Iljinskaja were collected and authenticated by Prof. Hu-Biao Chen from School of Chinese Medicine, Hong Kong Baptist University, and voucher specimens (No. CP20151201) was stored in our Research Laboratory. For the preparation of the extract of *C. paliurus* leaves (CP extract), the dried leaves of *C. paliurus* (5 kg) were soaked in boiled water (1:10 *m/v*) for 2 h twice. The solution was concentrated and dried under vacuum freezer to obtain crude extract. The crude extract was then extracted by 70% EtOH for 2 h (1:10 m/v) in an ultrasound bath. The refined solution was concentrated and dried under vacuum freezer again and the refined extract was stored in 4°C fridge until use. CP solution was prepared with 0.5% sodium carboxymethyl cellulose (CMC-Na) solution for animal oral administration and MeOH for phytochemical analysis.

Animal Studies

Animal Handling and Diets

Eight-week-old C57/BL6J mice were purchased from Laboratory Animal Services Centre, Chinese University of Hong Kong and raised in the Laboratory Animal Services Center, School of Chinese Medicine, Hong Kong Baptist University. The mice were raised in a 12 h light/dark cycle, temperature controlled (22°C) standard animal room provided with diet and water *ad libitum.* All experimental protocols were approved by the Animal Ethics Committees of Hong Kong Baptist University, in accordance with "Institutional Guidelines and Animal Ordinance" (Department of Health, Hong Kong Special Administrative Region) (Registration No. LIUYE/15-16/01-CLNC). Body weight, food consumption, and blood glucose level were monitored each week. Blood glucose level was determined by OMRON glucometer (Beijing, China) using blood samples collected from the tail vein.

Animal Groups

The diabetes mice model was induced by high-fat diet (adjusted Calories Diet, 42% from fat) (No. 881372) (Harlan Laboratories, Inc., Indianapolis, IN, United States) for 4 weeks and intraperitoneal (*i.p*) injection with STZ (25 mg/kg) three times in following 3 days. The mice with fasting glucose level higher than 11 mmol/L were considered as diabetic mice, and the diabetic mice with consecutive 7-day hyperglycemia (11 mmol/L or greater) were used for the experiment. An equal volume of vehicle was injected into the control mice. The diabetic mice were then divided into the diabetic group (model group), the CP treatment group (CP group) and glibenclamide treatment group (positive group). For the CP treatment group, the mice were orally administrated 2 g/kg/day CP until end of the experiment according to previous experimental data (**Supplementary Figure S1**). The normal mice were divided into two groups: vehicle control group (0.5% CMC-Na solution treated, named as blank group) and CP-treated control group (CP treated, named as control group). CP-treated control group mice were orally administered 2 g/kg/day CP extract and blank group mice were orally administered same volume 0.5% CMC-Na solution as CP solution. Glibenclamide was given at 15 mg/kg/day in 0.5% CNC-Na solution to mice in positive group according to the previous study (Xiao et al., 2017).

Blood Sample Collection and Preparation

For serum pharmacochemistry study, mice were orally administered CP solution and anesthesia by 3% chloral hydrate through intraperitoneal injection after 10 mins. About 1 mL blood was collected in heparin-tube. Plasma was obtained after 3,000 rpm centrifuge for 30 min at room temperature. A total of 900 μL MeOH was added to 100 μL plasma and centrifuged at 14,000 for 10 min at 4°C to precipitate protein. A total of 800 μL supernatant was dried under vacuum concentrator within 30 min and dissolved in 200 μL 70% methanol for LC-MS analysis.

For lipidomics study, about 1 mL blood was collected from mice under anesthesia, serum was obtained after centrifuging at 3,000 rpm for 30 min at room temperature. A total of 50 μL serum was used for lipidomics study. Briefly, 250 μL Folch solvent with the internal standard was added in 50 μL serum and vortexed vigorously. Two phases were formed after centrifugation at 5,000 rpm for 15 min. The bottom layer was dried under vacuum concentrator and dissolved in 200 μL of ACN/IPA/H2O (65:30:5 v/v/v) for analysis.

Another 100 μL serum was used for clinical index analysis including ALT, AST, ALP, CREA and BUN using a biochemical analyzer (Hitachi 902 Automatic Analyzer; Hitachi, Japan). TG, TCHO, LDL, and HDL were analyzed using assay kits purchased from Nanjing Jiancheng Bioengineering Institute (Nanjing, China) according to the manufacturers' instructions.

Hepatic Histopathology Analysis and Biochemical Analysis

At the end of the study, the mice were sacrificed, and liver tissue was collected for H&E staining to analyses histology changes. Liver tissue from sacrificed mice was soaked in 10% formalin solution (prepared by 1× phosphate-buffered saline, PBS) and fixed for 12 h. Samples were then made into paraffin sections as specimens and stained with hematoxylin and eosin (H&E) according to manufacturer's protocol (Mayer's Hematoxylin Solution, Sigma-Aldrich). The sections were observed and captured under microscopy. About other 50 mg liver tissues were homogenized in iced 1× PBS solution (1:10, *m/v*). The homogenized solution was used for TG and TCHO analysis following the protocol of Nanjing Jiancheng Bioengineering Institute (Nanjing, China).

Phytochemical and Metabolomics Study

Phytochemical Analysis

The chromatographic analysis was performed on an Agilent 1290 UPLC system equipped with an autosampler, binary gradient pump, and PDA detector. The system was operated at 30°C and a water ACQUITY UPLC HSS T3 column (150 mm × 2.1 mm,

1.7 μm) was used. The injection volume was 5 μL and the mobile phase flow rate was 0.4 mL/min. Solvents that constituted the mobile phase were (A) 0.2% aqueous acetic acid and (B) acetonitrile. The elution conditions were as follows: 0–5 min, linear gradient 2–5% B; 5–10 min, linear gradient 5–10% B; 10–15 min, linear gradient 10–25% B; 15–25 min, linear gradient 25–40% B; 25–28 min, linear gradient 40–90% B. Peaks were detected at 254 nm. The compounds of CP extracts were characterized by retention time, MS/MS information and related chemical standards in positive and negative modes.

Lipidomics Study

The liquid chromatogram was performed on an Agilent 1290 UPLC system. A waters ACQUITY UPLC HSS C18 column (2.1 mm × 100 mm, 1.8 μm particle size) was used for separation. The column temperature was maintained at 40°C and autosampler temperature was maintained at 8°C. The separation was performed with mobile phase A and B within 20 min per sample. Phase A consists of 60:40 water/ACN in 10 mM ammonium formate and 0.1% formic acid, and phase B is made by 90:10 IPA/ACN with 10 mM ammonium formate and 0.1% formic acid. The linear gradient was as follow: 32% B (0–1.5 min); 32–45% B (1.5–4 min); 45–52% B (4–5 min); 52–58% B (5–8 min); 58–66% B (8–11 min); 66–70% B (11–14 min); 70–75% B (14–18 min); 75–97% B (18–21 min); maintain 97% B (21–25 min); decrease to 32% B (25–30 min); maintained at 32% B (Gregory et al., 2013). The injection volume is 2 μL for the positive mode and 6 μL for the negative mode.

XCMS package in R was used to convert chromatograms intensity into raw data for multivariate statistical analysis using metaboanalyst (Huan et al., 2017). For lipid identification, the frame *m/z* values were used to search information on LIPID MAPS, Human Metabolome Database (HMDB) and Metlin database. The matches were confirmed by lipids' exact tandem mass (MS/MS) and retention time based on our internal standards (SPLASH™ Lipidomix® Mass Spec Standard, Avanti Polar Lipids, United States).

Bioinformatics and Statistical Analysis

Potential Targets Prediction and Linking Analysis

The detected chemical components of CP in plasma after oral administration were imported into our in-house target prediction tool "MOST" (Huang et al., 2017) to construct the target prediction database. Targets from the prediction database were then used to determine the relevance with diabetic dyslipidemia with literature review, and the relevant genes were considered as CP targets for diabetic dyslipidemia. The lipids data were imported into Cytoscape to generate a metabolites-reaction-enzyme-gene database. The genes of significantly changed lipids in CP treatment group were considered as lipid targets of CP. The predicted targets and lipids targets of CP were combined together to upload to STRING (Szklarczyk et al., 2014) for PPIs analysis to link the action of predicted targets with lipids targets of CP.

Target-Diabetic Dyslipidemia Link Analysis

All determined and predicted targets were searched on PubMed using key words: [targets name] AND [diabetes] AND [lipidemia]. The targets which were studied on lipid disorders in diabetes were also included.

Statistical Analysis

GraphPad was used for statistical analysis of the biochemical data. Statistically significant differences ($p < 0.05$) in mean values were calculated by Student's *t*-test or one-way ANOVA. The lipidomics data was processed by R package with XCMS. Metaboanalyst (Xia et al., 2015) was used for multivariate statistical analysis. Cytoscape was used trace associated gene-enzyme using KEGG database.

RESULTS

CP Attenuated Diabetic Dyslipidemia in Diabetic Mice Induced by High Fat Diet and STZ

As shown in **Table 1**, after high fat diet and STZ treatment, blood glucose levels of mice were significantly elevated whereas their body weight was significantly demoted compared with control and blank group, indicating that the diabetic mice model was well established. In contrast, those clinical signs were significantly rescued after CP treatment for 5 weeks. Since both hyperlipidemia and hepatic steatosis are characterized as

TABLE 1 | Blood glucose (mM) levels and body weight changes on week 0, 3, and 5.

	Blank	Control	Model	CP	Positive
Blood glucose (mM)					
Week 0	6.8 ± 1.2	6.1 ± 0.9	17.0 ± 3.5 ###	16.2 ± 4.3	16.5 ± 5.2
Week 3	6.7 ± 1.0	6.6 ± 1.4	17.5 ± 4.0 ###	12.7 ± 3.2 *	12.6 ± 3.5 *
Week 5	6.0 ± 1.0	5.1 ± 0.5	16.6 ± 3.0 ###	10.7 ± 1.5 ***	10.4 ± 2.0 ***
Body weight (g)					
Week 0	23.8 ± 0.8	23.5 ± 1.8	24.4 ± 1.0	24.4 ± 1.0	24.5 ± 0.9
Week 3	24.6 ± 1.0	25.0 ± 1.0	23.4 ± 1.8 #	24.1 ± 0.3	23.9 ± 1.3
Week 5	26.3 ± 1.2	26.2 ± 1.3	23.2 ± 1.8 ##	24.9 ± 0.6 *	24.6 ± 1.2 *

*The effects of CP extract on blood glucose levels and body weight of diabetic mice. All data are presented as means ± SD. Diabetic model group vs. control group: #p < 0.05, ##p < 0.01 and ###p < 0.001. CP or glibenclamide (positive) treatment group vs. diabetic model group: *p < 0.05, **p < 0.01, ***p < 0.001.*

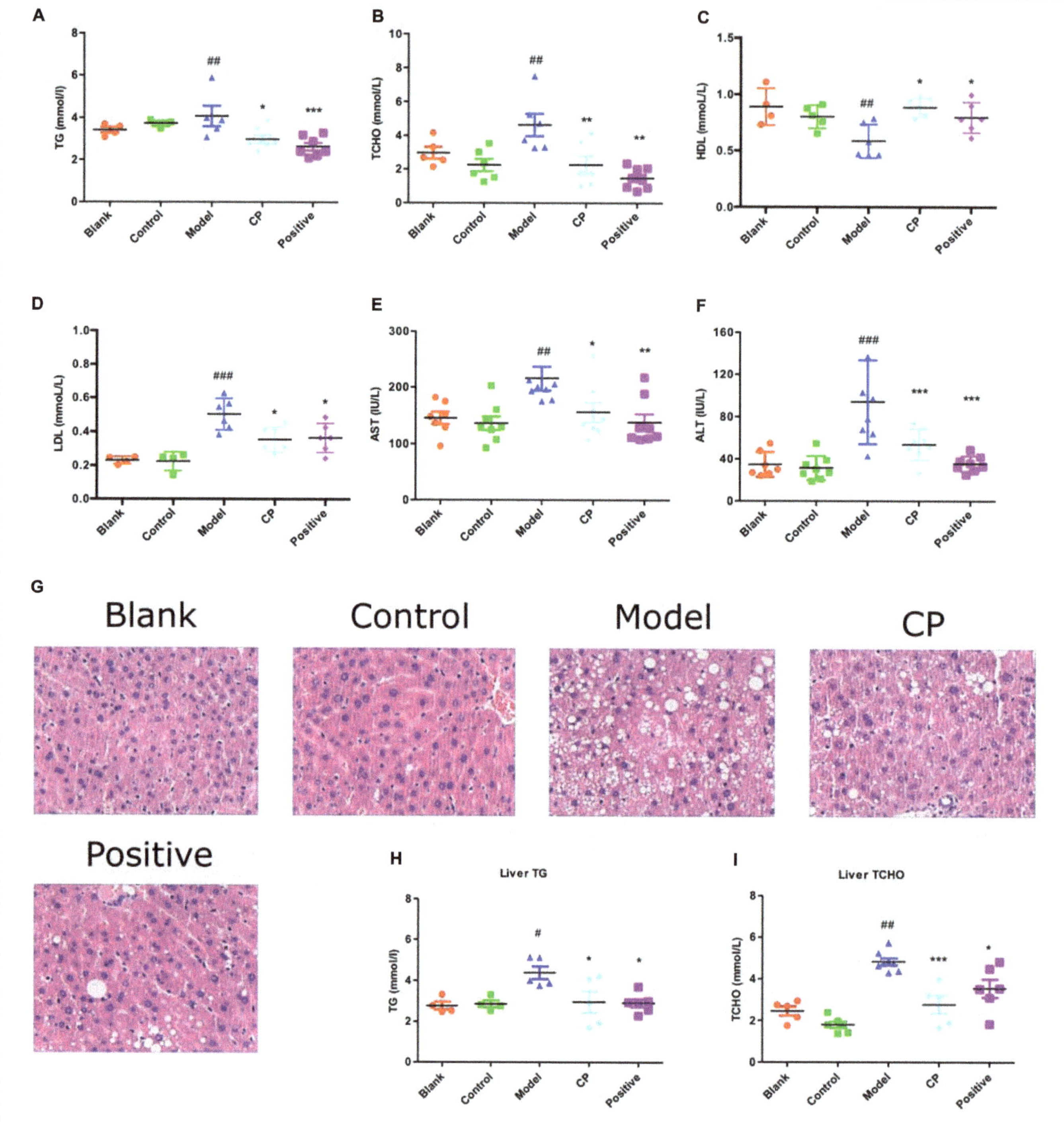

FIGURE 1 | *Cyclocarya paliurus* attenuated diabetic dyslipidemia and hepatic steatosis induced by high fat diet and STZ in mice. Blank: non-diabetic control group; Control: CP-treated non-diabetic control group; Model: STZ and high fat diet-induced diabetic model group; CP: CP treated model group; Positive: glibenclamide treated model group. **(A–F)** Serum TG, TCHO, HDL, LDL, AST, and ALT level. **(G)** Histology analysis of liver tissues by **H,E** staining. **(H,I)** Liver TG and TCHO level. All data are presented as means + SEM (n = 6~8). $^{\#}p < 0.05$, $^{\#\#}p < 0.01$, $^{\#\#\#}p < 0.001$ (comparison between control and model group); $^{*}p < 0.05$, $^{**}p < 0.01$, $^{***}p < 0.001$ (comparison between CP group, positive group, and model group).

substantial lipid disorders in diabetes, we determined serum TCHO, LDL, HDL, and TG levels, and hepatic AST, ALT, TG, and TCHO levels. Liver histopathological changes were also monitored. As shown in **Figure 1** and **Supplementary Figure S4**, compared to that of control and blank group, serum TG, TCHO, and LDL levels, as well as hepatic AST, ALT, TG, and TCHO levels of the model group were significantly increased, whereas serum HDL levels were significantly decreased, indicating that

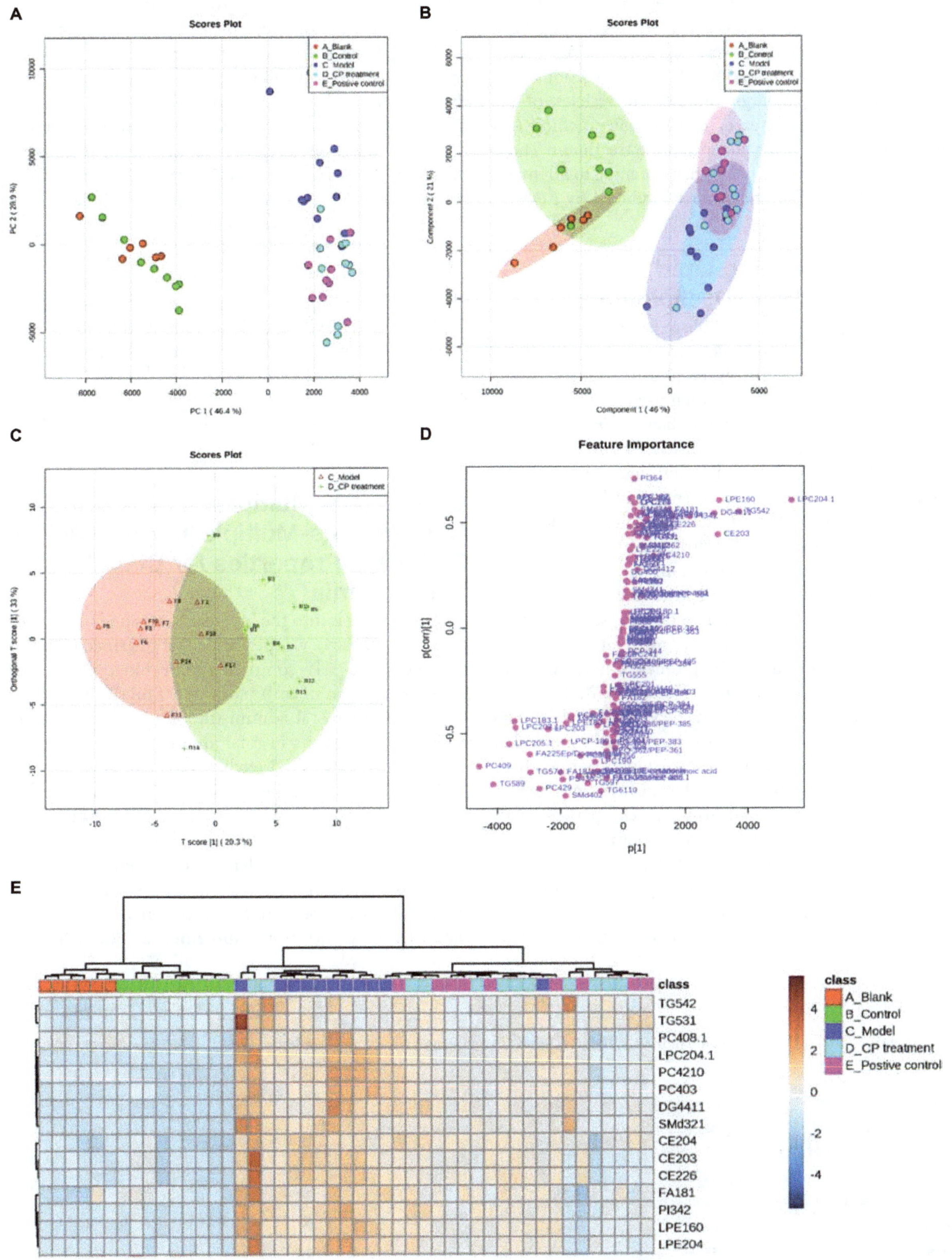

FIGURE 2 | The lipidomics study on serum from diabetic mice: Metabolic profiles and multivariate data analysis. **(A)** PCA score plot of the blank group (red color), control group (green color), model group (dark blue), CP group (light blue), and positive group (purple). **(B)** PLS-DA score plot with 95% confidence interval of all studied groups. **(C,D)** OPLS-DA score plot and S-plot between model group and CP treatment group. **(E)** Heatmap of selected metabolites was built based on one-way ANOVA rankings and hierarchical clustering. Each dot represents one mouse.

the hyperlipidemia and hepatic steatosis were developed in the model group. In CP or glibenclamide-treated groups, those altered lipids-associated indexes were significantly alleviated. In addition, histological examination of hepatic sections also revealed that there were a large number of vesicles of fat accumulating within hepatocytes of diabetic mice, which was significantly reduced after CP or glibenclamide treatment. These results suggested that CP extract has a great potential to attenuate diabetic dyslipidemia and hepatic steatosis induced by high fat diet and STZ in mice.

CP Improved Circulating Lipid Metabolism in Diabetic Dyslipidemia

To study the CP effect on lipid metabolism in diabetic mice, we performed a lipidomics study on mice serum. Fatty acyls (fatty acids), glycerolipids (DG and TG), glycerophospholipids (PC, PE, and PI), and sphingolipids (SM) were then used for multivariate statistical analysis as shown in **Supplementary Table S1.1**. As the PCA and PLS-DA are two effective multivariate analysis methods for large-scale data matrix, the combining data were analyzed using PCA and PLS-DA approaches. As shown in **Figures 2A,B**, PCA and PLS-DA score showed a clear classification between model group and control group, demonstrating that circulating lipids profiles are significantly different in the model group. As well, the CP-treated group or glibenclamide treated group also had its own distinctive classification, bearing some overlap. Considering the overlap between model group and CP-treated group, we further narrowed down the profiles of lipids in these two groups using OPLS-DA method. Notably, CE, DG, TG, PC, and SM were significantly distinguished between these two groups (**Figures 2C,D**), And then, we applied the hierarchal clustering analysis to segregate the lipid metabolites into three distinct groups (shown in **Figure 2E**). A significant number of lipids were up-regulated in model group in comparison with control or blank groups. After CP or glibenclamide treatment, the levels of these lipids were greatly down-regulated. The results suggest that CP or glibenclamide could significantly regulate lipid metabolism in diabetes. Interestingly, PCA and PLS-DA analysis result showed that the score plot of CP-treated group and glibenclamide-treated group were not separated, and the same result was observed in heat map of hierarchal clustering analysis (**Figures 2B,E**), suggesting CP and glibenclamide may share the similar metabolic pathways to improve the diabetic dyslipidemia.

Subsequently, we analyzed the changes of lipids between control (blank) groups and model groups, and found that 47 lipids were elevated and 53 lipids were reduced in model group. After CP treatment, 30 lipids including CE, DG, TG, PC, and SM species were significantly either up-regulated or down-regulated ($p < 0.05$) (**Figure 3**). After importing those CP-regulated lipids to Cytoscape, a network pathway was built based on KEGG database and revealed that metabolic pathways including arachidonic acid metabolism, bile acid biosynthesis, *de novo* fatty acid biosynthesis, glycerophospholipid metabolism, glycosphingolipid metabolism, linoleate metabolism and saturated fatty acids beta-oxidation are involved in the regulating function of CP in lipid metabolism (As shown in **Supplementary Figure S5**).

CP Possess Multiple Components-Multiple Targets-Multiple Pathways Properties for Diabetic Dyslipidemia

Since absorption into the bloodstream is one of the prerequisites for drug efficacy, we performed a pharmacochemistry study to detect the CP components in blood stream after oral administration in mice. As shown in **Table 2** and **Supplementary Figure S2**, after oral administration of CP to normal C57/BL6 mice, 13 compounds in total: quinic acid, neochlorogenic acid, chlorogenic acid, 4-hydroxybenzoic acid, gallic acid, quercetin-3-glucuronide, kaempferol, loganin 7-pentoside, astragalin, kaempferol-3-rhamnoside, quercetin, quadranoside IV, and asiatic acid were detected. Subsequently, we used in-house tools "MOST: most-similar ligand-based approach to target prediction" (Huang et al., 2017) to predict the protein targets of major potential active components of CP identified in bloodstream as shown in **Supplementary Table S1.2**. Sixty-nine

TABLE 2 | Constituents of CP identified in plasma.

No.	Compound	Classification	Blank plasma	Plasma after 10 min administration	Plasma after 30 min administration
1	Quinic acid	Organic acid	–	√	√
2	Neochlorogenic acid	Organic acid	–	√	–
3	Chlorogenic acid	Organic acid	–	√	√
4	4-Hydroxybenzoic acid	Organic acid	–	√	√
5	Gallic acid	Organic acid	–	√	–
6	Quercetin-3-glucuronide	Flavonoid	–	√	√
7	Astragalin	Flavonoid	–	√	√
8	Kaempferol	Flavonoid	–	√	√
9	Loganin 7-pentoside	Flavonoid	–	√	√
10	Kaempferol-3-rhamnoside	Flavonoid	–	√	√
11	Quercetin	Flavonoid	–	√	√
12	Quadranoside IV	Saponin	–	√	√
13	Asiatic acid	Saponin	–	√	√

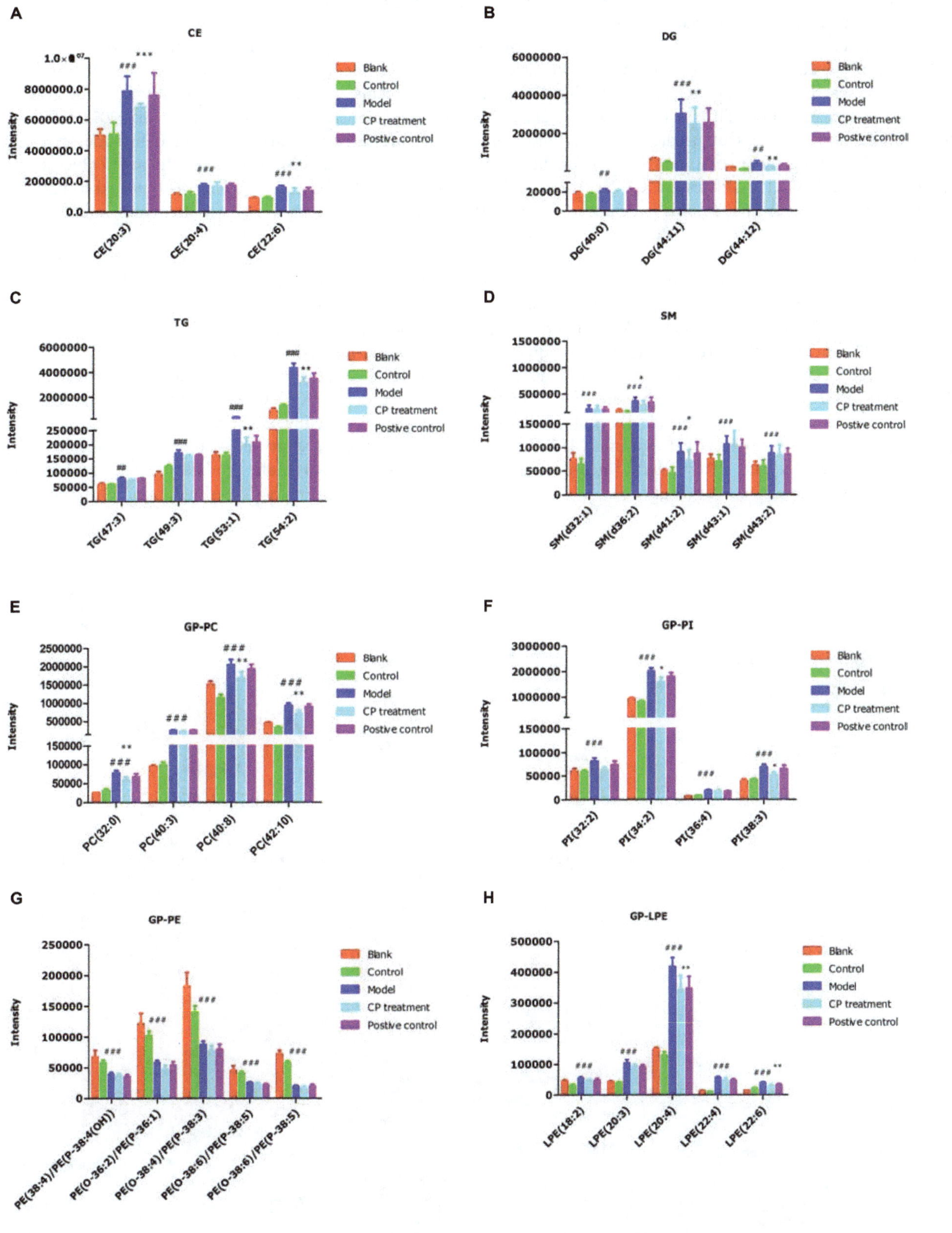

FIGURE 3 | *Cyclocarya paliurus* improved circulating lipids profiles in diabetic mice model. **(A)** Cholesterol ester (CE), **(B)** Diglyceride (DG); **(C)** Triglyceride (TG); **(D)** Sphingomyelin (SM); **(E)** Phosphatidylcholines (GP-PC); **(F)** Phosphatidylinositol (PI); **(G)** Phosphatidylethanolamine (GP-PE); **(H)** Lysophosphatidylethanolamine (GP-LPE). All data are presented as means ± SEM (n = 6~8). $^{\#}p < 0.05$, $^{\#\#}p < 0.01$, $^{\#\#\#}p < 0.001$ (comparison between control and model group); $^{*}p < 0.05$, $^{**}p < 0.01$, $^{***}p < 0.001$ (comparison between CP group and model group).

targets were matched for flavonoids, 59 targets were matched for organic acids, and 2 targets were matched for saponins. There targets were searched by related key words online to determine the relevance of diabetic dyslipidemia. Five targets were selected after reference searching. Finally, we linked the lipids targets with predicted targets using STRING (Szklarczyk et al., 2014) to build interaction networks of predicted targets and lipids targets via PPI. Among these compounds, the main predicted targets of CP were ALOX12, APP, BCL2, CYP2C9, and PTPN1 while the predicted-targets linked lipids targets via PPI analysis were PLA2G(s) and PI3K(s) families as shown in **Supplementary Figure S3**.

We then conducted reference searching to review the experiment study on these targets as shown in **Supplementary Table S2**. The ALOX, BCL-2, CYP 2C9, PLA2G(s) and PI3K(s) families, PLD2 and PTEN were determined as quercetin and kaempferol targets on diabetic dyslipidemia (Guo et al., 2017). PTPN1, PI3K(s) family and PLD2 were determined as targets of saponins such as quadranoside IV and asiatic acid (Ramachandran and Saravanan, 2015), whilst BCL-2, PI3K(s) family, PLD2 and PTEN were determined as action targets of gallic acid and 4-hydrobenzoic acids (**Figure 4**).

DISCUSSION

Hyperlipidemia is the most common form of dyslipidemia, refers to the abnormally elevated levels of any/all lipids or lipoproteins in the blood, frequently happened in long-term type II diabetes patients (Dixit et al., 2014). Recent studies have indicated that diabetic dyslipidemia may not only be the consequence but also the cause of disturbed glucose metabolism (Parhofer, 2015). Recently, CP was reported to improve insulin sensitivity (Jiang et al., 2014), attenuates inflammation (Wang Z. et al., 2017), and control hyperglycemic and hyperlipidemic abnormalities (Xu et al., 2017) both *in vitro* and *in vivo*, although the hypolipidemic mechanism has not been elucidated yet. In this study, we confirmed CP alleviated lipid dysfunction in diabetes, particularly diabetic dyslipidemia, as revealed by the clinical index, histological analysis, and lipidomics analysis. Mechanistically, we employed a network pharmacology approach to determine that CP's hypolipidemic effect involvement in PI3K and MAPK signaling pathways.

Lipidomics is a powerful tool to investigate lipid profiles changes. Previous studies indicated that circulating lipidomes were correlated with hyperlipidemia and hepatic steatosis

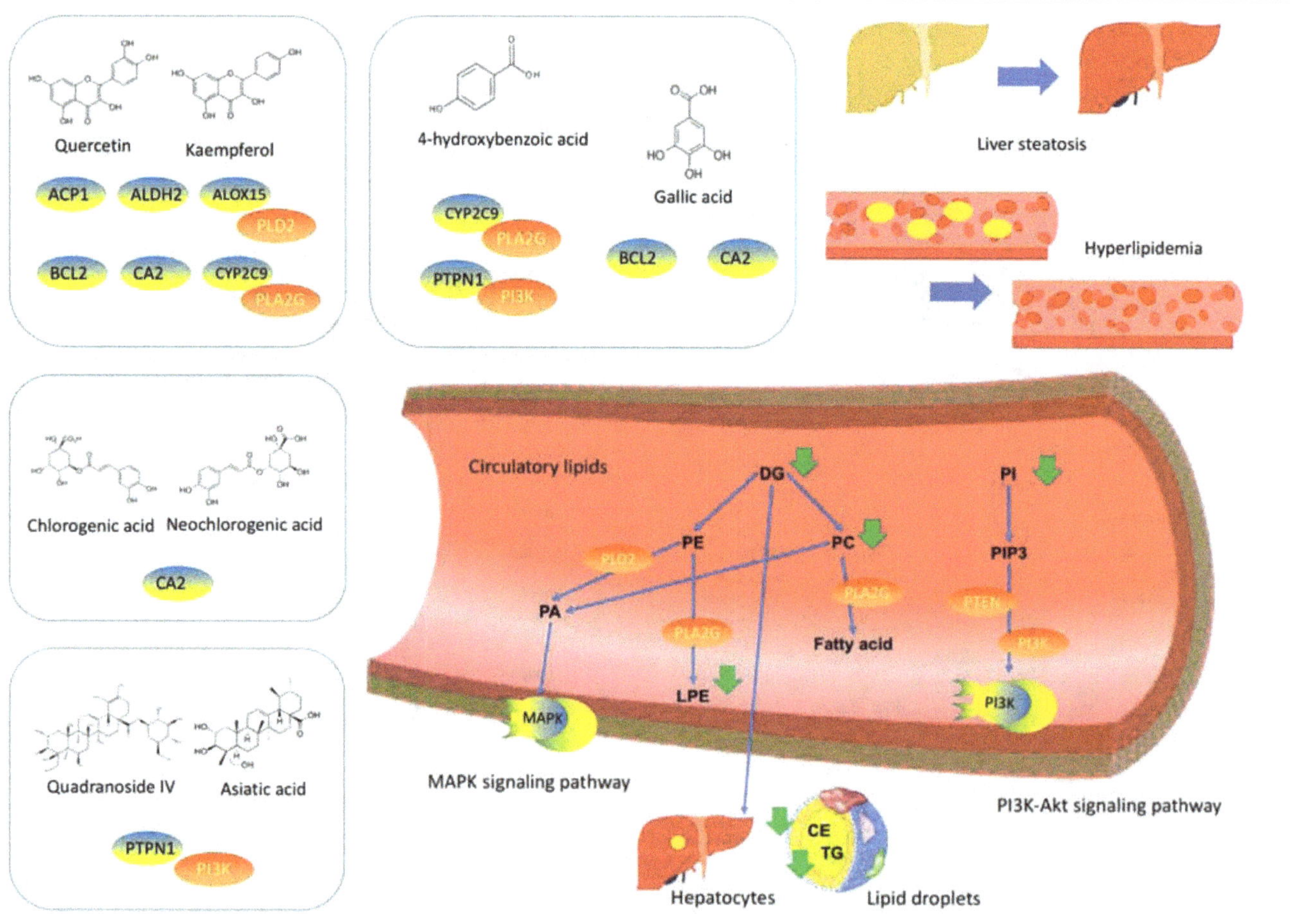

FIGURE 4 | *Cyclocarya paliurus* possess multiple components-multiple targets-multiple pathways properties for diabetic dyslipidemia. **Left** to **right:** The predicted targets based on CP constituents. The PPI network of predicted targets-linked lipid targets. The lipids regulated by CP in diabetic dyslipidemia.

(Wouters et al., 2008), therefore making lipids profiles an adequate indicator of CP effects in this study. Through the lipidomics study, it was shown that STZ and high-fat diet induced type 2 diabetic mice had lipid disorders due to lipid metabolism changes. Among the changed lipids, the majority lipids classes were DG, TG, CE, PC, SM, FA, PI, and PE. We found that CE, DG, TG, SM, PC, PI, and LPE were increased in the model group, while PE was decreased in the model group. CE is a dietary lipid involved in fat digestion and absorption as well as cholesterol metabolism. It directly affects LDL as well as HDL levels, and can be hydrolyzed by pancreatic enzymes to produce cholesterol and free fatty acids (Rosenson et al., 2016). DG and TG represent the main lipid components of fat deposits, which accumulated largely in lipid droplets of hepatocytes when in hepatic steatosis (Szczepaniak et al., 2005). Our results showed that CE, DG, and TG were downregulated after CP treatment which further indiacates the reduxction in fat accumulation in lipid droplets. PC (lecithin) are one class of glycerophospholipids with choline as a head group, which constitute major component of biological membranes, associating with the health benefits such as liver repair and lipolysis (Payne et al., 2014). Lipid absorption and utilization, particularly TG, is closely related to the PC content and its associated enzymes. Besides, PC can protect against steatosis in mice (Niebergall et al., 2011). Our results displayed that CP could reduce the palmitic acids levels and adjust PC content to improve lipid utilization and protect hepatic steatosis. PE is directly associated with diabetes and dyslipidemia and PC/PE ratio is closely correlated with the accumulation of hepatic TG content (Bradley et al., 2015; Ling et al., 2017). Our results showed that the levels of PE were elevated in CP-treated diabetic mice, indicating CP can reduce TG accumulation. SM contains either PC or PE as its head group. As lipid rafts, SM takes part in lipid microdomains and inhibition of SM synthesis would increase the ceramide level, a mediator of non-alcoholic fatty liver diseases (Kasumov et al., 2015). Our results showed that PC could increase SM content by reducing ceramide levels, possibly to alleviate hepatic steatosis. Our results indicate that CP has a great potential in the improvement of circulating lipid metabolism in diabetic dyslipidemia.

The beneficial function of CP on diabetic dyslipidemia can be deduced by its lipid regulating effect on circulatory system through multiple metabolic pathways. Therefore, it is important to identify the CP components and elucidate their biological activities to further define its use as a herbal product. Moreover, identifying the targets of CP's active components can lead to greater understanding of CP's mechanisms of action against diabetic dyslipidemia. By using lipidomics-based network pharmacology approach, we determined several CP targets for diabetic dyslipidemia based on its potential active components. Besides of ACP1, ALDH2, BCL2, and CA2 targets, the ALOX15, CYP2C9, and PTPN1 targets can interact with lipid targets PLD2, PTEN, PLA2G(s), and PI3K(s) family targets. BCL2, PTPN1, and PI3K alters expression of PI3K signaling pathway (Rahmani et al., 2013; Sugiyama et al., 2017). ALDH2, ALOX15, and BCL2 are involved in MAPK signaling pathway (De Chiara et al., 2006; Zhang et al., 2011; Zhao et al., 2011), and activation of MAPK can influence the expression of CYP2C9 (Bachleda et al., 2009). PLD2, and its product phosphatidic acid, can also activate MAPK (Grab et al., 2004). Therefore, the signaling pathway for its pharmacological mechanism may be related with PI3K and MAPK signaling pathway (Ma et al., 2015; Wu et al., 2017; Xiao et al., 2017). The multiple components of CP targeting multiple targets through multiple metabolic pathways to improve diabetic dyslipidemia in type 2 diabetic mice.

To our knowledge, we have provided a novel metabolomics-based network pharmacology approach to combine and link experimental targets and predicted targets together based on the bioactive components of herbal products. For a network pharmacology study, particularly on herbal medicine or herbal formula, the metabolomics-based network pharmacology strategy can integrate more comprehensive targets for targets prediction and linking their interactions. Integrating the analysis of systemic metabolic profiles based on metabolomics study with computational prediction based on serum pharmacochemistry information can result in more precise pharmacological mechanism associated targets prediction (Huang et al., 2018). It is also the first study to link lipids targets from lipidomics study with predicted targets from computational tools through PPI to improve the network pharmacology analysis. Up to now, there are some questions that still need to be answered: First, some of PPI between predicted targets and lipid targets have not been validated experimentally. Further experimental work can be performed to uncover the relationship between targets-targets. Next, the potential active compounds we identified in this study have been shown to be effective for anti-diabetic studies on animals, the systemic evaluation of combinatorial use on these compounds have not been conducted yet. Additional *in vitro* and *in vivo* studies in future will help to uncover the multiple pharmacological mechanisms found in herbal medicines.

CONCLUSION

In this study, we report CP attenuated diabetic dyslipidemia and hepatic streatosis in high fat diet and STZ-induced diabetic mice. The lipidomics study revealed CP improves circulatory lipids disorder, and the serum pharmacochemistry study revealed quinic acid, neochlorogenic acid, chlorogenic acid, 4-hydroxybenzoic acid, gallic acid, quercetin-3-glucuronide, kaempferol, loganin 7-pentoside, astragalin, kaempferol-3-rhamnoside, quercetin, quadranoside IV, and asiatic acid are potential active components of CP. Combining lipidomics and bioinformatics analysis, ALOX12, APP, BCL2, CYP2C9, and PTPN1 were predicted as direct targets of CP, whilst PLD2, PTEN and PLA2G(s) and PI3K(s) families were predicted as lipids linked targets of CP in diabetic hyperlipidemia. In conclusion, the CP was shown to be a multi-component and multi-targets herbal product with potent lipid regulation properties in dyslipidemia.

AUTHOR CONTRIBUTIONS

Z-xB and H-tX designed the study and revised the manuscript. Ht-X, BW, C-hL, LxZ, and Z-wN performed the animal experiment. LxZ performed the clinical index analysis, lipidomics analysis, bioinformatics analysis, and wrote the manuscript. Z-wN performed phytochemicals analysis of CP. TH performed bioinformatics analysis and revised the manuscript. LZ and C-yL provided technical support and advices toward study.

FUNDING

This work was kindly funded by grants from Kong Baptist University Research Grant (No. LIUYE/15-16/01-CLNC) and Shenzhen Science and Technology Innovation Committee Grant (No. JCYJ20170413170320959).

ACKNOWLEDGMENTS

We would like to thank Mr. Chan Chi Leung and Mr. Ho Hing Man for providing technical support for metabolomics study and Ms. Wang Jianying for providing some lipids reference standards. We also thank Dr. Anthony Booker for writing improvement.

REFERENCES

Andriankaja, O. M., and Joshipura, K. (2014). Potential association between prediabetic conditions and gingival and/or periodontal inflammation. *J. Diabetes Investig.* 5, 108–114. doi: 10.1111/jdi.12122

Association, A. D. (2015). Standards of medical care in diabetes—2015 abridged for primary care providers. *Clin. Diabetes* 33, 97–111. doi: 10.2337/diaclin.33.2.97

Bachleda, P., Vrzal, R., and Dvorák, Z. (2009). Activation of MAPKs influences the expression of drug-metabolizing enzymes in primary human hepatocytes. *Gen. Physiol. Biophys.* 28, 316–320. doi: 10.4149/gpb_2009_03_316

Beger, R. D., Dunn, W., Schmidt, M. A., Gross, S. S., Kirwan, J. A., Cascante, M., et al. (2016). Metabolomics enables precision medicine:"a white paper, community perspective.". *Metabolomics* 12:149. doi: 10.1007/s11306-016-1094-6

Bradley, R. M., Marvyn, P. M., Henao, J. J. A., Mardian, E. B., George, S., Aucoin, M. G., et al. (2015). Acylglycerophosphate acyltransferase 4 (AGPAT4) is a mitochondrial lysophosphatidic acid acyltransferase that regulates brain phosphatidylcholine, phosphatidylethanolamine, and phosphatidylinositol levels. *Biochim. Biophys. Acta* 1851, 1566–1576. doi: 10.1016/j.bbalip.2015.09.005

De Chiara, G., Marcocci, M. E., Torcia, M., Lucibello, M., Rosini, P., Bonini, P., et al. (2006). Bcl-2 phosphorylation by p38 MAPK Identification of target sites and biologic consequences. *J. Biol. Chem.* 281, 21353–21361. doi: 10.1074/jbc.M511052200

Dixit, A. K., Dey, R., Suresh, A., Chaudhuri, S., Panda, A. K., Mitra, A., et al. (2014). The prevalence of dyslipidemia in patients with diabetes mellitus of ayurveda Hospital. *J. Diabetes Metab. Disord.* 13:58. doi: 10.1186/2251-6581-13-58

Grab, L. T., Kearns, M. W., Morris, A. J., and Daniel, L. W. (2004). Differential role for phospholipase D1 and phospholipase D2 in 12-O-tetradecanoyl-13-phorbol acetate-stimulated MAPK activation, Cox-2 and IL-8 expression. *Biochim. Biophys. Acta* 1636, 29–39. doi: 10.1016/j.bbalip.2003.12.002

Gregory, K. E., Bird, S. S., Gross, V. S., Marur, V. R., Lazarev, A. V., Walker, W. A., et al. (2013). Method development for fecal lipidomics profiling. *Anal. Chem.* 85, 1114–1123. doi: 10.1021/ac303011k

Guo, C., Yang, R.-J., Jang, K., Zhou, X., and Liu, Y. (2017). Protective effects of pretreatment with quercetin against lipopolysaccharide-induced apoptosis and the inhibition of osteoblast differentiation via the mapk and wnt/β-catenin pathways in MC3T3-E1 cells. *Cell. Physiol. Biochem.* 43, 1547–1561. doi: 10.1159/000481978

Huan, T., Forsberg, E. M., Rinehart, D., Johnson, C. H., Ivanisevic, J., Benton, H. P., et al. (2017). Systems biology guided by XCMS Online metabolomics. *Nat. Methods* 14, 461–462. doi: 10.1038/nmeth.4260

Huang, T., Mi, H., Lin, C., Zhao, L., Zhong, L. L. D., Liu, F., et al. (2017). MOST: most-similar ligand based approach to target prediction. *BMC Bioinformatics* 18:165. doi: 10.1186/s12859-017-1586-z

Huang, T., Ning, Z., Hu, D., Zhang, M., Zhao, L., Lin, C., et al. (2018). Uncovering the mechanisms of Chinese Herbal Medicine (MaZiRenWan) for functional constipation by focused network pharmacology approach. *Front. Pharmacol.* 9:270. doi: 10.3389/fphar.2018.00270

Jiang, C., Wang, Q., Wei, Y., Yao, N., Wu, Z., Ma, Y., et al. (2015). Cholesterol-lowering effects and potential mechanisms of different polar extracts from *Cyclocarya paliurus* leave in hyperlipidemic mice. *J. Ethnopharmacol.* 176, 17–26. doi: 10.1016/j.jep.2015.10.006

Jiang, C., Yao, N., Wang, Q., Zhang, J., Sun, Y., Xiao, N., et al. (2014). *Cyclocarya paliurus* extract modulates adipokine expression and improves insulin sensitivity by inhibition of inflammation in mice. *J. Ethnopharmacol.* 153, 344–351. doi: 10.1016/j.jep.2014.02.003

Jung, U. J., and Choi, M.-S. (2014). Obesity and its metabolic complications: the role of adipokines and the relationship between obesity, inflammation, insulin resistance, dyslipidemia and nonalcoholic fatty liver disease. *Int. J. Mol. Sci.* 15, 6184–6223. doi: 10.3390/ijms15046184

Kasumov, T., Li, L., Li, M., Gulshan, K., Kirwan, J. P., Liu, X., et al. (2015). Ceramide as a mediator of non-alcoholic Fatty liver disease and associated atherosclerosis. *PLoS One* 10:e0126910. doi: 10.1371/journal.pone.0126910

Kurihara, H., Asami, S., Shibata, H., Fukami, H., and Tanaka, T. (2003). Hypolipemic Effect of *Cyclocarya paliurus* (Batal) Iljinskaja in lipid-loaded mice. *Biol. Pharm. Bull.* 26, 383–385. doi: 10.1248/bpb.26.383

Li, S., Fan, T.-P., Jia, W., Lu, A., and Zhang, W. (2014). Network pharmacology in traditional chinese medicine. *Evid. Based Complement. Altern. Med.* 2014:138460. doi: 10.1155/2014/138460

Lin, Z., Wu, Z.-F., Jiang, C.-H., Jiang, Q.-W., Ouyang, S., Che, C.-T., et al. (2016). The chloroform extract of *Cyclocarya paliurus* attenuates high-fat diet induced non-alcoholic hepatic steatosis in Sprague Dawley rats. *Phytomedicine* 23, 1475–1483. doi: 10.1016/j.phymed.2016.08.003

Ling, A. V., Gearing, M. E., Semova, I., Shin, D.-J., Clements, R., Lai, Z. W., et al. (2017). FoxO1 is required for most of the metabolic and hormonal perturbations produced by hepatic insulin receptor deletion in male mice. *Endocrinology* 159, 1253–1263. doi: 10.1210/en.2017-00870

Ma, Y., Jiang, C., Yao, N., Li, Y., Wang, Q., Fang, S., et al. (2015). Antihyperlipidemic effect of *Cyclocarya paliurus* (Batal.) Iljinskaja extract and inhibition of apolipoprotein B48 overproduction in hyperlipidemic mice. *J. Ethnopharmacol.* 166, 286–296. doi: 10.1016/j.jep.2015.03.030

Niebergall, L. J., Jacobs, R. L., Chaba, T., and Vance, D. E. (2011). Phosphatidylcholine protects against steatosis in mice but not non-alcoholic steatohepatitis. *Biochim. Biophys. Acta* 1811, 1177–1185. doi: 10.1016/j.bbalip.2011.06.021

Parhofer, K. G. (2015). Interaction between glucose and lipid metabolism: more than diabetic dyslipidemia. *Diabetes Metab. J.* 39, 353–362. doi: 10.4093/dmj.2015.39.5.353

Payne, F., Lim, K., Girousse, A., Brown, R. J., Kory, N., Robbins, A., et al. (2014). Mutations disrupting the Kennedy phosphatidylcholine pathway in humans with congenital lipodystrophy and fatty liver disease. *Proc. Natl. Acad. Sci. U.S.A.* 111, 8901–8906. doi: 10.1073/pnas.1408523111

Perry, R. J., Samuel, V. T., Petersen, K. F., and Shulman, G. I. (2014). The role of hepatic lipids in hepatic insulin resistance and type 2 diabetes. *Nature* 510, 84–91. doi: 10.1038/nature13478

Rahmani, M., Aust, M. M., Attkisson, E., Williams, D. C. J., Ferreira-Gonzalez, A., and Grant, S. (2013). Dual inhibition of Bcl-2 and Bcl-xL strikingly enhances

PI3K inhibition-induced apoptosis in human myeloid leukemia cells through a GSK3- and Bim-dependent mechanism. *Cancer Res.* 73, 1340–1351. doi: 10.1158/0008-5472.CAN-12-1365

Ramachandran, V., and Saravanan, R. (2015). Glucose uptake through translocation and activation of GLUT4 in PI3K/Akt signaling pathway by asiatic acid in diabetic rats. *Hum. Exp. Toxicol.* 34, 884–893. doi: 10.1177/0960327114561663

Richhariya, A., Fox, K. M., Punekar, R. S., Gandra, S. R., Fisher, M. D., Cziraky, M. J., et al. (2015). Gender Differences in Recurrent Cardiovascular Events Among High-risk Patients With Hyperlipidemia. *Circ. Cardiovasc. Qual. Outcomes* 8:A307. doi: 10.1161/circoutcomes.8.suppl_2.307

Rosenson, R. S., Brewer, H. B. Jr., Ansell, B. J., Barter, P., Chapman, M. J., Heinecke, J. W., et al. (2016). Dysfunctional HDL and atherosclerotic cardiovascular disease. *Nat. Rev. Cardiol.* 13, 48–60. doi: 10.1038/nrcardio.2015.124

Sattar, N., Preiss, D., Robinson, J. G., Djedjos, C. S., Elliott, M., Somaratne, R., et al. (2016). Lipid-lowering efficacy of the PCSK9 inhibitor evolocumab (AMG 145) in patients with type 2 diabetes: a meta-analysis of individual patient data. *Lancet Diabetes Endocrinol.* 4, 403–410. doi: 10.1016/S2213-8587(16)00003-6

Spence, J. D., Urquhart, B. L., and Bang, H. (2016). Effect of renal impairment on atherosclerosis: only partially mediated by homocysteine. *Nephrol. Dial. Transplant.* 31, 937–944. doi: 10.1093/ndt/gfv380

Stern, C., and Castera, L. (2017). Non-invasive diagnosis of hepatic steatosis. *Hepatol. Int.* 11, 70–78. doi: 10.1007/s12072-016-9772-z

Sugiyama, M., Banno, R., Mizoguchi, A., Tominaga, T., Tsunekawa, T., Onoue, T., et al. (2017). PTP1B deficiency improves hypothalamic insulin sensitivity resulting in the attenuation of AgRP mRNA expression under high-fat diet conditions. *Biochem. Biophys. Res. Commun.* 488, 116–121. doi: 10.1016/j.bbrc.2017.05.019

Szczepaniak, L. S., Nurenberg, P., Leonard, D., Browning, J. D., Reingold, J. S., Grundy, S., et al. (2005). Magnetic resonance spectroscopy to measure hepatic triglyceride content: prevalence of hepatic steatosis in the general population. *Am. J. Physiol. Metab.* 288, E462–E468. doi: 10.1152/ajpendo.00064.2004

Szklarczyk, D., Franceschini, A., Wyder, S., Forslund, K., Heller, D., Huerta-Cepas, J., et al. (2014). STRING v10: protein–protein interaction networks, integrated over the tree of life. *Nucleic Acids Res.* 43, D447–D452. doi: 10.1093/nar/gku1003

Wang, Q., Jiang, C., Fang, S., Wang, J., Ji, Y., Shang, X., et al. (2013). Antihyperglycemic, antihyperlipidemic and antioxidant effects of ethanol and aqueous extracts of *Cyclocarya paliurus* leaves in type 2 diabetic rats. *J. Ethnopharmacol.* 150, 1119–1127. doi: 10.1016/j.jep.2013.10.040

Wang, X., Zhang, A., Sun, H., and Han, Y. (2017). "Integrated serum pharmacochemistry of TCM and metabolomics strategies for innovative drug discovery," in *Serum Pharmacochemistry of Traditional Chinese Medicine*, eds X. Wang, A. Zhang, and H. Sun (New York, NY: Elsevier), 15–21.

Wang, Z., Xie, J., Yang, Y., Zhang, F., Wang, S., Wu, T., et al. (2017). Sulfated *Cyclocarya paliurus* polysaccharides markedly attenuates inflammation and oxidative damage in lipopolysaccharide-treated macrophage cells and mice. *Sci. Rep.* 7:40402. doi: 10.1038/srep40402

Wouters, K., van Gorp, P. J., Bieghs, V., Gijbels, M. J., Duimel, H., Lütjohann, D., et al. (2008). Dietary cholesterol, rather than liver steatosis, leads to hepatic inflammation in hyperlipidemic mouse models of nonalcoholic steatohepatitis. *Hepatology* 48, 474–486. doi: 10.1002/hep.22363

Wu, Z., Gao, T., Zhong, R., Lin, Z., Jiang, C., Ouyang, S., et al. (2017). Antihyperlipidaemic effect of triterpenic acid-enriched fraction from *Cyclocarya paliurus* leaves in hyperlipidaemic rats. *Pharm. Biol.* 55, 712–721. doi: 10.1080/13880209.2016.1267231

Xia, J., Sinelnikov, I. V., Han, B., and Wishart, D. S. (2015). MetaboAnalyst 3.0—making metabolomics more meaningful. *Nucleic Acids Res.* 43, W251–W257. doi: 10.1093/nar/gkv380

Xiao, H., Wen, B., Ning, Z., Zhai, L., Liao, C., Lin, C., et al. (2017). *Cyclocarya paliurus* tea leaves enhances pancreatic β cell preservation through inhibition of apoptosis. *Sci. Rep.* 7:9155. doi: 10.1038/s41598-017-09641-z

Xu, G., Yoshitomi, H., Sun, W., Guo, X., Wu, L., Guo, X., et al. (2017). *Cyclocarya paliurus* (Batal.) Ijinskaja aqueous extract (CPAE) ameliorates obesity by improving insulin signaling in the hypothalamus of a metabolic syndrome rat model. *Evid. Based Complement. Altern. Med.* 2017:4602153. doi: 10.1155/2017/4602153

Yan, G., Wang, X., Zhang, A., Shi, H., Zhou, Y., and Sun, H. (2017). "Serum pharmacochemistry of TCM for determining the active ingredients of shuanghuanglian formulae," in *Serum Pharmacochemistry of Traditional Chinese Medicine*, eds X. Wang, A. Zhang, and H. Sun (New York, NY: Elsevier), 155–169. doi: 10.1016/B978-0-12-811147-5.00011-X

Yang, Z.-W., Ouyang, K.-H., Zhao, J., Chen, H., Xiong, L., and Wang, W.-J. (2016). Structural characterization and hypolipidemic effect of *Cyclocarya paliurus* polysaccharide in rat. *Int. J. Biol. Macromol.* 91, 1073–1080. doi: 10.1016/j.ijbiomac.2016.06.063

Yao, X., Lin, Z., Jiang, C., Gao, M., Wang, Q., Yao, N., et al. (2015). *Cyclocarya paliurus* prevents high fat diet induced hyperlipidemia and obesity in Sprague–Dawley rats. *Can. J. Physiol. Pharmacol.* 93, 677–686. doi: 10.1139/cjpp-2014-0477

Yoshitomi, H., Tsuru, R., Li, L., Zhou, J., Kudo, M., Liu, T., et al. (2017). *Cyclocarya paliurus* extract activates insulin signaling via Sirtuin1 in C2C12 myotubes and decreases blood glucose level in mice with impaired insulin secretion. *PLoS One* 12:e0183988. doi: 10.1371/journal.pone.0183988

Zafrir, B., and Jain, M. (2014). Lipid-lowering therapies, glucose control and incident diabetes: evidence, mechanisms and clinical implications. *Cardiovasc. Drugs Ther.* 28, 361–377. doi: 10.1007/s10557-014-6534-9

Zhang, P., Xu, D., Wang, S., Fu, H., Wang, K., Zou, Y., et al. (2011). Inhibition of aldehyde dehydrogenase 2 activity enhances antimycin-induced rat cardiomyocytes apoptosis through activation of MAPK signaling pathway. *Biomed. Pharmacother.* 65, 590–593. doi: 10.1016/j.biopha.2009.12.001

Zhao, J., O'Donnell, V. B., Balzar, S., Croix, C. M. S., Trudeau, J. B., and Wenzel, S. E. (2011). 15-Lipoxygenase 1 interacts with phosphatidylethanolamine-binding protein to regulate MAPK signaling in human airway epithelial cells. *Proc. Natl. Acad. Sci. U.S.A.* 108, 14246–14251. doi: 10.1073/pnas.1018075108

Zhao, X., Zheng, X., Fan, T.-P., Li, Z., Zhang, Y., and Zheng, J. (2015). A novel drug discovery strategy inspired by traditional medicine philosophies. *Science* 347, S38–S40.

13

Network Pharmacology–Based Analysis and Experimental Exploration of Antidiabetic Mechanisms of Gegen Qinlian Decoction

Yu Xu[1†], Jihan Huang[2†], Ning Wang[1], Hor-Yue Tan[1], Cheng Zhang[1], Sha Li[1], Guoyi Tang[1] and Yibin Feng[1]*

[1]School of Chinese Medicine, Li Ka Shing Faculty of Medicine, The University of Hong Kong, Hong Kong, China, [2]Center for Drug Clinical Research, Shanghai University of Traditional Chinese Medicine, Shanghai, China

***Correspondence:**
Yibin Feng
yfeng@hku.hk

[†]These authors have contributed equally to this work

Type-2 diabetes mellitus (T2DM) and therapy options have been studied increasingly due to their rising incidence and prevalence. The trend of applying traditional Chinese medicine (TCM) to treat T2DM is increasing as a crucial medical care for metabolic dysfunctions. Gegen Qinlian decoction (GQL), a well-known classical TCM formula used in China, has been clinically applied to treat various types of chronic metabolic diseases. However, antidiabetic effects of GQL administration during T2DM have never been studied systematically. We assessed physiological and molecular targets associated with therapeutic effects of GQL by evaluating network topological characteristics. The GQL-related biological pathways are closely associated with antidiabetic effects, including the TNF and PI3K–AKT signaling pathways. Associated primary biological processes such as RNA polymerase II promoter transcription participate in the inflammatory response, oxidative stress reduction, and glucose metabolic process, thereby exerting multiple biological effects on the antidiabetic mechanism. Furthermore, our results showed that GQL can affect blood glycemic levels and ameliorate inflammatory symptoms, and liver and pancreas tissue injury in high-fat diet plus streptozotocin-induced diabetic mice. *In vivo* and *in vitro* experiments confirmed that antidiabetic effects of GQL were associated with a modulation of the TNF and PI3K–AKT–MTOR pathways.

Keywords: type 2 diabetes mellitus, network analysis, herbal medicine, Gegen Qinlian decoction, multi-pathways

INTRODUCTION

Type-2 diabetes mellitus (T2DM) is a chronic metabolic disease which constitutes a severe threat to global public health (Chan et al., 2009). T2DM is a chronic hyperglycemia and inflammatory disease which may lead to macrovascular and microvascular degenerative complications, including cardiovascular diseases, diabetic nephropathy, and retinopathy (Usuelli and La Rocca, 2015). Metabolic dysfunction and inflammatory responses are partly responsible for islet function loss and irreversible host organ damage during pathological progression of T2DM and its associated complications. The World Health Organization estimated the number of deaths caused by diabetes mellitus and its related complications at approximately 1,600,000 in 2016. Severe diabetic complications and the lack of comprehensive therapy of T2DM and its associated afflictions require identification of novel effective treatment avenues (Kalra et al., 2018). As a crucial healthcare and alternative medicinal complement avenue, many traditional Chinese medicines (TCMs) have shown superior success regarding treatment of human metabolic disorders in China, Korea, and Japan. The remarkable efficacy and safety of TCMs with low toxicity have been acknowledged after several hundred years of practical clinical application in chronic metabolic disorder therapy (Pang et al., 2015).

As an alternative medicinal application, TCM has been demonstrated to exert excellent clinical effects on T2DM due to its rich herbal plant resources, many of which have been developed and are commonly used alone or in combination with adjuvant hypoglycemic agents for T2DM therapy (Covington, 2001). Gegen QinLian decoction (GQL) is a well-known classical TCM which has been used to treat chronic diarrhea and damp-heat syndrome, according to ancient records (Shang Han Lun) (Li et al., 2016). GQL is composed of four herbal drugs at a weight ratio of 5:3:3:2, for example, 15 g Puerariae Lobatae Radix (Gegen, *Pueraria lobata* (Wild.) Ohwi), 9 g Scutellariae Radix (Huangqin, *Scutellaria baicalensis* Georgi), 9 g Coptidis Rhizoma (Huanglian, *Coptis chinensis* Franch.), and 6 g Glycyrrhizae Radix et Rhizoma (zhi gan cao, *Glycyrrhiza uralensis* Fisch.). Modern clinical research has shown that GQL can normalize hyperglycemia and hyperlipidemia in T2DM patients (Ryuk et al., 2017), and its practical therapeutic application during diabetes mellitus has been assessed for more than ten years (Zeng et al., 2006). GQL was also used to treat T2DM-related complications with promising results (Han et al., 2017). However, the different constituents of GQL may exert various effects, which obscures the underlying molecular mechanisms; therefore, the respective antidiabetic chemical and pharmacological processes must be elucidated.

Systems pharmacology can help identify novel strategies and useful methods for discovering TCMs to treat complex diseases (Li and Zhang, 2013). In recent years, new network pharmacology combined with gene ontology (GO) enrichment analysis has become a useful tool to systemically determine interactions among TCM compounds, gene or protein targets, and pathways of diseases, which implies a holistic concept of TCM therapy (Li et al., 2014; Guo et al., 2019). Based on systemic bioinformatics, network pharmacology facilitates evaluation of feasibility and applicability of TCM for treating complex diseases through compound-target and target-signaling network analysis. Network pharmacology was successfully established in our laboratory for investigating complex herbal formulas used to treat human cancers (Wang et al., 2018b; Guo et al., 2019; Huang et al., 2020a). Meanwhile, previous ingredient–drug networks combined with GO biological analysis has showed that 4-hydroxymephenytoin from Puerariae Lobatae Radix can improve insulin metabolism in islet cells and adipocytes (Li et al., 2014). In the current study, we examined the pharmacological mechanisms of GQL and its effects on T2DM using network pharmacology analysis and experimental confirmation. Network pharmacology analysis was performed to identify the protective drug targets and the essential signaling pathways affected by GQL during T2DM. Furthermore, we examined GQL-related antidiabetic mechanisms using *in vivo* and *in vitro* experiments. Our results suggest the potential underlying mechanism of GQL and provide strong evidence for this therapeutic avenue of treating T2DM.

MATERIALS AND METHODS

Ultrahigh-Performance Liquid Chromatography Analysis of Gegen Qinlian Decoction Constituents

Nong's GQL formula (A190049310) was commercially purchased from PuraPharm (Hong Kong, China), and its constituents were identified using UHPLC analysis. GQL powder (1 g) was extracted using methanol (10 ml) in a 15-ml centrifuge tube, and the methanol solution was sonicated and centrifuged at 35,000 rpm. The supernatant solution was then filtered through a 0.45-μm membrane before UHPLC analysis. Chromatographic analysis was performed using a reverse-phase ACE Excel C18 column (100 mm × 2.1 mm) at a flow rate of 0.379 ml/min at 35 C. The elution media with 0.15% trifluoroacetic acid (B) and methanol (A) were used with a gradient protocol as follows: 77–70% B for 0–4.4 min, 70%–65% B for 4.4–4.576 min, 65%–42% B for 4.576–6.864 min, 42%–45% B for 6.864–7.040 min, 45%–45% B for 7.04–9.68 min, 45%–30% B for 9.68–12 min, and 30–30% B for 12–15 min.

Interaction Network of Gegen Qinlian Decoction Constituents and T2DM Target Genes

We collected information on the GQL chemical constituents from previous studies (An et al., 2014; Wang et al., 2016; Qiao et al., 2016; Qiao et al., 2018). Forty-two active chemical GQL constituents were identified, including eight compounds from Puerariae Lobatae *Radix*, 14 compounds from Scutellariae Radix, seven compounds from Coptidis Rhizoma, and 13 compounds from Glycyrrhizae Radix et Rhizoma. Some chemical compounds of GQL show some properties of absorption, distribution, metabolism, and excretion (ADME) and the standard of drug-likeness (DL), and potentially druggable compounds were selected as active constituents for further target prediction of GQL. Information on oral bioavailability (OB) and DL index of the 42 compounds is shown in **Supplementary Table S1**. Bioinformatic data of protein targets of bioactive GQL constituents were analyzed based on the online TCMSP database (http://tcmspw.com/) (**Supplementary Table S2**). Next, T2DM-associated target genes were compiled using the TTD (http://db.idrblab.net/ttd/), KEGG (http://www.kegg.jp/), and CTD (http://ctdbase.org/) databases to identify corresponding T2DM-associated protein targets (Zhou et al., 2019). The complex network diagrams of active GQL constituents and identified anti-T2DM targets were plotted as an ingredient–target interaction network to be mapped using Cytoscape 3.6.1 software (Shannon et al., 2003). To illustrate GQL-related target protein interactions in T2DM, highly connected target proteins were screened based on protein–protein interaction information using STRING software (http://string-db.org). We used a high confidence threshold (>0. 9) to ensure reliability, and protein–protein interaction data with high node degrees obtained from STRING were selected for establishing a protein–protein interaction network.

Target Proteins Analysis

To identify potential target proteins affected by GQL, GO biological function and KEGG pathway enrichment searches were carried out using the annotation database of DAVID biological information (Huang et al., 2007) to determine the predicted target protein function affected by GQL and their important role in signaling transduction. The top 10 significantly enriched terms for the predicted proteins regarding biological process (BP), cellular components (CC), and molecular functions (MF) were produced using the Benjamini–Hochberg procedure (Haynes, 2013).

Establishment and Treatment of a T2DM Mouse Model

All animal experiments were approved by the Committee on the Use of Live Animals in Teaching and Research of the University of Hong Kong. After adaptive feeding for one week, six-week-old C57BL/6J male mice were fed a high-fat diet (HFD, Research Diets, D12492) to induce obesity. After four weeks, HFD-fed mice were intraperitoneally injected with streptozotocin solution (STZ; Sigma-Aldrich, St. Louis, MO, United States) at 50 mg/kg on two consecutive days (Srinivasan et al., 2005). Next, mice with high-fasting blood glucose levels (≥11.0 mmol/L) were randomly selected as T2DM models. The diabetic mice were assigned to a GQL treatment and a control group (n = 5, each). Following the best practice in pharmacological research (Heinrich et al., 2020), we used a common criterion of drug dosage, body surface area (BSA) formulas (Reagan-Shaw et al., 2008), to calculate the drug doses in mice. With respect to previous studies on GQL in clinical (Tong et al., 2011) and animal studies (Blanchard and Smoliga, 2015; Lv et al., 2019; Wu et al., 2019), we orally administered GQL at 1 g/kg (GQL-L group) and 2 g/kg (GQL-H group) to T2DM mice for six weeks. An oral glucose tolerance test (OGTT) was used to assess glucose tolerance. After an initial glucose gauge (2 g/kg), blood glucose levels were monitored using a glucometer at various time points. The glucose plot area under the curve (AUC) was used to evaluate glucose tolerance in T2DM mice after GQL treatment. The calculation of the glucose AUC was performed using Prism 8.3.1 software. Serum samples were used to measure insulin, HbA1c, ALT, and AST levels.

Cell Culture

AML12 hepatocytes (obtained from the American Type Culture Collection, Manassas, VA, United States) were cultured in DMEM/F12 medium (10% FBS plus 100 mg/ml streptomycin and 100 U/mL penicillin) and were incubated at 37 C in an incubator continuously supplying 5% CO_2. To assess antidiabetic effects of GQL, we cultured AML12 cells in a palmitate plus high-glucose (33 mM) medium at 37 C for 24 h and treated the cells without or without GQL (100 μg/ml).

Immunoblotting

Protein was extracted by adding RIPA solution, and supernatant containing proteins was collected after centrifugation. After protein quantification using a Bio-Rad Protein Assay Kit II (5000002), protein separation was performed by SDS-PAGE gel electrophoresis, and separated proteins were transferred to a membrane and blocked using 5% BSA solution to prevent nonspecific protein binding. After blocking, the immunoblot membrane was incubated with primary antibodies against the target proteins such as GAPDH, iNOS, P-65, SOCS 2, P-ERK, P-AKT, P-MTOR, and P-JNK. After washing three times, the membrane was incubated with secondary antibody (1: 2,500). Protein expression was visualized using the ECL system and was analyzed using the Chemidoc chemiluminescent platform (Guo et al., 2019).

RT-PCR Analysis

Total RNA was isolated by using an RNeasy Mini Kit (Qiagen, Hilden, Germany), and concentration was measured at a 260 / 280-nm ratio. First-strand cDNA was transcribed from total RNA using a First Strand Synthesis Kit (Takara, Japan). PCR was conducted using SYBR Green reagent, specific primers (**Table 1**), and a Light Cycler 480 (Roche, Basel, Switzerland).

Hematoxylin and Eosin and Oil Red O Staining

Tissue samples of HFD + STZ mice were fixed in 4% paraformaldehyde buffer, and tissue sections (5 μm thickness) were stained using H&E and Oil Red O for general histology (Lucchesi et al., 2015).

Data Analyses

Statistical analysis was conducted using an ANOVA or Student's two-tailed t-test with Prism Software 8.3.1. Statistical significance is reported at $p < 0.05$.

RESULTS

Interaction Analysis of Gegen Qinlian Decoction and Type-2 Diabetes Mellitus Target Proteins

TCM was administered orally to examine its efficacy after the ADME process, and OB of the 42 active ingredients in GQL has been indicated to determine potentially druggable active compounds (Qiao et al., 2018). By screening the OB and DL index (**Supplementary Table S1**), we identified 12 candidate compounds from four herbs that contributed active compounds, including wogonin, oroxylin A, baicalein, baicalin, coptisine, epiberberine, berberine, palmatine, isoliquiritigenin, liquiritigenin, glycyrol, and formononetin (**Supplementary Figure S1**). Based on previous studies, GQL formula constituents were determined using UPLC analysis (**Figure 1A**), and puerarin (MOL07), daidzin (MOL01), berberine (MOL24), palmitane (MOL25), baicalin (MOL17),

TABLE 1 | PCR primer sequences and target genes.

Genes	Forward (5′-3′)	Reverse (5′-3′)
TNFα	CTACCTTGTTGCCTCCTCTTT	GAGCAGAGGTTCAGTGATGTAG
IL-6	AGGATACCACTCCCAACAGACCT	CAAGTGCATCATCGTTGTTCATAC
IL1β	CTTCAGGCAGGCAGTATCACTCAT	TCTAATGGGAACGTCACACACCAG
Caspase-8	CTCCGAAAAATGAAGGACAGA	CGTGGGATAGGATACAGCAGA
Caspase-3	AAGGAGCAGCTTTGTGTGTGT	AAGAGTTTCGGCTTTCCAGTC
β-actin	ACGGCCAGGTCATCACTATTG	TGGAAAAGAGCCTCAGGGC

and baicalein (MOL12) were identified as the major active constituents of the GQL formula. GQL contained puerarin at 1.038%, which meets the quality standard requirement of GQL formula according to the China Pharmacopeia 2015. We explored the therapeutic targets of the 42 active GQL constituents, and SMILES structural similarity of the selected active GQL constituents (**Supplementary Table S3**) was used to investigate the drug–target interaction prediction through the similarity ensemble approach, in which 38 different ingredients of GQL with practical pharmacological activities were closely associated with the 468 target proteins shown in **Supplementary Table S4**. Accordingly, the component–target–disease network showed that 38 active ingredients interacting with 148 T2DM-related target genes were generated using a therapeutic target database (Wang et al., 2020), and the network visualization was analyzed using Cytoscape 3.6.1 (**Figure 1B**). The compound–target network comprising 715 edges and 186 nodes showed that six high-degree compounds were associated with multiple target proteins, that is, MOL18 (chrysin, 38), MOL12 (baicalein, 44), MOL03 (daidzein, 58), MOL07 (puerarin, 41), MOL08 (wogonin, 53), and MOL28 (isoliquiritigenin, 46). Critical target proteins or ingredients with a high degree of connection in the interaction network may be responsible for essential antidiabetic effects of GQL.

Gegen Qinlian Decoction Type-2 Diabetes Mellitus Target Protein Identification

Highly connected subnetworks with 53 gene nodes were identified using the MCODE module analysis (Zhang et al., 2019) (**Figure 2A**). The Venn diagram results (**Figure 2B**) suggested 11 overlapping genes which were identified by matching the four herbal compounds-related genes with each other, including AR, ESR1, PTGS2, PIM1, CDK2, ESR2, HSP90AA1, NOS2, NOS3, PTGS1, and RXRA. This interaction network contained 296 edges and 52 nodes (**Figure 3C**), of which edges represent interactions between the proteins and nodes represent target proteins. MAPK14, JUN, STAT3, IL-2, JAK2, TP53, CCND1, AKT1, FOS, RELA,MMP9, SIRT1, PPARG, IL-6, EGFR, TGFB1, VEGFA, JAK2, PTGS2, IL1B, TNF, and NFKB1 were centrally located in the interaction network with high node degrees, suggesting that these high-degree proteins may be the key antidiabetic targets of GQL during T2DM treatment.

Identification of Potential Signaling Pathways

Among the GO enriched categories, the BP ontology (101 records), CC ontology (14 records), and MF ontology (19 records) consisted of 75.4, 14.2, and 10.4%, respectively (**Figure 3A**). Target proteins of the BP category were mostly associated with RNA polymerase II promoter transcription and were relevant to the inflammatory response, oxidative stress reduction, and glucose metabolic process (**Figure 3B**). Target proteins in the MF category were predominantly associated with heme binding and cytokine activity (**Figure 3C**), and CC target proteins were categorized as belonging to extracellular space or cytosol (**Figure 3D**). The results showed that GQL may thus bind kinase in plasma or in the cell membrane during inflammatory response, oxidative stress, and glucose metabolism. To further elucidate the association of target proteins with signaling pathways, a target–pathway interaction network was produced based on GQL-related target proteins (**Figure 4A**). Furthermore, the top 30 KEGG pathways were screened out (Benjamini–Hochberg corrected $p < 0.05$) to generate a target–pathway signaling network involving 33 target proteins (**Figure 4B**). KEGG analysis indicated that these target proteins mostly participated in the regulation of TNF, NOD-like receptor, PI3K–AKT, FoxO, TLR, and apoptosis. GO and KEGG enrichment analyses suggested that bioactive ingredients of GQL affecting the TNF inflammatory signaling and PI3K/AKT pathways were responsible for the main therapeutic effects during T2DM.

Antidiabetic Effects of Gegen Qinlian Decoction in Diabetic Mice

Curative effects of the GQL formula on HFD + STZ-induced diabetic mice were evaluated, and GQL treatment showed promising hyperglycemic effects, as evidenced by the reduction in fasting blood glucose levels (**Figure 5A**). Compared with the controls, the GQL-L and GQL-H treatment mice showed significantly reduced glucose levels during the six-week treatment. Moreover, improvements regarding body weight (**Figure 5B**), triglycerides (**Figure 5C**), cholesterol (**Figure 5D**), HbA1C (**Figure 5E**), and insulin levels (**Figure 5F**) were also observed in the GQL treatments. The OGTT assay showed lower AUC values in GQL-L GQL-H mice than in the controls (**Figures 5G,H**). GQL treatment significantly reduced the levels of ALT and AST in the serum of HFD + STZ

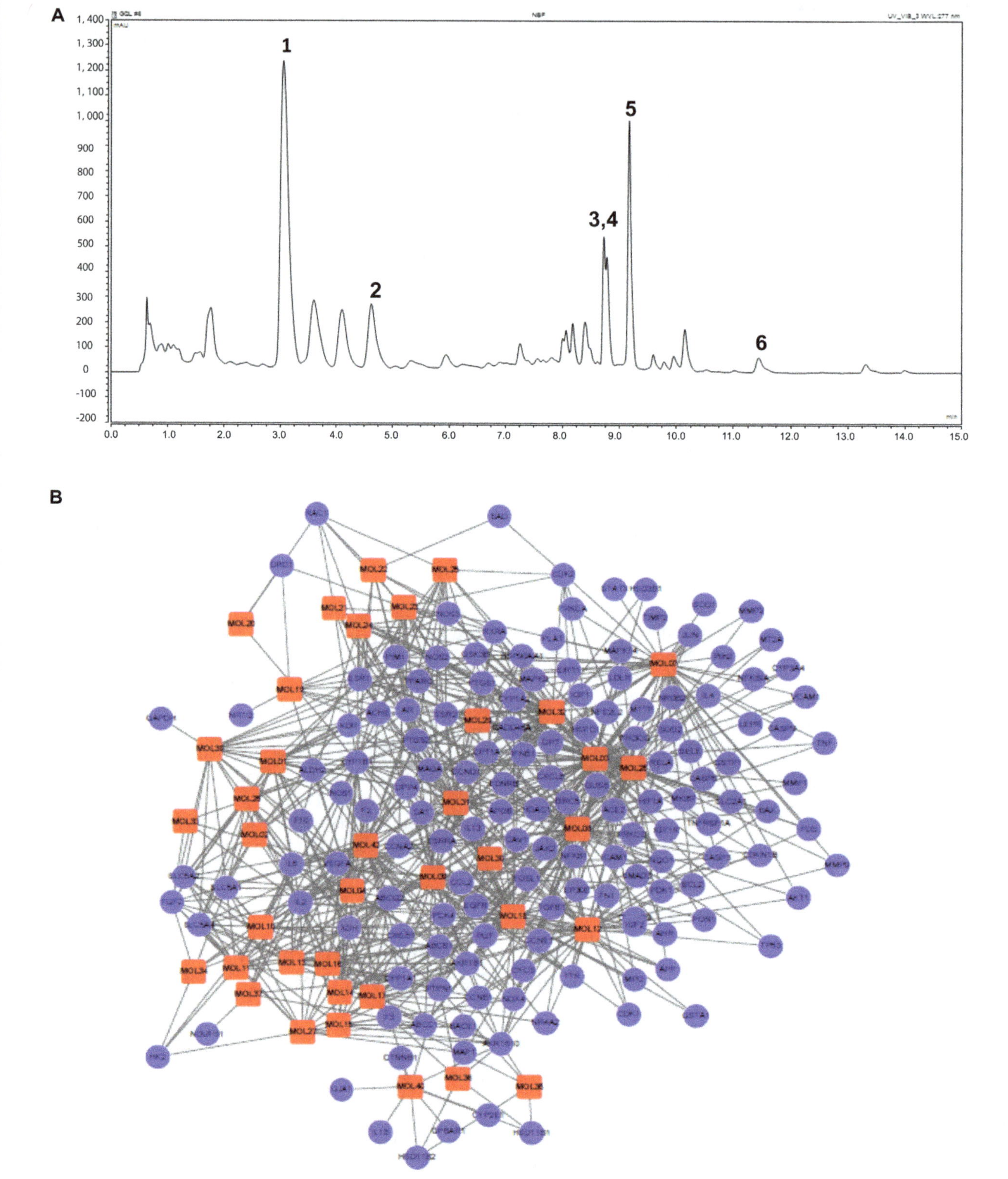

FIGURE 1 | (A) UPLC-UV profiles of GQL. (1) Puerarin (MOL07), (2) daidzin (MOL01), (3) berberine (MOL24), (4) palmitane (MOL25), (5) baicalin (MOL17), and (6) baicalein (MOL12). **(B)** Compound–target network with 715 edges and 186 nodes. Red squares indicate antidiabetic active compounds (13) of GQL. Purple circles indicate 80 common target proteins of active GQL constituents and T2DM targets. Edges indicate interactions between targets and ingredients.

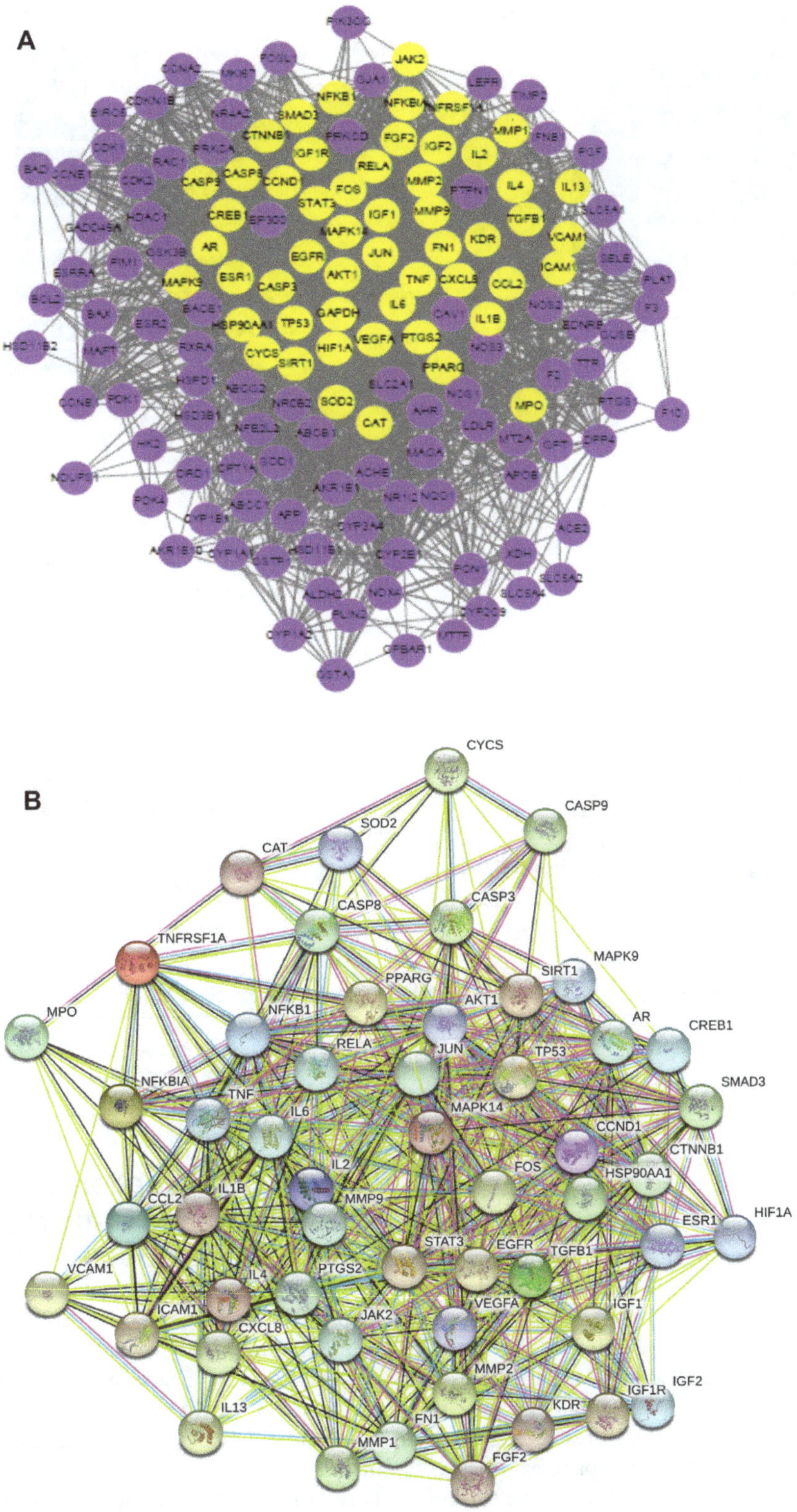

FIGURE 2 | (A) Highly connected subnetworks (53 nodes, 1,120 edges) produced using Cytoscape 3.6.0, **(B)** a Venn diagram of the four herb compound-related gene numbers, and **(C)** protein–protein interaction network (52 nodes, 296 edges) produced using STRING.

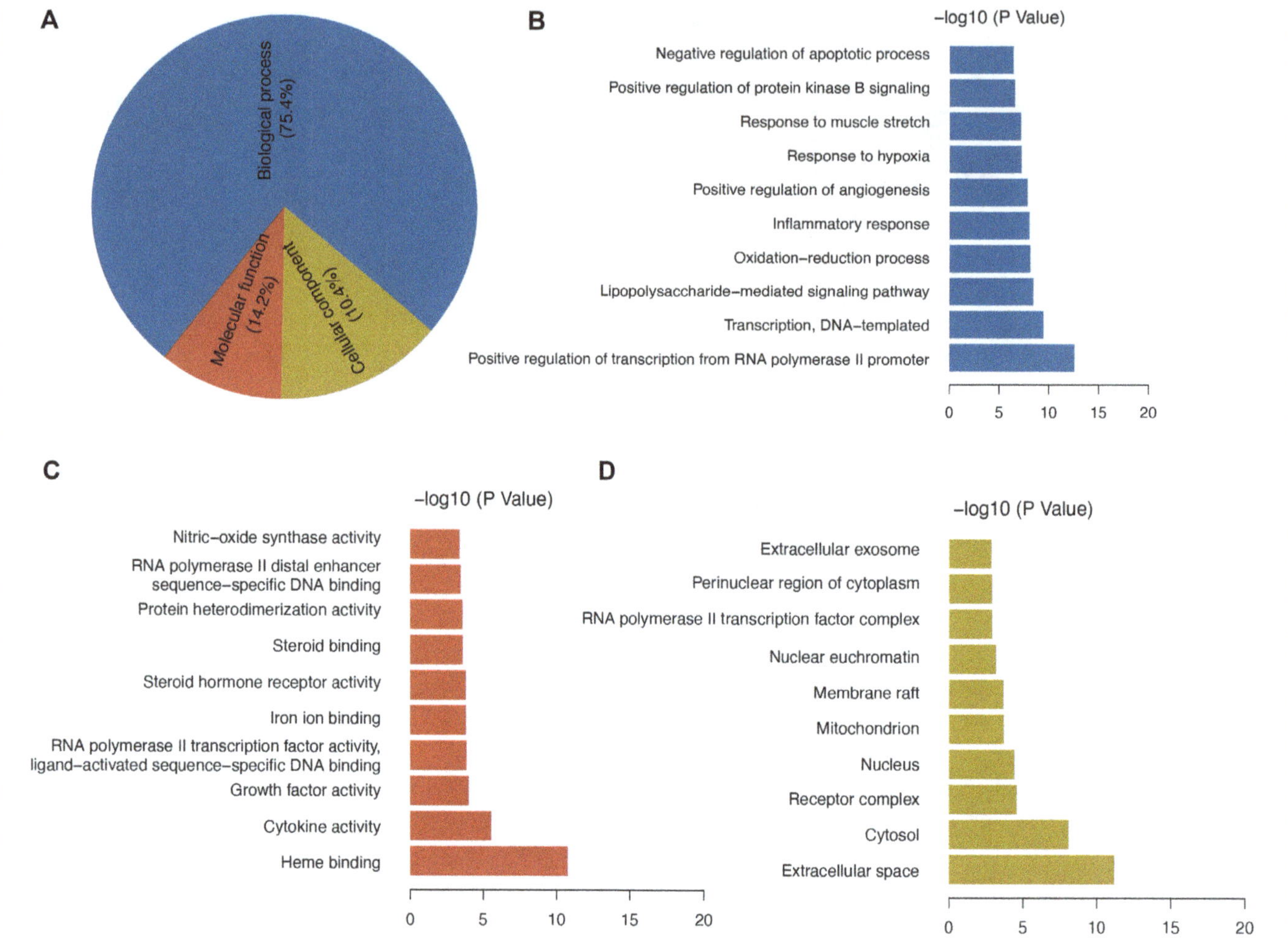

FIGURE 3 | (A) GO enrichment analysis, and **(B–D)** top 10 significant GO enrichment terms in categories BP, MF, and CC.

mice (**Figures 5I,J**). Severe steatosis and cytoplasmic vacuoles were observed in hepatocytes of HFD + STZ mice, in addition to inflammatory infiltration. Oral administration of GQL prevented fat deposition in liver tissues, as shown by Oil Red O staining (**Figure 5K**). Compared with the controls, liver structures were significantly altered in GQL-L and GQL-H mice, as indicated by smaller amounts of fatty vacuoles and less interlobular mononuclear inflammation (**Figure 5K**). Under hyperglycemic conditions, the pancreatic tissue of HFD + STZ model mice showed severe necrotic changes and a reduction in the size of islets, especially around large vessels (Pandey et al., 2019). GQL supplementation prevented histomorphological changes in pancreatic tissues of HFD + STZ mice. These results suggested that GQL alleviates liver and islet cell damage in pancreatic tissues caused by diabetes mellitus. By examining antidiabetic effects of GQL in HFD + STZ mice, we found that GQL reduced the serum levels of TNFα and IL-1β (**Figure 6A**) and the levels of TNF-α, IKKα, IL-6, IL-1β, CASP 8, and CASP three mRNA (**Figure 6B**), which confirmed that antidiabetic effects of GQL were associated with TNF-α signaling. Additionally, GQL increased the levels of phosphorylated AKT, MOTR, ERK, and JNK in liver tissue (**Figures 6C,D**), confirming activation of AKT/mTOR signaling in GQL-treated diabetic mice.

In vitro Confirmation of PI3K/AKT and TNF-α Signaling Pathway Activation by Gegen Qinlian Decoction

PI3K/AKT and TNF-α–related target proteins and signaling pathways were assessed in AML12 hepatocytes exposed to palmitate and high glucose levels. The TNF signaling pathway was examined by measuring TNFα, IKKα, IL-6, IL-1β, CASP 8, and CASP 3 mRNA (**Figure 7A**), showing that GQL treatment significantly reduced TNF-related inflammatory proteins, including TNFα, IKKα, IL-6, and IL-1β (**Figure 7B**). Furthermore, GQL-induced inflammation reduction was associated with reduced levels of phosphorylated NF-κB protein and increased phosphorylated JNK and ERK1/2 production (Smith et al., 2007), as well as SOCS3 protein expression, which contributed to apoptosis (**Figures 7C,D**). To confirm activation of the PI3K/AKT signaling pathway (**Figure 8A**), we measured AKT and MTOR proteins in

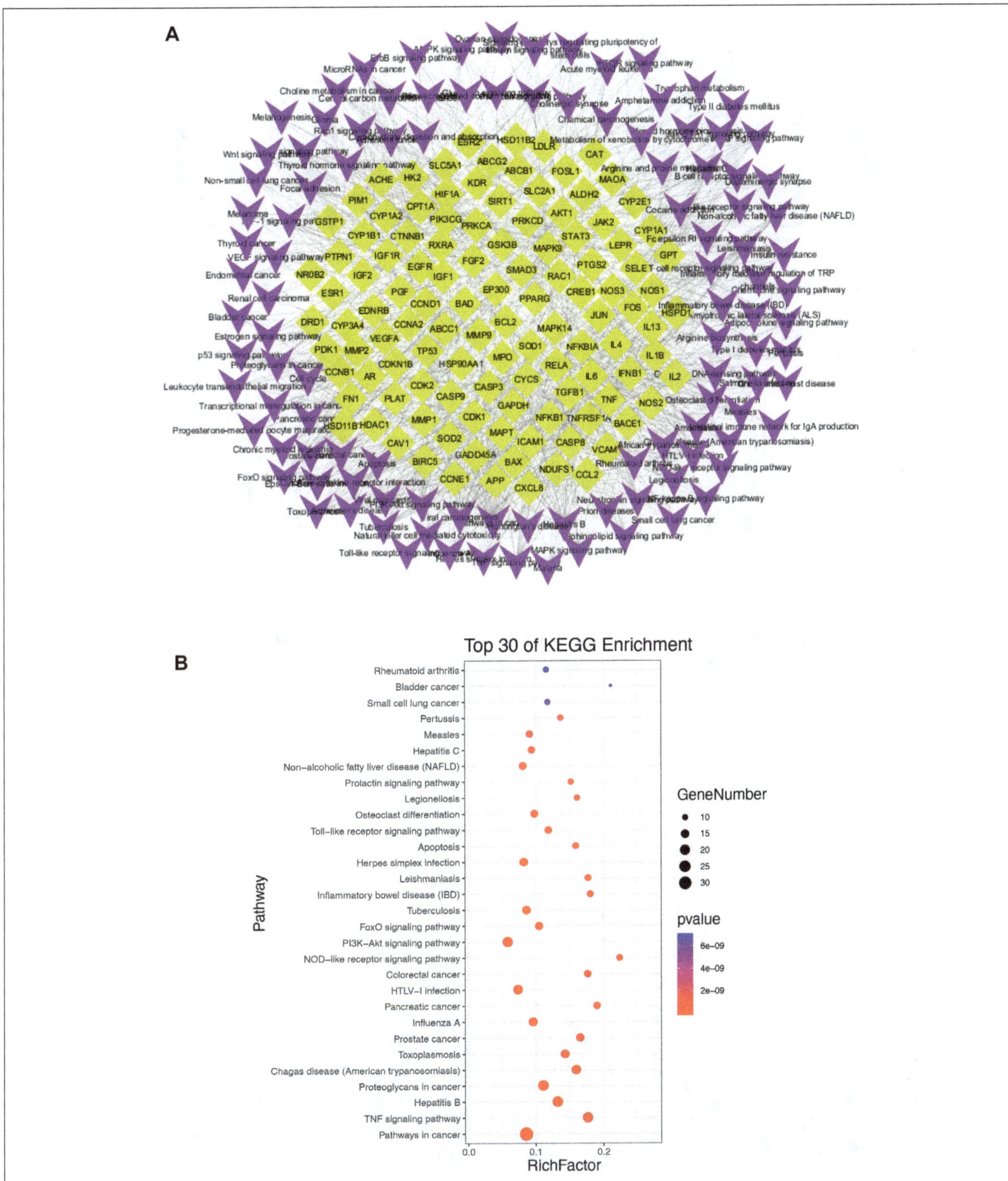

FIGURE 4 | (A) Target–pathway interaction network and **(B)** KEGG enrichment analysis.

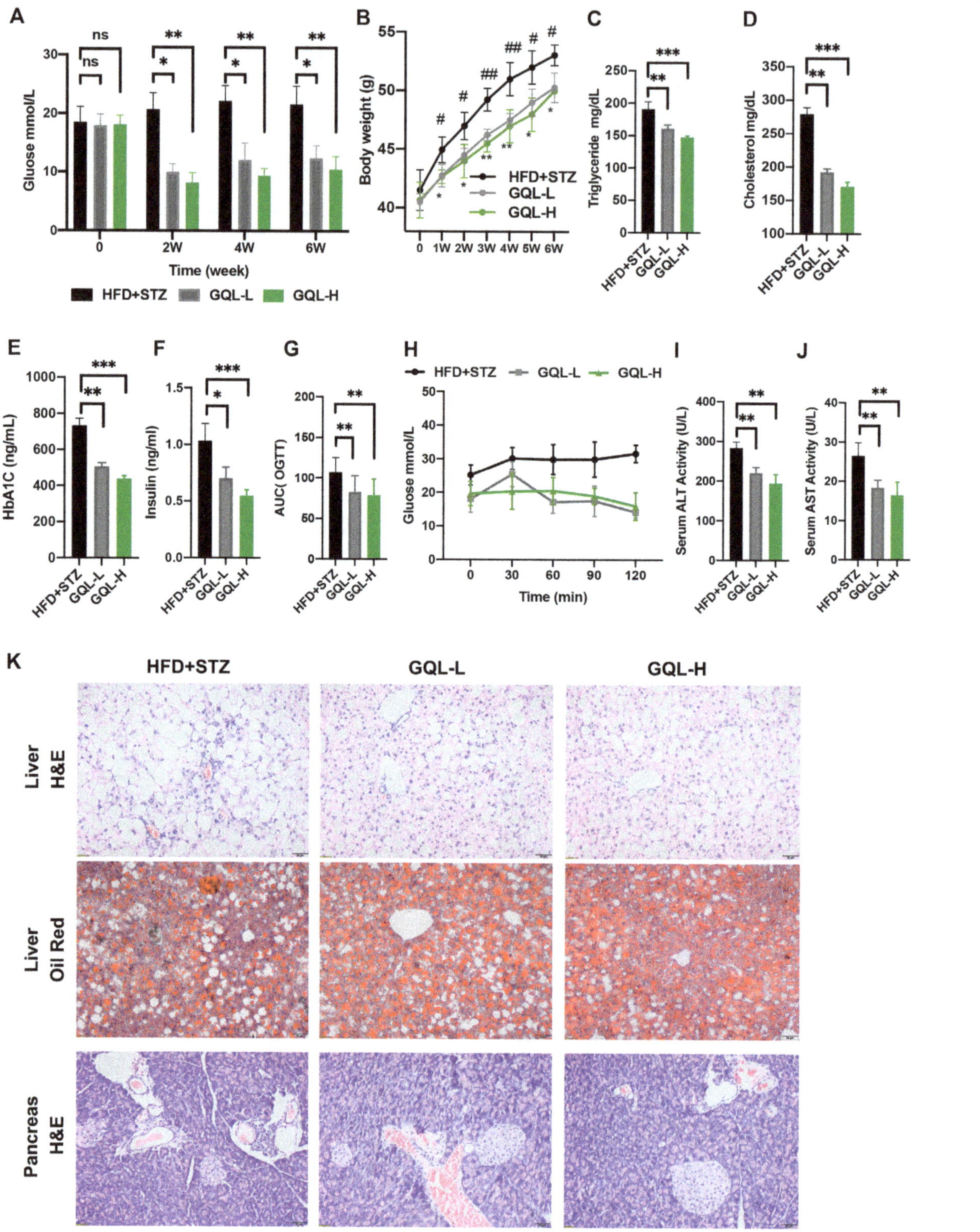

FIGURE 5 | (A) Fasting blood glucose changes in HFD + STZ-treated C57BL/6 mice after GQL treatment; **(B)** body weight elevation; **(C,D)** triglyceride and cholesterol levels; **(E,F)** HbA1c and insulin levels; **(G)** glucose AUC during OGTT; **(H)** glucose levels during OGTT measured 0, 30, 60, 90, and 120 min after oral administration of glucose solution (2 g/kg); **(I,J)** serum ALT and AST levels.

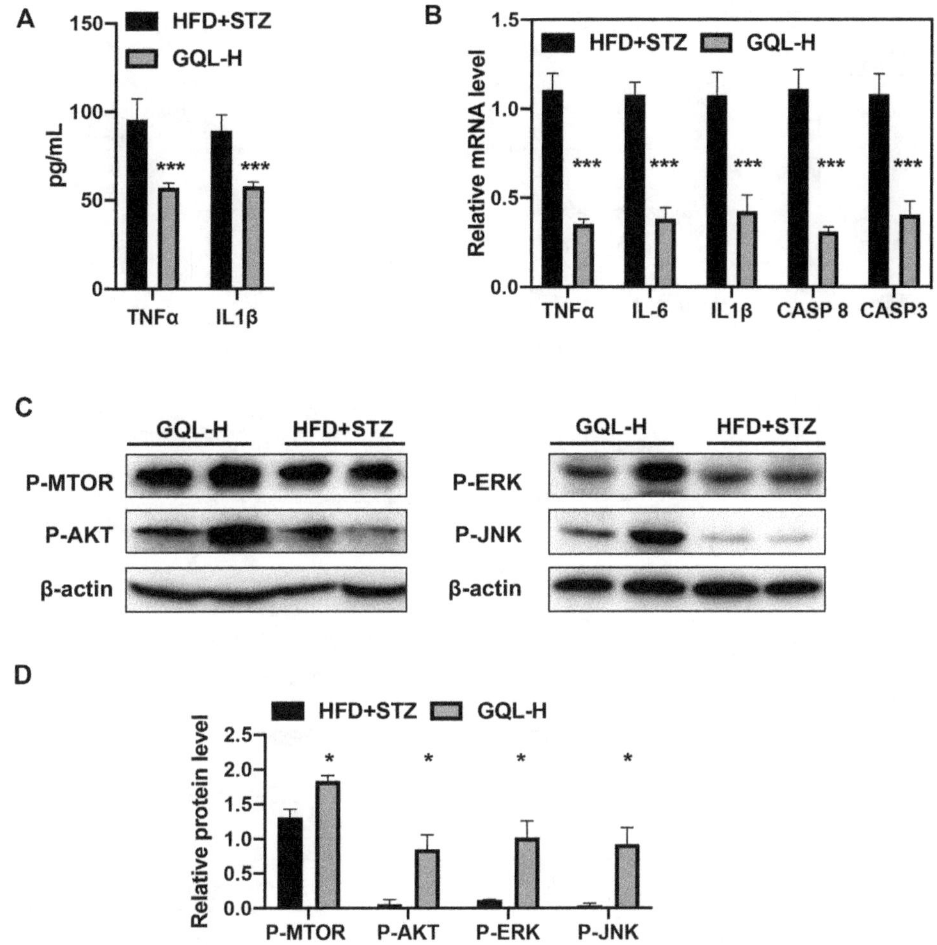

FIGURE 6 | (A) Serum TNFα and IL1β; **(B)** levels of TNFα, IKKα, IL-6, IL1β, CASP 8, CASP3, and AP-1 mRNA in diabetic mice determined using RT-PCR; **(C,D)** relative levels of P-AKT, P-MTOR, -JNK, and P-ERK proteins detected by immunoblotting.

AML12 cells using Western blotting. GQL treatment increased AKT and mTOR phosphorylation (**Figures 8B–D**), suggesting that GQL may activate AKT/mTOR signaling.

DISCUSSION

T2DM is a heterogeneous disease with high morbidity and complex associated afflictions. Thus, development of diabetes is associated with multiple target proteins or pathways. TCMs composed of multiple indigents may exert various pharmacological effects *via* multiple targets and signaling pathways, which may aid in T2DM treatment. However, the complexity of TCMs may complicate in-depth research to elucidate the underlying mechanisms. Due to extensive clinical application of GQL to treat T2DM in China (Ryuk et al., 2017), network pharmacology is important to verify the pharmacological mechanism by which GQL attenuates T2DM.

Our study explored the mechanisms of a multicomponent, multigene-targeting GQL formula by establishing a T2DM association network. This analysis was based on therapeutic effects of GQL formula relevant to 148 antidiabetic target genes, and GQL regulated binding kinase in plasma or cell membranes and modulated inflammatory responses, oxidative reduction, and glucose metabolic process by 38 significant proteins and signaling pathways, that is, the PI3–AKT (Huang et al., 2018), insulin (Brännmark et al., 2013), and TNF signaling pathways (Alipourfard et al., 2019). Based on KEGG pathway analysis, PI3-AKT and TNF signaling pathways were among the top 30 significant pathways, and GO enrichment highlighted the main biological processes of RNA polymerase II promoter transcription for modulating insulin metabolism, glucose homeostasis, and inflammation, thereby exerting multicomponent, multi-target, multichannel, and antidiabetic effects. Chronic low-grade inflammation is a common characteristic of T2DM, with primary alterations occurring in the liver and pancreatic islets. The NF-κB and JNK signaling pathways contribute to chronic inflammation during T2DM. GQL can be used to treat inflammation and oxidative stress so as to reduce the severity of colitis by inhibiting TLR4/NF-κB activation (Li et al., 2016). Our experiments indicated that GQL suppressed activation of NF-κB and of two major mitogen-

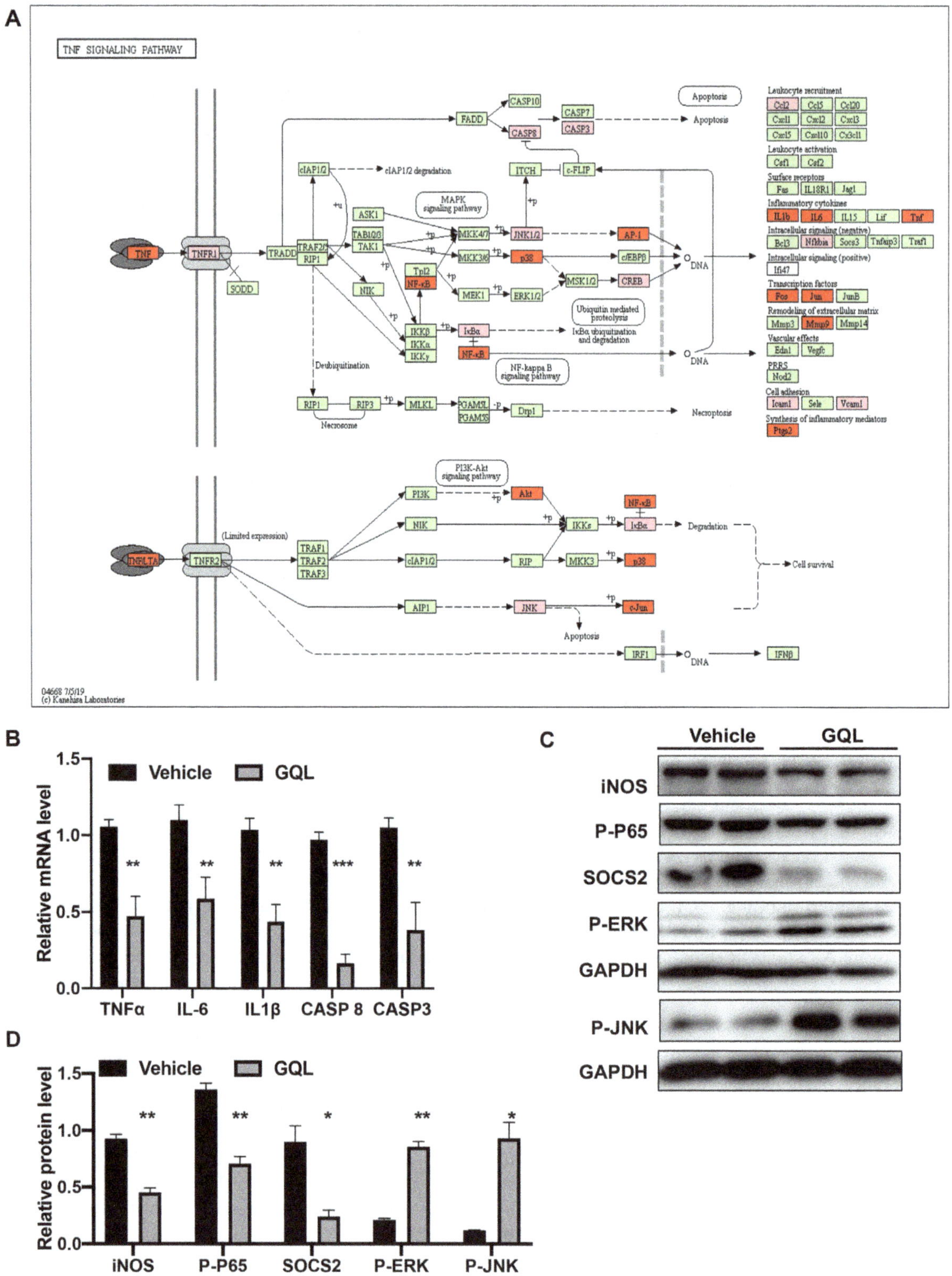

FIGURE 7 | (A) KEGG pathway map of the TNFα signaling pathway; **(B)** levels of TNFα, IKKα, IL-6, IL1β, CASP 8, CASP3, and AP-1 mRNA determined using RT-PCR; **(C,D)** relative expression of iNOS, P-P65, SOCS2, P-JNK, and P-ERK as detected by immunoblotting.

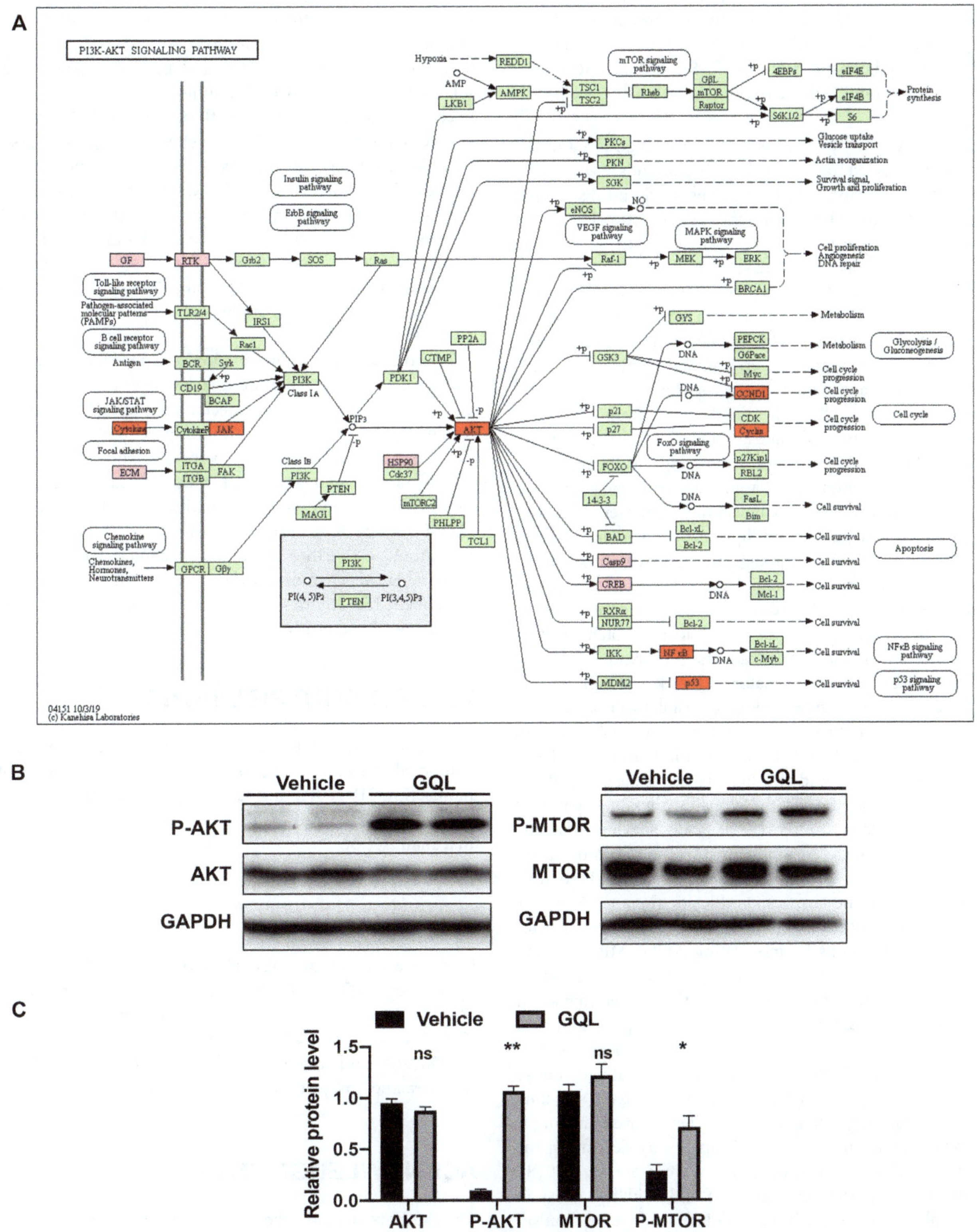

FIGURE 8 | (A) KEGG pathway map of the AKT signaling pathway, and **(B)** relative levels of P-AKT, AKT, P-MTOR, and MTOR proteins as evaluated by immunoblotting.

activated protein kinases (ERK1/2 and JNK). Inhibition of NF-κB and ERK1/2 ameliorated TNF-α–induced inflammation induced by high glucose exposure (Smith et al., 2007). Our results showed that GQL promoted phosphorylation of AKT and mTOR *in vitro* and *in vivo* to inhibit T2DM development.

In the current study, GQL constituents with high OB and DL indices were selected as bioactive compounds with high pharmacokinetics because they may be absorbed and distributed in the patient's body. Our compound–target network analysis showed 12 potential candidate compounds with high node degrees, that is, wogonin, oroxylin A, baicalein, baicalin, coptisine, epiberberine, berberine, palmatine, isoliquiritigenin, liquiritigenin, glycyrol, and formononetin, all of which may be associated with the marked antidiabetic effect of GQL on T2DM. These bioactive compounds exert antihyperlipidemic, anti-inflammatory, and anti-oxidative effects during diabetes and diabetic complications. Bioactive isoflavones from Puerariae Lobatae Radix, puerarin, and daidzin showed antidiabetic effects in animal studies, such as puerarin improving insulin resistance and islet damage by inhibiting inflammation and oxidative stress during diabetes and diabetic complications (Chen et al., 2018). Daidzin can modulate glucose and lipid metabolism and reduces the inflammatory response through the TNFα/JNK signaling pathway in macrophages during T2DM (Das et al., 2018). Wogonin, baicalin, and baicalein are active ingredients of Scutellariae Radix, which have been considered potential anti-oxidative and anti-inflammatory agents for treating obesity, insulin resistance, and inflammatory disorders (Fang et al., 2020). Wogonin can increase glucose cellular absorption to reduce hyperglycemia through the AKT and GLUT4 pathways (Khan and Kamal, 2019), and it exerts anti-inflammatory effects through NF-κB signaling and anti-fibrosis effects against diabetic nephropathy through the TGF-β1/Smad3 signaling pathway (Zheng et al., 2020); moreover, it can alleviate diabetic cardiomyopathy through anti-inflammatory and anti-oxidative activities (Khan et al., 2016a). Alkaloids, especially berberine, palmatine, and coptisine, are responsible for therapeutic effects of *Rhizoma coptidis*, which can have beneficial effects on diabetes and diabetic complications by modulating AKT/AMPK–NF-κB/MAPK/PI3K and oxidative stress signaling pathways (Wang et al., 2018a). Specifically, berberine acts as an antihyperglycemic agent during T2DM treatment through increased phosphorylation of AKT, thereby improving insulin resistance through AMPK activation (Chang et al., 2015). Coptisine ameliorates oxidative injury in diabetic nephropathy by regulating the Nrf2 signaling pathway, and liquiritigenin inhibits diabetes-induced mesangial matrix accumulation in diabetic nephropathy by decreasing the NF-κB and NLRP3 inflammasome (Zhu et al., 2018). Isoliquiritigenin attenuates inflammation and oxidative stress in diabetic renal injuries through an SIRT1-dependent mechanism (Huang et al., 2020b). These previous studies on bioactive compounds and the results of the present study support the use of pharmacological network prediction. In the exploration of the potential underlying mechanism, network pharmacology has shaped its own analytical rules and evaluation of rationality (Li, 2021). Our results suggested successful network pharmacology for screening the mechanism of action of TCMs with respect to a specific disease. Anti-inflammation and PI3K-AKT/MTOR activation (Khan et al., 2016b) and multiple active ingredients of GQL that can synergize with numerous target proteins result in diverse beneficial mechanisms in the treatment T2DM. Our results showed that the antihyperglycemic effects of GQL were associated with alleviation of liver and pancreas injury, which is common during T2DM (Loria et al., 2013). Moreover, our results indicated that GQL in T2DM treatment may affect the TNF/NF-κB and PI3K/AKT/MTOR pathways to reduce inflammation and improve hyperglycemia. Furthermore, detailed pharmacological mechanisms by which GQL ameliorates T2DM will be investigated in our future study.

In conclusion, a combination of pharmacology network analysis and experimental approaches may be a useful research tool to elucidate antidiabetic mechanisms of TCMs in detail. The development of T2DM is a complex pathological process involving multiple signaling pathways and multiple targets. Our results suggest that GQL can modulate multiple target proteins in multiple signaling pathways and can be used for T2DM therapy. The antidiabetic effects of GQL *in vitro* and *in vivo* should be further examined in clinical trials with T2DM patients. However, more evidence is needed to further validate antidiabetic bioactivities of the active compounds and to evaluate their respective contributions.

AUTHOR CONTRIBUTIONS

YF and NW initiated the idea and designed the experiments. YX conducted the *in vivo* and *in vitro* experiments and wrote the manuscript. HYT, JH, and CZ analyzed the experimental data, and SL and GT revised the manuscript. All authors approved the final manuscript.

FUNDING

This research was partially supported by the Research Grants Committee (RGC) of Hong Kong, HKSAR (project code: 17121419), Health Medical Research Fund (project codes: 15162961 and 16172751), Wong's donation (project code: 200006276), and a donation from the Gaia Family Trust of New Zealand (project code: 200007008).

ACKNOWLEDGMENTS

The authors would like to express great thanks to Keith Wong, Cindy Lee, and Alex Shek for their technical support.

REFERENCES

Alipourfard, I., Datukishvili, N., and Mikeladze, D. (2019). TNF-α Downregulation Modifies Insulin Receptor Substrate 1 (IRS-1) in Metabolic Signaling of Diabetic Insulin-Resistant Hepatocytes. *Mediators Inflamm.* 2019, 3560819. doi:10.1155/2019/3560819

An, R., You, L., Zhang, Y., Wang, X., and Ma, Y. (2014). A Rapid UPLC Method for Simultaneous Determination of Eleven Components in 'Ge-Gen-Qin-Lian' Decoction. *Pharmacogn. Mag.* 10, 464. doi:10.4103/0973-1296.141821

Bak, E. J., Kim, J., Choi, Y. H., Kim, J. H., Lee, D. E., Woo, G. H., et al. (2014). Wogonin Ameliorates Hyperglycemia and Dyslipidemia via PPARα Activation in Db/db Mice. *Mol. Cel Endocrinol* 33, 156. doi:10.1016/j.clnu.2013.03.013

Blanchard, O. L., and Smoliga, J. M. (2015). Translating Dosages from Animal Models to Human Clinical Trials-Revisiting Body Surface Area Scaling. *FASEB j.* 29, 1629–1634. doi:10.1096/fj.14-269043

Brännmark, C., Nyman, E., Fagerholm, S., Bergenholm, L., Ekstrand, E.-M., Cedersund, G., et al. (2013). Insulin Signaling in Type 2 Diabetes. *J. Biol. Chem.* 288, 9867–9880. doi:10.1074/jbc.m112.432062

Chan, J. C. N., Malik, V., Jia, W., Kadowaki, T., Yajnik, C. S., Yoon, K.-H., et al. (2009). Diabetes in Asia. *JAMA* 301, 2129–2140. doi:10.1001/jama.2009.726

Chang, W., Chen, L., and Hatch, G. M. (2015). Berberine as a Therapy for Type 2 Diabetes and its Complications: From Mechanism of Action to Clinical Studies. *Biochem. Cel Biol* 93, 479. doi:10.1139/bcb-2014-0107

Chen, X., Yu, J., and Shi, J. (2018). Management of Diabetes Mellitus with Puerarin, a Natural Isoflavone FromPueraria Lobata. *Am. J. Chin. Med.* 46, 1771–1789. doi:10.1142/s0192415x18500891

Covington, M. B. (2001). Traditional Chinese Medicine in the Treatment of Diabetes. *Diabetes Spectr.* 14, 154–159. doi:10.2337/diaspect.14.3.154

Das, D., Sarkar, S., Bordoloi, J., Wann, S. B., Kalita, J. a.-O., and Manna, P. a.-O. (2018). Daidzein, its Effects on Impaired Glucose and Lipid Metabolism and Vascular Inflammation Associated with Type 2 Diabetes. *Biofactors* 44, 407. doi:10.1002/biof.1439

Fang, P., Yu, M., Shi, M., Bo, P., Gu, X., and Zhang, Z. (2020). Baicalin and its Aglycone: a Novel Approach for Treatment of Metabolic Disorders. *Pharmacol. Rep.* 72, 13–23. doi:10.1007/s43440-019-00024-x

Guo, W., Huang, J., Wang, N., Tan, H.-Y., Cheung, F., Chen, F., et al. (2019). Integrating Network Pharmacology and Pharmacological Evaluation for Deciphering the Action Mechanism of Herbal Formula Zuojin Pill in Suppressing Hepatocellular Carcinoma. *Front. Pharmacol.* 10, 1185. doi:10.3389/fphar.2019.01185

Han, J., Wang, Z., Xing, W., Yuan, Y., Zhang, Y., Lv, T., et al. (2017). Effect of Gegen Qinlian Decoction on Cardiac Gene Expression in Diabetic Mice. *Int. J. Genomics* 2017, 7421761. doi:10.1155/2017/7421761

Haynes, W. (2013). "Benjamini-Hochberg Method," in *Encyclopedia of Systems Biology*. Editors W. Dubitzky, O. Wolkenhauer, K.-H. Cho, and H. Yokota (New York, NY: Springer New York), 78. doi:10.1007/978-1-4419-9863-7_1215

Heinrich, M., Appendino, G., Efferth, T., Fürst, R., Izzo, A. A., Kayser, O., et al. (2020). Best Practice in Research - Overcoming Common Challenges in Phytopharmacological Research. *J. Ethnopharmacology* 246, 112230. doi:10.1016/j.jep.2019.112230

Huang, D., Sherman, B. T., Tan, Q., Collins, J. R., Alvord, W. G., Roayaei, J., et al. (2007). The DAVID Gene Functional Classification Tool: a Novel Biological Module-Centric Algorithm to Functionally Analyze Large Gene Lists. *Genome Biol.* 8, R183. doi:10.1186/gb-2007-8-9-r183

Huang, X., Liu, G., Guo, J., and Su, Z. (2018). The PI3K/AKT Pathway in Obesity and Type 2 Diabetes. *Int. J. Biol. Sci.* 14, 1483–1496. doi:10.7150/ijbs.27173

Huang, J., Chen, F., Zhong, Z., Tan, H. Y., Wang, N., Liu, Y., et al. (2020a). Interpreting the Pharmacological Mechanisms of Huachansu Capsules on Hepatocellular Carcinoma Through Combining Network Pharmacology and Experimental Evaluation. *Front. Pharmacol.* 11, 414. doi:10.3389/fphar.2020.00414

Huang, X., Shi, Y., Chen, H., Le, R., Gong, X., Xu, K., et al. (2020b). Isoliquiritigenin Prevents Hyperglycemia-Induced Renal Injuries by Inhibiting Inflammation and Oxidative Stress via SIRT1-dependent Mechanism. *Cell Death Dis* 11, 1040. doi:10.1038/s41419-020-03260-9

Kalra, S., Jena, B. N., and Yeravdekar, R. (2018). Emotional and Psychological Needs of People with Diabetes. *Indian J. Endocrinol. Metab.* 22, 696–704. doi:10.4103/ijem.ijem_189_17

Khan, S., and Kamal, M. A. (2019). Wogonin Alleviates Hyperglycemia Through Increased Glucose Entry into Cells Via AKT/GLUT4 Pathway. *Curr. Pharm. Des.* 25, 2602. doi:10.2174/1381612825666190722115410

Khan, K. H., Wong, M., Rihawi, K., Bodla, S., Morganstein, D., Banerji, U., et al. (2016a). Hyperglycemia and Phosphatidylinositol 3-Kinase/Protein Kinase B/Mammalian Target of Rapamycin (PI3K/AKT/mTOR) Inhibitors in Phase I Trials: Incidence, Predictive Factors, and Management. *Oncologist* 21, 855. doi:10.1634/theoncologist.2015-0248

Khan, S., Zhang, D., Zhang, Y., Li, M., Wang, C., Zheng, Z. a.-O., et al. (2016b). Wogonin Attenuates Diabetic Cardiomyopathy through its Anti-inflammatory and Anti-oxidative Properties. *Mol. Cell Endocrinol.* 428. 101. doi:10.1016/j.mce.2016.03.025

Li, S., and Zhang, B. (2013). Traditional Chinese Medicine Network Pharmacology: Theory, Methodology and Application. *Chin. J. Nat. Medicines* 11, 110–120. doi:10.1016/s1875-5364(13)60037-0

Li, H., Zhao, L., Zhang, B., Jiang, Y., Wang, X., Guo, Y., et al. (2014). A Network Pharmacology Approach to Determine Active Compounds and Action Mechanisms of Ge-Gen-Qin-Lian Decoction for Treatment of Type 2 Diabetes. *Evid. Based Complement. Alternat Med.* 2014, 495840. doi:10.1155/2014/495840

Li, R., Chen, Y., Shi, M., Xu, X., Zhao, Y., Wu, X., et al. (2016). Gegen Qinlian Decoction Alleviates Experimental Colitis via Suppressing TLR4/NF-κB Signaling and Enhancing Antioxidant Effect. *Phytomedicine* 23, 1012–1020. doi:10.1016/j.phymed.2016.06.010

Li, S. (2021). Network Pharmacology Evaluation Method Guidance - Draft. *World J. Traditional Chin. Med.* 7, 146–154. doi:10.4103/wjtcm.wjtcm_11_21

Loria, P., Lonardo, A., and Anania, F. (2013). Liver and Diabetes. A Vicious circle. *Hepatol. Res. : official J. Jpn. Soc. Hepatol.* 43, 51–64. doi:10.1111/j.1872-034x.2012.01031.x

Lucchesi, A. N., Cassettari, L. L., and Spadella, C. T. (2015). Alloxan-Induced Diabetes Causes Morphological and Ultrastructural Changes in Rat Liver that Resemble the Natural History of Chronic Fatty Liver Disease in Humans. *J. Diabetes Res.* 2015, 494578. doi:10.1155/2015/494578

Lv, J., Jia, Y., Li, J., Kuai, W., Li, Y., Guo, F., et al. (2019). Gegen Qinlian Decoction Enhances the Effect of PD-1 Blockade in Colorectal Cancer with Microsatellite Stability by Remodelling the Gut Microbiota and the Tumour Microenvironment. *Cel Death Dis* 10, 415. doi:10.1038/s41419-019-1638-6

Pandey, M. K., Kumar, R., Pandey, A. K., Soni, P., Gangurde, S. S., Sudini, H. K., et al. (2019). Mitigating Aflatoxin Contamination in Groundnut through A Combination of Genetic Resistance and Post-Harvest Management Practices. *Toxins (Basel)* 11, 315. doi:10.3390/toxins11060315

Pang, B., Zhou, Q., Zhao, T.-Y., He, L.-S., Guo, J., Chen, H.-D., et al. (2015). Innovative Thoughts on Treating Diabetes from the Perspective of Traditional Chinese Medicine. *Evidence-Based Complement. Altern. Med.* 2015, 905432. doi:10.1155/2015/905432

Qiao, X., Wang, Q., Wang, S., Miao, W. J., Li, Y. J., Xiang, C., et al. (2016). Compound to Extract to Formulation: a Knowledge-Transmitting Approach for Metabolites Identification of Gegen-Qinlian Decoction, a Traditional Chinese Medicine Formula. *Sci. Rep.* 6, 39534. doi:10.1038/srep39534

Qiao, X., Wang, Q., Wang, S., Kuang, Y., Li, K., Song, W., et al. (2018). A 42-Markers Pharmacokinetic Study Reveals Interactions of Berberine and Glycyrrhizic Acid in the Anti-diabetic Chinese Medicine Formula Gegen-Qinlian Decoction. *Front. Pharmacol.* 9, 622. doi:10.3389/fphar.2018.00622

Reagan-Shaw, S., Nihal, M., and Ahmad, N. (2008). Dose Translation from Animal to Human Studies Revisited. *FASEB J.* 22, 659–661. doi:10.1096/fj.07-9574LSF

Ryuk, J. A., Lixia, M., Cao, S., Ko, B.-S., and Park, S. (2017). Efficacy and Safety of Gegen Qinlian Decoction for Normalizing Hyperglycemia in Diabetic Patients: A Systematic Review and Meta-Analysis of Randomized Clinical Trials. *Complement. Therapies Med.* 33, 6–13. doi:10.1016/j.ctim.2017.05.004

Shannon, P., Markiel, A., Ozier, O., Baliga, N. S., Wang, J. T., Ramage, D., et al. (2003). Cytoscape: a Software Environment for Integrated Models of Biomolecular Interaction Networks. *Genome Res.* 13, 2498–2504. doi:10.1101/gr.1239303

Smith, M. V., Lee, M. J., Islam, A. S., Rohrer, J. L., Goldberg, V. M., Beidelschies, M. A., et al. (2007). Inhibition of the PI3K-Akt Signaling Pathway Reduces Tumor Necrosis Factor-α Production in Response to Titanium Particles *In Vitro*. *JBJS* 89, 1019–1027. doi:10.2106/jbjs.f.00615

Srinivasan, K., Viswanad, B., Asrat, L., Kaul, C. L., and Ramarao, P. (2005). Combination of High-Fat Diet-Fed and Low-Dose Streptozotocin-Treated Rat:

a Model for Type 2 Diabetes and Pharmacological Screening. *Pharmacol. Res.* 52. 313. doi:10.1016/j.phrs.2005.05.004

Tong, X.-l., Zhao, L.-h., Lian, F.-m., Zhou, Q., Xia, L., Zhang, J.-c., et al. (2011). Clinical Observations on the Dose-Effect Relationship of Gegen Qin Lian Decoction () on 54 Out-Patients with Type 2 Diabetes. *J. Traditional Chin. Med.* 31, 56–59. doi:10.1016/s0254-6272(11)60013-7

Usuelli, V., and La Rocca, E. (2015). Novel Therapeutic Approaches for Diabetic Nephropathy and Retinopathy. *Pharmacol. Res.* 98, 39–44. doi:10.1016/j.phrs.2014.10.003

Wang, Q., Song, W., Qiao, X., Ji, S., Kuang, Y., Zhang, Z. X., et al. (2016). Simultaneous Quantification of 50 Bioactive Compounds of the Traditional Chinese Medicine Formula Gegen-Qinlian Decoction Using Ultra-high Performance Liquid Chromatography Coupled with Tandem Mass Spectrometry. *J. Chromatogr. A.* 1454, 15. doi:10.1016/j.chroma.2016.05.056

Wang, J., Ran, Q., Zeng, H. R., Wang, L., Hu, C. J., and Huang, Q. W. (2018a). Cellular Stress Response Mechanisms of Rhizoma Coptidis: a Systematic Review. *Chin. Med.* 13, 27. doi:10.1186/s13020-018-0184-y

Wang, N., Yang, B., Zhang, X., Wang, S., Zheng, Y., Li, X., et al. (2018b). Network Pharmacology-Based Validation of Caveolin-1 as a Key Mediator of Ai Du Qing Inhibition of Drug Resistance in Breast Cancer. *Front. Pharmacol.* 9, 1106. doi:10.3389/fphar.2018.01106

Wang, Y., Zhang, S., Li, F., Zhou, Y., Zhang, Y., Wang, Z., et al. (2020). Therapeutic Target Database 2020: Enriched Resource for Facilitating Research and Early Development of Targeted Therapeutics. *Nucleic Acids Res.* 48, D1031, doi:10.1093/nar/gkz981

Wu, Y., Wang, D., Yang, X., Fu, C., Zou, L., and Zhang, J. (2019). Traditional Chinese Medicine Gegen Qinlian Decoction Ameliorates Irinotecan Chemotherapy-Induced Gut Toxicity in Mice. *Biomed. Pharmacother.* 109, 2252–2261. doi:10.1016/j.biopha.2018.11.095

Zeng, Y. P., Huang, Y. S., and Hu, Y. G. (2006). Effect of gegen qinlian decoction combined with short-term intensive insulin treatment on patients with type 2 diabetes mellitus of dampness-heat syndrome. *Zhongguo Zhong Xi Yi Jie He Za Zhi* 26, 514–520.

Zhang, S., Wang, L., and Zan, L. (2019). Investigation into the Underlying Molecular Mechanisms of white Adipose Tissue through Comparative Transcriptome Analysis of Multiple Tissues. *Mol. Med. Rep.* 19, 959–966. doi:10.3892/mmr.2018.9740

Zheng, Z. C., Zhu, W., Lei, L., Liu, X. Q., and Wu, Y. G. (2020). Wogonin Ameliorates Renal Inflammation and Fibrosis by Inhibiting NF-κB and TGF-β1/Smad3 Signaling Pathways in Diabetic Nephropathy. *Drug Des. Devel Ther.* 14. 4135. doi:10.2147/DDDT.S274256

Zhou, J., Wang, Q., Xiang, Z., Tong, Q., Pan, J., Wan, L., et al. (2019). Network Pharmacology Analysis of Traditional Chinese Medicine Formula *Xiao Ke Yin Shui* Treating Type 2 Diabetes Mellitus. *Evidence-Based Complement. Altern. Med.* 2019, 4202563. doi:10.1155/2019/4202563

Zhu, X., Shi, J., and Li, H. (2018). Liquiritigenin Attenuates High Glucose-Induced Mesangial Matrix Accumulation, Oxidative Stress, and Inflammation by Suppression of the NF-κB and NLRP3 Inflammasome Pathways. *Biomed. Pharmacother.* 106, 976, doi:10.1016/j.biopha.2018.07.045

14

Mechanisms Underlying the Action of Ziziphi Spinosae Semen in the Treatment of Insomnia: A Study Involving Network Pharmacology and Experimental Validation

Zhenhua Bian[1,2], Wenming Zhang[2], Jingyue Tang[2], Qianqian Fei[2], Minmin Hu[2], Xiaowei Chen[2], Lianlin Su[1], Chenghao Fei[1], De Ji[1], Chunqin Mao[1], Huangjin Tong[1], Xiaohang Yuan[2] and Tulin Lu[1]**

[1]College of Pharmacy, Nanjing University of Chinese Medicine, Nanjing, China, [2]Department of Pharmacy, Wuxi TCM Hospital Affiliated to Nanjing University of Chinese Medicine, Wuxi, China

***Correspondence:**
Xiaohang Yuan
13861759928@126.com
Tulin Lu
ltl2021@njucm.edu.cn

Purpose: This study aimed to investigate the potential mechanisms and related bioactive components of ZSS for the treatment of insomnia.

Method: The insomnia model of rat induced by PCPA was established. After oral administration of ZSS extract, the general morphological observation, pentobarbital sodium-induced sleep test and histopathological evaluation were carried out. Network pharmacology, assisted by UHPLC-Q-Exactive-MS/MS analysis, was developed to identify the targets of ZSS in the treatment of insomnia, as well as the corresponding signaling pathways. In addition, we validated the identified targets and pathways by RT-qPCR and immunohistochemical analysis.

Results: The pentobarbital sodium-induced sleep test, determination of 5-HT and GABA levles in hypothalamic tissues and HE staining showed that ZSS extract was an effective treatment for insomnia. Network pharmacology analysis identified a total of 19 candidate bioactive ingredients in ZSS extract, along with 433 potentially related targets. Next, we performed protein-protein interaction (PPI), MCODE clustering analysis, GO functional enrichment analysis, KEGG pathway enrichment analysis, and ingredient-target-pathway (I-T-P) sub-networks analysis. These methods allowed us to investigate the synergistic therapeutic effects of crucial pathways, including the serotonergic and GABAergic synapse pathways. Our analyses revealed that palmitic acid, coclaurine, jujuboside A,

Abbreviations: 5-HT, 5-hydroxytryptamine; ANOVA, Analysis of Variance; BATMAN-TCM, a bioinformatics analysis tool for molecular mechanism of traditional Chinese medicine; Con, control; DAB, 3,3′-diaminobenzidine; ESI-MS, electrospray ionization tandem mass spectrometry; Est, estazolam; GABA, Gamma-aminobutyric acid; GABRA1, Gamma-aminobutyric acid receptor subunit alpha-1; GABRG2, Gamma-aminobutyric acid receptor subunit gamma-2; GC-MS, gas chromatography-mass spectrometry; GO, gene ontology; HCD, high energy collision dissociation; HE, hematoxylin-eosin; HTR1A, 5-hydroxytryptamine receptor 1A; HTR2A, 5-hydroxytryptamine receptor 2A; IOD, integrated optical density; KEGG, Kyoto Encyclopedia of Genes and Genomes; LC-MS, liquid chromatography-mass spectrometry; MCODE, Molecular Complex Detection; mean ± SD, mean ± Standard deviation; PCPA, p-chlorophenylalanine; RT-qPCR, Real Time Quantitative PCR; TCMSP, traditional Chinese medicine systems pharmacology database and analysis platform; UHPLC-Q-Exactive-MS/MS, Ultra high performance liquid chromatography-quadrupole-exactive-mass spectrometry/mass spectrometry.

N-nornuciferine, caaverine, magnoflorine, jujuboside B, and betulinic acid, all played key roles in the regulation of these crucial pathways. Finally, we used the PCPA-induced insomnia in rats to validate the data generated by network pharmacology; these *in vivo* experiments clearly showed that pathways associated with the serotonergic and GABAergic system were activated in the rats model. Furthermore, ZSS treatment significantly suppressed high levels of HTR1A, GABRA1, and GABRG2 expression in the hypothalamus and reduced the expression levels of HTR2A.

Conclusion: Based on the combination of comprehensive network pharmacology and *in vivo* experiments, we successfully identified the potential pharmacological mechanisms underlying the action of ZSS in the treatment of insomnia. The results provide a theoretical basis for further development and utilization of ZSS, and also provide support for the development of innovative drugs for the treatment of insomnia.

Keywords: Ziziphi Spinosae Semen, insomnia, network pharmacology, targets, pharmacological mechanisms

INTRODUCTION

Insomnia is a common sleep disorder that is characterized by sustained difficulty initiating or maintaining sleep. The global prevalence of insomnia symptoms range from 8 to 40% (Vgontzas and Fernandez-Mendoza, 2013). Research has shown that insomnia frequently causes other psychological and physical disorders, including depression, anxiety, hypertension, diabetes, cardiovascular diseases, and cerebrovascular diseases (Morin et al., 2014; Horsch et al., 2017). Numerous sedative-hypnotic drugs have been used in the clinic, including benzodiazepines, antihistamines, and antidepressants; however, these drugs have common side effects, such as dizziness, lethargy, and physical dependence (Zhou et al., 2018). In addition, Chinese herbal medicine has been historically used to treat insomnia and is now a recognized therapeutic used across the world (Shi et al., 2014).

Ziziphi Spinosae Semen (ZSS), known as suan zao ren in China, has been widely used to manage insomnia and palpitations in Traditional Chinese Medicine (Yeung et al., 2012; Rodríguez Villanueva and Rodríguez Villanueva, 2017; Shergis et al., 2017; Zhou et al., 2018). Modern pharmacological research indicates that ZSS exhibits good sedative and hypnotic effects on the central nervous system (Xiao et al., 2018). There are many prescriptions containing ZSS as a raw medical material in the Chinese Pharmacopoeia; these are commonly used to treat palpitations and insomnia. Over 150 different components have been separated and identified from ZSS, including saponins, flavonoids, alkaloids, and polysaccharides. Total saponins and compounds from ZSS are well known for their significant sedative and hypnotic effects (Du et al., 2020). Until now, the pharmacological investigation of total saponins for the treatment of insomnia has mainly focused on jujubosides, jujuboside A, jujuboside B, and other monomers. A previous research study showed that jujubosides, the main saponins of ZSS, significantly reduced the spontaneous activity of mice by regulating the serotonin system (He et al., 2020). It has also been reported that jujuboside A can inhibit the formation of the hippocampus *via* a glutamate-mediated excitatory signaling pathway (Zhang et al., 2003). Jujubosides can also modulate the expression of γ-amino-butyric acid A ($GABA_A$) receptor subunits in hippocampal neurons (You et al., 2010). Other studies have shown that jujuboside B can up-regulate the expression of $GABA_A$ receptors and increase the frequency of chloride channel opening, thus creating a hypnotic effect (Song et al., 2017). It has been shown that the total flavonoids of ZSS can extensively reduce the spontaneous activity of mice and prolong their sleep time (Jiang et al., 2007). Spinosin, the main flavonoid of ZSS, can enhance pentobarbital-induced sleep by regulating the serotonergic system (Wang et al., 2008). However, it is important that we identify potential mechanisms for the overall effects of ZSS if we are to create advanced approached for treating insomnia.

In this study, we used network pharmacology assisted by UHPLC-Q-Exactive-MS/MS analysis to predict the active ingredients and candidate targets fo ZSS. We also used network construction to investigate the active mechanisms underlying the effect of ZSS treatment on insomnia. Finally, we validated the proposed active mechanisms of ZSS in a PCPA-induced insomnia rat model by RT-qRCR and immunohistochemical analysis. The research procedure is shown in **Figure 1**.

MATERIALS AND METHODS

Chemicals and Reagents

Ziziphi Spinosae Semen (ZSS) was purchased from Jiangsu Yabang Chinese Herbal Medicine Co., Ltd. (Changzhou, China). Jujuboside A (batch number P13J9S65562), Jujuboside B (batch number C28A10S87087), Spinosin (batch number P09D11F133853), 6‴-Feruloylspinosin (batch number P04J12S136476), Betulinic acid (batch number R17F11F108704) were obtained from Shanghai yuanye Biological Technology Co., Ltd. (Shanghai, China). Pentobarbital sodium was purchased from Tianjin Yifang

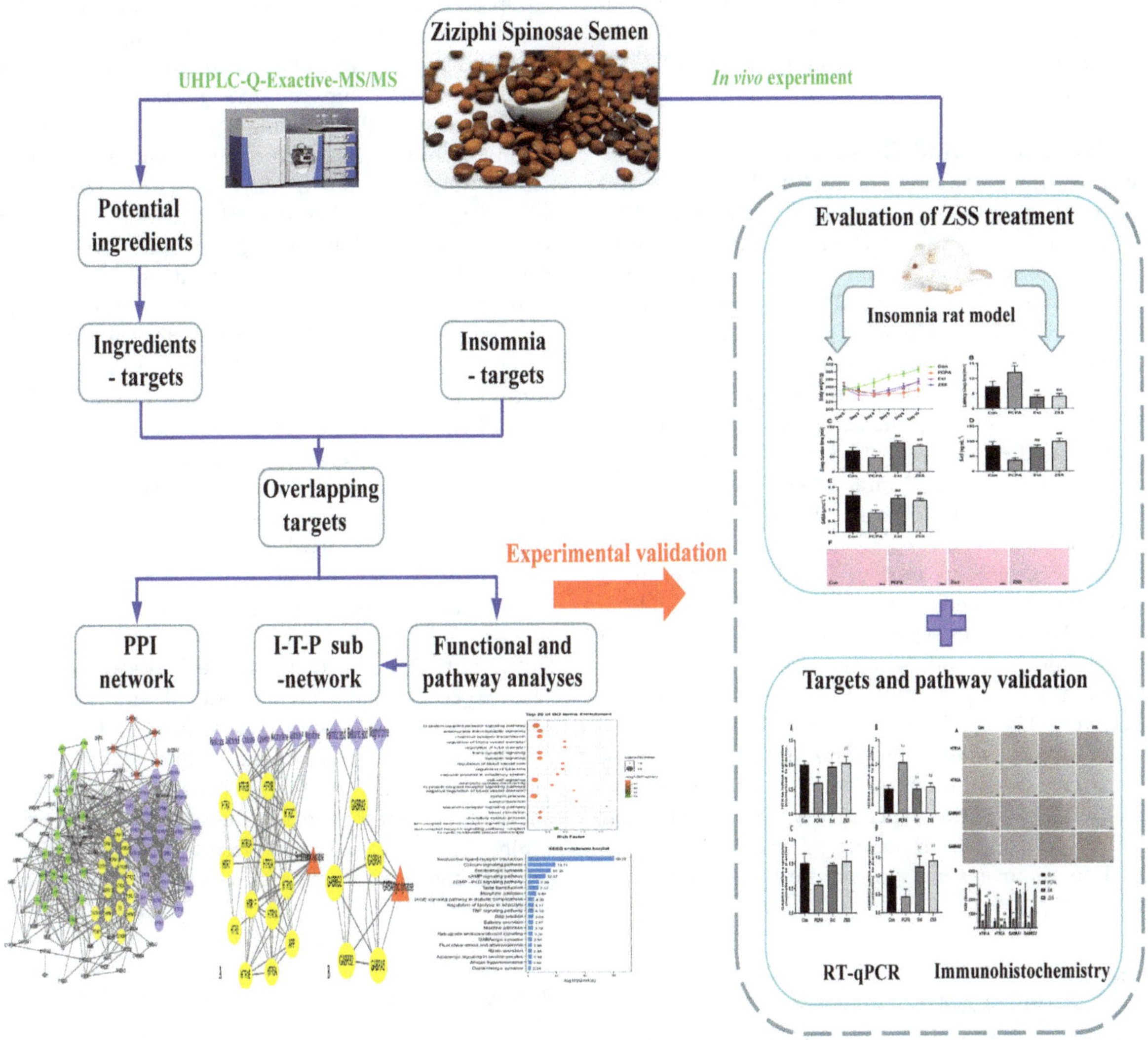

FIGURE 1 | The workflow plan used to investigate the effects of ZSS on insomnia using network pharmacology and an experimental validation approach.

Technology Co., Ltd. (Tianjin, China). *p*-chlorophenylalanine (PCPA) was supplied by Sinopharm Chemical Reagent Co., Ltd. (Shanghai, China). Acetonitrile, Formic acid and methanol (LC-MS grade) were obtained from Thermo Fisher Scientific (New Jersey, United States). Ammonium formate (LC-MS grade) was purchased from Sigma Aldrich (St. Louis, United States) while 2-chlorobenzalanine was purchased from Shanghai Aladdin Biochemical Technology Co., Ltd. (Shanghai, China). Ultrapure water was purified with a Milli-Q purification system (Milford, MA, United States). Other chemicals and reagents were all analytical grade.

Plant Extract Preparation

ZSS was formally identified as *Ziziphus jujuba* Mill. var. *spinosa* (Bunge) Hu ex H. F. Chou by Professor Tu-Lin Lu (Nanjing University of Chinese Medicine). The ZSS voucher specimen (ZSS-19121601) was deposited in the Traditional Chinese Medicine laboratory, Wuxi Traditional Chinese Medicine Hospital Affiliated to Nanjing University of Chinese Medicine under closed and dry conditions at 25 ± 5°C. A dried sample of ZSS was crushed and extracted with petroleum ether (60–90°C) for 2 h and the extraction repeated two further times. After degreasing, we added 8 volumes of 70% alcohol to the ZSS; the mixture was then fluxed three times (1.5 h each time) and the final filtrates were combined. The filtered extract was concentrated under a vacuum and then dried by a rotary evaporator (Shang et al., 2020). The total yield of alcohol extract from ZSS was 14.94% (w/w).

UHPLC-Q-Exactive-MS/MS Analysis of ZSS Extract

Sample Preparation

First, we weighed 6.9 mg of ZSS extract and mixed this with 5 ml of methanol. This was then ultrasonicated at room temperature for 15 min (300 W, 40 KHZ) and centrifuged for 10 min at 12,000 rpm. Finally, the supernatants were filtered through a 0.22 μm membrane to obtain prepared samples for UHPLC-Q-Exactive-MS analysis.

UHPLC-Q-Exactive-MS/MS Conditions

Chromatographic separation was accomplished in a Vanquis UHPLC system (Thermo Fischer Scientific, Waltham, MA, United States) equipped with a Thermo Fischer Scientific Hypersll GOLD (100 × 2.1 mm, 1.8 μm) column maintained at 35°C with a flow rate of 0.3 ml/min. The temperature of the autosampler was 5°C. Gradient elution of analytes was carried out with 0.1% acetic acid in 10 mM ammonium acetate buffer solution (A) and acetonitrile (B). We injected 1 μl of each sample after equilibration. An increasing linear gradient of solvent B (v/v) was then applied, as follows: 0–10 min, 5–20% B; 10–14 min, 20–25% B; 14–25 min, 25–35% B; 25–30 min, 35–100% B; 30–31 min, 100–100% B; 31–32 min, 100–5% B; 32–35 min, 5–5% B.

The ESI-MS^n experiments were executed on a Thermo Q Exactive mass spectrometer (Thermo Fischer Scientific, Massachusetts, United States) with spray voltages of 3.5 and −3.0 kV in positive and negative modes, respectively. Sheath gas and auxiliary gas were set at 40 and 15 arbitrary units, respectively. The capillary temperature was 320°C. The analyzer scanned over a mass range of m/z 150–2,000 Da for a full scan at a mass resolution of 70,000. Data dependent acquisition (DDA) MS/MS experiments were performed with HCD scans. Dynamic exclusion was implemented to remove some unnecessary information in MS/MS spectra.

Data Processing

The analysis of UHPLC-MS data was performed using Thermo Xcalibur Version 4.1 software (Thermo Fischer Scientific, Massachusetts, United States). We tentatively identified the compounds of ZSS by considering a range of factors, including molecular weight, retention time, fragment information obtained from the MS/MS model, further matching annotation in our in-house database of compounds, along with previous literature and standard references.

Animal Experimentation

Male Sprague-Dawley rats (200 ± 20 g) were obtained from SPF (Beijing) Biotechnology Co., Ltd (Permission No. SCXK (jing) 2019–0010). All animals were housed in a breeding environment (12 h light-dark cycle, 25 ± 2°C, and 55 ± 5% relative humidity). All rats had free access to water and food. This animal research was approved by the Ethics Committee of Wuxi Hospital of Traditional Chinese Medicine (Approval ID: SKJJ2020011707) and conformed to animal welfare regulations and the ethical principles for animal protection and the relevant provisions put forward by the National Experimental Animal Welfare Ethics guidelines.

After 7 days of acclimation, the rats were randomly divided into four groups (6 rats per group): a normal group, a model group, an estazolam group, and a ZSS group. The PCPA-induced model of insomnia was established using a method that was described previously (Si et al., 2020). Rats in the model group, the estazolam group, and the ZSS group, were intraperitoneally injected with PCPA (350 mg/kg) once a day for 3 days. The normal group received the same amount of physiological saline. On the fourth day, the ZSS group was orally administered with ZSS alcohol extract (dissolved in normal saline) at a dose of 403.38 mg/kg (equivalent to a crude drug dose of 2.7 g/kg) once a day for 7 days (Du et al., 2019; Hua et al., 2021). The human equivalent dose (HED) of the dose is 0.43 g/kg, which is 2 times of the clinical dosage (Food and Drug Administration, 2005). The estazolam group was administered with 0.5 mg/kg of estazolam (dissolved in normal saline) once a day for 7 days. Rats in the other two groups were treated with an equal volume of physiological saline. At the end of the animal experiment and after fasting for 12 h, all rats were anaesthetized by an intraperitoneal injection of pentobarbital sodium (45 mg/kg). Blood samples were then collected from the abdominal aorta and hypothalamic tissues were quickly removed.

Pentobarbital Sodium-Induced Sleep Test

This experiment was carried out 30 min after the last drug administration. Rats were placed on their backs following an intraperitoneal injection of pentobarbital sodium (35 mg/kg), and then monitored the rats for signs of sleeping. Our main criterion for sleep was that the rats lost their righting reflex for more than 1 min. Sleep latency was recorded as the time between pentobarbital sodium injection and the loss of the righting reflex. Sleep duration was recorded from the loss of the righting reflex until recovery (Xu et al., 2019).

Assay for Hypothalamic 5-HT and GABA

The hypothalamic samples were homogenized with ice-cold PBS (w/v, 1:9). The homogenate was centrifuged at 3,000 rpm for 10 min at 4°C. The supernatant was collected. The levels of 5-HT and GABA in hypothalamic tissues were measured using ELISA kits according to the manufacturer's instructions (Nanjing JinTing Biotechnology Co., Ltd. Nanjing, China).

Histopathological Examination

Hypothalamic tissues were fixed in 4% paraformaldehyde, dehydrated, embedded in paraffin, and then sectioned. Sections (4 μm thick) were then dewaxed to water, and stained with hematoxylin and eosin (HE). Finally, hypothalamic lesions were observed by microscopy, as described previously (Shen et al., 2020).

Network Pharmacology

The Screening of Candidate Ingredients

The phytochemicals identified by UHPLC-Q-Exactive-MS/MS were used for network pharmacology investigations. We used Lipinski's rule of five related parameters to screen the active compounds: a molecular weight (MW) ≤ 500, an octanol-water partition coefficient log P (ALogP) ≤ 5, a hydrogen bond donor count (Hdon) ≤ 5, and a hydrogen bond acceptor count (Hacc) ≤

10. The principle of screening candidate ingredients was to meet at least two of the parameters (Wang et al., 2020). Some compounds (e.g., jujuboside A) exhibited low values with explicit pharmacological effects; these were also selected for further study.

Analysis of Putative Targets

We used BATMAN-TCM (http://bionet.ncpsb.org.cn/batman-tcm/) (Ji et al., 2019) and the SwissTargetPrediction database (http://www.swisstargetprediction.ch/) (Gfeller et al., 2014) to identify the relevant biological targets of candidate ingredients from ZSS. We also retrieved disease-associated targets from the GeneCards database (https://www.genecards.org/) by using "insomnia" and "sedation and hypnosis" as keywords (Hu et al., 2020). Then, the overlapping targets between ingredient- and insomnia-associated targets were then visualized by creating Venn diagrams (https://bioinfogp.cnb.csic.es/tools/venny/index.html) (Huang et al., 2020). In addition, these overlapping targets were introduced into the STRING database (https://www.string-db.org/) to investigate protein-protein interaction (PPI) relationships; this allowed us to identify targets that were closely related to insomnia (Liang et al., 2021); the protein interaction selection score was set to >0.6. Cytoscape version 3.6.1 software (Free Software Foundation, Inc., Boston, MA, United States) was used to visualize the PPI network. Then, we used the MCODE plugin to conduct cluster analysis of the targets showing high levels of interaction (Zhang et al., 2019).

GO and KEGG Pathway Enrichment Analyses

Next, the core targets obtained from MCODE cluster analysis were imported into Omicshare tools (https://www.omicshare.com/). We then performed Gene Ontology (GO) and Kyoto Encyclopedia of Genes and Genomes (KEGG) pathway enrichment analyses for the core targets and identified the key biological functions (biological processes, molecular functions, and cellular components) and related signaling pathways (Wu et al., 2020). Finally, an ingredient-target-pathway (I-T-P) network was generated by Cytoscape version 3.6.1 software, which featured a number of relationships, including the active chemical ingredients of ZSS, the core targets, and the enriched signaling pathways (An et al., 2020).

Experimental Validation

RT-qPCR Experiment

Total RNA was extracted from the rat hypothalamus with Trizol reagent (Invitrogen, Carlsbad, CA, United States). cDNA was then synthetized with a reverse transcription kit (TaKaRa, Dalian, China) by GeneExplorer PCR (Bioer Technology, Hangzhou, China). Next, the cDNA was used as a target for amplification using the TB Green Premix PCR Kit (TaKaRa, Dalian, China) and a LightCycler 480 II (Roche, Rotkreuz, Switzerland). The real-time PCR thermal cycling protocol was as follows: 95°C for 5 min, followed by 50 cycles of 95°C for 10 s, 60°C for 10 s and 72°C for 10 s. The primer sequences were synthesized by Sangon Biotech Co., Ltd. (Shanghai, China), as follows: β-actin (Forward) 5′-CCT CACTGTCCACCTTCCA-3′ and (Reverse) 5′-GGGTGTAAA ACGCAGCTCA-3′; HTR1A (Forward) 5′-GGGCAACTCCAA AGAGCA-3′ and (Reverse) 5′-TCACCGTCTTCCTTTCACG-3′; HTR2A (Forward) 5′-TTCCTTGTCATGCCTGTGT-3′ and (Reverse) 5′-ATAGCGGTCCAGGGAGAT-3′; GABRA1 (Forward) 5′-GACTATCTTTGGGCCTGGA-3′ and (Reverse) 5′-CATCTTGGGAGGGCTGT-3′; GABRG2 (Forward) 5′-ACAATGCCACCCACCTT-3′ and (Reverse) 5′-TATCCTCCCGTGTCTCCA-3′. The relative expression of the target genes were normalized to the threshold cycle (CT) value of β-actin, and the data analysis was performed using the $2^{-\triangle\triangle Ct}$ method (Poh et al., 2017). Real-time PCR was performed for each sample in three replicates.

Immunohistochemistry

Paraffin-embedded rat hypothalamic tissues were sectioned and dewaxed to water. Then, high pressure boiling was used for antigen retrieval and endogenous catalase was blocked by 3% H_2O_2. Next, sections (4 μm thick) were incubated overnight at 4°C with HTR1A (PA5-75267, 1:200) (Invitrogen, Carlsbad, CA, United States), HTR2A (PA5-95288, 1:200) (Invitrogen, Carlsbad, CA, United States), GABRA1 (ab94585, 1:200) (Abcam, United Kingdom) and GABRG2 (ab87328, 1:200) (Abcam, United Kingdom) antibodies. The following morning, sections were washed and then incubated for 20 min at 37°C with HRP-conjugated secondary antibodies (goat anti-rabbit IgG H&L, ab205718, Abcam, 1:2,000), followed by DAB and hematoxylin staining. Finally, the stained sections were imaged and observed by NIKON ECLIPSE CI microscopy (Nikon, Japan). The integrated optical density (IOD) of the expression levels of target proteins/positive cells were then quantified with Image Pro Plus version 7.0 software (Media Cybernetics, Inc., MD, United States) (Jin et al., 2020).

Statistics

Experimental data are shown as mean ± standard deviation (SD). One-way analysis of variance (ANOVA) was used for all statistical analysis followed by a Dunnett's test and performed in GraphPad Prism version 8 (GraphPad Software Inc., San Diego, CA, United States). p-values < 0.05 was considered to be statistically significant.

RESULTS

UHPLC-Q-Exactive-MS Analysis of ZSS Extract

UHPLC-Q-Exactive-MS identified a total of 34 phytochemicals in ZSS extract, including twenty-four flavonoids, two triterpenoid saponins, two triterpene acids, four alkaloids, and two fatty acids (**Table 1**). Five of these compounds (spinosin, 6‴-feruloylspinosin, jujuboside A, jujuboside B, and betulinic acid) were identified by comparison to standard references; the others were identified by comparison with literature.

General Status

Twelve to 48 h after the injection of PCPA, most of the rats began to show hyperactivity; they also showed increased levels of

TABLE 1 | Identified ingredients in ZSS extract.

NO.	RT (min)	Compound name	Formula	MS	Error (ppm)	MS/MS
1	7.07	Magnoflorine	$C_{20}H_{24}NO_4$	342.1697 [M]$^+$	−0.877	297.1119,282.0885,265.0858,58.0660
2	7.29	Coclaurine	$C_{17}H_{19}NO_3$	286.1432 [M + H]$^+$	−2.097	269.1170,237.0908,219.0807,175.0753,107.0495
3	7.50	Vicenin II	$C_{27}H_{30}O_{15}$	593.1527 [M-H]$^-$	2.697	503.1214,473.1101,383.0780,353.0673
4	9.31	6‴-(4‴′-O-glc)-vanilloylspinosin	$C_{42}H_{48}O_{23}$	921.2646 [M + H]$^+$	−0.217	351.0860,327.0861,297.0757,151.0390
5	9.45	Isovitexin-2″-O-β-D-glucopy-ranoside	$C_{27}H_{30}O_{15}$	593.1536 [M-H]$^-$	4.215	413.0886,293.0460
6	9.93	Zivulgarin	$C_{28}H_{32}O_{15}$	609.1801 [M + H]$^+$	−2.134	447.1288,351.0871,327.0861,297.0755,285.0757
7	10.05	Camelliaside B	$C_{32}H_{38}O_{19}$	725.194 [M-H]$^-$	0.827	575.1411,284.0331,255.0297
8[a]	10.09	Spinosin	$C_{28}H_{32}O_{15}$	609.1799 [M + H]$^+$	−2.462	447.1291,429.1185,411.1071,393.0966,381.0961, 351.0862,327.0862,297.0757,285.0757
9	10.11	Isospinosin	$C_{28}H_{32}O_{15}$	607.1682 [M-H]$^-$	2.306	487.1257,445.1151,427.1041,324.0644,307.0617,292.0380
10	10.14	Isovitexin	$C_{21}H_{20}O_{10}$	433.1115 [M + H]$^+$	−3.463	397.0923,379.0818,337.0707,313.0707,283.0600
11	10.69	Swertisin	$C_{22}H_{22}O_{10}$	445.1144 [M-H]$^-$	0.899	325.0724,297.0410,282.0539
12	11.11	Caaverine	$C_{17}H_{17}NO_2$	268.1327 [M + H]$^+$	−1.865	251.1065,219.0804,191.0854
13	11.14	6‴-Pyridyloylspinosin	$C_{34}H_{35}NO_{16}$	714.2020 [M + H]$^+$	−1.260	351.0865, 327.0862, 323.0930,297.0759,124.0395
14	11.46	Kaempferol-3-rutinoside	$C_{27}H_{30}O_{15}$	593.1524 [M-H]$^-$	2.192	285.0407
15	11.73	6‴-*p*-Hydroxylbenzoylspinosin	$C_{35}H_{36}O_{17}$	727.1891 [M-H]$^-$	1.650	427.1042,325.0724,307.0616,239.0563,179.0345,137.0236
16	11.79	Isovitexin-2″-O-(6-feruloyl)-glucopyranoside	$C_{37}H_{38}O_{18}$	769.1995 [M-H]$^-$	1.300	413.0883,341.0675,311.0566,293.0462,235.0613,193.0500
17	12.00	6‴-O-(3S-1-N-β-D-glucopyranosyl -2-oxo-3-hydroxy-indole-3-acetyl) spinosin	$C_{44}H_{49}NO_{23}$	958.2634 [M-H]$^-$	1.252	649.1790,607.1710,487.1236,469.1152,307.0618,146.0238
18	12.31	6‴-O-(3R-1-N-β-D-glucopyranosyl -2-oxo-3-hydroxy-indole-3-acetyl) spinosin	$C_{44}H_{49}NO_{23}$	958.2631 [M-H]$^-$	0.939	649.1757,607.1664,427.1036,307.0636
19	12.34	6‴-Sinapoylspinosin	$C_{39}H_{42}O_{19}$	813.2258 [M-H]$^-$	1.230	427.1042,307.0616
20	12.70	6‴-*p*-Coumaloylspinosin	$C_{37}H_{38}O_{17}$	753.2056 [M-H]$^-$	2.655	633.1624,607.1690,445.1169,427.1041,325.0724, 307.0610,265.0721,205.0504
21[a]	12.72	6‴-Feruloylspinosin	$C_{38}H_{40}O_{18}$	785.2261 [M + H]$^+$	−3.311	505.7764,411.1066,393.0963,351.0869,327.0859, 321.0950,297.0747,177.0547
22	13.44	6‴-(N-β-D-glucopyranosyl)-2‴′,3‴′-dihydro-2‴′-oxo-3‴′-yl-acetate spinosin	$C_{44}H_{49}NO_{22}$	944.2802 [M + H]$^+$	6.460	393.0969,351.0863,327.0862,297.0765
23	13.67	Isomer of NO.22	$C_{44}H_{49}NO_{22}$	944.2805 [M + H]$^+$	6.778	393.0960,351.0872,327.0860,297.0756
24	14.30	6-(−) -phaseolspinosin	$C_{43}H_{50}O_{19}$	869.2889 [M-H]$^-$	1.841	779.7828,607.1709,545.9795,510.7946,477.1872,427.1047
25	14.71	6‴-benzoylspinosin	$C_{35}H_{36}O_{16}$	713.2072 [M + H]$^+$	−0.561	327.0860,351.0859,297.0739
26	15.46	N-nornuciferine	$C_{18}H_{19}NO_2$	282.1481 [M + H]$^+$	−2.835	265.1221,250.0986,234.1037
27	15.48	6″-O-(3-glc-indole-acetyl)-6‴-feruloylspinosin	$C_{54}H_{57}NO_{25}$	1120.3273 [M + H]$^+$	−1.696	393.0963,351.0861,327.0860,297.0745,285.0760, 177.0546,146.0601,145.0285
28	15.65	Isomer of NO.27	$C_{54}H_{57}NO_{25}$	1120.3273 [M + H]$^+$	−1.696	393.0963,351.0861,327.0860,297.0745,285.0760, 177.0546,146.0601,145.0285
29[a]	23.98	Jujuboside A	$C_{58}H_{94}O_{26}$	1205.5967 [M-H]$^-$	0.498	1073.5563,911.5052,749.4493,603.3905
30[a]	26.58	Jujuboside B	$C_{52}H_{84}O_{21}$	1043.5446 [M-H]$^-$	1.342	911.5043,749.4492, 603.3910
31	29.38	Ceanothic acid	$C_{30}H_{46}O_5$	485.3280 [M-H]$^-$	1.648	423.3280
32[a]	31.19	Betulinic acid	$C_{30}H_{48}O_3$	455.3538 [M-H]$^-$	1.757	
33	32.29	Palmitic acid	$C_{16}H_{32}O_2$	255.2332 [M-H]$^-$	1.175	
34	32.35	Oleic acid	$C_{18}H_{34}O_2$	281.2491 [M-H]$^-$	1.778	

[a]-*identified by standard references.*

sensitivity and aggressiveness. Their fur became dry and dull and the color of their toenails began to turn white or yellow. Over time, the rats in the model group began to show fatigue, characteristic dullness developed in their fur, and they showed a slow response to external stimulation. Eventually, the rats showed serious fatigue and had begun to gain weight gradually. We found that the fur color and response to external stimulation were improved in the ZSS group and the estazolam group. Rats in the normal control group showed a normal state throughout the entire experiment. There was a significant difference in weight gain when compared between the control group and the PCPA group ($p < 0.05$) (**Figure 2A**). The weight of rats in the ZSS and estazolam treatment groups were significantly higher than that in the PCPA group ($p < 0.05$).

Effects of ZSS on Pentobarbital Sodium-Induced Sleep

The latency sleep time of rats in the estazolam group and the ZSS group was significantly lower ($p < 0.01$) than that in the PCPA group (**Figure 2B**). Treatment with estazolam or ZSS extract significantly prolonged the total sleep time ($p < 0.01$) when compared with the PCPA group (**Figure 2C**).

Effects of ZSS on Hypothalamic 5-HT and GABA in PCPA-Induced Insomnia Rat

As shown in **Figures 2D,E**, the levels of 5-HT and GABA in the hypothalamus of the PCPA group were significantly decreased as compared to the control group ($p < 0.01$). Compared with the PCPA group, oral administration of SCE remarkably increased the levels of 5-HT and GABA ($p < 0.01$).

Histopathological Observation

In the control group, there was an abundance of hypothalamic nerve cells; these had a clear shape and were evenly distributed. In the PCPA group, cells were deformed, loosely arranged; some had even disappeared. These pathological changes were restored when rats were treated with ZSS extract and estazolam (**Figure 2F**).

Network Pharmacology

Candidate Ingredients and Potential Targets of ZSS

According to Lipinski's rule, our network pharmacology study identified 21 candidate compounds (**Table 2**). Using associated databases, we failed to identify related targets for 6‴-Sinapoylspinosin and 6‴-*p*-Coumaloylspinosin. Ultimately, we identified 19 active compounds and 433 compound-related targets (**Supplementary Table S1**). In total, 504 insomnia-associated targets were acquired from the GeneCards database (**Supplementary Table S2**). After overlapping the ZSS-associated targets and the insomnia-associated targets, we identified 118 targets potential targets for ZSS in the treatment of insomnia (**Supplementary Table S3**). Next, we created a PPI network and performed MCODE clustering analysis in Cytoscape to identify the way the potential targets interacted and to identify kernel targets. We identified 111 nodes and 787 edges in the PPI network (**Figure 3**). The clustering coefficient and average neighborhood number were 0.611 and 14.180, respectively. MCODE clustering analysis identified 4 clusters. As shown in **Table 3**, 65 key targets were identified from 4 clusters, thus representing potential core targets for ZSS in the treatment of insomnia. Most of these targets were neuroactive ligand receptors, including serotonin receptors (e.g., HTR1A, HTR1B, HTR1E, HTR1D, HTR1F, HTR2A, HTR2B, HTR2C, HTR3A and HTR5A), $GABA_A$ receptors (e.g., GABRA1, GABRA2, GABRA5, GABRB2 and GABRG2), dopamine receptors (e.g., DRD1, DRD2, DRD3, DRD4 and DRD5), adrenergic receptor (e.g., ADRA1A, ADRA1B, ADRA1D, ADRA2A, ADRA2B and ADRA2C), cannabinoid signaling (e.g. CNR1 and CNR2), and muscarinic acetylcholine receptors (e.g. CHRM1 and CHRM3).

GO and KEGG Pathway Enrichment Analysis

GO enrichment analysis demonstrated that the core targets were associated with various neural-associated biological processes, including G protein-coupled receptor signaling pathways, anterograde *trans*-synaptic signaling, chemical synaptic transmission, *trans*-synaptic signaling, and synaptic signaling (**Figure 4**). Next, we applied KEGG enrichment analysis to identify the overall regulation of ZSS in the treatment of insomnia with regards to specific signaling pathways. The targets identified overlapped between neuroactive ligand-receptor interaction, serotonergic synapse, and GABAergic synapse (**Figure 5**).

Next, we used ingredient-target-pathway (I-T-P) sub-networks to construct serotonergic synapse and GABAergic synapse pathways and reveal the synergistic effects of ZSS to treat insomnia (**Figures 6A,B**). As shown in the two networks, palmitic acid, coclaurine, jujuboside A, N-nornuciferine, caaverine, magnoflorine, jujuboside B, and betulinic acid, all played roles in pathways associated with the serotonergic synapse and the GABAergic synapse.

Recent studies have shown that multiple subtypes of serotonin (5-HT) receptors In the central nervous system are mainly involved in the modulation of sleep (Cui et al., 2011). In addition, 5-HT_{1A} (HTR1A) and 5-HT_{2A} (HTR2A) have been identified as common targets for the treatment of insomnia, in both clinical and basic studies (Jiang et al., 2016; Ohno et al., 2018; Shao et al., 2020; Lv et al., 2021), as well as prevenient studies of ZSS for the treatment of insomnia (Shen et al., 2020). $GABA_AR\alpha1$ (GABRA1) and $GABA_AR\gamma2$ (GABRG2) are two significant subunits of GABA receptors, and are known to play an important role in the first line treatment of insomnia (Zhong et al., 2020; Lv et al., 2021). Based on our preliminary results, we preferentially selected HTR1A, HTR2A, GABRA1, and GABRG2, as potential therapeutic targets of ZSS for further experimental validation.

Experimental Validation

RT-qPCR Experiments

Network pharmacology demonstrated that neuroactive ligand-receptor interaction (important-related targets: HTR1A, HTR2A, GABRA1 and GABRG2), serotonergic synapse (important-related targets: HTR1A and HTR2A), and GABAergic synapse (important-related targets: GABRA1 and GABRG2) signaling pathways were involved in the effects of ZSS on insomnia. We determined the expression levels of hypothalamic-related genes (**Figures 7A–D**). The administration of PCPA led to a significant reduction in the gene expression of *HTR1A*, *GABRA1*, and *GABRG2* (both $p < 0.05$), and an increase in the expression levels of *HTR2A* mRNA ($p < 0.01$). We found that ZSS treatment significantly elevated the gene expression levels of *HTR1A* ($p < 0.01$), *GABRA1* ($p < 0.05$) and *GABRG2* ($p < 0.01$) and decreased the expression levels of *HTR2A* mRNA ($p < 0.01$).

Immunohistochemistry

We also used immunohistochemistry analysis to investigate the expression levels of related targets in the hypothalamus (**Figures 8A,B**). The injection of PCPA induced a significant reduction in the number of HTR1A-, GABRA1-, and GABRG2-positive cells ($p < 0.01$), and an increase in the number of HTR2A-positive cells in the hypothalamus ($p < 0.01$). Following ZSS treatment, the number of HTR1A-, GABRA1-, and GABRG2-positive cells increased significantly ($p < 0.01$); however, the number of HTR2A-positive cells decreased significantly ($p < 0.01$).

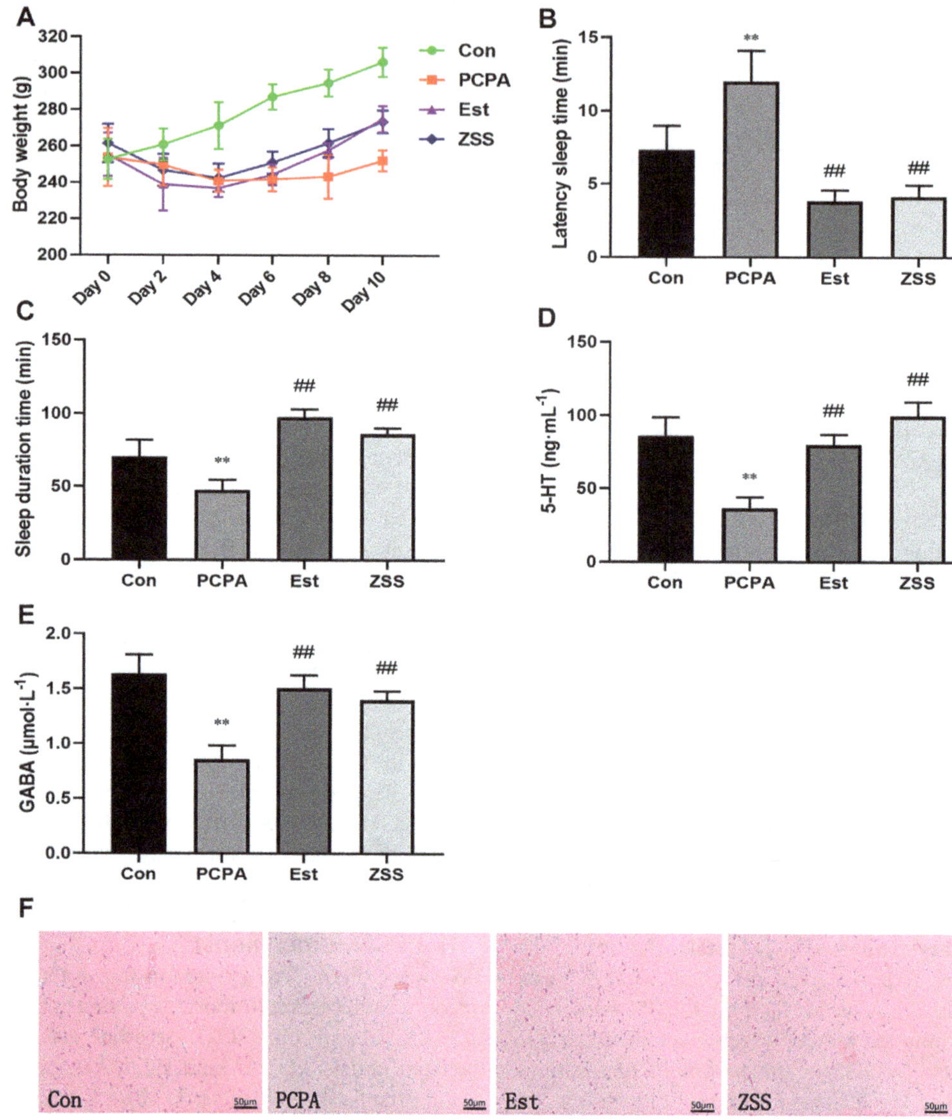

FIGURE 2 | The effects of ZSS extract on body weight **(A)**, pentobarbital sodium-induced sleep latency **(B)** and sleep duration **(C)**, the levels of 5-HT **(D)** and GABA **(E)**. Histopathological observation of the hypothalamus at ×200 magnification **(F)**. Con, control group; PCPA, PCPA-induced insomnia model group; Est, estazolam-positive group; ZSS, alcohol extract of Ziziphi Spinosae Semen group. $^{**}p < 0.01$ compared with the control group, $^{\#\#}p < 0.01$ compared with the model group. Data shows mean ± SD values and n = 6.

DISCUSSION

Previous research involving ZSS mostly focused on the pharmacodynamics of certain components, but failed to address the specific mechanisms underlying the pharmacodynamics of ZSS from an overall material basis. In this study, we employed network pharmacology and *in vivo* validation experiments to identify the specific mechanisms underlying the actions of ZSS in the treatment of insomnia. The identification of specific components of herbal materials identified by network pharmacology should be more accurate than when simply retrieved from databases of herbal ingredients (e.g., TCMSP, https://old.tcmsp-e.com/tcmsp.php; BATMAN-TCM, http://bionet.ncpsb.org.cn/batman-tcm/). The chemical composition of herbal materials may often change during the processes used for extraction and concentration. Research has shown that modern analytical techniques, such as GC-MS and UPLC-MS, should be used as supplementary tools to obtain more accurate results relating to chemical compositions (Ren et al., 2020; Tian et al., 2020; Oh et al., 2021). In the current study, UPLC-Q-Exactive-MS/MS identified a series of triterpenoid saponins and flavonoids from ZSS extract; some of these were spinosin derivatives, including 6‴-(4⁗-O-glc)-vanilloylspinosin, 6‴-pyridyloylspinosin, 6‴-*p*-hydroxylbenzoylspinosin, 6‴-O-(3S-1-N-β-D-glucopyranosyl-2-oxo-3-hydroxy-indole-3-acetyl) spinosyn, 6‴-sinapoylspinosin,

TABLE 2 | The parameters of drug-likeness of candidate compounds.

NO.	Compound	Molecular weight	ALogP	Hydrogen bond donor count	Hydrogen bond acceptor count
1	Magnoflorine	342.4	2.7	2	4
2	Coclaurine	285.34	2.6	3	4
3	Vicenin II	594.5	−2.3	11	15
4	Zivulgarin	608.5	−1.6	9	15
5	Camelliaside B	726.6	−2.5	11	19
6	Spinosin	608.5	−1.1	9	15
7	Isospinosin	608.5	−1.1	9	15
8	Isovitexin	432.4	0.2	7	10
9	Swertisin	446.4	0.5	6	10
10	Caaverine	267.32	2.6	2	3
11	Kaempferol-3-rutinoside	594.5	−0.9	9	15
12	6‴-Sinapoylspinosin	814.7	0.6	9	19
13	6‴-*p*-Coumaloylspinosin	754.7	0.7	9	17
14	6‴-Feruloylspinosin	784.7	0.7	9	18
15	N-nornuciferine	281.3	3	1	3
16	Jujuboside A	1207.3	−1.6	14	26
17	Jujuboside B	1045.2	0.5	11	21
18	Ceanothic acid	486.7	7.6	3	5
19	Betulinic acid	456.7	8.2	2	3
20	Palmitic acid	256.42	6.4	1	2
21	Oleic acid	282.5	6.5	1	2

6‴-*p*-coumaloylspinosin, 6‴-feruloylspinosin, 6‴-(N-β-D-glucopyranosyl)-2‴',3‴'-dihydro-2‴'-oxo-3‴'-yl-acetate spinosin, 6-(-)-phaseolspinosin, 6‴-benzoylspinosin, and 6″-O-(3-glc-indole-acetyl)-6‴-feruloylspinosin; these are rare in other plants. According to Lipinski's rule of five, we selected compounds with good drug-likeness in ZSS for our network pharmacology research. In addition, we also included compounds with good activity but poor properties of drug-likeness.

Previous research identified that the serotonin (5-HT) system plays an active role in sleep disorders, depression, anxiety disorders, and other disorders of the central nervous system (Novati et al., 2008; Babson et al., 2017; Van Dalfsen and Markus, 2019). According to amino acid sequence, gene structure, second messengers, and pharmacological activity, the serotonin receptors can be divided into seven categories (HTR1-7) (Domínguez-Soto et al., 2017). The HTR1A and HTR2A subtypes are the most noteworthy receptors; this is because of their highly specific and important role in the brain. These receptor subtypes have been used to investigate the pathogenesis of nervous system diseases and research focused on anti-insomnia and anti-depressant drugs (Antypa et al., 2013; Dong et al., 2016). HTR1A receptor agonists, buspirone, and eptapirone, have all been shown to reduce REMS (rapid eyes movement sleep), increase REMS latency, and elevate the levels of 5-HT in brain (Wilson et al., 2005). This may be one of the reasons why HTR1A receptor agonists can ameliorate sleep symptoms. HTR1A receptors are mainly expressed on the axons of serotonergic neurons in the raphe nucleus, but are also expressed in the hypothalamus, thalamus, frontal cortex, amygdala and hippocampus (Polter and Li, 2010). The regulation of HTR1A receptors during sleep, emotion, self-cognition, and other physiological activities, involves the precise coordination of presynaptic and postsynaptic receptors (Albert et al., 2014). The results of both experimental and clinical studies have proven the effect of HTR2A receptor antagonists in the treatment of insomnia (Cohrs et al., 2005). HTR2A receptor antagonists (e.g., ketanserin, seganserinm, and ritanserin) can increase SWS (slow wave sleep) and NREMS (non-rapid eye movement sleep), reduce the number of awakenings, but has no effect on REMS. Therefore, HTR2A receptor antagonists are considered to be ideal drugs for insomnia (Fish et al., 2005; Yi et al., 2007; Monti, 2010). Similarly, our systems biology investigations showed that the serotonergic synapse signaling pathway plays a dominant role in the therapeutic effect of ZSS. Our RT-qPCR and immunohistochemistry experiments also demonstrated that ZSS extract had a significant regulatory effect on the expression of HTR1A and HTR2A.

GABA produces a neuroinhibitory effect by binding with its receptor GABA (A-C) (Bormann, 2000). Of the different forms of GABA receptor, the $GABA_A$ receptor is the one that is most used in insomnia research. GABA acts on the GABA site of the $GABA_A$ receptor; this increases the permeability of chloride ions in the membranes of nerve cells (Olsen and Sieghart, 2008). Chloride ions can then enter into cells along a concentration gradient; the negative potential in cell membranes increases further, from a polarized state to a hyperpolarized state (Dela Peña et al., 2015). Depolarization is very difficult and causes a reduction in excitability, thus resulting in sedation, hypnosis, and antianxiety (Succol et al., 2012). Of the $GABA_A$ receptor subunits, GABRA1 and GABRG2 have been frequently reported to mediate insomnia (Tochitani and Kondo, 2013; Dixon et al., 2015). In this study, RT-qPCR and immunohistochemistry revealed that an extract of ZSS led

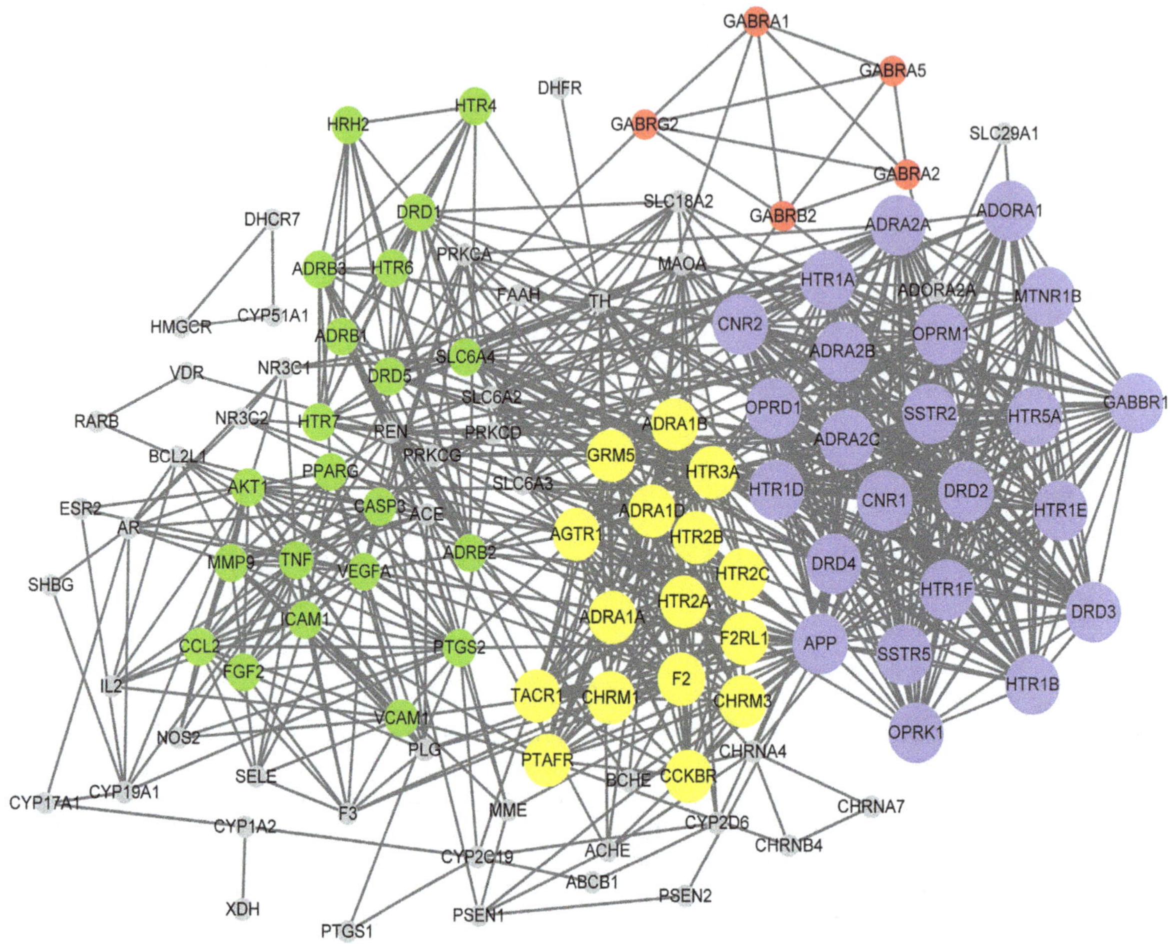

FIGURE 3 | PPI network of the potential targets for ZSS in the treatment of insomnia. Different clusters are represented by different colors. For each cluster, node size is directly proportional to the MCODE score.

TABLE 3 | Targets clustering analysis using MOCDE from PPI network.

Cluster	Score	Nodes number	Edges number	Targets
1	23	23	253	APP, CNR2, CNR1, HTR1E, HTR1F, ADORA1, SSTR2, SSTR5, HTR1B, ADRA2B, ADRA2C, ADRA2A, OPRM1, HTR1D, HTR5A, MTNR1B, DRD4, GABBR1, HTR1A, DRD3, DRD2, OPRD1, OPRK1
2	14.933	16	112	CHRM1, CHRM3, AGTR1, TACR1, ADRA1A, HTR3A, HTR2C, PTAFR, F2, ADRA1B, GRM5, HTR2B, ADRA1D, CCKBR, HTR2A, F2RL1
3	9.1	21	91	FGF2, HRH2, MMP9, HTR4, ADRB3, PPARG, ICAM1, ADRB2, ADRB1, TNF, AKT1, CASP3, DRD1, DRD5, HTR6, HTR7, VCAM1, SLC6A4, CCL2, PTGS2, VEGFA
4	5	5	10	GABRA1, GABRG2, GABRA2, GABRA5, GABRB2

to an increase in the expression of GABRA1 and GABRG2 receptors in the hypothalamus of rats suffering from insomnia. Systems biology analysis further indicated that the $GABA_A$ receptor signaling pathway is a crucially important pathway involved in the therapeutic effect of ZSS.

The active ingredients of Chinese herbal materials (CHM) are the material basis for their pharmacological actions. In addition, these ingredients, with good biological activities and measurability, are considered as the quality markers (Q-markers) for CHM. Q-markers for CHM represent a new concept for the quality control of herbal medicines (Kang et al., 2019). As shown in our ingredients-target-pathway (I-T-P) sub-networks, two triterpenoid saponins (jujuboside A, jujuboside B), four alkaloids (coclaurine, N-nornuciferine, caaverine, magnoflorine), one triterpene

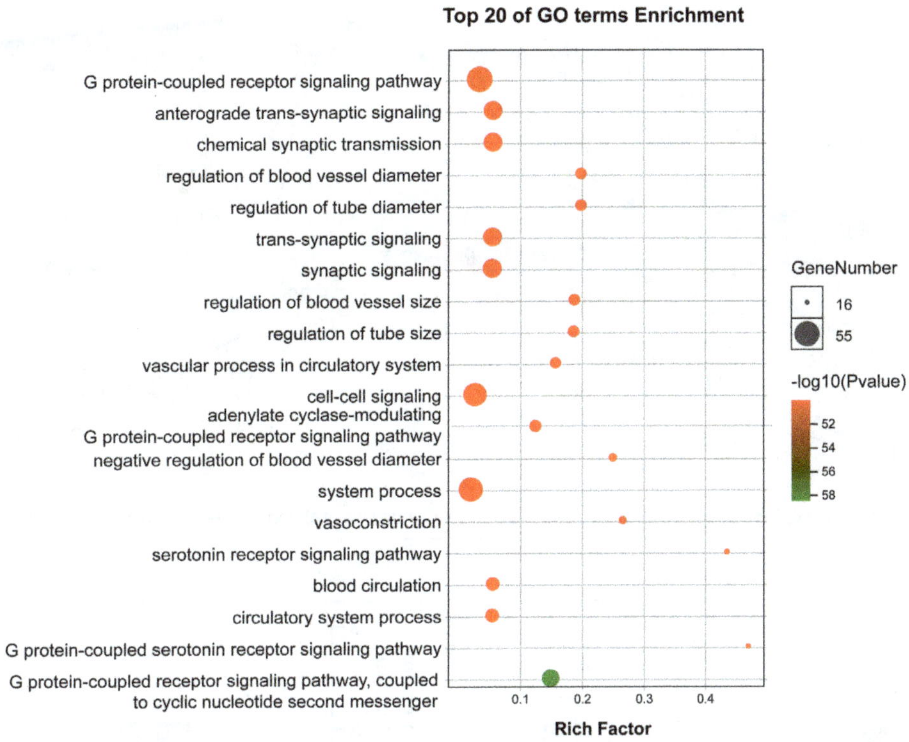

FIGURE 4 | GO enrichment analysis of targets for ZSS in the treatment of insomnia.

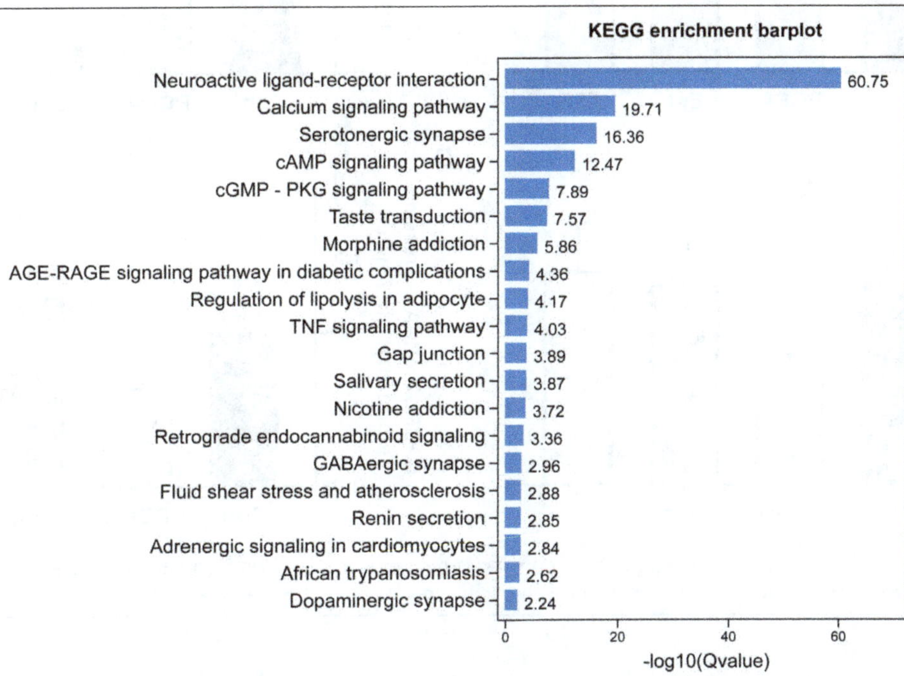

FIGURE 5 | KEGG enrichment analysis of targets for ZSS in the treatment of insomnia.

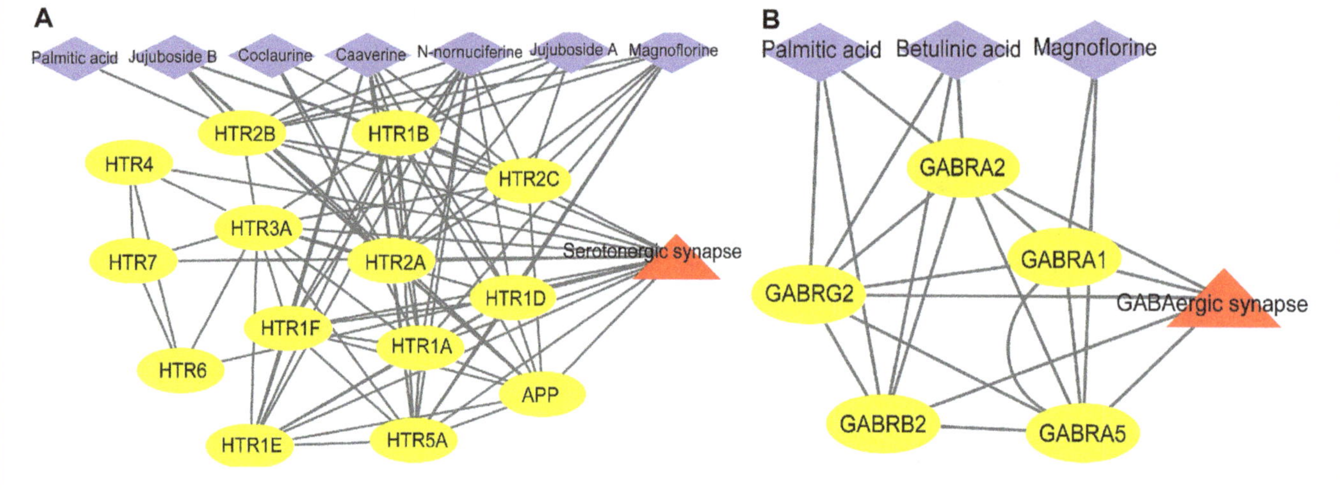

FIGURE 6 | Ingredient-target-pathway (I-T-P) sub-networks of the serotonergic synapse pathway **(A)** and the GABAergic synapse pathway **(B)**.

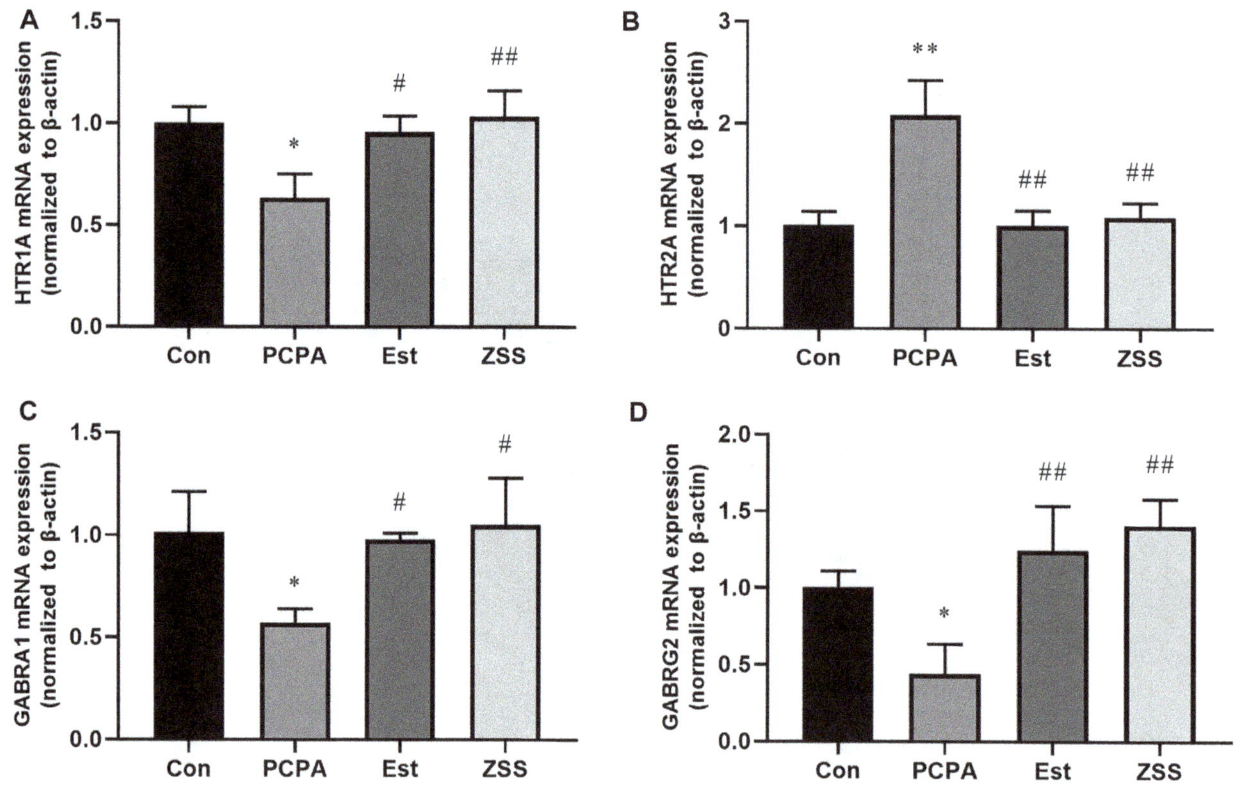

FIGURE 7 | The effects of ZSS on the mRNA expression levels of *HTR1A* **(A)**, *HTR2A* **(B)**, *GABRA1* **(C)** and *GABRG2* **(D)** in the hypothalamus. $^{*}p < 0.05$, $^{**}p < 0.01$ compared with the control group, $^{\#}p < 0.01$, $^{\#\#}p < 0.01$ compared with the model group. Data are shown as mean ± SD values and n = 3.

acid (betulinic acid), and one fatty acid (palmitic acid), participated in regulating the serotonergic synapse and GABAergic synapse pathways. These components can therefore be regarded as the important material basis of ZSS for the treatment of insomnia, thus expanding our understanding of natural drugs for the treatment of insomnia. In addition to jujuboside A and spinosin as quality control indicators for Chinese Pharmacopoeia (Edition 2020), it is also important that we focus on alkaloids (coclaurine, N-nornuciferine, caaverine, and magnoflorine), and other core components (betulinic acid and palmitic acid), as candidate Q-markers.

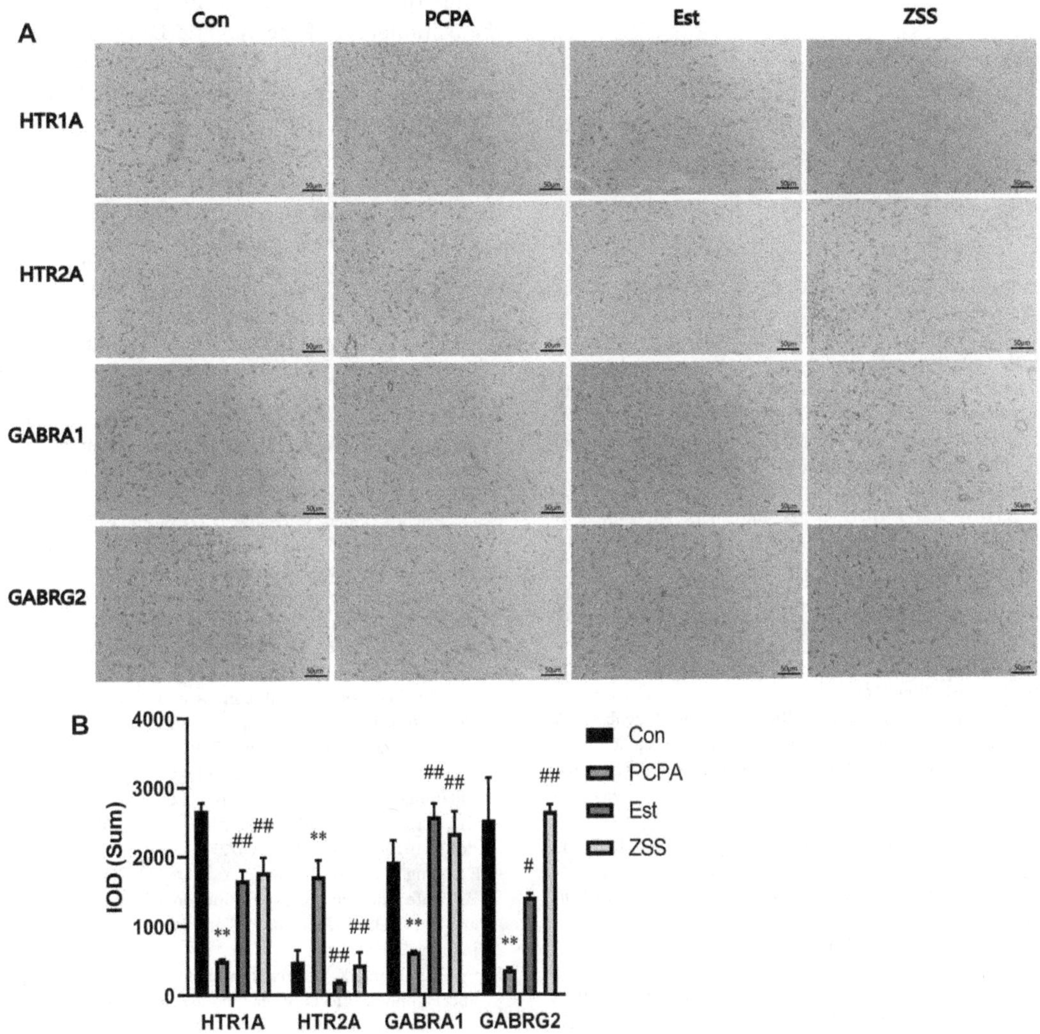

FIGURE 8 | The effects of ZSS on the expression of HTR1A, HTR2A, GABRA1 and GABRG2 in the hypothalamus **(A)** and immunohistochemistry results (the sum of the IOD) **(B)**. $^{**}p < 0.01$ compared with the control group, $^{\#\#}p < 0.01$ compared with the model group. Data are shown as mean ± SD values and n = 3.

CONCLUSION

Our research indicated that the mechanism underlying the action of ZSS in the treatment of insomnia is mainly related to the modulation of 5-HT and GABAergic synapse pathways. We also demonstrated that the regulation of HTR1A, HTR2A, GABRA1, and GABRG2, plays significant roles in these pathways. Jujuboside A, jujuboside B, coclaurine, N-nornuciferine, caaverine, magnoflorine, betulinic acid, and palmitic acid, were all identified in ZSS and shown to contribute to the modulation of 5-HT and GABAergic synapse pathways. This research systematically investigated the role of multiple components in the effects of ZSS on insomnia and provided a new basis for the improvement of quality control standards. However, further in-depth preclinical studies are needed to validate the results obtained from the current analysis. These selected phytochemicals may be used as potential candidate drugs for the treatment of insomnia and deserve further research attention.

AUTHOR CONTRIBUTIONS

XY, MH, CM, and TL designed the research. ZB, WZ, JT, QF, LS, CF, DJ, HT, and XC performed the experiments and analyzed the data. ZB drafted the manuscript.

FUNDING

This research was supported by Wuxi Science and Technology Development Fund Projects (Reference: N20192038), Top Talent Support Program for Young and Middle-aged People of Wuxi Health Committee (Reference: HB2020059), the National Key Research and Development Plan (Reference: 2018YFC1707000) and Postgraduate Research and Practice Innovation Program of Jiangsu Province (Reference: KYCX20_1513).

REFERENCES

Albert, P. R., Vahid-Ansari, F., and Luckhart, C. (2014). Serotonin-Prefrontal Cortical Circuitry in Anxiety and Depression Phenotypes: Pivotal Role of Pre- and Post-Synaptic 5-HT1A Receptor Expression. *Front. Behav. Neurosci.* 8, 199. doi:10.3389/fnbeh.2014.00199

An, H. M., Huang, D. R., Yang, H., Liu, X. G., Du, J., Li, Y., et al. (2020). Comprehensive Chemical Profiling of Jia-Wei-Qi-Fu-Yin and its Network Pharmacology-Based Analysis on Alzheimer's Disease. *J. Pharm. Biomed. Anal.* 189, 113467. doi:10.1016/j.jpba.2020.113467

Antypa, N., Calati, R., Souery, D., Pellegrini, S., Sentissi, O., Amital, D., et al. (2013). Variation in the HTR1A and HTR2A Genes and Social Adjustment in Depressed Patients. *J. Affect. Disord.* 150 (2), 649–652. doi:10.1016/j.jad.2013.02.036

Babson, K. A., Sottile, J., and Morabito, D. (2017). Cannabis, Cannabinoids, and Sleep: a Review of the Literature. *Curr. Psychiatry Rep.* 19 (4), 23. doi:10.1007/s11920-017-0775-9

Bormann, J. (2000). The 'ABC' of GABA Receptors. *Trends Pharmacol. Sci.* 21 (1), 16–19. doi:10.1016/s0165-6147(99)01413-3

Cohrs, S., Meier, A., Neumann, A. C., Jordan, W., Rüther, E., and Rodenbeck, A. (2005). Improved Sleep Continuity and Increased Slow Wave Sleep and REM Latency during Ziprasidone Treatment: A Randomized, Controlled, Crossover Trial of 12 Healthy Male Subjects. *J. Clin. Psychiatry* 66 (8), 989–996. doi:10.4088/jcp.v66n0805

Cui, S. Y., Cui, X. Y., Zhang, J., Wang, Z. J., Yu, B., Sheng, Z. F., et al. (2011). Diltiazem Potentiates Pentobarbital-Induced Hypnosis via 5-HT1A and 5-HT2A/2C Receptors: Role for Dorsal Raphe Nucleus. *Pharmacol. Biochem. Behav.* 99 (4), 566–572. doi:10.1016/j.pbb.2011.06.001

dela Peña, I. J. I., Hong, E., Kim, H. J., de la Peña, J. B., Woo, T. S., Lee, Y. S., et al. (2015). Artemisia Capillaris Thunberg Produces Sedative-Hypnotic Effects in Mice, Which Are Probably Mediated through Potentiation of the GABAA Receptor. *Am. J. Chin. Med.* 43 (4), 667–679. doi:10.1142/s0192415x1550041x

Dixon, C. L., Harrison, N. L., Lynch, J. W., and Keramidas, A. (2015). Zolpidem and Eszopiclone Prime α1β2γ2 GABAA Receptors for Longer Duration of Activity. *Br. J. Pharmacol.* 172 (14), 3522–3536. doi:10.1111/bph.13142

Domínguez-Soto, Á., Usategui, A., Casas-Engel, M. D. L., Simón-Fuentes, M., Nieto, C., Cuevas, V. D., et al. (2017). Serotonin Drives the Acquisition of a Profibrotic and Anti-Inflammatory Gene Profile through the 5-Ht7r-PKA Signaling axis. *Sci. Rep.* 7 (1), 14761. doi:10.1038/s41598-017-15348-y

Dong, Z. Q., Li, X. R., He, L., He, G., Yu, T., and Sun, X. L. (2016). 5-HTR1A and 5-HTR2A Genetic Polymorphisms and SSRI Antidepressant Response in Depressive Chinese Patients. *Neuropsychiatr. Dis. Treat.* 12, 1623–1629. doi:10.2147/ndt.s93562

Du, C., Pei, X., Zhang, M., Yan, Y., and Qin, X. (2019). $_1$H-NMR Based Metabolomic Study of Sedative and Hypnotic Effect of Ziziphi Spinosae Semen in Rats. *Chin. Traditional Herbal Drugs* 50 (10), 2405–2412. doi:10.7501/j.issn.0253-2670.2019.10.022

Du, C., Yan, Y., Shen, C., Cui, X., Pei, X., and Qin, X. (2020). Comparative Pharmacokinetics of Six Major Compounds in normal and Insomnia Rats after Oral Administration of Ziziphi Spinosae Semen Aqueous Extract. *J. Pharm. Anal.* 10 (4), 385–395. doi:10.1016/j.jpha.2020.03.003

Fish, L. R., Gilligan, M. T., Humphries, A. C., Ivarsson, M., Ladduwahetty, T., Merchant, K. J., et al. (2005). 4-Fluorosulfonylpiperidines: Selective 5-HT2A Ligands for the Treatment of Insomnia. *Bioorg. Med. Chem. Lett.* 15 (16), 3665–3669. doi:10.1016/j.bmcl.2005.05.104

Food and Drug Administration (2005). Guidance for Industry: Estimating the Maximum Safe Starting Dose in Initial Clinical Trials for Therapeutics in Adult Healthy Volunteers. Available at: https://www.fda.gov/media/72309 (Accessed May 05, 2015).

Gfeller, D., Grosdidier, A., Wirth, M., Daina, A., Michielin, O., and Zoete, V. (2014). SwissTargetPrediction: A Web Server for Target Prediction of Bioactive Small Molecules. *Nucleic Acids Res.* 42, W32–W38. doi:10.1093/nar/gku293

He, S. R., Zhao, C. B., Zhang, J. X., Wang, J., Wu, B., and Wu, C. J. (2020). Botanical and Traditional Uses and Phytochemical, Pharmacological, Pharmacokinetic, and Toxicological Characteristics of Ziziphi Spinosae Semen: A Review. *Evid. Based Complement. Alternat. Med.* 2020, 5861821. doi:10.1155/2020/5861821

Horsch, C. H., Lancee, J., Griffioen-Both, F., Spruit, S., Fitrianie, S., Neerincx, M. A., et al. (2017). Mobile Phone-Delivered Cognitive Behavioral Therapy for Insomnia: A Randomized Waitlist Controlled Trial. *J. Med. Internet Res.* 19 (4), e70. doi:10.2196/jmir.6524

Hu, L., Chen, Y., Chen, T., Huang, D., Li, S., and Cui, S. (2020). A Systematic Study of Mechanism of Sargentodoxa Cuneata and Patrinia Scabiosifolia against Pelvic Inflammatory Disease with Dampness-Heat Stasis Syndrome via Network Pharmacology Approach. *Front. Pharmacol.* 11, 582520. doi:10.3389/fphar.2020.582520

Hua, Y., Guo, S., Xie, H., Zhu, Y., Yan, H., Tao, W. W., et al. (2021). Ziziphus Jujuba Mill. Var. Spinosa (Bunge) Hu Ex H. F. Chou Seed Ameliorates Insomnia in Rats by Regulating Metabolomics and Intestinal Flora Composition. *Front. Pharmacol.* 12, 653767. doi:10.3389/fphar.2021.653767

Huang, X. F., Zhang, J. L., Huang, D. P., Huang, A. S., Huang, H. T., Liu, Q., et al. (2020). A Network Pharmacology Strategy to Investigate the Anti-inflammatory Mechanism of Luteolin Combined with *In Vitro* Transcriptomics and Proteomics. *Int. Immunopharmacol.* 86, 106727. doi:10.1016/j.intimp.2020.106727

Ji, E., Wang, T., Guo, F., Zhang, Y., Tang, C., Tang, D., et al. (2019). Xiaoerfupi Alleviates the Symptoms of Functional Dyspepsia by Regulating the HTR3A and C-FOS. *Biomed. Pharmacother.* 120, 109442. doi:10.1016/j.biopha.2019.109442

Jiang, J. G., Huang, X. J., Chen, J., and Lin, Q. S. (2007). Comparison of the Sedative and Hypnotic Effects of Flavonoids, Saponins, and Polysaccharides Extracted from Semen Ziziphus Jujube. *Nat. Prod. Res.* 21 (4), 310–320. doi:10.1080/14786410701192827

Jiang, Y., Cui, C., Ge, H., Guan, S., Lian, Y., and Liu, J. (2016). Effect of 5-HT2A Receptor Polymorphisms and Occupational Stress on Self-Reported Sleep Quality: A Cross-Sectional Study in Xinjiang, China. *Sleep Med.* 20, 30–36. doi:10.1016/j.sleep.2015.12.007

Jin, S., Kim, K. K., Park, B. S., Kim, D. H., Jeong, B., Kang, D., et al. (2020). Function of Astrocyte MyD88 in High-Fat-Diet-Induced Hypothalamic Inflammation. *J. Neuroinflammation* 17 (1), 195. doi:10.1186/s12974-020-01846-w

Kang, T., Dou, D., and Xu, L. (2019). Establishment of a Quality Marker (Q-Marker) System for Chinese Herbal Medicines Using Burdock as an Example. *Phytomedicine* 54, 339–346. doi:10.1016/j.phymed.2018.04.005

Liang, J., Huang, Y., Mai, Z., Zhan, Q., Lin, H., Xie, Y., et al. (2021). Integrating Network Pharmacology and Experimental Validation to Decipher the Mechanism of Action of Huanglian Jiedu Decoction in Treating Atherosclerosis. *Drug Des. Devel. Ther.* 15, 1779–1795. doi:10.2147/dddt.s304911

Lv, Y. B., Zhou, Q., Yan, J. X., Luo, L. S., and Zhang, J. L. (2021). Enzymolysis Peptides from Mauremys Mutica Plastron Improve the Disorder of Neurotransmitter System and Facilitate Sleep-Promoting in the PCPA-Induced Insomnia Mice. *J. Ethnopharmacol.* 274, 114047. doi:10.1016/j.jep.2021.114047

Monti, J. M. (2010). Serotonin 5-HT(2A) Receptor Antagonists in the Treatment of Insomnia: Present Status and Future Prospects. *Drugs Today (Barc)* 46 (3), 183–193. doi:10.1358/dot.2010.46.3.1437247

Morin, C. M., Leblanc, M., Ivers, H., Bélanger, L., Mérette, C., Savard, J., et al. (2014). Monthly Fluctuations of Insomnia Symptoms in a Population-Based Sample. *Sleep* 37 (2), 319–326. doi:10.5665/sleep.3406

Novati, A., Roman, V., Cetin, T., Hagewoud, R., Den Boer, J. A., Luiten, P. G., et al. (2008). Chronically Restricted Sleep Leads to Depression-Like Changes in Neurotransmitter Receptor Sensitivity and Neuroendocrine Stress Reactivity in Rats. *Sleep* 31 (11), 1579–1585. doi:10.1093/sleep/31.11.1579

Oh, K. K., Adnan, M., and Cho, D. H. (2021). Active Ingredients and Mechanisms of Phellinus Linteus (Grown on Rosa Multiflora) for Alleviation of Type 2 Diabetes Mellitus through Network Pharmacology. *Gene* 768, 145320. doi:10.1016/j.gene.2020.145320

Ohno, R., Miyagishi, H., Tsuji, M., Saito, A., Miyagawa, K., Kurokawa, K., et al. (2018). Yokukansan, a Traditional Japanese Herbal Medicine, Enhances the Anxiolytic Effect of Fluvoxamine and Reduces Cortical 5-HT2A Receptor Expression in Mice. *J. Ethnopharmacol.* 216, 89–96. doi:10.1016/j.jep.2018.01.032

Olsen, R. W., and Sieghart, W. (2008). International Union of Pharmacology. LXX. Subtypes of Gamma-Aminobutyric Acid(A) Receptors: Classification on the Basis of Subunit Composition, Pharmacology, and Function. Update. *Pharmacol. Rev.* 60 (3), 243–260. doi:10.1124/pr.108.00505

Poh, A. R., Love, C. G., Masson, F., Preaudet, A., Tsui, C., Whitehead, L., et al. (2017). Inhibition of Hematopoietic Cell Kinase Activity Suppresses Myeloid Cell-Mediated Colon Cancer Progression. *Cancer Cell* 31 (4), 563–575. doi:10.1016/j.ccell.2017.03.006

Polter, A. M., and Li, X. (2010). 5-HT1A Receptor-Regulated Signal Transduction Pathways in Brain. *Cell Signal* 22 (10), 1406–1412. doi:10.1016/j.cellsig.2010.03.019

Ren, Y., Ai, J., Liu, X., Liang, S., Zheng, Y., Deng, X., et al. (2020). Anticoagulant Active Ingredients Identification of Total Saponin Extraction of Different Panax Medicinal Plants Based on Grey Relational Analysis Combined with UPLC-MS and Molecular Docking. *J. Ethnopharmacol.* 260, 112955. doi:10.1016/j.jep.2020.112955

Rodríguez Villanueva, J., and Rodríguez Villanueva, L. (2017). Experimental and Clinical Pharmacology ofZiziphus jujubaMills. *Phytother. Res.* 31 (3), 347–365. doi:10.1002/ptr.5759

Shang, J., Chen, X. L., Li, L., Zhang, H., Yang, L., Yang, B., et al. (2020). Identification of the Absorptive Constituents and Their Metabolites *In Vivo* of Ziziphi Spinosae Semen by UPLC-ESI-Q-TOF-MS/MS. *Biomed. Chromatogr.* 34 (12), e4965. doi:10.1002/bmc.4965

Shao, J., Zheng, X., Qu, L., Zhang, H., Yuan, H., Hui, J., et al. (2020). Ginsenoside Rg5/Rk1 Ameliorated Sleep via Regulating the GABAergic/serotoninergic Signaling Pathway in a Rodent Model. *Food Funct.* 11 (2), 1245–1257. doi:10.1039/c9fo02248a

Shen, C. Y., Wan, L., Zhu, J. J., and Jiang, J. G. (2020). Targets and Underlying Mechanisms Related to the Sedative and Hypnotic Activities of Saponin Extracts from Semen Ziziphus Jujube. *Food Funct.* 11 (5), 3895–3903. doi:10.1039/d0fo00098a

Shergis, J. L., Ni, X., Sarris, J., Zhang, A. L., Guo, X., Xue, C. C., et al. (2017). Ziziphus Spinosa Seeds for Insomnia: A Review of Chemistry and Psychopharmacology. *Phytomedicine* 34, 38–43. doi:10.1016/j.phymed.2017.07.004

Shi, R., Han, Y., Yan, Y., Qiao, H. Y., He, J., Lian, W. W., et al. (2019). Loganin Exerts Sedative and Hypnotic Effects via Modulation of the Serotonergic System and GABAergic Neurons. *Front. Pharmacol.* 10, 409. doi:10.3389/fphar.2019.00409

Shi, Y., Dong, J. W., Zhao, J. H., Tang, L. N., and Zhang, J. J. (2014). Herbal Insomnia Medications that Target GABAergic Systems: A Review of the Psychopharmacological Evidence. *Curr. Neuropharmacol.* 12 (3), 289–302. doi:10.2174/1570159x11666131227001243

Si, Y., Wang, L., Lan, J., Li, H., Guo, T., Chen, X., et al. (2020). Lilium Davidii Extract Alleviates P-Chlorophenylalanine-Induced Insomnia in Rats through Modification of the Hypothalamic-Related Neurotransmitters, Melatonin and Homeostasis of the Hypothalamic-Pituitary-Adrenal axis. *Pharm. Biol.* 58 (1), 915–924. doi:10.1080/13880209.2020.1812674

Song, P., Zhang, Y., Ma, G., Zhang, Y., Zhou, A., and Xie, J. (2017). Gastrointestinal Absorption and Metabolic Dynamics of Jujuboside A, A Saponin Derived from the Seed of Ziziphus Jujuba. *J. Agric. Food Chem.* 65 (38), 8331–8339. doi:10.1021/acs.jafc.7b02748

Succol, F., Fiumelli, H., Benfenati, F., Cancedda, L., and Barberis, A. (2012). Intracellular Chloride Concentration Influences the GABAA Receptor Subunit Composition. *Nat. Commun.* 3, 738. doi:10.1038/ncomms1744

Tian, D., Yang, Y., Yu, M., Han, Z. Z., Wei, M., Zhang, H. W., et al. (2020). Anti-Inflammatory Chemical Constituents of Flos Chrysanthemi Indici Determined by UPLC-MS/MS Integrated with Network Pharmacology. *Food Funct.* 11 (7), 6340–6351. doi:10.1039/d0fo01000f

Tochitani, S., and Kondo, S. (2013). Immunoreactivity for GABA, GAD65, GAD67 and Bestrophin-1 in the Meninges and the Choroid Plexus: Implications for Non-neuronal Sources for GABA in the Developing Mouse Brain. *PLoS One* 8 (2), e56901. doi:10.1371/journal.pone.0056901

Van Dalfsen, J. H., and Markus, C. R. (2019). The Serotonin Transporter Gene-Linked Polymorphic Region (5-HTTLPR) and the Sleep-Promoting Effects of Tryptophan: A Randomized Placebo-Controlled Crossover Study. *J. Psychopharmacol.* 33 (8), 948–954. doi:10.1177/0269881119855978

Vgontzas, A. N., and Fernandez-Mendoza, J. (2013). Insomnia with Short Sleep Duration: Nosological, Diagnostic, and Treatment Implications. *Sleep Med. Clin.* 8 (3), 309–322. doi:10.1016/j.jsmc.2013.04.009

Wang, L. E., Bai, Y. J., Shi, X. R., Cui, X. Y., Cui, S. Y., Zhang, F., et al. (2008). Spinosin, a C-Glycoside Flavonoid from Semen Zizhiphi Spinozae, Potentiated Pentobarbital-Induced Sleep via the Serotonergic System. *Pharmacol. Biochem. Behav.* 90 (3), 399–403. doi:10.1016/j.pbb.2008.03.022

Wang, W., Zhang, Y., Luo, J., Wang, R., Tang, C., and Zhang, Y. (2020). Virtual Screening Technique Used to Estimate the Mechanism of Adhatoda Vasica Nees for the Treatment of Rheumatoid Arthritis Based on Network Pharmacology and Molecular Docking. *Evid. Based Complement. Alternat. Med.* 2020, 5872980. doi:10.1155/2020/5872980

Wilson, S. J., Bailey, J. E., Rich, A. S., Nash, J., Adrover, M., Tournoux, A., et al. (2005). The Use of Sleep Measures to Compare a New 5HT1A Agonist with Buspirone in Humans. *J. Psychopharmacol.* 19 (6), 609–613. doi:10.1177/0269881105058775

Wu, L., Chen, Y., Yi, J., Zhuang, Y., Cui, L., and Ye, C. (2020). Mechanism of Action of Bu-Fei-Yi-Shen Formula in Treating Chronic Obstructive Pulmonary Disease Based on Network Pharmacology Analysis and Molecular Docking Validation. *Biomed. Res. Int.* 2020, 1–12. doi:10.1155/2020/9105972

Xiao, H. B., Wang, Y. S., Luo, Z. F., and Lu, X. Y. (2018). SZSJ Protects Against Insomnia by a Decrease in ADMA Level and an Improvement in DDAH Production in Sleep-Deprived Rats. *Life Sci.* 209, 97–102. doi:10.1016/j.lfs.2018.07.044

Yeung, W. F., Chung, K. F., Poon, M. M., Ho, F. Y., Zhang, S. P., Zhang, Z. J., et al. (2012). Chinese Herbal Medicine for Insomnia: A Systematic Review of Randomized Controlled Trials. *Sleep Med. Rev.* 16 (6), 497–507. doi:10.1016/j.smrv.2011.12.005

Yi, P. L., Lin, C. P., Tsai, C. H., Lin, J. G., and Chang, F. C. (2007). The Involvement of Serotonin Receptors in Suanzaorentang-Induced Sleep Alteration. *J. Biomed. Sci.* 14 (6), 829–840. doi:10.1007/s11373-007-9197-8

You, Z. L., Xia, Q., Liang, F. R., Tang, Y. J., Xu, C. L., Huang, J., et al. (2010). Effects on the Expression of GABAA Receptor Subunits by Jujuboside A Treatment in Rat Hippocampal Neurons. *J. Ethnopharmacol.* 128 (2), 419–423. doi:10.1016/j.jep.2010.01.034

Zhang, M., Ning, G., Shou, C., Lu, Y., Hong, D., and Zheng, X. (2003). Inhibitory Effect of Jujuboside A on Glutamate-Mediated Excitatory Signal Pathway in hippocampus. *Planta Med.* 69 (8), 692–695. doi:10.1055/s-2003-42786

Zhang, R., Guo, H., Yang, X., Li, Z., Zhang, D., Li, B., et al. (2019). Potential Candidate Biomarkers Associated with Osteoarthritis: Evidence from a Comprehensive Network and Pathway Analysis. *J. Cel. Physiol.* 234 (10), 17433–17443. doi:10.1002/jcp.28365

Zhong, Y., Zheng, Q., Hu, P., Huang, X., Yang, M., Ren, G., et al. (2020). Sedative and Hypnotic Effects of Perilla Frutescens Essential Oil through GABAergic System Pathway. *J. Ethnopharmacol.* 279, 113627. doi:10.1016/j.jep.2020.113627

Zhou, Q. H., Zhou, X. L., Xu, M. B., Jin, T. Y., Rong, P. Q., Zheng, G. Q., et al. (2018). Suanzaoren Formulae for Insomnia: Updated Clinical Evidence and Possible Mechanisms. *Front. Pharmacol.* 9, 76. doi:10.3389/fphar.2018.00076

15

Anti-Inflammatory Effect of a TCM Formula Li-Ru-Kang in Rats with Hyperplasia of Mammary Gland and the Underlying Biological Mechanisms

Yingying Wang[1,2], Shizhang Wei[2], Tian Gao[3], Yuxue Yang[1,2], Xiaohua Lu[1,2], Xuelin Zhou[2], Haotian Li[2], Tao Wang[1,2], Liqi Qian[4], Yanling Zhao[2] and Wenjun Zou[1]**

[1] College of Pharmacy, Chengdu University of Traditional Chinese Medicine, Chengdu, China, [2] Department of Pharmacy, 302 Military Hospital of China, Beijing, China, [3] Affiliated Hospital of Chengdu University of Traditional Chinese Medicine, Chengdu, China, [4] Department of Traditional Chinese Medicine, First Affiliated Hospital of Chinese People's Liberation Army General Hospital, Beijing, China

***Correspondence:**
Yanling Zhao
zhaoyl2855@126.com
Wenjun Zou
zouwenjun@163.com

Li-Ru-Kang (LRK), a formula of eight traditional Chinese medicines (TCM), has been used to treat hyperplasia of mammary gland (HMG) in TCM clinics. However, how LRK works in HMG patients is unclear. To explore the possible mechanisms of LRK against HMG, the network pharmacology was used to screen the potential targets and possible pathways that involved in LRK treated HMG. Rat HMG model induced by estrogen and progesterone was used to further verify the effects of the key molecules of LRK selected from the enriched pathways on HMG. Nipple heights and diameters were measured and uterus index was calculated. The histopathological changes of mammary gland tissue were detected by hematoxylin-eosin (H&E) staining. Western blot was used to detect the phosphorylation of ERK, JNK, and P38. And immunohistochemistry staining was performed to evaluate the levels of estrogen receptor α (ERα), progesterone receptor (PR), nuclear factor-(NF-)κB (p65), interleukin-1β (IL-1β), tumor necrosis factor α (TNF-α), cyclooxygenases 2 (COX-2), inducible nitric oxide synthase (iNOS), 8-hydroxy-2′deoxyguanosine (8-OHdG), and nitrotyrosine (NT). Our results indicate that LRK treatment rescues significantly nipples height and diameter, decreases uterus index and ameliorates HMG. LRK treatment also markedly attenuates the over-expression of IL-1β, TNF-α, COX-2, and iNOS, and suppressed the formation of 8-OHdG and NT. Furthermore, LRK treatment significantly inhibits the phosphorylation of JNK, ERK, and p38 and expression of NF-κB (p65), interestingly, LRK treatment has no effect on the expression of ERα and PR. Our data suggest that the LRK treatment protects the mammary glands from the damage of oxidative stress and inflammation induced by estrogen and progesterone, via suppresses of MAPK/NF-κB signaling pathways without affecting on the expression of ERα and PR.

Keywords: Li-Ru-Kang (LRK), hyperplasia of mammary gland (HMG), inflammatory responses, oxidative stress, MAPK

INTRODUCTION

Hyperplasia of mammary gland (HMG), a common disease, occurs among middle-aged women with high frequency (Jia et al., 2017). It is a kind of pathological hyperplasia of lobules of mammary gland induced by the disorder of estrogen and progesterone (Bennett et al., 1990; Zhang et al., 2016). The morbidity of HMG is increasing nowadays with a risk of breast cancer (Chen et al., 2015). Tamoxifen is an estrogen antagonist with antiproliferative effects. It has been widely used for breast cancer as well as HMG (Cline et al., 1998; Li et al., 2018). However, some women do not tolerate tamoxifen and have a risk of side effects (Kleinberg et al., 2011; Martinez de Dueñas et al., 2014). Therefore, it is important to discovery safer and more effective drugs with minimum side effects for HMG.

Traditional Chinese medicine (TCM) has been frequently used as alternative treatments for various types of diseases. For complicated or multi-factorial diseases, emerging evidence indicates that multiple drugs that have common or different pharmacological targets often display better therapeutic efficacy than a single medication (Roth et al., 2002). The formulae with multiple herbs exert therapeutic efficacies through the synergistic effects of their multiple ingredients via multiple targets (Che et al., 2013; Shao and Zhang, 2013).

Li-Ru-Kang (LRK) consisted of Ostreae Concha (Ostrea gigas Thunberg.), Cervi Cornu [Alpinia aquatica (Retz.) Roscoe.], Polygoni Multiflori Radix [Polygoni Multiflori (Thunb.) Moldenke.], Curcumae Radix (Curcuma aromatica Salisb.), Cremastrae Pseudobulbus Pleiones Pseudobulbus [Cremastra appendiculate (D. Don) Makino.], Bupleuri Radix (Bupleurum chinense DC.), Prunellae Spica (Prunellae vulgaris L.) and Glycyrrhizae Radix et rhizoma (Glycyrrhizae uralensis Fish. ex DC). LRK is a Chinese preparation formulated through TCM principles of tonifying the kidney, smoothing the liver, dissipating nodule and activating blood circulation. LRK has an overall regulatory effect on HMG. The randomized trials of LRK showed that LRK had favorable effect in the treatment of HMG (Qian et al., 2007; Li et al., 2013). Studies showed that LRK could improve the histological lesions in mammary gland, uterus and ovaries (Qian et al., 2005). LRK also affects abnormal secretion of sex hormones in model of HMG induced by estradiol benzoate. The serum levels of estradiol (E2) and prolactin (PRL) were decreased and progesterone (P) was increased remarkably by LRK (Qian et al., 2004). Our previous study explained the modulatory properties of LRK treatment on HMG using metabolomics and network pharmacology analyses, showed the therapeutic effects of LRK on HMG (Wei et al., 2018). However, the biological mechanisms of LRK for HMG are still blur.

Network pharmacology, a technology for system biology study, could clarify the potential mechanisms of complicated ingredients through large data set analysis. In that TCM formula has been thought to be multi-ingredients and multi-targets, network pharmacology is a suitable approach to meeting this challenge and determining the mechanism on LRK for treating HMG (Che et al., 2013; Tao et al., 2013; Mao et al., 2017).

Therefore, in the present study, network pharmacology approach combined with molecular biology was performed to further investigate the active ingredients and the underlying mechanism of LRK for the treatment of HMG.

MATERIALS AND METHODS

Database Construction

The chemical structures of the compounds in LRK were obtained from TCM Database@Taiwan (TDT)[1] (Chen, 2011) and Traditional Chinese Medicine Systems Pharmacology (TCMSP) database[2]. All compounds were selected according to selection criteria [oral bioavailability (OB) $\geq$ 30 and drug-likeness (DL) $\geq$ 0.18], as suggested by TCMSP (Liu et al., 2013). Known compound targets were collected from Herbal Ingredients' Targets Database (HIT)[3] (Ye et al., 2011), and the putative targets from these were screened out from Therapeutic Targets Database (TTD)[4] through structural similarity comparison (Chen et al., 2002). Gene and protein targets associated with HMG therapy were collected from the Online Mendelian Inheritance in Man (OMIM)[5] database. Other interaction proteins of the aforementioned targets were obtained from Database of Interacting Proteins (DIP)[6], and different ID types of the proteins were converted to UniProt IDs.

Network Construction and Analysis

To provide the scientific and reasonable interpretation of the complex relationships between the compounds and targets associated with HMG, network analysis was carried out. The compound-target-disease network was constructed using candidate compounds, potential targets and HMG significant targets. The network was performed using Cytoscape 3.5.1 software (National Institute of General Medical Sciences, United States). The topological features of each node in the network were calculated by "Degree", "Betweenness centrality", and "Closeness centrality" ("Degree" values twofold greater than the median value of all the network nodes, "Betweenness centrality" and "Closeness centrality" value greater than the median value of all the network nodes) (Wang J.B. et al., 2018). Targets with higher value were screened as the candidates for HMG.

Plant Material

LRK consisted of *Ostreae Concha* (*Ostrea gigas* Thunberg.), *Cervi Cornu* [*Alpinia aquatica* (Retz.) Roscoe.], *Polygoni Multiflori Radix* [*Polygoni Multiflori* (Thunb.) Moldenke.], *Curcumae Radix (Curcuma aromatica* Salisb.), *Cremastrae*

[1] http://tcm.cmu.edu.tw/
[2] http://lsp.nwu.edu.cn/
[3] http://lifecenter.sgst.cn/hit/
[4] http://bidd.nus.edu.sg/group/cjttd/
[5] https://www.omim.org/
[6] http://dip.doe-mbi.ucla.edu/dip/Main.cgi

Pseudobulbus Pleiones Pseudobulbus [*Cremastra appendiculate* (D. Don) Makino.], *Bupleuri Radix (Bupleurum chinense* DC.), *Prunellae Spica (Prunellae vulgaris* L.) and *Glycyrrhizae Radix et rhizoma (Glycyrrhizae uralensis* Fish. ex DC) which were purchased from Heyanling, Co., Ltd. (Beijing, China). The origin and quality of the 8 herbs were identified according to the Chinese Pharmacopeia (2015 Edition). The eight TCMs of LRK were composited with the weight ratio of 30: 12: 12: 10: 10: 9: 9: 6. At first, *Cervi Cornu* slice were smashed into powder. Then it was decocted with appropriate amount of water and kept slightly boiling for 1 h. Next, the filtrate of *Cervi Cornu* was obtained and combined with the rest of TCM proportionally, followed by another 1 h heat extraction with boiled water (1/10, weight/volume) three times. The final yield of powder to raw materials was about 9.2%.

Reagents

The antibodies of phosphorylation-MAPK Family Antibody Sampler Kit used for western blot were purchased from Cell Signaling (United States) (#9910). And nuclear factor-(NF-)κB (p65) (XCJ36131), cyclooxygenases 2 (COX2) (06416080202), inducible nitric oxide synthase (iNOS) (16716110102), interleukin-1β (IL-1β) (01016051201), tumor necrosis factor α (TNF-α) (60291-1-Ig), estrogen receptor α (ERα) (AF6058), and progesterone receptor (PR) (37917011102) for immunohistochemistry were purchased from Wu han goodbio technology Co., Ltd (China). Antibodies of 8-hydroxy-2′deoxyguanosine (8-OHdG) (GR3173165-3), nitrotyrosine (NT) (GR174728-22), GAPDH (AC001) were purchased from Abcam (the United States).

Animals and Administration

Female SD rats weighting 180–220 g [license number: SCXK-(A) 2012–0004] were obtained from the laboratory animal center of the Military Medical Science Academy of the People's Liberation Army (PLA). They were maintained separately at animal experimental center of 302 Hospital of People's Liberation Army (Beijing) with a specific pathogen free (SPF) environment (24°C, 65% humidity, 12 h day/night). The rats were randomly divided into six groups. All rats except for control group were intramuscularly injected with estrogen at a dose of 0.5 mg/kg/d for consecutive 25 days. All rats but control group were intramuscularly injected with progesterone at a dose of 5 mg/kg/d in the following 5 days (Wang et al., 2011). LRK (0.056, 0.112, 0.224 g/kg/d for the low, medium and high dose, respectively) and tamoxifen (Yangtze River Pharmaceutical Co., Ltd. 5 mg/kg/d) were dissolved in normal saline and intragastrically administered to rats, respectively, except for control and model group for 30 days. The rats were sacrificed 12 h after the last administration. All animal studies have been approved by the Ethical Committee of 302 Military hospital of China. The blood, mammary gland and uterus were collected. The blood was centrifuged at 3500 rpm for 15 min to separate the serum without hemolysis. Serum and the rest of mammary gland tissue for hematoxylin-eosin staining were stored at -80°C.

Measurement of Body Weight, Nipple Height and Diameter, and Uterus Indexes

Body weight, nipple height and diameter of all rats were recorded after administration. Uterus index (Wang et al., 2011) was calculated by the following formulae:

$$\text{Uterus index} = W_{\text{uterus}}\,(\text{mg})/W_{\text{body}}\,(\text{g})$$

W_{uterus} and W_{body} stand for the average weight of uterus and body weight of rats.

Histopathological Evaluations and Immunohistochemical Observation

The mammary gland tissues obtained from the experimental rats were fixed in the 10% neutral buffered formalin and then embedded in paraffin. Subsequently, the embedded mammary gland tissues were cut into thin slices and disposed using hematoxylin-eosin (H&E) staining.

Immunohistochemical analysis was performed using deparaffinized mammary sections. The sections were immersed in freshly prepared 2% H_2O_2 at room temperature for 25 min and blocked with 5% rabbit serum for 30 min. Then the primary antibody [NF-κB (p65) (1:100), -COX-2 (1:1000), -TNF-α (1:200), -IL-1β (1:400), -iNOS (1:1000), -NT (1:100), -8-OHdG (1:100), -ERα (1:200), or -PR (1:200)] was added and incubated at 4°C overnight. After being washed with PBS, the sections were treated with the secondary antibody conjugated with horseradish peroxidase at room temperature for 50 min. Then, they were immersed in diaminobenzidine (DAB) for 3 min. The hematoxylin-stained sections were dehydrated by ethanol. Stained areas of the sections were visualized using an optical microscope at ×200. Image analysis software Image-Pro Plus 6.0 was used to select the yellow area of the immunohistochemical reactant on the image and then the mean integrated optical density (IOD) of these areas was measured.

Western Blot Analysis

The mammary expressions of p-P38 p-JNK and p-ERK were evaluated by western blot analysis. Mammary gland tissue of rats was homogenized and subsequently lysed by tissuelyser (Shanghai Jingxin Industrial Development Co., Ltd, Shanghai, China) with RIPA buffer containing a protease inhibitor mixture. The protein was distilled and then centrifugated at 12,000 rpm and 4°C for 10 min to separate debris. Protein concentration was determined using the BCA protein assay kit. Protein samples (25 μg) were separated by SDS-polyacrylamidegel electrophoresis and transferred to a PVDF membrane by electrophoretic transfer. Transferred membranes were blocked for 1 h at room temperature with 2% BSA in Tris-buffered saline containing 0.1% Tween 20 (TBST), and then incubated overnight at 4°C with different primary antibodies [anti-p-P38 (1:1000), p-JNK (1:1000) and p-ERK (1:1000)]. After washes with TBST 4 times, the membranes were incubated with horseradish peroxidase-conjugated secondary antibody (1:3000) in TBST with 2.5% nonfat milk for 1 h at room temperature.

Western blots were developed on films using the enhanced chemiluminescence technique. Quantification of bands was determined by densitometric analysis using Bio-Rad Quantity One. The data were normalized using GAPDH (1:3000) as an internal control.

Statistical Analysis

Data were presented as means ± SD. and were analyzed using the IBM SPSS Statistics 21. Data among groups were analyzed with ANOVA. $P < 0.05$ and $P < 0.01$ were considered statistically significant.

RESULTS

Prediction for the Direct Targets of LRK on HMG

A total of 72 chemical constituents of LRK, 351 drug targets, 213 HMG targets and 358 interacting proteins were obtained from TDT, HIT, TTD, OMIM, and DIP. Then, the ingredients, drug targets, disease targets and interacting proteins were connected for interaction network of "compound-target-disease" construction, which was presented with color-coded nodes (**Figure 1A**). In the network, the yellow squares represented the direct targets which were the common targets of LRK and HMG. The common targets were the key targets for LRK on treating HMG as well as the relatively important targets screened for further research.

Subsequently, the topological parameters values of each target in the network including "Degree", "Betweenness centrality", and "Closeness centrality" were analyzed for the important key protein targets and related signaling pathways screening. The results showed that 13 direct targets were selected according to their Degree twice greater than the median (>14), Betweenness Centrality and Closeness Centrality greater than the median (Betweenness Centrality value >0.004; Closeness Centrality value >0.28) (**Table 1**). Additionally, COX2 and NF-κB might be the most important targets of LRK on treating HMG due to their highest degree.

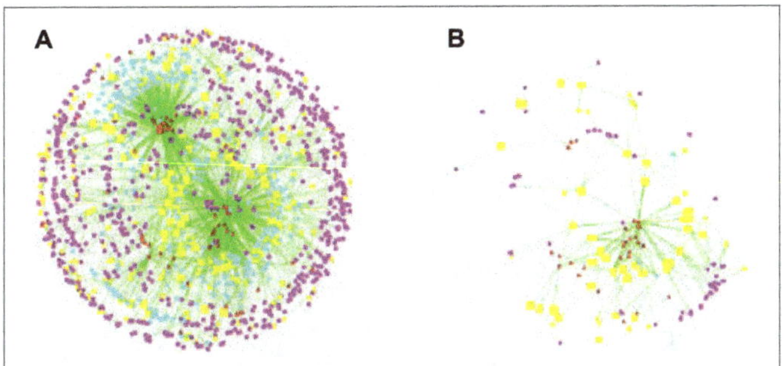

FIGURE 1 | Compound-target-disease network of LRK. **(A)** The main network of "compound-target-disease" of LRK. **(B)** The sub-network with direct targets and the corresponding ingredients. Notes: The red triangles represent active chemical constituents of LRK, the blue dots represent the indirect targets for drugs, the yellow dots represent the targets of the specific disease of HMG, the yellow squares represent the common targets of herbs and HMG, and the purple dots represent the interactional proteins with the targets of HMG and drugs.

Prediction of Active Ingredients in LRK

Furthermore, active ingredients from LRK were explored be network pharmacology prediction. As shown in **Figure 1B**, 24 potential active ingredients directly related to LRK on HMG. According to the OB ≥ 30 and DL ≥ 0.18, 19 active ingredients including saikosaponin c_qt, quercetin, kaempferol, chrysazin, luteolin, beta-sitosterol, isorhamnetin, curcolactone, stigmasterol, 2-methoxy-9,10-dihydrophenanthrene-4,5-diol, areapillin, morin, 3,5,6,7-tetramethoxy-2-(3,4,5-trimethoxyphenyl) chromone, delphinidin, troxerutin, cubebin, α-spinasterol, linoleyl acetate, and vulgaxanthin-I might be responsible for the effect of LRK on HMG, and they were listed in **Table 2**.

Pathway Analysis of LRK on HMG

The results above showed that 19 active ingredients related to 13 direct targets played the key role of LRK in treating HMG. However, the key pathways still unknown. Therefore, the pathways of the direct target proteins were enriched. The analysis of KEGG pathways indicated that there were five pathways enriched related to HMG, including MAPK signaling pathway, Toll-like receptor signaling pathway, TNF signaling pathway, NOD-like receptor signaling pathway and Chemokine signaling pathway, which were directly involved in inflammation. The proteins like NF-κB (p65), COX2 were involved in major pathways (**Table 3**). According to the count of relative targets and the percentage on all pathways, MAPK signaling pathway might play the key role in LRK treating HMG. These results indicated that the protect effect of LRK on HMG might associate to MAPK pathway, regulate NF-κB, anti-inflammatory, and anti-oxidative stress.

Therapeutic Effect of LRK on HMG

In order to assess the therapeutic effect of LRK, the height and diameter of nipples (left 2 and right 2) and uterus index of rats were measured. As shown in **Figure 2**, both of the left and right nipples were markedly decreased by LRK treatment compared to the HMG model group. Similarly, the diameter of nipples (left 2 and right 2) of rat were also significantly decreased compared to the model group ($P < 0.01$) (**Figures 2A,B**). And the result showed that the effect of LRK is comparable to the tamoxifen treatment. Uterus is the main target organ of estrogen, the high level of exogenous estrogen will induce the obviously increased of uterus index (Jia et al., 2017). Thereby, the uterus index was examined. It showed that the uterus index was decreased in a dose-dependent manner by LRK treatment (**Figure 2C**).

Subsequently, hematoxylin and eosin (H&E) staining was performed to visualized the pathological changes of mammary gland sections. As shown in **Figure 2D**, Estrogen and progesterone stimulation induced severe HMGs in rats, reveled by histological abnormalities, including significant

TABLE 1 | Topological parameters of Li-Ru-Kang (LRK) on HMG obtained from network pharmacology analysis.

UniProt ID	Direct target	Degree	Betweenness centrality	Closeness centrality
P35354	PTGS2 COX2	34	0.020	0.302
Q04206	RELA NFKB	28	0.026	0.303
P23219	PTGS1 COX1	27	0.014	0.301
P31749	AKT1 PKB, RAC	25	0.032	0.328
P00533	EGFR ERBB, ERBB1, HER1	23	0.026	0.296
P37231	PPARG NR1C3	22	0.019	0.327
P05412	JUN	22	0.011	0.309
P25963	NFKBIA IKBA, MAD3, NFKBI	22	0.017	0.293
P09211	GSTP1 FAEES3, GST3	21	0.021	0.326
O15111	CHUK IKKA, TCF16	21	0.019	0.304
O14920	IKBKB IKKB	17	0.007	0.283
P00441	SOD1	17	0.015	0.282
P15692	VEGFA VEGF	16	0.011	0.284

TABLE 2 | Information of active ingredients of LRK and their topological parameters.

Compounds	Herbs	PK parameters		Betweenness centrality	Closeness centrality	Degree
		OB (%)	DL			
Saikosaponin c_qt	*Bupleuri Radix*	30.5	0.63	0.1429255	0.3728633	158
Quercetin	*Prunellae Spica*	46.43	0.28	0.1330894	0.3710792	154
Kaempferol	*Bupleuri Radix*, *Prunellae Spica*	41.88	0.24	0.0283762	0.311816	63
Chrysazin	*Polygoni Multiflori Radix*	28.74	0.19	0.0430047	0.3024919	62
Luteolin	*Prunellae Spica*	36.16	0.25	0.0664633	0.3213628	57
Beta-sitosterol	*Cremastrae Pseudobulbus Pleiones Pseudobulbus Cremastrae Pseudobulbus Pleiones Pseudobulbus*, *Curcumae Radix*, *Prunellae Spica*	36.91	0.75	0.0080004	0.2876571	38
Isorhamnetin	*Bupleuri Radix*	49.6	0.31	0.0217248	0.2926011	37
Curcolactone	*Curcumae Radix*	51.51	0.2	0.0473816	0.288728	37
Stigmasterol	*Prunellae Spica*, *Bupleuri Radix*, *Cremastrae Pseudobulbus Pleiones Cremastrae Pseudobulbus Pleiones Pseudobulbus*	43.83	0.76	0.0054813	0.274641	31
2-methoxy-9,10-dihydrophenanthrene-4,5-diol	*Cremastrae Pseudobulbus Pleiones Pseudobulbus*	44.97	0.18	0.0094876	0.2827056	30
Areapillin	*Bupleuri Radix*	48.96	0.41	0.0035804	0.2766548	17
Morin	*Prunellae Spica*	46.23	0.27	0.0068017	0.2666157	17
3,5,6,7-tetramethoxy-2-(3,4,5-trimethoxyphenyl) chromone	*Bupleuri Radix*	31.97	0.59	0.0022551	0.2751281	12
Delphinidin	*Prunellae Spica*	40.63	0.28	0.0016301	0.2708576	8
Troxerutin	*Bupleuri Radix*	31.6	0.28	3.50E-05	0.2329384	7
Cubebin	*Bupleuri Radix*	57.13	0.64	4.26E-05	0.2329773	5
α-spinasterol	*Bupleuri Radix*	42.98	0.76	3.13E-05	0.2601565	4
Linoleyl acetate	*Bupleuri Radix*	42.1	0.2	3.13E-05	0.2601565	4
Vulgaxanthin-I	*Prunellae Spica*	56.14	0.26	1.33E-05	0.2363298	2

proliferative lesions, mammary ducts ectasia expansion of mammary lumens, significant increase of acinars and lobules. Conversely, the administration of LRK significantly improved the morphological changes of HMGs dose-dependently. Above all, the results indicated the specific therapeutic effect of LRK on HMG.

TABLE 3 | Potential pathways and the target proteins in KEGG analysis.

Terms	Count	%	*P*-value	Benjamini	Target protein
MAPK signaling pathway	6	46.2	4.20E-05	2.10E-04	NFKB, JUN, AKT1, IKKA, IKKB, EGFR
TNF signaling pathway	6	46.2	9.70E-09	5.40E-07	NF-κB, AKT1, IKBA, IKKA, IKKB, COX2
Toll-like receptor signaling pathway	6	31.2	5.60E-07	5.70E-06	AKT1, IKKB, IKKA, NF-κB, IKBA, JUN
Chemokine signaling pathway	5	38.5	2.10E-04	7.70E-04	AKT, IKKA, IKKB, NF-κB, IKBA
NOD-like receptor signaling pathway	4	30.8	1.00E-04	4.70E-04	IKKA, IKKB, NF-κB, IKBA

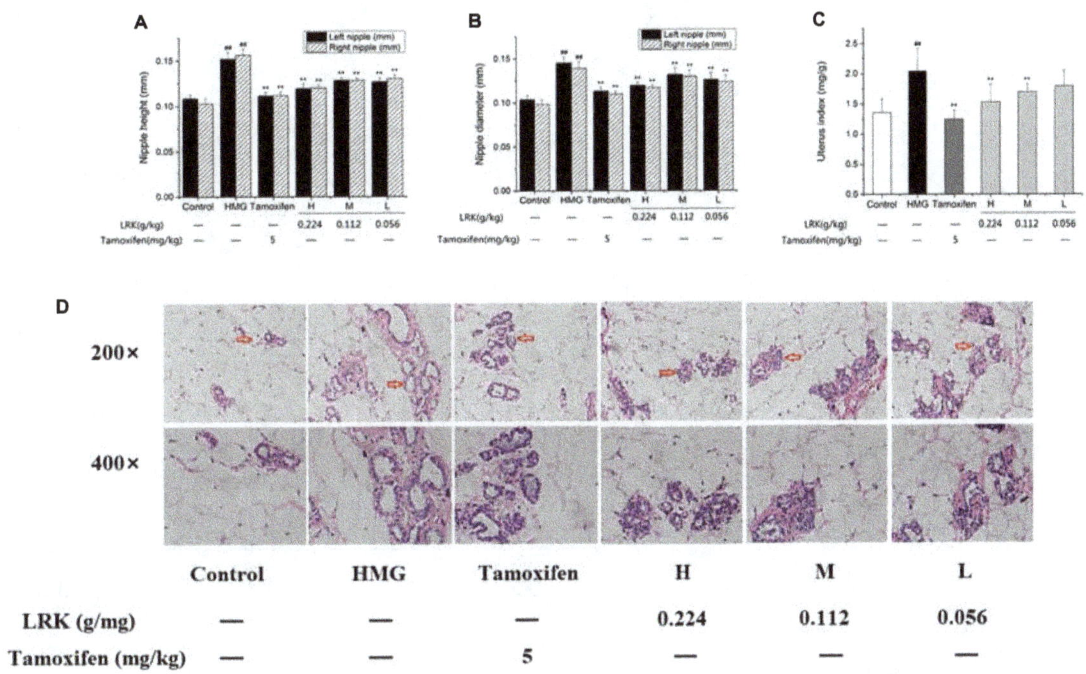

FIGURE 2 | Height and diameter of left and right nipples, uterus index in different group. **(A)** Height of left and right nipples. **(B)** Diameter of left and right nipples. **(C)** Uterus index; $N = 9$; **(D)** The effect of LRK on the pathological features of mammary gland tissues. $^{\#\#}P < 0.01$ vs. Control group; $^{**}P < 0.01$ vs. HMG model group.

Effect of LRK on the Expression of Inflammatory Cytokines (COX-2, IL-1β, iNOS, and TNF-α)

Previously studies reported that inflammatory cytokines such as COX-2, IL-1β, iNOS, and TNF-α play important role in the development of HMG (Yang et al., 2013; Chen et al., 2015; Guo et al., 2017). IL-1β and TNF-α, pro-inflammatory cytokines, were significantly increased in model group induced by estrogen and progesterone. While, the LRK treatment could notably decrease the expression of TNF-α and IL-1β compared to model group. COX-2 and iNOS, acted as pro-inflammatory enzymes. LRK treatment significantly inhibited the over-expressions of COX-2 and iNOS in rats induced by estrogen and progesterone in a dose-dependent manner ($P < 0.01$) (**Figure 3**). In summary, the results showed the significant anti-inflammatory effect of LRK.

Effect of LRK on Oxidative Stress [8-OHdG and Nitrotyrosine (NT)]

As shown in **Figure 4**, there was an obvious oxidative stress injury in model group, reveled by the high expression of 8-OHdG and NT, markers of oxidative stress, compared to the control group. In the LRK groups, the high expression of 8-OHdG and NT were significantly inhibited in a dose-dependent elevation, which indicated the anti-oxidative stress effect of LRK (**Figure 4**).

Effect of LRK on Expression of ERα and PR

The expression of estrogen receptor and progesterone receptor in mammary gland plays an important role in the physiological and pathological changes of mammary gland. So, we examined the expression of ERα and PR. As shown in **Figure 5**, LRK could not affect the expression of ERα and PR.

Effect of LRK on Expression of p-JNK, p-P38, p-ERK, and NF-κB (p65)

The pathway analysis results in this study indicated that LRK may play anti-inflammatory and anti-oxidative stress role through MAPK/ NF-κB signaling pathways. To determine whether LRK could affect MAPK, we examined the expressions of p-JNK, p-P38, p-ERK. The results showed that p-P38, p-ERK, and p-JNK

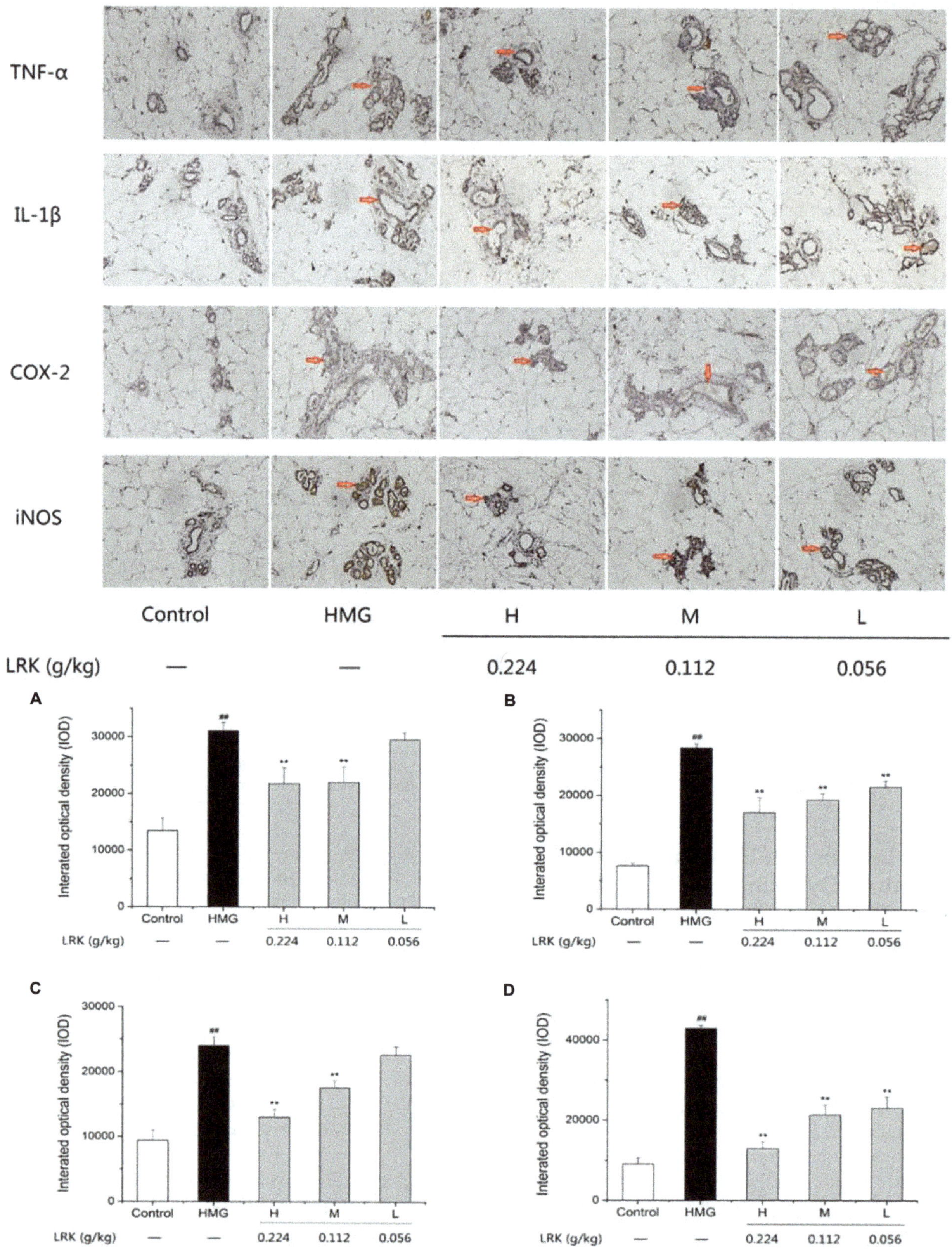

FIGURE 3 | The effect of LRK on the expression of TNF-α, IL-1β, COX-2, and iNOS. The integrated optical density of positive expression of **(A)** TNF-α, **(B)** IL-1β, **(C)** COX-2, **(D)** iNOS; $N = 3$; $^{\#\#}P < 0.01$ vs. Control group; $^{**}P < 0.01$ vs. HMG model group.

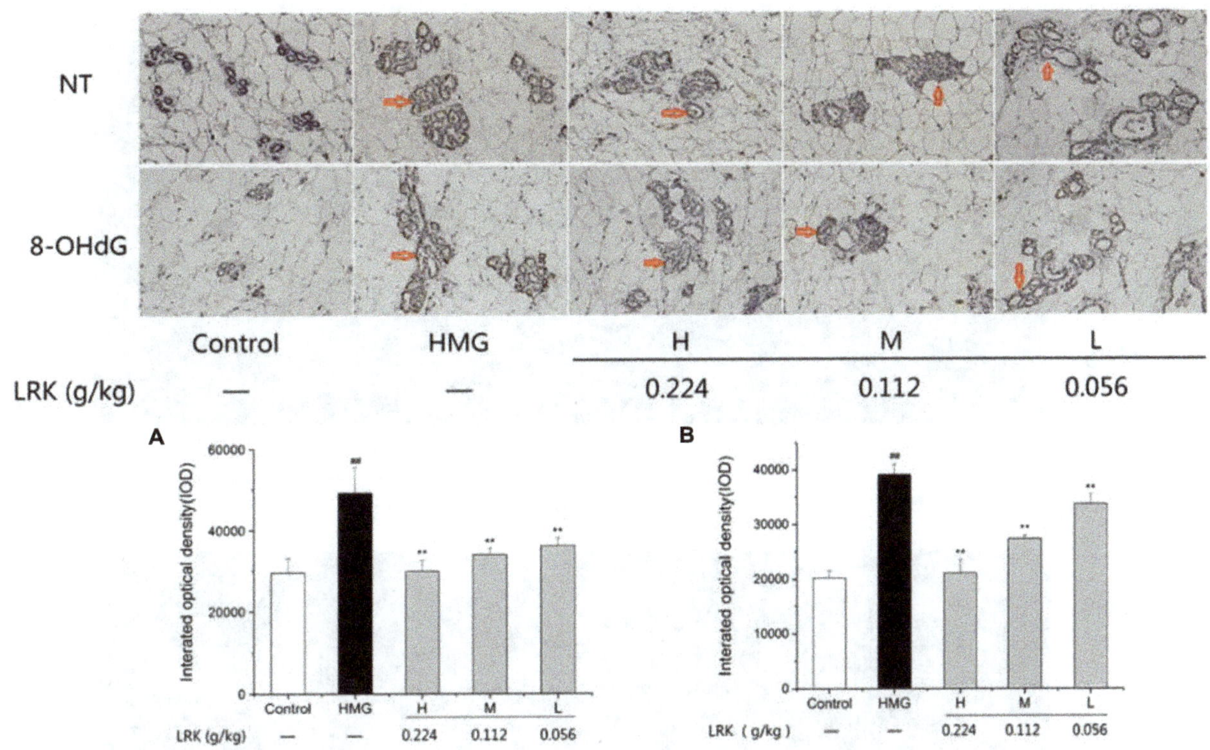

FIGURE 4 | The effect of LRK on the expression of NT and 8-OHdG. The integrated optical density of positive expression of **(A)** NT, **(B)** 8-OHdG in different group; $N = 3$; $^{\#\#}P < 0.01$ vs. Control group; $^{**}P < 0.01$ vs. HMG model group.

were slightly expressed in normal mammary cells. In HMG model group, expressions of p-P38, p-ERK, and p-JNK were notably increased. LRK administration significantly suppressed the over-expressions of p-P38, p-ERK, and p-JNK versus the model group (**Figure 6**).

There existed a large degree of cross-talk within the MAPK cascades and other signaling networks. For example, there were interactions between mediators of the MAPK and NF-κB pathway (Chen et al., 2015). The expression of NF-κB (p65) was examined by immunohistochemical analysis. NF-κB (p65) was increased significantly in the HMG model group. LRK treatment significantly and dose-dependently suppressed the mammary over-expressions of NF-κB (p65) when compared to the model ones (**Figure 7**).

DISCUSSION

HMG, a common disease in middle-aged women has severe cancerous tendencies, and poses a significant public health challenge to women (Marchant, 2002). It is reported that HMG, especially atypical HMG, leads to higher risk of breast cancer. (Wang et al., 2011; Zhang et al., 2012). Studies showed that HMG is related to endocrine disorders, the most of that are caused by the imbalance of estrogen and progestin. (Liu et al., 2012; You et al., 2017) The treatment of HMG has become a heated topic in the world. HMG is mainly treated by surgery and medication (Henry, 2014; Chen et al., 2015). Tamoxifen, as the main therapeutic drug of HMG could improve the overall survival for patients. However, adherence to and persistence with the medications is poor in part because of bothersome side effects that can negatively affect quality of life (Henry, 2014). Thus, it is important and urgency to find more effective and few side effects drug to block development of HMG.

LRK, a TCM formula, has been clinically used for the treatment of HMG for several years. The First Affiliated Hospital of the General Hospital of PLA conducted clinical trials and demonstrated that LRK could inhibit HMG (Li et al., 2013). Previous study showed high effective rate (88.0%) in the treatment of HMG. Meanwhile the patients' symptoms and abnormalities of gonadal hormone was obvious improved (Qian et al., 2007). However, the underlying mechanisms of LRK for HMG are still unclear. Thus, the aim of this study is to explore the underlying mechanism of LRK on HMG.

To clarify the effect of LRK on HMG in rats, we established HMG model in rats induced by estrogen and progesterone. The decreasing of nipple heights and diameters, uterus index and ameliorate of histopathological in LRK groups indicated that LRK could improving HMG in rats. Then, we further explore the active ingredients and underlying mechanism of LRK on HMG.

To reveal the therapeutic mechanisms of LRK on HMG, we firstly predicted the active ingredients and potential targets of LRK against HMG through network pharmacology. We found 19 potential compounds, including saikosaponin

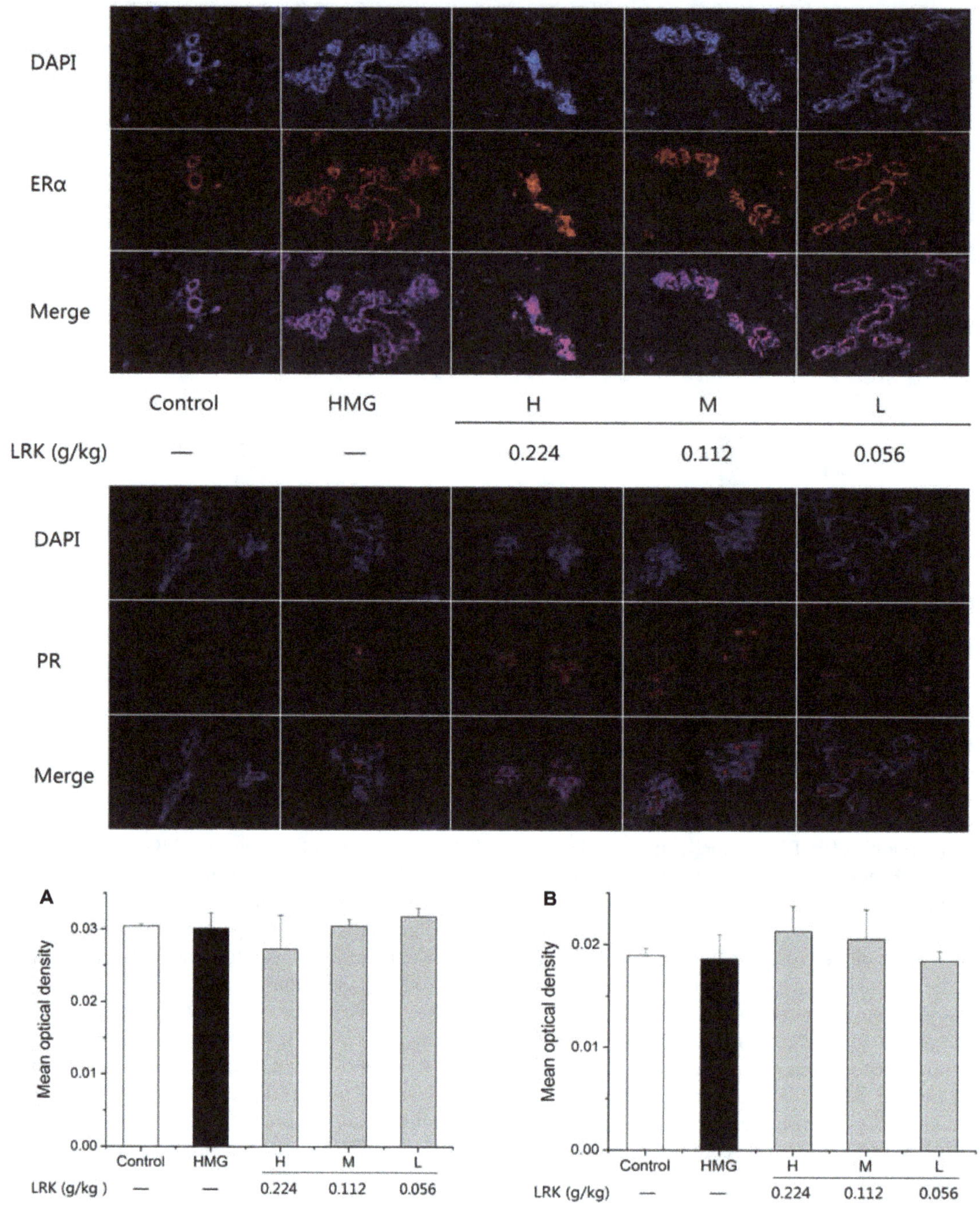

FIGURE 5 | The effect of LRK on the expression of ERα and PR. The mean optical density of positive expression of **(A)** ERα, **(B)** PR in different groups; $N = 3$.

c_qt, quercetin, kaempferol and chrysazin, Luteolin, beta-sitosterol, isorhamnetin, curcolactone, stigmasterol, 2-methoxy-9,10-dihydrophenanthrene-4,5-diol, areapillin, morin, 3,5,6,7-tetramethoxy-2-(3,4,5-trimethoxyphenyl) chromone, delphinidin, troxerutin, cubebin, α-spinasterol, linoleyl acetate and vulgaxanthin-I might play the key role in LRK-treated HMG. Studies showed that most of those potential active ingredients have anti-inflammatory or anti-oxidative effects, such as quercetin, (Song et al., 2018, kaempferol (Huang et al., 2018; Wang J. et al., 2018), Luteolin (Aziz et al., 2018), beta-sitosterol (Liao et al., 2018), isorhamnetin (Qiu et al., 2016), delphinidin (Wang et al., 2017), troxerutin (Najafi et al., 2018), cubebin (Bastos et al., 2001), morin (Athira et al., 2016), linoleyl acetate (Peana et al., 2002) have anti-inflammatory effects. Compounds like quercetin (Sherif, 2018), kaempferol (Kouhestani et al., 2018), Luteolin (Yang et al., 2018), beta-sitosterol (Yin et al., 2018),

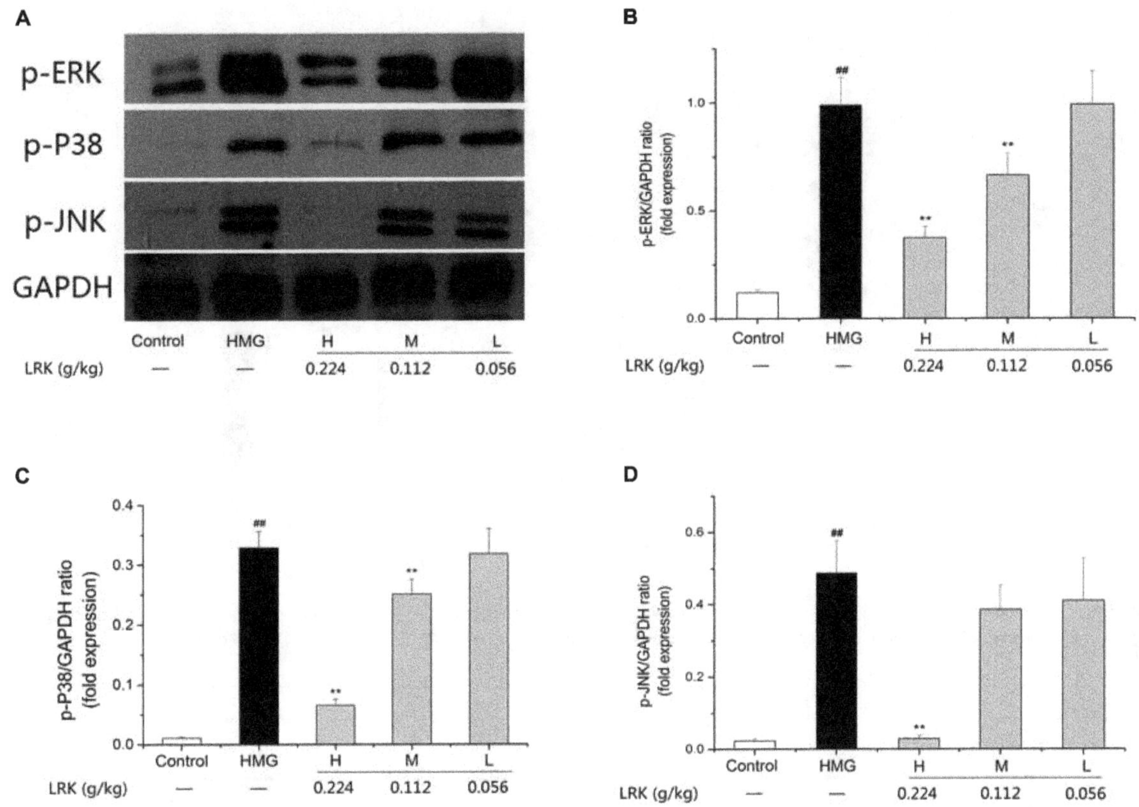

FIGURE 6 | Alterations of the mitogen-activated protein kinase (MAPK) pathways in the mammary glands of LRK-treated rats. **(A)** Expression of p-ERK, p-P38, and p-JNK by western blot analysis; **(B)** The p-ERK/GAPDH ratio; **(C)** the p-P38/GAPDH ratio; **(D)** the p-JNK /GAPDH ratio. Sample loading was normalized by GAPDH. $N = 3$; $^{\#\#}P < 0.01$ vs. Control group; $^{**}P < 0.01$ vs. HMG model group.

delphinidin (Cheol et al., 2016), troxerutin (Farajdokht et al., 2017), morin (Ma et al., 2016), linoleyl acetate (Peng et al., 2014) showed anti-oxidative stress effect. Studies indicated that HMG was related to inflammatory and oxidative stress (Chen et al., 2015). Therefore, those active ingredients predicted by network pharmacology might play important role in LRK treat HMG.

Meanwhile, KEGG analysis indicated that MAPK signaling pathway contributes the most for the therapeutic effect of LRK on HMG, it might be the essential pathway for our research. Additionally, Toll-like receptor signaling pathway and TNF signaling pathway were either directly involved in inflammation or played other important roles.

Simultaneously, there were studies proved that MAPK signaling pathway is essential in regulating many cellular processes including inflammation, cell stress response, cell differentiation, cell proliferation, metabolism, motility and apoptosis (Arthur and Ley, 2013). There were four distinct MAPK cascades including the extracellular signal-regulated kinase (p42/44 ERK)/MAPK, the p38 pathway, the c-jun N-terminal kinase (JNK)/stress-activated protein kinase (SAPK) pathway and the Big MAP kinase-1 (BMK-1) pathway (Burotto et al., 2014). P38, ERK, and JNK pathway was the most important signaling pathways involving the regulation of many physiological functions of cells and playing an important role in the anthogenesis and pathophysiological process of many kinds of diseases, such as regulating the proliferations and differentiations of cells, participation in oxidative stress reaction (Li et al., 2017). Currently, more and more researches proved that TCM have the protective effect against HMG via the possible mechanism of regulating endocrine, inflammatory and oxidative stress (Wang et al., 2011; Zhang et al., 2012). And studies indicated that TCM can significantly inhibit and improve HMG in a large degree via ERK, JNK signaling pathway, as well as regulating NF-κB (Squires et al., 2003; Chen et al., 2013; Wu, 2015). It is well-known that NF-κB can activate the inflammatory cytokines like IL-1, TNF-α, and COX2 (May and Ghosh, 1998). Researches indicated that MAPK and NF-κB signaling pathway play an important role in HMG treated by TCM while NF-κB building a link among oxidative stress and inflammatory responses in HMG (Chen et al., 2015). Therefore, we verified the MAPK and NF-κB signaling pathway for further experiments.

The experimental results showed that the phosphorylation of P38, ERK, and JNK in HMG rats was significantly increased after stimulation of estrogen and progesterone. While the overexpression of p-p38, p-ERK, and p-JNK were decreased after the treatment of LRK. As the downstream of MAPK signaling pathway and an important inflammatory

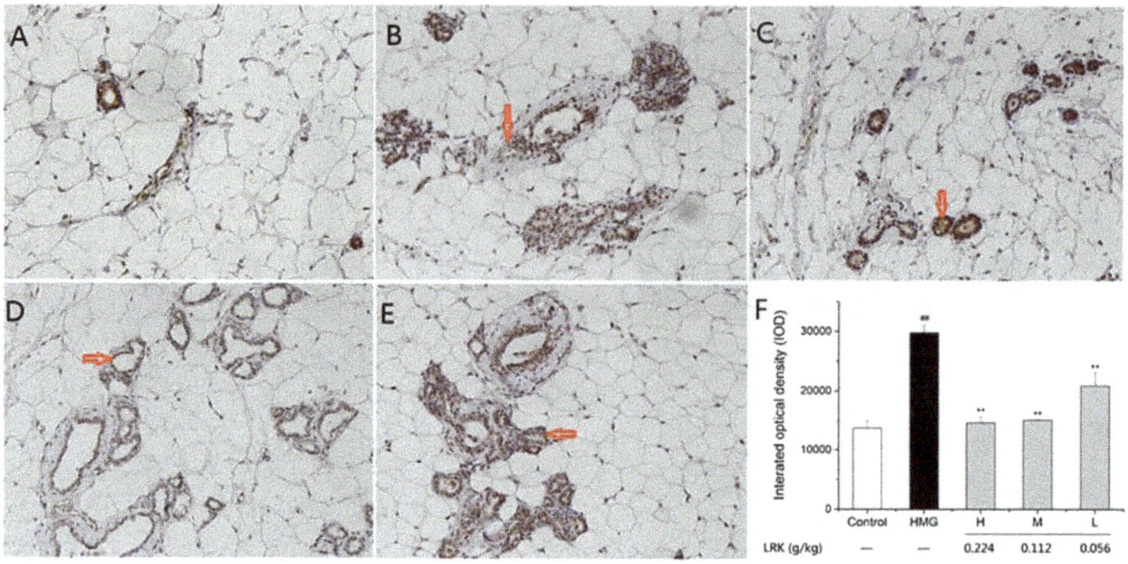

FIGURE 7 | The effect of LRK on the expression of NF-κB (p65). Immunohistochemical analysis of NF-κB (p65) in **(A)** Control group, **(B)** HMG Model group, **(C)** H group, **(D)** M group, **(E)** L group, **(F)** The integrated optical density of positive expression of P65; $N = 3$; $^{\#\#}P < 0.01$ vs. Control group; $^{**}P < 0.01$ vs. HMG model group.

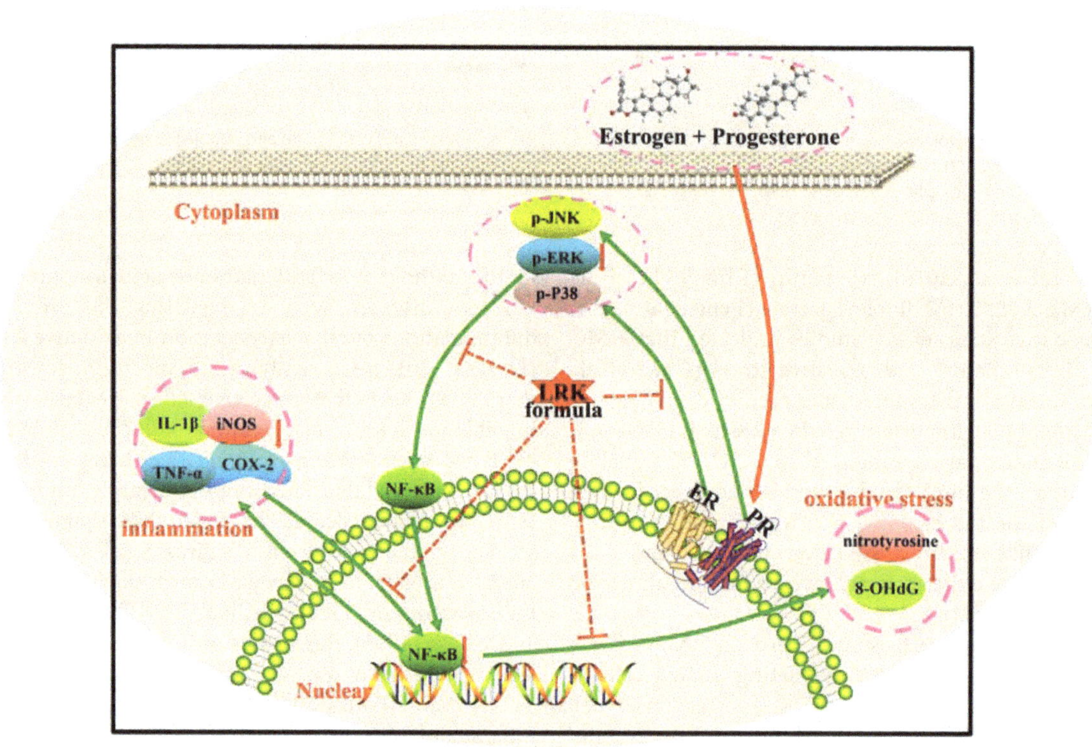

FIGURE 8 | The probable protection mechanism of LRK in HMG.

transcription factor, NF-κB was decreased after LRK treated. And the expression of inflammatory mediators (including IL-1, and TNF-α) and pro-inflammatory cytokines (such as COX2 and iNOS) were down-regulated after LRK treated. Those results indicated LRK could reduce inflammation in HMG.

ER and PR, as the receptor of estrogen and progestin, and studies showed PR and ERα could active the MAPK signaling pathway (Liu, 2012). The present study showed that LRK treatment has no effect on the expression of ERα and PR. Those results indicate that LRK might plays therapeutic effect on HMG by activating MAPK signaling pathways directly, rather than through ERα and PR to activating MAPK signaling pathways.

8-OHdG is a predominant form of free radical-induced oxidative lesions in nuclear and mitochondrial DNA. Therefore, 8-OHdG is widely used as a biomarker for oxidative stress (Wu et al., 2004; Arulselvan et al., 2016). Nitrotyrosine (NT) is mainly formed by the reaction of superoxide radicals with NO, which is used to detect peroxynitrite (Fitri et al., 2017). NT formation has been detected in a variety of systemic inflammatory diseases and is considered as a marker of NO-derived species. Estrogen can generate considerable reactive oxygen species (ROS) and lead to high level of oxidative stress (Chen et al., 2015; Das Gupta et al., 2015). Activation of NF-κB could upregulated the expression of NO, further promote ROS and oxidative stress indexes (Qi, 2014). In the present study, LRK treatment significantly reduced the expression of 8-OHdG and NT. Hence, LRK may also act as an anti-oxidative agent on HMG treatment.

Our data indicated that LRK treatment protects the mammary glands from the damage of oxidative stress and inflammation via suppresses of MAPK/NF-κB signaling pathways without affecting on the expression of ERα and PR.

In this study, there were some limitations that several pathways were predicted related to the therapeutic effect of LRK on HMG via network pharmacology, however, parts of pathway were demonstrated by our experiment. Although, 19 potential active compounds were predicted by network pharmacology, and literatures reported showed anti-inflammatory and anti-oxidative effect of those ingredients, the effect of those active ingredients on HMG were still unknown. Maker clear the active ingredients is necessary for the formula research. Accordingly, in the next work of our group, we will have a comprehensive study to illuminate the active ingredients and the mechanisms of LRK against HMG.

Previous study verified the effect of MAPK inhibitor (UO126) in mammary epithelial cells (HC11 and EpH4) and breast cancer cells (MC4-L2), indicated that MAPK inhibitor could inhibit the activation of ERK signaling and suppress the proliferation, to inhibiting hyperplasia and growth (Cotrim et al., 2013). Our research group will further validate the effect of MAPK/NF-κB signaling pathway in LRK treat HMG by using the MAPK inhibitors to mimic the function of LRK, to proving the importance of MAPK/NF-κB signaling pathway for LRK work in HMG rat. Furthermore, we will comprehensively explicit the active ingredients of LRK by screening the active ingredients of LRK *in vitro* alternative model, and testing the active components to see whether they could achieve the similar effects as LRK treatment subsequently.

CONCLUSION

Summarily, the present study demonstrated that there was a therapeutic effect of LRK on HMG by reducing pathological lesions in mammary gland tissue attenuating the over-activation of inflammation cytokines such as IL-1β, TNF-α, COX-2, iNOS, and suppressing the expression of 8-OHdG and NT. Furthermore, the combination of network pharmacology and experiment verification illustrated that the protect effect of LRK on HMG in rats might be associated with MAPK/NF-κB signaling pathways (**Figure 8**).

AUTHOR CONTRIBUTIONS

YW was responsible for primary data generation, analysis and writing the manuscript. SW, XZ, LQ, YZ, and WZ participated in the design of the study. YY, XL, and TW were involved the *in vivo* experimentation and technical work. SW and YY were responsible for the extensive statistical analyses. HL, TG, WZ, and XZ gave advice on the writing.

FUNDING

This study was supported by the Project of Chinese Medicine Education Association (No. 2016SKT-M035).

ACKNOWLEDGMENTS

We thank YZ and WZ for kindly revising this manuscript.

REFERENCES

Arthur, J. S., and Ley, S. C. (2013). Mitogen-activated protein kinases in innate immunity. *Nat. Rev. Immunol.* 13, 679–692. doi: 10.1038/nri3495

Arulselvan, P., Fard, M. T., Tan, W. S., Gothai, S., Fakurazi, S., Norhaizan, M. E., et al. (2016). Role of antioxidants and natural products in inflammation. *Oxid. Med. Cell. Longev.* 2016:5276130. doi: 10.1155/2016/5276130

Athira, K. V., Madhana, R. M., Kasala, E. R., Samudrala, P. K., Lahkar, M., and Gogoi, R. (2016). Morin hydrate mitigates cisplatin-induced renal and hepatic injury by impeding oxidative/nitrosative stress and inflammation in mice. *J. Biochem. Mol. Toxicol.* 30, 571–579. doi: 10.1002/jbt.21817

Aziz, N., Kim, M. Y., and Cho, J. Y. (2018). Anti-inflammatory effects of luteolin: a review of in vitro, in vivo, and in silico studies. *J. Ethnopharmacol.* 225, 342–358. doi: 10.1016/j.jep.2018.05.019

Bastos, J. K., Carvalho, J. C., de Souza, G. H., Pedrazzi, A. H., and Sarti, S. J. (2001). Anti-inflammatory activity of cubebin, a lignan from the leaves of zanthoxyllum naranjillo griseb. *J. Ethnopharmacol.* 75, 279–282. doi: 10.1016/S0378-8741(01)00171-4

Bennett, I. C., Mccaffrey, J. F., Mccaffrey, E., and Wyatt, B. (1990). Serum oestradiol in women with and without breast disease. *Br. J. Cancer* 61, 142–146. doi: 10.1038/bjc.1990.29

Burotto, M., Chiou, V. L., Lee, J. M., and Kohn, E. C. (2014). The MAPK pathway across different malignancies: a new perspective. *Cancer* 120, 3446–3456. doi: 10.1002/cncr.28864

Che, C. T., Wang, Z. J., Chow, M. S., and Lam, C. W. (2013). Herb-herb combination for therapeutic enhancement and advancement: theory, practice and future perspectives. *Molecules* 18, 5125–5141. doi: 10.3390/molecules18055125

Chen, C. Y. (2011). Tcm database@taiwan: the world's largest traditional Chinese medicine database for drug screening in silico. *PLoS One* 6:e15939. doi: 10.1371/journal.pone.0015939

Chen, H., Mo, X., Yu, J., and Huang, Z. (2013). Alpinetin attenuates inflammatory responses by interfering toll-like receptor 4/nuclear factor kappa b signaling pathway in lipopolysaccharide-induced mastitis in mice. *Int. Immunopharmacol.* 17, 26–32. doi: 10.1016/j.intimp.2013.04.030

Chen, T., Li, J., Chen, J., Song, H., and Yang, C. (2015). Anti-hyperplasia effects of rosa rugosa polyphenols in rats with hyperplasia of mammary gland. *Environ. Toxicol. Pharmacol.* 39, 990–996. doi: 10.1016/j.etap.2015.02.014

Chen, X., Ji, Z. L., and Chen, Y. Z. (2002). TTD: therapeutic target database. *Nucleic Acids Res.* 30, 412–415. doi: 10.1093/nar/30.1.412

Cheol, N. D., Sool, H. Y., Been, N. J., Jeong, K. R., and Bin, P. H. (2016). Cytoprotective mechanism of cyanidin and delphinidin against oxidative stress-induced tenofibroblast death. *Biomol. Ther.* 24, 426–432. doi: 10.4062/biomolther.2015.169

Cline, J. M., Soderqvist, G., Schoultz, E. V., Skoog, L., and Bo, V. S. (1998). Effects of conjugated estrogens, medroxyprogesterone acetate, and tamoxifen on the mammary glands of macaques. *Breast Cancer Res. Treat.* 48, 221–229. doi: 10.1023/A:1005984932268

Cotrim, C. Z., Fabris, V., Doria, M. L., Lindberg, K., Gustafsson, J. Å, Amado, F., et al. (2013). Estrogen receptor beta growth-inhibitory effects are repressed through activation of mapk and pi3k signalling in mammary epithelial and breast cancer cells. *Oncogene* 32, 2390–2402. doi: 10.1038/onc.2012.261

Das Gupta, S., So, J. Y., Wall, B., Wahler, J., Smolarek, A. K., Saetan, S., et al. (2015). Tocopherols inhibit oxidative and nitrosative stress in estrogen-induced early mammary hyperplasia in aci rats. *Mol. Carcinog.* 54, 916–925. doi: 10.1002/mc.22164

Farajdokht, F., Amani, M., Bavil, F. M., Alihemmati, A., Mohaddes, G., Babri, S., et al. (2017). Troxerutin protects hippocampal neurons against amyloid beta-induced oxidative stress and apoptosis. *Excli J.* 16, 1081–1089. doi: 10.17179/excli2017-526

Fitri, L. E., Rosmarwati, E., Rizky, Y., Budiarti, N., Samsu, N., and Mintaroem, K. (2017). Strong renal expression of heat shock protein 70, high mobility group box 1, inducible nitric oxide synthase, and nitrotyrosine in mice model of severe malaria. *Rev. Soc. Bras. Med. Trop.* 50, 489–498. doi: 10.1590/0037-8682-0049-2017

Guo, Y., Zhang, B., Yan, S., Shi, B., and Guo, X. (2017). Protective effects of selenium on oxidative damage induced by lipopolysaccharide in dairy cow mammary epithelial cells. *Chin. J. Animal Nutr.* 29, 3375–3384.

Henry, N. L. (2014). Endocrine therapy toxicity: management options. American society of clinical oncology educational book / ASCO. *Am. Soc. Clin. Oncol.* 34, e25–e30. doi: 10.14694/EdBook_AM.2014.34.e25

Huang, X., Pan, Q., Mao, Z., Wang, P., Zhang, R., Ma, X., et al. (2018). Kaempferol inhibits interleukin-1β stimulated matrix metalloproteinases by suppressing the mapk-associated erk and p38 signaling pathways. *Mol. Med. Rep.* 18, 2697–2704. doi: 10.3892/mmr.2018.9280

Jia, Y., Liu, X., Jia, Q., Zhang, W., Sun, C., Yuan, D., et al. (2017). The anti-hyperplasia of mammary gland effect of protein extract hss from tegillarca granosa. *Biomed. Pharmacother.* 85, 1–6. doi: 10.1016/j.biopha.2016.11.109

Kleinberg, D. L., Ameri, P., and Singh, B. (2011). Pasireotide, an igf-i action inhibitor, prevents growth hormone and estradiol-induced mammary hyperplasia. *Pituitary* 14, 44–52. doi: 10.1007/s11102-010-0257-0

Kouhestani, S., Jafari, A., and Babaei, P. (2018). Kaempferol attenuates cognitive deficit via regulating oxidative stress and neuroinflammation in an ovariectomized rat model of sporadic dementia. *Neural Regen. Res.* 13, 1827–1832. doi: 10.4103/1673-5374.238714

Li, H. T., Liu, H. H., Yang, Y. X., Wang, T., Zhou, X. L., Yu, Y., et al. (2018). Therapeutic effects of a traditional chinese medicine formula plus tamoxifen vs. tamoxifen for the treatment of mammary gland hyperplasia: a meta-analysis of randomized trials. *Front. Pharmacol.* 9:45. doi: 10.3389/fphar.2018.00045

Li, S. N., Qian, L. Q., Ma, J. L., Xia, Z. Y., Li, B. Y., Gao, F., et al. (2013). A randomized trial of chinese medicine lirukang granule combined with psychological intervention for cyclomastopathy and menoxenia. *Chin. J. Integr. Med.* 19, 22–28. doi: 10.1007/s11655-013-1321-6

Li, X., Xin, P., Wang, C., Wang, Z., Wang, Q., and Kuang, H. (2017). Mechanisms of traditional chinese medicine in the treatment of mammary gland hyperplasia. *Am. J. Chin. Med.* 45, 443–458. doi: 10.1142/S0192415X17500276

Liao, P. C., Lai, M. H., Hsu, K. P., Kuo, Y. H., Chen, J., Tsai, M. C., et al. (2018). Identification of β-sitosterol as in vitro anti-inflammatory constituent in *Moringa oleifera*. *J. Agric. Food Chem.* 66, 10748–10759. doi: 10.1021/acs.jafc.8b04555

Liu, C., Yue, Y. H., and Hao, X. L. (2012). Progress of research into the pathogenesis of breast hyperplasia. *Med. Recapit.* 58, 1703–1721.

Liu, H., Wang, J., Zhou, W., Wang, Y., and Yang, L. (2013). Systems approaches and polypharmacology for drug discovery from herbal medicines: an example using licorice. *J. Ethnopharmacol.* 146, 773–793. doi: 10.1016/j.jep.2013.02.004

Liu, Y. (2012). The mechanism and regulation factors of progesterone receptor activation. *J. Int. Obstet. Gynecol.* 39, 570–573.

Ma, Y., Ge, A., Zhu, W., Liu, Y. N., Ji, N. F., Zha, W. J., et al. (2016). Morin attenuates ovalbumin-induced airway inflammation by modulating oxidative stress-responsive mapk signaling. *Oxid. Med. Cell. Longev.* 2016:5843672. doi: 10.1155/2016/5843672

Mao, Y., Hao, J., Jin, Z. Q., Niu, Y. Y., Yang, X., Liu, D., et al. (2017). Network pharmacology-based and clinically relevant prediction of the active ingredients and potential targets of chinese herbs in metastatic breast cancer patients. *Oncotarget* 8, 27007–27021. doi: 10.18632/oncotarget.15351

Marchant, D. J. (2002). Benign breast disease. *Obstet. Gynecol. Clin. North Am.* 29, 1–20. doi: 10.1016/S0889-8545(03)00048-2

Martinez de Dueñas, E., Ochoa, A. E., Lopez-Barajas, I. B., Ferrer, M. T., Bandrés, M. F., Chicharro García, L. M., et al. (2014). Adjusting the dose of tamoxifen in patients with early breast cancer and cyp2d6 poor metabolizer phenotype. *Breast* 23, 400–406. doi: 10.1016/j.breast.2014.02.008

May, M. J., and Ghosh, S. (1998). Nf- kappab and rel proteins:evolutionarily conserved medators of immune responses. *Immunology* 16, 225–260. doi: 10.1146/annurev.immunol.16.1.225

Najafi, M., Noroozi, E., Javadi, A., and Badalzadeh, R. (2018). Anti-arrhythmogenic and anti-inflammatory effects of troxerutin in ischemia/reperfusion injury of diabetic myocardium. *Biomed. Pharmacother.* 102, 385–391. doi: 10.1016/j.biopha.2018.03.047

Peana, A. T., D'Aquila, P. S., Panin, F., Serra, G., Pippia, P., and Moretti, M. D. (2002). Anti-inflammatory activity of linalool and linalyl acetate constituents of essential oils. *Phytomedicine* 9, 721–726. doi: 10.1078/09447110232162 1322

Peng, H. Y., Lin, C. C., Wang, H. Y., Ying, S., and Chou, S. T. (2014). The melanogenesis alteration effects of achillea millefolium l. essential oil and linalyl acetate: involvement of oxidative stress and the jnk and erk signaling pathways in melanoma cells. *Plos One* 9:e95186. doi: 10.1371/journal.pone.0095186

Qi, Y. (2014). *Mechanism Research of Xinfeng Capsule on Improving Cardiopulmonary Function in Patients with Ankylosing Spondylitis Based on the Signal Path of NF-κB-iNOS-NO*. Doctoral dissertation, Anhui University of traditional Chinese Medicine, Hefei.

Qian, L. Q., Pan, C., Feng, Z. Q., Leng, J., and Zhi-Yin, X. U. (2005). Effect of lirukang liquid on morphology of mammary gland, uterus and ovary of models with hyperplasia of mammary glands. *J. Nanjing Univ. Tradit. Chin. Med.* 21, 255–257.

Qian, L. Q., Pei, X. H., and Chen, R. M. (2004). Effect of lirukang on the level of serum sex hormones in the model of galactophore hyperplasia. *Chin. J. Inf. TCM* 11, 684–686.

Qian, L. Q., Pei, X. H., Xu, Z. Y., and Wang, C. (2007). Clinical observation on treatment of hyperplasia of mammary gland by lirukang granule. *Chin. J. Integr. Med.* 13, 120–124. doi: 10.1007/s11655-007-0120-y

Qiu, S., Sun, G., Zhang, Y., Xiangling, L. I., and Wang, R. (2016). Involvement of the nf-κb signaling pathway in the renoprotective effects of isorhamnetin in a type 2 diabetic rat model. *Biomed. Rep.* 4, 628–634. doi: 10.3892/br.2016.636

Roth, B. L., Baner, K., Westkaemper, R., Siebert, D., Rice, K. C., Steinberg, S. A., et al. (2002). Salvinorin a: a potent naturally occurring nonnitrogenous κ opioid selective agonist. *Proc. Natl. Acad. Sci. U.S.A.* 99, 11934–11939. doi: 10.1073/pnas.182234399

Shao, L. I., and Zhang, B. (2013). Traditional chinese medicine network pharmacology: theory, methodology and application. *Chin. J. Nat. Med.* 11, 110–120.

Sherif, I. O. (2018). Uroprotective mechanism of quercetin against cyclophosphamide-induced urotoxicity: effect on oxidative stress and inflammatory markers. *J. Cell. Biochem.* 119, 7441–7448. doi: 10.1002/jcb.27053

Song, J. Y., Truong, D. V., and Yang, B. S. (2018). Quercetin shows the pharmacological activity to simultaneously downregulate the inflammatory and fibrotic responses to tissue injury in association with its ability to target multi-kinases. *Pharmacology* 102, 142–153. doi: 10.1159/000490417

Squires, M. S., Hudson, E. A., Howells, L., Sale, S., Houghton, C. E., Jones, J. L., et al. (2003). Relevance of mitogen activated protein kinase (mapk) and phosphotidylinositol-3-kinase/protein kinase b (pi3k/pkb) pathways to induction of apoptosis by curcumin in breast cells. *Biochem. Pharmacol.* 65, 361–376. doi: 10.1016/S0006-2952(02)01517-4

Tao, W., Xu, X., Wang, X., Li, B., Wang, Y., Li, Y., et al. (2013). Network pharmacology-based prediction of the active ingredients and potential targets of chinese herbal radix curcumae formula for application to cardiovascular disease. *J. Ethnopharmacol.* 145, 1–10. doi: 10.1016/j.jep.2012.09.051

Wang, C. H., Zhu, L. L., Ju, K. F., Liu, J. L., and Li, K. P. (2017). Anti-inflammatory effect of delphinidin on intramedullary spinal pressure in a spinal cord injury rat model. *Exp. Ther. Med.* 14, 5583–5588. doi: 10.3892/etm.2017.5206

Wang, J., Fang, X., Ge, L., Cao, F., Zhao, L., Wang, Z., et al. (2018). Antitumor, antioxidant and anti-inflammatory activities of kaempferol and its corresponding glycosides and the enzymatic preparation of kaempferol. *PLoS One* 13:e0197563. doi: 10.1371/journal.pone.0197563

Wang, J. B., Cui, H. R., Wang, R. L., Zhang, C. E., Niu, M., Bai, Z. F., et al. (2018). A systems pharmacology-oriented discovery of a new therapeutic use of the tcm formula liuweiwuling for liver failure. *Sci. Rep.* 8:5645. doi: 10.1038/s41598-018-21515-6

Wang, L., Zhao, D., Di, L., Cheng, D., Zhou, X., Yang, X., et al. (2011). The anti-hyperplasia of mammary gland effect of thladiantha dubia root ethanol extract in rats reduced by estrogen and progestogen. *J. Ethnopharmacol.* 134, 136–140. doi: 10.1016/j.jep.2010.11.071

Wei, S., Qian, L., Niu, M., Liu, H., Yang, Y., Wang, Y., et al. (2018). The modulatory properties of li-ru-kang treatment on hyperplasia of mammary glands using an integrated approach. *Front. Pharmacol.* 9:651. doi: 10.3389/fphar.2018.00651

Wu, H. Y. (2015). *Experimental Study on Effect of Dangguishaoyao Modified Decotion on ERK Gene Expression in Rats.* Fuzhou: Fujian University of Traditional Chinese Medicine.

Wu, L. L., Chiou, C. C., Chang, P. Y., and Wu, J. T. (2004). Urinary 8-ohdg: a marker of oxidative stress to dna and a risk factor for cancer, atherosclerosis and diabetics. *Clin. Chim. Acta* 339, 1–9. doi: 10.1016/j.cccn.2003.09.010

Yang, G., Yu, M., Fan, W., Xu, T., and Chen, H. (2013). Expression of nuclear factor kappa B and correlations with tumor necrosis factor-α in breast cancer. *Prog. Mod. Biomed.* 13, 5860–5863.

Yang, S. C., Chen, P. J., Chang, S. H., Weng, Y. T., Chang, F. R., Chang, K. Y., et al. (2018). Luteolin attenuates neutrophilic oxidative stress and inflammatory arthritis by inhibiting raf1 activity. *Biochem. Pharmacol.* 154, 384–396. doi: 10.1016/j.bcp.2018.06.003

Ye, H., Ye, L., and Kang, H. (2011). HIT: linking herbal active ingredients to targets. *Nucleic Acids Res.* 39, D1055–D1059. doi: 10.1093/nar/gkq1165

Yin, Y., Liu, X., Liu, J., Cai, E., Zhu, H., Li, H., et al. (2018). Beta-sitosterol and its derivatives repress lipopolysaccharide/d-galactosamine-induced acute hepatic injury by inhibiting the oxidation and inflammation in mice. *Bioorg. Med. Chem. Lett.* 28, 1525–1533. doi: 10.1016/j.bmcl.2018.03.073

You, Z., Sun, J., Xie, F., Chen, Z., Zhang, S., Chen, H., et al. (2017). Modulatory effect of fermented papaya extracts on mammary gland hyperplasia induced by estrogen and progestin in female rats. *Oxid. Med. Cell. Longev.* 2017:8235069. doi: 10.1155/2017/8235069

Zhang, G., Zeng, X., Peng, Z., Si, H., Zheng, Y., Li, D., et al. (2012). Modulation of expression of p16 and her2 in rat breast tissues of mammary hyperplasia model by external use of rupifang extract. *J. Tradit. Chin. Med.* 32, 651–656. doi: 10.1016/S0254-6272(13)60087-4

Zhang, Z. Y., Cheng, H. Z., and Pharmacy, D. O. (2016). Research advances in pathogenesis of mammary gland hyperplasia and medication and its establishment of animal model. *Anti Infect. Pharm.* 13, 966–969.

Permissions

All chapters in this book were first published by Frontiers; hereby published with permission under the Creative Commons Attribution License or equivalent. Every chapter published in this book has been scrutinized by our experts. Their significance has been extensively debated. The topics covered herein carry significant findings which will fuel the growth of the discipline. They may even be implemented as practical applications or may be referred to as a beginning point for another development.

The contributors of this book come from diverse backgrounds, making this book a truly international effort. This book will bring forth new frontiers with its revolutionizing research information and detailed analysis of the nascent developments around the world.

We would like to thank all the contributing authors for lending their expertise to make the book truly unique. They have played a crucial role in the development of this book. Without their invaluable contributions this book wouldn't have been possible. They have made vital efforts to compile up to date information on the varied aspects of this subject to make this book a valuable addition to the collection of many professionals and students.

This book was conceptualized with the vision of imparting up-to-date information and advanced data in this field. To ensure the same, a matchless editorial board was set up. Every individual on the board went through rigorous rounds of assessment to prove their worth. After which they invested a large part of their time researching and compiling the most relevant data for our readers.

The editorial board has been involved in producing this book since its inception. They have spent rigorous hours researching and exploring the diverse topics which have resulted in the successful publishing of this book. They have passed on their knowledge of decades through this book. To expedite this challenging task, the publisher supported the team at every step. A small team of assistant editors was also appointed to further simplify the editing procedure and attain best results for the readers.

Apart from the editorial board, the designing team has also invested a significant amount of their time in understanding the subject and creating the most relevant covers. They scrutinized every image to scout for the most suitable representation of the subject and create an appropriate cover for the book.

The publishing team has been an ardent support to the editorial, designing and production team. Their endless efforts to recruit the best for this project, has resulted in the accomplishment of this book. They are a veteran in the field of academics and their pool of knowledge is as vast as their experience in printing. Their expertise and guidance has proved useful at every step. Their uncompromising quality standards have made this book an exceptional effort. Their encouragement from time to time has been an inspiration for everyone.

The publisher and the editorial board hope that this book will prove to be a valuable piece of knowledge for researchers, students, practitioners and scholars across the globe.

List of Contributors

Yun Huang
Shenzhen Key Laboratory of Edible and Medicinal Bioresources, Shenzhen Research Institute, Shenzhen, China

Ping Yao and Long Wang
Division of Life Science and Center for Chinese Medicine, The Hong Kong University of Science and Technology, Clear Water Bay, Hong Kong

Ka Wing Leung, Huaiyou Wang, Xiang Peng Kong, Tina Ting Xia Dong and Karl Wah Keung Tsim
Shenzhen Key Laboratory of Edible and Medicinal Bioresources, Shenzhen Research Institute, Shenzhen, China
Division of Life Science and Center for Chinese Medicine, The Hong Kong University of Science and Technology, Clear Water Bay, Hong Kong

Yicun Chen
Division of Life Science and Center for Chinese Medicine, The Hong Kong University of Science and Technology, Clear Water Bay, Hong Kong
Department of Pharmacology, Shantou University Medical College, Shantou, China

Pengqian Wang
Institute of Chinese Materia Medica, China Academy of Chinese Medical Sciences, Beijing, China

Yanan Yu, Jun Liu, Qiong Liu and Zhong Wang
Institute of Basic Research in Clinical Medicine, China Academy of Chinese Medical Sciences, Beijing, China

Bing Li
Institute of Basic Research in Clinical Medicine, China Academy of Chinese Medical Sciences, Beijing, China
Institute of Information on Traditional Chinese Medicine, China Academy of Chinese Medical Sciences, Beijing, China

Yingying Zhang and Dongfeng Li
Dongzhimen Hospital, Beijing University of Chines Medicine, Beijing, China

Wenjuan Xu
School of Mathematical Sciences, Peking University, Beijing, China

Xiaoyi Wei, Weixin Hou, Jiajun Liang, Peng Fang, Bo Dou, Chongyang Ma and Qiuyun Zhang
School of Traditional Chinese Medicine, Capital Medical University, Beijing, China

Zisong Wang
Department of Traditional Chinese Medicine, Beijing Chaoyang Hospital, Capital Medical University, Beijing, China

Jiayang Sai
Department of Oncology, The Third Affiliated Hospital, Beijing University of Chinese Medicine, Beijing, China

Tian Xu, Fafeng Cheng, Xueqian Wang and Qingguo Wang
School of Traditional Chinese Medicine, Beijing University of Chinese Medicine, Beijing, China

Tianduanyi Wang, Zengrui Wu, Lixia Sun, Weihua Li, Guixia Liu and Yun Tang
Shanghai Key Laboratory of New Drug Design, School of Pharmacy, East China University of Science and Technology, Shanghai, China

Yingying Yang and Tingting Bao
Graduate College, Beijing University of Chinese Medicine, Beijing, China
Institute of Metabolic Diseases, Guang'anmen Hospital, China Academy of Chinese Medical Sciences, Beijing, China

Lu Ding, Daqing Zhao and Xiangyan Li
Jilin Ginseng Academy, Key Laboratory of Active Substances and Biological Mechanisms of Ginseng Efficacy, Ministry of Education, Jilin Provincial Key Laboratory of Bio-Macromolecules of Chinese Medicine, Changchun University of Chinese Medicine, Changchun, China

Yaxin Li, Siyu Song and Jiachao Zhao
College of Integrated Traditional Chinese and Western Medicine, Changchun University of Chinese Medicine, Changchun, China

Jing Ma, Jing Wang and Ziyuan Wang
Affiliated Hospital of Changchun University of Chinese Medicine, Changchun, China

Qingwei Li, Zezheng Gao, Linhua Zhao and Xiaolin Tong
Institute of Metabolic Diseases, Guang'anmen Hospital, China Academy of Chinese Medical Sciences, Beijing, China

Zeyu Wang
Department of Scientific Research, Changchun University of Chinese Medicine, Changchun, China

Runzhi Zhang, Xue Zhu, Hong Bai and Kang Ning
School of Life Science and Technology, Huazhong University of Science and Technology, Wuhan, China

Guosong Zhu, Jiaqiang Zhang, Yali Yang, Haoran Zhang and Kaiwei Wang
Department of Anesthesia and Perioperative Medicine, Henan Provincial People's Hospital, People's Hospital of Zhengzhou University, Zhengzhou, China

Wenwen Jin, Fangchu Su and Jianhua Zhang
Medical Engineering Technology and Data Mining Institute, Zhengzhou University, Zhengzhou, China

Junting Liang and Chuanliang Chen
Clinical Bioinformatics Experimental Center, Henan Provincial People's Hospital, People's Hospital of Zhengzhou University, Zhengzhou, China

Wenjuan Zhang, Ying Huai, Zhiping Miao and Airong Qian
Lab for Bone Metabolism, Key Lab for Space Biosciences and Biotechnology, School of Life Sciences, Northwestern Polytechnical University, Xi'an, China
Research Center for Special Medicine and Health Systems Engineering, School of Life Sciences, Northwestern Polytechnical University, Xi'an, China
NPU-UAB Joint Laboratory for Bone Metabolism, School of Life Sciences, Northwestern Polytechnical University, Xi'an, China

Yonghua Wang
Lab of Systems Pharmacology, College of Life Sciences, Northwest University, Xi'an, China

Xin Ba, Pan Shen, Yao Huang, Liang Han, Wei Ji Lin, Hui Jia Yan and Li Jun Xu
Institute of Integrated Traditional Chinese and Western Medicine, Tongji Hospital, Tongji Medical College, Huazhong University of Science and Technology, Wuhan, China

Ying Huang, Zhe Chen and Sheng Hao Tu
Institute of Integrated Traditional Chinese and Western Medicine, Tongji Hospital, Tongji Medical College, Huazhong University of Science and Technology, Wuhan, China
Department of Integrated Traditional Chinese and Western Medicine, Tongji Hospital, Tongji Medical College, Huazhong University of Science and Technology, Wuhan, China

Hui Wang
Rehabilitation and Sports Medicine Research Institute of Zhejiang Province, Zhejiang Provincial People's Hospital, People's Hospital of Hangzhou Medical College, Hangzhou, China

Kai Qin
Department of Integrated Traditional Chinese and Western Medicine, Tongji Hospital, Tongji Medical College, Huazhong University of Science and Technology, Wuhan, China

Yi Chen, Jiahui Wei, Ying Zhang, Wenwei Sun, Zhuoheng Li, Xiaoyu Xu and Panhong Li
College of Pharmaceutical Sciences and Chinese Medicine, Southwest University, Chongqing, China
Chongqing Key Laboratory of New Drug Screening from Traditional Chinese Medicine, Chongqing, China
Pharmacology of Chinese Materia Medica - the Key Discipline Constructed by the State Administration of Traditional Chinese Medicine, Chongqing, China

Qin Wang
Department of Traditional Chinese Medicine and Pharmacy, Chongqing Hospital of Traditional Chinese Medicine, Chongqing, China

Cong Li
Department of Obstetrics and Gynecology, First Affiliated Hospital of Chongqing Medical University, Chongqing, China

Shu-Yue Qu, Xia Heng, Yi-Yu Qi, Ping-Yuan Ge, Nian-Yun Yang and Hua-Xu Zhu
Jiangsu Key Laboratory for High Technology Research of TCM Formulae, Nanjing University of Chinese Medicine, Nanjing, China

Xiao-Yue Li, Sai-jia Ni, Zeng-Ying Yao and Qi-Chun Zhang
Jiangsu Key Laboratory for Pharmacology and Safety Evaluation of Chinese Materia Medica, School of Pharmacy, Nanjing University of Chinese Medicine, Nanjing, China

Rui Guo
School of Medicine and Holistic Integrative Medicine, Nanjing University of Chinese Medicine, Nanjing, China

Yi Cao
Institute of Literature in Chinese Medicine, Nanjing University of Chinese Medicine, Nanjing, China

Lixiang Zhai, Zi-wan Ning and Tao Huang
School of Chinese Medicine, Hong Kong Baptist University, Kowloon, Hong Kong

Bo Wen and Zhao-xiang Bian
School of Chinese Medicine, Hong Kong Baptist University, Kowloon, Hong Kong
Shenzhen Research Institute and Continuing Education, Hong Kong Baptist University, Shenzhen, China

Cheng-hui Liao
Shenzhen Research Institute and Continuing Education, Hong Kong Baptist University, Shenzhen, China

Cheng-yuan Lin and Ling Zhao
School of Chinese Medicine, Hong Kong Baptist University, Kowloon, Hong Kong

Jihan Huang
Center for Drug Clinical Research, Shanghai University of Traditional Chinese Medicine, Shanghai, China

Yu Xu, Ning Wang, Hor-Yue Tan, Cheng Zhang, Sha Li, Guoyi Tang and Yibin Feng
School of Chinese Medicine, Li Ka Shing Faculty of Medicine, The University of Hong Kong, Hong Kong, China

Zhenhua Bian
College of Pharmacy, Nanjing University of Chinese Medicine, Nanjing, China
Department of Pharmacy, Wuxi TCM Hospital Affiliated to Nanjing University of Chinese Medicine, Wuxi, China

Wenming Zhang, Jingyue Tang, Qianqian Fei, Minmin Hu, Xiaowei Chen and Xiaohang Yuan
Department of Pharmacy, Wuxi TCM Hospital Affiliated to Nanjing University of Chinese Medicine, Wuxi, China

Lianlin Su, Chenghao Fei, De Ji, Chunqin Mao, Huangjin Tong and Tulin Lu
College of Pharmacy, Nanjing University of Chinese Medicine, Nanjing, China
Department of Pharmacy, Wuxi TCM Hospital Affiliated to Nanjing University of Chinese Medicine, Wuxi, China

Yingying Wang, Yuxue Yang, Xiaohua Lu and Tao Wang
College of Pharmacy, Chengdu University of Traditional Chinese Medicine, Chengdu, China
Department of Pharmacy, 302 Military Hospital of China, Beijing, China

Shizhang Wei, Xuelin Zhou, Haotian Li and Yanling Zhao
Department of Pharmacy, 302 Military Hospital of China, Beijing, China

Tian Gao
Affiliated Hospital of Chengdu University of Traditional Chinese Medicine, Chengdu, China

Hai-tao Xiao
School of Pharmaceutical Sciences, Health Science Center, Shenzhen University, Shenzhen, China

Liqi Qian
Department of Traditional Chinese Medicine, First Affiliated Hospital of Chinese People's Liberation Army General Hospital, Beijing, China

Wenjun Zou
College of Pharmacy, Chengdu University of Traditional Chinese Medicine, Chengdu, China

Index

A

Acute Lung Injury, 64, 93-94, 101-102, 141

Alzheimer's Disease, 47-48, 60-62, 80, 84, 159, 172, 214

Anti-oxidative Activity, 1-2, 15

Autoimmune Disease, 93, 127, 142

B

Berberine, 84, 158-160, 165-168, 170, 172, 188, 190, 198-199

Bioactive Compounds, 35-37, 42, 82, 94, 104, 106, 108, 113, 115-117, 119, 124, 198, 200

C

Cell Culture, 5, 66, 95, 188

Cell Cycle, 31, 93, 231, 240

Cell Proliferation, 97, 126, 131-132, 134, 139-140, 225

Cell Viability, 5, 12, 66, 71, 99, 126, 128

Cellular Component, 37, 70, 136

Chemokine Signaling Activation, 18, 30

Chronic Obstructive Pulmonary Disease, 64, 124

Cirrhosis, 34, 89-91

Combination Index, 113

Cyclocarya Paliurus, 174-176, 178, 181-182, 184-185

Cytokines, 37, 43, 46, 57, 64, 101, 116, 127, 139, 221, 225-227

D

Depression, 61, 83, 91, 115, 157-160, 162, 165-166, 168-173, 202, 209, 214-215

Depressive Disorder, 60, 157-158, 165, 170-172

Diabetes, 46, 48, 61, 80, 83-84, 90-91, 115, 174-178, 180, 182-189, 192, 195, 198-200, 202, 215

Diabetic Dyslipidemia, 174-175, 177-178, 180, 182-184

Diglyceride, 174, 181

Drug Discovery, 19, 30, 32, 40, 61-62, 80, 89, 91, 102, 104-105, 110, 113-114, 123-125, 141, 170, 172, 185, 228

Drug-target Interactions, 48, 60, 105, 109-111, 123, 125

E

Endometrial Tissue, 143-144, 156

Endometriosis, 143-146, 150-153, 155-156

Epithelial-mesenchymal Transition, 63-64, 143-144, 151-156

Extracellular Matrix, 63, 76, 153

F

False Positive Rate, 50

Ferulic Acid, 8, 143-146, 149, 154, 156

Force Swimming Test, 157

Formic Acid, 37, 65-66, 161-162, 177, 203

G

Gene Microarray, 18

Gene Ontology, 37, 39-40, 50-51, 66, 130, 145, 148, 162, 165, 187, 201, 205

Gene Set, 21, 37, 40, 49-51, 53, 59

H

Hepatic Steatosis, 42, 174-175, 177-178, 180, 182-185

Hepatocellular Carcinoma, 83, 155, 199

Histopathological Staining, 126

Hormone Releasing, 18, 28, 30

Hyperlipidemia, 33, 42, 100, 174-175, 177, 180, 182-183, 185, 187

Hyperplasia, 126, 131-132, 136, 139-140, 216-217, 227-230, 236

Hypertension, 48-51, 53, 57-60, 62, 64, 83-84, 100, 158, 202

I

Immunofluorescence, 126, 129, 131, 133, 135, 137-138

In Vivo Experiments, 19, 23, 30, 35, 128, 139, 171, 202

Ischemic Stroke, 18, 30-31, 46, 140, 159

J

Jiawei Foshou San, 143-146, 149-153

L

Liver Steatosis, 33-34, 185

M

Mass Spectrometer, 5, 7, 66, 162, 204

Menstruation, 143, 153

Mesenchymal Cells, 64, 77

Molecular Docking, 66, 74-76, 123, 157, 162, 168, 215

Multiple Genetic Dysfunctions, 18

Myofibroblast, 64, 75, 77

N

Network Pharmacology, 33, 44-46, 48, 60-61, 63-64, 69, 73, 76-77, 79-84, 86-94, 97, 101-102, 113, 123, 125-127, 129, 133, 136, 141-144, 155-159, 161, 170, 172-175, 182-184, 186-187, 195, 198-204, 207-209, 214-217, 219-220, 223, 227

Non-alcoholic Fatty Liver Disease, 33-35, 39, 184

Non-alcoholic Steatohepatitis, 33-34

P

Phenolic Acid, 2

Phosphoric Acid, 128, 176

Platelet Aggregation, 94, 116

Principle Component Analysis, 1, 10

Protein-protein Interaction, 31, 33, 35, 40, 42, 48, 50, 53, 56, 58, 66, 77, 91, 93, 143-145, 147, 155, 162, 174, 185, 188, 191, 201, 205

Pulmonary Fibrosis, 63, 76-78

Q

Qimai Feiluoping Decoction, 63-64

R

Rna Isolation, 146

S

Scutellaria Baicalensis Georgi, 61, 93-94, 96, 100, 159-161, 165, 187

Serotonergic Synapse, 47, 53, 56, 160, 171, 207, 209, 212

Sinisan, 33-35, 37, 39, 42-43, 45, 83

Sphingomyelin, 174, 181

Structured-based Virtual Screening, 105, 110

Synergistic Effect, 39, 59, 104, 113

Synergistic Index, 113

Synovial Tissue, 127, 129, 131-133

Systems Pharmacology, 35, 47-48, 53, 56, 60-62, 82, 90-91, 104-106, 113, 115-117, 120, 122, 124-125, 141, 144-145, 172, 187, 201, 217

T

Target Genes, 47, 53, 56-57, 59, 93, 95, 97, 130, 187, 189, 205

Tetrahydropalmatine, 143-146, 149, 154-156

Total Triglyceride, 33, 41-42, 174

Traditional Chinese Medicine, 16-18, 33, 45-47, 60-65, 76-77, 79, 81, 89-90, 104, 114, 123-125, 127, 130, 140-141, 143-145, 154, 159, 161, 173, 184-186, 199-202, 204, 216-217, 228-229

True Positive Rate, 50

Tryptophan Metabolism, 56, 157-158, 160, 162, 165-171

U

Ursodeoxycholic Acid, 18-19

W

Western Blot, 23, 28-29, 68, 71, 73-74, 95, 100, 129, 131, 134, 147, 216, 218, 225

Wutou Decoction, 126-129, 131-137

www.ingramcontent.com/pod-product-compliance
Lightning Source LLC
LaVergne TN
LVHW082158200926
848484LV00008B/2182